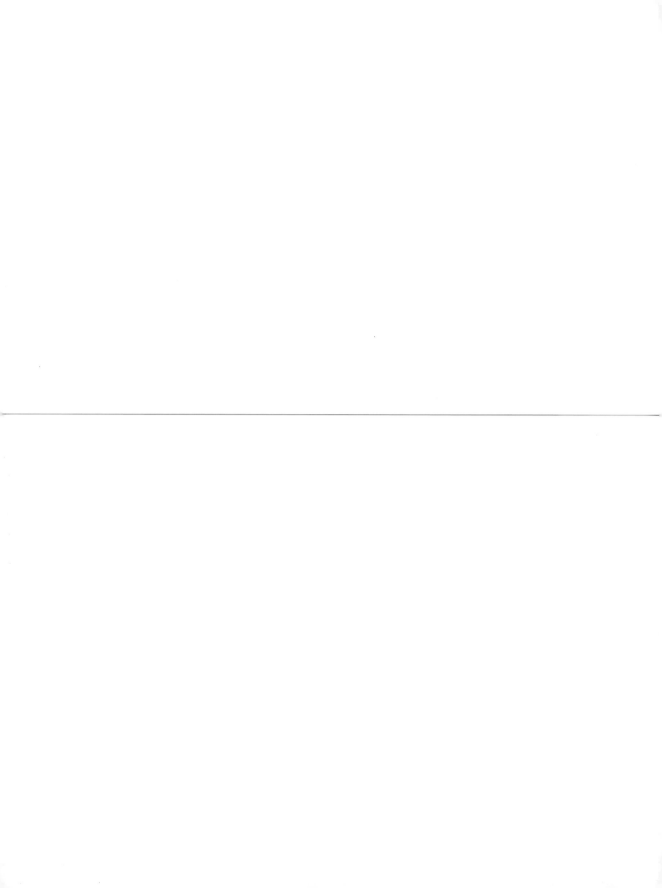

High-Risk Cardiac Revascularization
and Clinical Trials

High-Risk Cardiac Revascularization and Clinical Trials

Edited by

DOUGLASS A MORRISON MD, FACC, FSCAI
Professor of Medicine and Radiology,
University of Arizona
Director, Cardiac Catheterization Laboratory
Southern Arizona VA Health Care System (SAVAHCS)
Tucson, Arizona, USA

PATRICK W SERRUYS MD, PhD, FACC, FESC
Professor of Interventional Cardiology,
Erasmus University
Head of Interventional Department,
Heartcenter Rotterdam
University Hospital Rotterdam-Dijkigt
Rotterdam, The Netherlands

MARTIN DUNITZ

First published in the United Kingdom in 2002
by Martin Dunitz Ltd, The Livery House, 7–9 Pratt Street, London NW1 0AE

Tel.: +44 (0) 20 74822202
Fax.: +44 (0) 20 72670159
E-mail: info@dunitz.co.uk
Website: http://www.dunitz.co.uk

A CIP record for this book is available from the British Library.

ISBN 1 84184 185 4

Distributed in the USA by
Fulfilment Center
Taylor & Francis
7625 Empire Drive
Florence, KY 41042, USA
Toll Free Tel.: +1 800 634 7064
E-mail: cserve@routledge_ny.com

Distributed in Canada by
Taylor & Francis
74 Rolark Drive
Scarborough, Ontario M1R 4G2, Canada
Toll Free Tel.: +1 877 226 2237
E-mail: tal_fran@istar.ca

Distributed in the rest of the world by
Thomson Publishing Services
Cheriton House
North Way
Andover, Hampshire SP10 5BE, UK
Tel.: +44 (0)1264 332424
E-mail: salesorder.tandf@thomsonpublishingservices.co.uk

Composition by Wearset Ltd, Boldon, Tyne and Wear
Printed and bound in Great Britain by Biddles Ltd., Guildford & King's Lynn

Contents

Contributors ix

Introduction

An interventionalist's perspective   *Spencer B King III* 3

A cardiac surgeon's perspective   *Robert H Jones* 5

Section I: Is the medical management optimal?

1.   What constitutes medically refractory in the new millennium?   11
     Douglass A Morrison and Jerome Sacks

2.   Beta-blocking agents   *Jason R Wollmuth and Douglass A Morrison* 25

3.   Statins and other lipid-lowering agents   *Douglass A Morrison and Stephen P Thomson* 43

4.   Angiotensin-converting enzyme inhibitors   *Hoang M Thai and Douglass A Morrison* 61

5.   Anticoagulants in unstable angina and acute myocardial infarction   *Kodangudi B Ramanathan* 73

6.   Antiplatelet therapy   *H Daniel Lewis, Jr* 85

Section II: The benefits of revascularization

7.   To prolong a life: summary of the coronary bypass trials   *Robert C Brooks and Katherine M Detre* 97

8.   To improve a life: relief of symptoms, exercise tolerance, ACME and RITA-2   *Edward D Folland* 107

9.   Rationale and design for the Clinical Outcomes Utilizing Revascularization and Aggressive druG
     Evaluation (COURAGE) trial   *William E Boden* 121

10. Results of randomized controlled trials in patients with non-ST segment elevation acute
     coronary syndromes (TIMI-IIIB, VANQWISH, FRISC-II, TACTICS TIMI-18)   *William E Boden* 135

Section III: Comparative trials of CABG versus PCI

11. Bypass Angioplasty Revascularization Investigation (BARI)   *Martial G Bourassa* 145

12. The RITA trials   *Robert A Henderson* 163

13. Emory angioplasty versus surgery trial *Spencer B King III* 177

14. Percutaneous coronary intervention and coronary bypass surgery in high-risk patients: a look from the South *Alfredo E Rodriguez* 187

15. The MASS trials *Luiz A Machado César and Whady A Hueb* 203

16. The AWESOME trial *Douglass A Morrison, Jerome Sacks, William G Henderson and Gulshan Sethi* 217

17. Randomized comparison of coronary artery bypass surgery and stenting for the treatment of multi-vessel disease *Patrick W Serruys and Felix Unger* 235

Section IV: Differential risks/differential benefits: patient subsets

18. Re-operative revascularization *Bruce W Lytle* 257

19. Elective stenting of left main coronary artery disease *Seung-Jung Park* 265

20. Coronary interventions in acute myocardial infarction *Vincent S DeGeare and Cindy L Grines* 283

21. Acute myorcardial infarction: SMASH perspective *Jean-Christophe E Stauffer and Philip M Urban* 311

22. Cardiogenic shock: SHOCK trial perspective *Debabrata Mukherjee, Eric R Bates and Judith S Hochman* 327

23. Cardiogenic shock: a VA perspective *Douglass A Morrison and Jerome Sacks* 337

24. Chronic occlusions *Haresh Mehta and Bernhard Meier* 347

Section V: Comorbidity

25. Chronic pulmonary disease *Darryl Weiman, Kodangudi B Ramanathan and Douglass A Morrison* 363

26. Cerebrovascular and peripheral vascular co-morbidity *Douglass A Morrison, Gumpanart Veerakul and Krisada Sastravaha* 373

27. Liver disease *Edmund J Bini and Chris E Lascarides* 387

28. Renal function and high-risk coronary artery procedures *Stuart B Pett Jr* 415

29. High-risk coronary interventions in diabetic patients *Steven P Sedlis and Jeffrey D Lorin* 425

Section VI: Adding value to the revascularization option

30. Off-pump coronary artery bypass in high-risk patients *Rick A Esposito* 453

31. Support for percutaneous coronary interventions: IABP, CPS and beyond *Carl L Tommaso* 469

32. Stents and high-risk cardiac revascularization *David R Holmes Jr and Douglass A Morrison* 479

33. Pharmacologic support for PCI: glycoprotein IIb/IIIa receptor blockers *Douglass A Morrison* 489

34. Myocardial protection for high-risk coronary surgery
Vladimir Birjiniuk and Diane Panton Lapsley 503

Section VII: What can be done after the revascularization to discourage recidivism?

35. Cardiac rehabilitation   *Shefali Vora and Victor Froelicher* 511

Section VIII: Medicine vs PCI vs CABG in 2001 for high-risk unstable angina

36. Cost comparisons of PCI vs CABG   *Kevin T Stroupe* 549

37. High-risk myocardial ischemia in 2002: medicine, PCI and CABG
Douglass A Morrison and Jerome Sacks 559

Index 565

Contributors

Eric R Bates MD
Professor of Internal Medicine
University of Michigan
University Hospital
Ann Arbor, MI, USA

Edmund J Bini MD, FACP, FACG
Staff Physician, Gastroenterology and Hepatology
VA New York Harbour Healthcare System
Assistant Professor of Medicine
New York University Medical Center
New York, NY, USA

Vladimir Birjiniuk MD
Clinical Director, Cardiac Surgery
Surgical Service
VA Boston Healthcare System
West Roxbury, MA, USA

William E Boden MD, FACC
Professor of Medicine, University of Connecticut
Director of Cardiology
Hartford Hospital
Hartford, CT, USA

Martial G Bourassa MD
Senior Cardiologist
Department of Medicine
Montreal Heart Institute
Montreal, QC, Canada

Robert C Brooks MD, PhD
Department of Medicine
University of Pittsburgh
Pittsburgh, PA, USA

Vincent S DeGeare MD, FACC, FACP
Interventional Cardiologist
Keesler Air Force Medical Center
Keesler AFB, MS, USA

Katherine M Detre MD Dr PH, FACC
Department of Epidemiology
Graduate School of Public Health
University of Pittsburgh
Pittsburgh, PA, USA

Rick A Esposito MD
Associate Professor of Clinical Surgery
New York University School of Medicine
New York, NY, USA

Edward D Folland MD, FACC, FSCAI
Co PI, VA ACME
U Mass Memorial Medical Group
Worcester, MA, USA

Victor Froelicher MD, FACC
Professor of Medicine
Stamford University
Cardiology
VA Palo Alto Healthcare System
Palo Alto, CA, USA

Cindy L Grines MD, FAC
Director, Cardiac Catheterization Laboratories
Director, Interventional Fellowship Program
William Beaumont Hospital
Royal Oak, MI, USA

Robert A Henderson DM, FRCP, FESC
Consultant Cardiologist
Nottingham City Hospital NHS Trust
Nottingham, UK

William G Henderson PhD
Visiting Professor
University of Colorado
Health Outcomes Program
Fitzsimons Campus
Aurora, CO, USA

Judith S Hochman MD
Director, Cardiac Care and Stepdown Units
Director of Cardiac Research
St Luke's Roosevelt Hospital
Professor of Medicine
Columbia University
New York, NY, USA

David R Holmes Jr MD, FACC, FSCAI
Director, Cardiac Catheterization Laboratory
Mayo Clinic
Rochester, MN, USA

Whady A Hueb MD, PhD
Professor of Cardiology
Assistant Physician, Chronic Coronary Disease Unit
Heart Institute (InCor), Clinical Division
University of Sao Paulo Medical School
Sao Paolo, Brazil

Robert H Jones MD, FACC
Mary and Deryl Hart Professor of Surgery
Department of Surgery
Duke University Medical Center
Durham, NC, USA

Spencer B King III MD, MACC, FSCAI
Fuqua Chair of Interventional Cardiology
The Fuqua Heart Center of Piedmont Hospital
Co-Director, Atlanta Cardiovascular Research
Institute
Atlanta, GA, USA

Diane Panton Lapsley RN, MS, CS
Cardiovascular Clinical Specialist
Cardiology Service
VA Boston Healthcare System
West Roxbury, MA, USA

Chris E Lascarides MD
Gastroenterology Fellow
New York University Medical Center
New York, NY, USA

H Daniel Lewis Jr MD, FACC
Professor Emeritus
University of Kansas School of Medicine
Kansas City, KS, USA

Jeffrey D Lorin MD, FACC
Assistant Professor of Clinical Medicine
New York University School of Medicine
Staff Cardiologist
VA New York Harbor Healthcare System
Manhattan Campus
New York, NY, USA

Bruce W Lytle MD
Surgeon, Department of Thoracic and
Cardiovascular Surgery
The Cleveland Clinic Foundation
Cleveland, OH, USA

Luiz A Machado Cesar MD
Professor of Cardiology
Director, Chronic Coronary Disease Unit
Heart Institute (InCor), Clinical Division
University of Sao Paulo Medical School
Sao Paolo, Brazil

Haresh Mehta MD
Consultant Cardiologist
PD Hinduja National Hospital and Medical
Research Center
Mahim
Mumbai, India

Bernhard Meier MD, FACC, FESC
Professor of Cardiology
Chairman, Swiss Cardiovascular Center Bern
University Hospital
Bern, Switzerland

Douglass A Morrison MD, FACC, FSCAI
Professor of Medicine and Radiology
University of Arizona
Director, Cardiac Catheterization Laboratory
Southern Arizona VA Health Care System
(SAVAHCS)
Tucson, AZ, USA

Debabrata Mukherjee MD
Assistant Professor, Division of Cardiology
University of Michigan
University Hospital
Ann Arbor, MI, USA

Seung-Jung Park MD, PhD
Chief, Division of Cardiology
Director, Interventional Cardiology
Cardiac Center, Asian Medical Center
University of Ulsan
Seoul, Korea

Stuart B Pett Jr MD
Associate Professor of Surgery
University of New Mexico Health Science Center
Chief, Cardiothoracic Surgery
New Mexico Federal Regional Medical Center
Albuquerque, NM, USA

Kodangudi B Ramanathan MD, MRCP (UK)
Professor of Medicine
University of Tennessee
Chief Cardiology
VA Medical Center
Memphis, TN, USA

Alfredo E Rodriguez MD, PhD, FACC
Director, Cardiac International Unit and
Cardiology Unit
Otamendi Hospital
Buenos Aires, Argentina

Jerome Sacks PhD
Biostatistician, AWESOME
CSPCC Hines VA Hospital
Hines, IL, USA

Krisada Sastravaha MD
Cardiology
Bhumibol Adulyadej Hospital
Royal Thai Air Force
Bangkok, Thailand

Steven P Sedlis MD, FACC, FSCAI
Associate Profesor of Clinical Medicine
New York University School of Medicine
Chief, Cardiology
VA New York Harbor Healthcare System
Manhattan Campus
New York, NY, USA

Patrick W Serruys MD, PhD, FACC, FESC
Professor of Interventional Cardiology, Erasmus
University
Head of Interventional Department, Heartcenter
Rotterdam
Thoraxcenter
University Hospital Rotterdam Dijkigt
Rotterdam, The Netherlands

Gulshan Sethi MD, FACC
Cardiology and Cardiothoracic Surgery
SAVAHCS and University of Arizona
Tucson, AZ, USA

Jean-Christophe E Stauffer MD
Division de Cardiologie – CHUV
Lausanne, Switzerland

Kevin T Stroupe PhD
Health Economist
Midwest Center for Health Services and Policy
Research
Cooperative Studies Program Coordinating Center
Edward Hines Jr VA Hospital
Hines, IL, USA

Hoang M Thai MD, FACC
Assistant Professor of Medicine
Director, Echocardiography Laboratory
SAVAHCS
Sarver Heart Center
University of Arizona
Tucson, AZ, USA

Stephen P Thomson MD
Endocrinology
SAVAHCS
Tucson, AZ, USA

Carl L Tommaso MD, FACC, FCAI
9669 N Kenton St Suite 601
Skokie, IL, USA

Felix Unger MD
Chief, Surgery
Klinik fur Herzchirurgie
Salzburg, Austria

Philip M Urban MD, FACC, FESC
Division de Cardiologie – CHUV
Lausanne, Switzerland

Gumpanart Veerakul MD, FSCAI
Chief, Cardiology
Bhumibol Adulyadej Hospital
Royal Thai Air Force
Bangkok, Thailand

Shefali Vora MD
Cardiology
VA Palo Alto Healthcare System
Palo Alto, CA, USA

Darryl Weiman MD
Professor of Surgery
Chief of Cardiothoracic Surgery
University of Tennessee
Memphis, TN, USA

Jason R Wollmuth MD
Cardiology Research Fellow
SAVAHCS and University of Arizona
Tucson, AZ, USA

Introduction

An interventionalist's perspective

Spencer B King III

When Andreas Gruentzig performed the first coronary angioplasty procedure on September 16, 1977, he was extending a method that had been developed for the peripheral circulation and extensively tested in animal models. The first patients selected were those who were significantly symptomatic, had documented myocardial ischemia, and had predominantly single-vessel disease. Although some multi-vessel patients were treated in the early days, the procedure was designed to address severely stenotic arteries with relatively discrete lesions that could be managed with the equipment available at that time. Our assessment of the patients Gruentzig treated showed the technique to be successful in alleviating angina, and the 10-year follow-up was also impressive. Single-vessel patients had a 95% survival; however the small number of patients with multi-vessel disease had a survival of 81%. As the technique began to evolve, more patients with multi-vessel disease were selected for angioplasty. A number of people, including Geoffrey Hartzler, began to push the competition with surgery. In the early 1980s after Andreas Gruentzig had joined our group at Emory University, it became evident that for angioplasty to be an accepted therapy with documented benefit, it would have to be compared to the gold standard, namely coronary bypass surgery.

By 1987, we were successful in convincing the National Heart, Lung and Blood Institute to support a randomized trial comparing angioplasty to surgery in multi-vessel disease

patients. The Emory Angioplasty Surgery Trial (EAST) began enrollment in June, 1977 and was followed one year later by the first enrollment in the Bypass Angioplasty Revascularization Investigation (BARI). CABRI and other trials in Europe were also started. The lessons from a number of these trials will be delineated in this volume but they all were instructive in that survival and freedom from myocardial infarction were relatively equivalent; however repeat procedures in these multi-vessel patients were very common in the angioplasty groups. The principal reason for this early re-intervention was the restenosis phenomenon, which increased dramatically when multiple vessels were approached. The advent of stenting in the late 1980s provided a platform that would promise to change that. The first observation was that stenting provided a bail-out option so that urgent bypass surgery was no longer necessary for most patients undergoing acute closure during the procedure. The first coil stent was placed by our group at Emory in 1987. The same year, the Palmaz-Schatz stent was implanted in Sao Paulo, Brazil; however, the era of stenting would not begin until several years later after extensive clinical trials had been carried out. In the mid 1990s there was a dramatic increase in the use of stents, so that in the late 1990s stenting had become the dominant percutaneous interventional procedure. Observational studies and randomized trials documented that stenting would have a lower restenosis rate than balloon angioplasty (i.e. STRESS and BENESTENT). There was also the question of whether this benefit would extend to improved survival for patients, especially those with multi-vessel disease undergoing percutaneous intervention (PCI). Three trials have now been completed in patient subsets that are somewhat similar to EAST, BARI and CABRI. These are the ARTS trial, SOS trial, and the ERACI trial. These trials will be described in some detail in this volume but suffice it to say that, taking these trials together, there is no compelling evidence that survival is different with one strategy or the other. In ARTS, the one-year mortality is almost identical between PCI and surgery. In SOS, surgery is slightly better than PCI, and in ERACI, PCI is somewhat better than surgery. The differences, however, are not striking.

All of the previous balloon angioplasty and surgery trials selected patients who were felt to be at reasonable risk from the perspective of angioplasty and surgery and indeed the in-hospital mortality in most of these trials hovered around 1%, suggesting that the highest risk patients may not have been included. A recent survey of the STS (Society for Thoracic Surgery) database shows that, among 149,000 patients undergoing isolated coronary bypass surgery, the overall mortality rate is 2.7%. There are, of course, patients with much higher risk, of which some of the defining features are older age, decreased left ventricular function and, especially, prior bypass surgery.

It was courageous for the AWESOME investigators to design a trial to look specifically at this high-risk group of patients to establish whether percutaneous intervention could be an alternative to high-risk surgery. The outcome of that trial is a vindication of the quality of care provided by the Veterans Administration surgeons and the PTCA operators. During a time when surgery and percutaneous intervention are benefiting from technologic advances, it appears that patients are also benefiting. The multiple analyses of the results of the AWESOME trial will go far toward influencing practice and will stimulate many new questions that will need to be investigated.

The vision of Gruentzig to apply non-invasive therapies for patients with obstructive coronary artery disease had little hope of going beyond the relatively ideal lesions, given the status of technology. At present, however, with technologies that can be applied very extensively throughout the coronary tree, the question remains what will be the long-term outcome of patients having such procedures? The AWESOME trial has given us significant insight into the early and intermediate term risks for such patients, and it is hoped that longer term follow-up will provide additional insights. Undoubtedly, both surgery and percutaneous intervention have benefited from the efforts of the investigators who carried out this trial as they refined and developed their techniques. As the continuum of medical care for these patients also develops, it is hoped that those undergoing surgery and interventional therapies will also benefit in the long run.

A cardiac surgeon's perspective

Robert H Jones

Death by procedure is feared by patient, family, and physician. Only the hope for pay back of greater long-term survival motivates a patient to consent to procedures with substantial risk. In the early years of surgical myocardial revascularization, patients with abnormal heart function were known to have the greatest chance of dying during operation and, therefore, were thought to be poor surgical candidates. Fear of high operative mortality during the developmental era of coronary artery bypass graft (CABG) surgery caused initial randomized trials conducted from 1972 to 1978 comparing CABG to medical treatment to be designed to exclude most high-risk patients. Even the last of these trials, the CASS trial, included only 160 patients with a left ventricular ejection fraction (LVEF) < 0.50. The ten-year survival was 61% in the 82 medically-treated patients and 79% in the 78 patients who underwent CABG ($p = 0.01$ [1]. This survival advantage of CABG was not related to the presence or severity of heart failure or angina symptoms. A meta-analysis by Yusuf [2] combined individual patient data from the CASS trial with those enrolled in the six other early randomized trials. Only 191 (7.2%) of the 2649 total patients had an LVEF < 0.40, and only 106 (4.0%) of these patients who were primarily symptomatic with angina also had heart failure symptoms. Coronary artery bypass grafts improved survival among all patients with proximal left anterior descending (LAD) stenosis, three-vessel, or left main coronary artery disease (CAD), regardless of left ventricular function. In these patients with

a survival benefit from CABG, a low LVEF increased the absolute benefit but did not change the relative benefit of CABG. A literature search of 326 published reports on results of CABG in patients with heart failure or left ventricular dysfunction identified three well-designed cohort studies [3]. Mortality benefit of CABG over medical therapy was 10 and 20 lives per 100 patients at three years in two of the three studies and 29 lives per 100 patients at five years in the third study.

The therapy known as medical treatment in all randomized trials and most observational comparisons with CABG really only reflected the natural history of CAD since it rarely included drugs now known to be life prolonging, such as angiotensin-converting enzyme (ACE) inhibitors, beta-blockers, lipid lowering, and anti-platelet agents. Refinement of operative and post-operative surgical management has also steadily improved CABG results over the past two decades. The paucity of modern data available to clinicians who must daily make high-risk management decisions in patients with advanced ischemic heart disease emphasizes the need for a properly-designed randomized comparison of these therapies commonly used in clinical practice.

In the absence of randomized clinical trial data, large cardiovascular databases have been an important source of outcome information for patients with advanced ischemic heart disease. Relatively few characteristics identify high short-term risk for revascularization by percutaneous coronary intervention (PCI) [4] or

CABG [5]. Moreover, most patient characteristics that increase the short-term operative risk also predict the greatest long-term survival benefit from the procedure [6]. This surgical revascularization advantage occurs because clinical variables that increase short-term mortality with CABG predict even greater mortality over time in medically-treated patients.

The distribution of prognostic characteristics always differs among treatment groups in unrandomized patient cohorts because clinicians must use baseline clinical characteristics to select the treatment that appears most likely to improve survival for individual patients. Therefore, statistical adjustment for these baseline differences is essential. The most robust multiple-step statistical modeling approach to adjust for these differences is to first separate data corresponding to each treatment group for multivariable modeling of all baseline variables found to be significant in univariate comparisons against the end-point of survival. Thereafter, patients in all treatment groups should be collapsed into a common data set for multivariable modeling of those variables found to be significant in any of the preliminary multivariable models developed for individual treatment groups. Treatment interaction terms with all significant baseline variables should then be added to develop the final multivariable model. Illustrative comparison of Kaplan–Meier survival curves is generated only on treatment subgroups defined by clinical characteristics that interact with treatment in Cox models.

Using this modeling approach in the Duke Databank for Cardiovascular Diseases, the severity of coronary atherosclerosis is the only baseline clinical characteristic that strongly interacts with the three treatment strategies of medicine, PCI, and CABG [6]. The severity of coronary atherosclerosis is best defined by a CAD index that weights prognostic information derived from the location and severity of coronary atherosclerosis into a single number ranging from 0–100. Multivariable Cox models developed in a large population of patients

with CAD amenable to treatment by PCI, CABG, or medicine, show the CAD index to predict death most strongly in medically-treated patients, weakly in PCI-treated patients, and not at all in CABG-treated patients. Using the CAD index to subset for Kaplan–Meier comparisons, PCI provides better survival than CABG or medical therapy in patients with a CAD index below 45. Coronary artery bypass graft provides better survival than PCI or medical treatment in patients with a CAD index above 70, and PCI and CABG provide equivalent survival advantage over medical therapy in patients with a CAD index between 45 and 70. Although some clinical indicators of high risk, such as diabetes and advanced age, weakly interact with PCI or CABG treatment, the power of these interactions is sufficiently small to be of little clinical consequence. Therefore, the CAD index identifies the therapy most likely to benefit an individual patient. The other baseline information that is associated with high risk, but not interacting with treatment, multiplies the absolute survival benefit expected for an individual high-risk patient receiving the optimal therapy in comparison to the population average. The greatest absolute survival benefit would be expected for high-risk patients assigned to the most efficacious treatment strategy.

The New York State Database has been used to evaluate treatment-related outcomes at three years in a single state experience with PCI and CABG [7]. Multivariable modeling in this large data set shows no treatment-related interaction with any baseline clinical variable other than coronary anatomy. The BARI randomized and registry populations, when combined into a single data set and analyzed by multivariable modeling, showed no strong interaction between coronary anatomy and CABG or PCI. However, this data set included only 3610 patients who reflected a narrow range of coronary anatomy. A treatment interaction on survival was observed between the baseline characteristics of diabetes and of ST segment elevation. Patients with diabetes had better survival with CABG than PCI. This survival difference was totally confined to the randomized population and not seen in the registry population who were eligible but had declined randomization. BARI patients with ST-elevation on admission had better long-term survival if treated by PCI in comparison with CABG. However, the numbers of patients with ST-segment elevation was small and the clinical significance of this observation needs to be confirmed in additional studies.

Extrapolating outcome models derived from these populations of patients treated by physician selection leads to the conclusion that all high-risk patients will benefit from aggressive therapy. This conclusion is overly simplistic and counter-intuitive. Clearly, a point is reached where some patients have such advanced disease that aggressive intervention will cause greater short-term risk than the expected long-term benefit. Moreover, recent demonstration of improvement in survival of medical treatment that incorporates modern pharmaceutical regimens in the high-risk patient emphasizes the urgent need for well-designed randomized comparisons of modern medical treatment and revascularization strategies.

A Surgical Treatment for IsChemic Heart Failure (STICH) trial has been funded by the NHLBI to compare modern medical and surgical therapy in those patients for whom equipoise of anticipated benefit now exists between medical and surgical therapy. The design of this trial excludes only patients for whom medicine is the reasonable therapeutic alternative, such as those with advanced dementia or other debilitating disease and those who are heart transplant candidates. Although PCI is not included as an option in the trial, the trial will address the impact of revascularization on survival that can be used to infer benefit from PCI. Moreover, this trial will relate continuous quantitative relationships between a number of physiologic measurements of the magnitude of ischemia and viability as predictors of survival with a revascularization strategy. Patients in this cohort who have anterior akinesia or dyskinesia will also be randomly assigned to receive revascularization with or without surgical ventricular restoration to a more normal size. If this trial is conducted as proposed, results are not anticipated to be available until 2008. In the interim, compilation of information on outcomes of the high-risk patient, such as represented in this book, will remain the best source of decision-making for the clinician regarding this common clinical dilemma.

REFERENCES

1. Alderman EL, Bourassa MG, Cohen LS et al for the CASS Investigators. Ten-year follow-up of survival and myocardial infarction in the randomized Coronary Artery Surgery Study, *Circulation* 1990; **82:** 1629–1646.
2. O'Connell JB, Bristow MR. Economic impact of heart failure in the United States: time for a different approach, *Heart Lung Transplant* 1993; **13**:S107–S112.
3. Kaesemeyer WH. Holding smokers accountable for heart disease costs, *Circulation* 1994; **90**:1029–1032.
4. Block PC, Peterson EC, Krone R et al. Identification of variables needed to risk adjust outcomes of coronary interventions evidence-based guidelines for efficient data collection, *J Am Coll Cardiol* 1998; **32**:275–282.
5. Jones RH, Hannan EL, Hammermeister KE et al. Identification of preoperative variables needed for risk adjustment of short-term mortality after coronary artery bypass graft surgery, *J Am Coll Cardiol* 1996; **28**:1478–1487.
6. Jones RH. In search of the optimal surgical mortality, *Circulation* 1989; **79** (suppl I):I-132–I-136.
7. Hannan EL, Racz MJ, McAllister BD et al. A comparison of three-year survival after coronary artery bypass graft surgery and percutaneous transluminal coronary angioplasty, *J Am Coll Cardiol* 1999; **33**:63–72.
8. Brooks MM, Jones RH, Bach RG et al for the BARI Investigators. Predictors of mortality and mortality from cardiac causes in the Bypass Angioplasty Revascularization Investigation (BARI) Randomized Trial and Registry, *Circulation* 2000; **101**:2682–2689.

Section I: Is the medical management optimal?

1

What constitutes medically refractory in the new millennium?

Douglass A Morrison and Jerome Sacks

CONTENTS • What's so important about medically refractory? • Medically refractory prior to revascularization • Medically refractory after revascularization

WHAT'S SO IMPORTANT ABOUT MEDICALLY REFRACTORY?

It is important to clarify objectives before discussing strategy [1]. Most patients with acute coronary syndromes (ACS) can be medically stabilized; that is, their symptoms (objectively documented ischemia, hemodynamic or electrical instability) can be controlled by medicines [2]. Those patients who cannot be medically stabilized are called medically refractory. Medically refractory patients:

- have a higher risk of adverse outcomes (such as death, myocardial infarction or emergency revascularization); and
- constitute a group for whom aggressive therapy (catheterization and revascularization by either coronary bypass graft surgery or percutaneous coronary intervention) is likely to impart a significant clinical benefit.

This text was designed to review the evidence regarding the role of cardiac revascularization, by either percutaneous coronary intervention (PCI) or coronary artery bypass graft surgery (CABG), in the treatment of patients with higher than 'usual' risk of adverse outcomes,

particularly death. The book is based on the notion of a hierarchy of evidence. At the top of this hierarchy stands the randomized clinical trial (RCT). Two or more RCTs are required for a Class A recommendation in the American College of Cardiology/American Heart Association (ACC/AHA) guidelines, which have been produced for nearly two decades by these organizations to provide guidance for caregivers of heart disease patients [3–5].

As outlined in the first section of this text, the accumulated weight of hundreds of RCTs, involving hundreds of thousands of patients, support 'hard endpoint' clinical benefits (survival; reduction in myocardial infarction; reduction in stroke; increased exercise capacity) for a number of medical therapies, specifically:

- Antiplatelet agents such as aspirin and clopidogrel [6–11].
- Lipid-lowering agents, especially statins [12–31].
- Beta-blocking drugs [32–66].
- Angiotensin-converting enzyme inhibition (ACE-I) [67–93].
- Platelet glycoprotein IIb/IIIa receptor inhibitor infusions [94–102].
- Anticoagulants [103–109].

As outlined in the second section of this text, the objective data is far more limited for hard endpoint clinical benefits with revascularization by either CABG or PCI. Additionally, what evidence there is for hard endpoint clinical benefit is limited to higher risk patients. Both high- and low-risk patients can achieve excellent symptomatic relief with CABG or PCI; but symptoms are 'soft', both in terms of being subjective and individual as well as being non-specific (patients can experience severe symptoms from non-cardiac etiologies).

This is why the concept medically refractory is important. It is the attempt to objectively define where the benefit/risk consideration begins to favor an attempt at revascularization. After that point, we can debate (and through this text, we shall!) which revascularization method should be utilized, PCI or CABG. But until we reach that point, most would agree to treat patients with the medical therapy that relieves symptoms and is supported by RCTs.

In designing the AWESOME trial (chapter 16), which compared PCI and CABG in five high-risk groups, we felt that it was ethically appropriate to limit enrollment to patients who had symptoms (ischemia, hemodynamics, or electrical instability) that were refractory to medical therapy. This design feature formed the basis of our attempts to define medically refractory prior to revascularization [1, 110, 111]. One of the important surprises of the trial was that, by having very high proportions of revascularized patients who were receiving proven medical therapies (aspirin, heparin, beta-blockers), we had substantially lower short- and long-term mortalities than previous registry results had predicted [110, 111]. This led to the development of another underlying theme of this text, namely that continuing to give patients appropriate medical therapy after revascularization is associated with improved outcomes.

MEDICALLY REFRACTORY PRIOR TO REVASCULARIZATION

Sackett and colleagues remind us that a rational approach to therapeutic decisions depends upon the clarity with which three goals are defined: identifying the ultimate objectives of therapy, selection of the specific treatments, and specifying the treatment targets [1].

In our text, *Medically refractory rest angina*, we attempted to define medically refractory, based on the assumption that the primary objective of therapy was relief of symptoms [2]. The specific treatments available for relief of symptoms were antianginals such as beta-blockers, calcium blockers and nitrates. The use of aspirin and heparin were predicated in data from randomized clinical trials (RCT) that these drugs were associated with a reduction in adverse outcomes. What seemed to be controversial in 1992 was the specification of targets, and specifically whether categories of drugs, dosages of drugs, or physiological targets (such as resting heart rate and blood pressure) were adequate [2]. For our text, and subsequent randomized clinical trial (AWESOME; chapter 16) [110, 111], we chose physiologic targets.

Since 1992 the situation has changed dramatically. Numerous RCTs have demonstrated a far greater importance of therapy directed at the treatment goal of reducing adverse outcomes (specifically prolonging survival and reducing the frequency of MI, stroke or heart failure). To be clinically useful, the term 'medically refractory' needs to be reconsidered. The objective of preventing adverse outcomes and even prolonging survival is supported by RCTs of post-myocardial infarction (MI) patients by means of aspirin, beta-blockers, lipid-lowering statins and angiotension-converting enzyme inhibition [3–93]. CT data even supports the use of statin drugs among patients who have yet to manifest coronary artery disease [12–31].

The categories of drugs, and the evidence for their use (now primarily emphasizing reduction in adverse outcomes) are summarized in the three American College of Cardiology/

American Heart Association (ACC/AHA) guidelines on ST elevation MI, unstable angina and non-ST elevation MI, and stable angina [3–5]. These guidelines do not specify dosages or targets. Clearly, one is on the firmest ground in applying RCT data if one is applying the study results to patients who might have been included in the trials and if one uses the same drugs and dosages that were used in the trial. Unfortunately, many patients would be excluded and many patients will not tolerate the dosages used in the trials.

Caveats in the use of physiologic targets for developing a definition of medically refractory:

- Patient age, and the drug excretory function, either renal or hepatic, must be considered.
- Physiologic targets such as heart rate may have to be applied differently in patients with a range of left and/or right ventricular systolic and diastolic functions.
- Patient age, symptoms (for example dizziness), conduction system function, and cerebrovascular function may influence what levels of heart rate and blood pressure (BP) a given patient may be able to tolerate.
- There is data to push low density lipoprotein (LDL) cholesterol down to 100 with statins in patients with prior myocardial events, but only to 130 if the patient has risk factors but has not had a cardiac event.

Mechanisms of unstable coronary syndromes cannot, currently, be used as measures, or even surrogates, of medical refractoriness even when they are readily quantifiable [112–126].

- Thrombus on a pre-existing plaque is the most widely accepted mechanism for both ST elevation (occlusive) and non-ST elevation (non-occlusive) myocardial infarction. Treating or preventing thrombus is a legitimate objective of both antiplatelet and antithrombin drug therapies. But without a reproducible measure of thrombus formation, we are left defining the dose of the drug based on trial doses such as 75 or 325 mg for most aspirin studies, or some surrogate functional target such as activated clotting time (ACT) or partial thromboplastin time (PTT) for intravenous heparin.

Table 1.1 Therapeutic objectives and specific drug treatments

- Prolongation of life and prevention of myocardial infarction, and other adverse cardiac events:
  - Antiplatelet agents [6–11, 103–110].
  - Lipid-lowering agents, particularly statins [12–31].
  - Beta-blockers [32–66].
  - Angiotensin-converting enzyme inhibition [67–93].
  - Glycoprotein IIb/IIIa receptor blockers [94–101].
- Relief of symptoms and improved quality of life:
  - Aspirin [6–11, 104–107] and/or clopidogrel [10–11].
  - Anticoagulants including low molecular weight heparins [103–110].
  - Nitrates [2].
  - Beta-blockers [32–66].
  - Calcium-channel blockers.

- Dynamic obstruction, or vasospasm, is a reason to use intravenous nitroglycerin but it does not provide us with an objective target dose. In the Veterans Affairs surgical consultant's database, any dose of intravenous nitroglycerin (even 5 μg/min!) is a risk factor. Although it is 'intuitive' that symptoms at 200 μg/min are likely to be more refractory than symptoms of 10 μg/min, there is no cross patient threshold for this or most drugs.
- Progressive mechanical obstruction can occur as a result of spasm, thrombus, recoil or progression of atherosclerosis but does not lend itself to a measure of refractoriness.
- If inflammation turns out to be an important component of acute ischemia, this could be a part of how aspirin 'works', and 'measuring' antiplatelet function would be even further from a clinically usable definition of refractory.
- Secondary unstable angina also complicates the use of pathophysiologic surrogates for refractoriness.

Table 1.2 Drug target doses based upon randomized clinical trials

	Drug	Target dose	Trials
I. Antiplatelet agents [6–11]	Aspirin	325 mg	Antiplatelet trialists
	Clopidogrel	75 mg	CAPRIE, CURE
II. Lipid-lowering, particularly statins [12–31]	Prevastatin	40 mg	WOSCOPS, LIPID, CARE
	Simvastatin	20–40 mg	4S, MAAS
	Lovastatin	20–40 mg	AFCAPS/TexCAPS
	Atorvastatin	80 mg	MIRACL
	Gemfibrozil	600 BID	Helsinki Heart, VAHIT
	Clofibrate	1500 mg	Newcastle
	Niacin	3 gm	Stockholm, CDP, CLAS
III. Beta-blockers [32–66]	Atenolol iv	5 mg	ISIS-1, Yusuf et al
	Atenolol po	50–100 mg	ISIS-1
	Metoprolol po	50–100 BID	MIAMI, TIMI IIb
	Metoprolol iv	5 mg × 3 doses	MIAMI, TIMI IIb
	Propranolol iv	0.1 mg/kg	Norris et al; Peter et al
	Propranolol po	320 mg/day in 4 doses	Norris et al; Peter et al
	Carvedilol iv	2.5 mg	Basu et al
	Carvedilol po	12.5–50 BID	
IV. Angiotensin-converting enzyme inhibitors [67–93]	Lisinopril	10 QD	GISSI-3
	Captopril	25–50 TID	ISIS-4
	Enalapril	20 QD	CONSENSUS, SOLVD, V-HeFT II
	Zofenopril	30 TID	SMILE
	Ramipril	10 QD	AIRE
	Trandaloopril	4 QD	TRACE

QD, once per day; BID, two times per day; TID, three times per day; SQ, subcutaneous; IV, intravenous.

- It may be that in the future, markers of inflammation, or hypercoagulability, or enzymes indicative of small amounts of injury ('necrolettes') may become therapeutic targets, but the data is not yet available.

Redefinition of medically refractory for 2002, taking into account the above-listed principles.

Goal 1: Prevent adverse events including death.

- Antiplatelet therapy: aspirin 75–325 mg or clopidogrel 75 mg if significant contraindication to aspirin.
- Beta-blocker therapy for all post-MI patients and hypertensive patients or heart-failure patients: to RCT doses unless limited by symptomatic bradycardia, or hypotension or idiosyncratic issues such as bronchospasm.
- Angiotensin-converting enzyme inhibition for all patients with a left ventricular ejection fraction (LVEF) of 0.40; to RCT doses unless limited by symptomatic hypotension.
- Lipid-lowering to LDL < 160 for all patients, < 130 for all patients with risk factors, and < 100 for all prior MI and post-revascularization patients.

Goal 2: Relief of symptoms.

- Antiplatelet therapy: as above.
- Anticoagulant therapy; either unfractionated heparin with target PTT or ACT or low molecular weight heparin using RCT doses.
- Nitrates tolerated to tolerance.
- Beta-blockers to RCT doses, unless proscribed or limited, as above.
- Calcium blockers to RCT doses unless limited by symptomatic bradycardia and/or hypotension.
- Glycoprotein IIb/IIIa receptor blockers: it is controversial, even with RCT data, whether this should be included as part of 'medically refractory' at this time.

Table 1.3 Summary of recommended care appropriate in year 2002

- Patients with stable or unstable coronary syndromes should receive 75–325 mg oral aspirin unless there is a major contraindication, in which case, clopidogrel is an acceptable alternative.
- Patients with prior MI should receive oral beta-blockers titrated to RCT dosages unless symptomatic bradycardia or hypotension, or significant idiosyncratic response to beta blockade precludes.
- Patients with LVEF < 0.40 and/or history of symptomatic heart failure, or prior MI, especially anterior MI, should receive titrated dosing of angiotensin converting enzyme inhibition toward RCT dosages unless proscribed by hypotension or other objective side-effect.
- Coronary artery disease (CAD) patients should have blood pressure reduced to resting < 140/90.
- CAD patients should have a fasting lipid panel and statin drugs or alternatives with a goal of < 130 mg/dL for asymptomatic subjects with risk factors, and < 100 for patients with prior ML, revascularization or angina.
- CAD patients should have counseling to stop smoking.

The above considerations specify settings where either beta-blocker or ACE-I agents are 'first-line'. Otherwise either calcium blockers or vasodilators are acceptable alternatives as either antihypertensive or antianginal agents. In subjects who continue to have angina or angina equivalents after the above conditions are met, further titration of beta-blockers, calcium blockers and nitrates are directed towards a resting heart rate in the 50s (without symptoms) or a resting blood pressure in the region of 100 mmHg (without symptoms). Patients with symptoms, despite the above therapies and targets, are medically refractory.

What regimen should patients be receiving before even taking them to the catheterization laboratory for diagnostic study?

(A) For acute ST segment elevation myocardial infarct patients going to laboratory for primary intervention, most authorities would agree patients should receive:

- Oral aspirin 75–325 mg; if sensitivity precludes this option, clopidogrel is an alternative with 300 mg loading dose and 75 QD (once daily) having pharmacokinetic advantages.
- Intravenous heparin bolus or subcutaneous (SQ) low molecular weight heparin; heparin needs to be adjusted based on weight and physiologic action as measured by activated partial thromboplastin time or activated clotting time. Low molecular weight heparin does not require adjustment but is dose-based.
- Provided heart rate and blood pressure is adequate and the patient is not in shock or acute pulmonary edema, then IV metoprolol 5 mg in three doses, or comparable doses of atenolol, propranolol, or esmolol can be applied. The RCT data for these drugs admittedly comes largely from the pre-fibrinolytic era, but it has physiologic plausibility and is RCT data.
- One of the glycoprotein IIb/IIIa receptor blockers as adjunct to acute MI intervention, which usually includes a stent. The bulk of the data and even one head to head comparison favor abciximab (Reopro).
- Clopidogrel 300 mg load and then 75 QD for approximately one month after percutaneous coronary intervention (PCI)/stent.
- Lipid panel at time of admission with discharge on dose sufficient to lower LDL < 100 mg.
- If LVEF < 0.40, titration of angiotensin-converting enzyme inhibitor (ACE-I) post-procedure to target dose of one of the large RCTs.

- If BP remains > 140/90 after above procedure, continue up-titration of beta blockade or calcium blocker.

(B) For non-ST elevation acute myocardial infarction and unstable angina, patients should receive:

- Oral aspirin 75–325 mg; if sensitivity precludes this option, clopidogrel is an alternative with 300 mg loading dose and 75 QD having pharmacokinetic advantages.
- Intravenous heparin bolus or SQ low molecular weight heparin; heparin needs to be adjusted based on weight and physiologic action as measured by activated partial thromboplastin time or activated clotting time. Low molecular weight heparin does not require adjustment but is dose-based.
- Up-titration of beta-blockade (unless patient is in shock, pulmonary edema, bronchospasm or advanced heart block.) For patients with ongoing pain, an iv dosing schedule used for ST elevation MI is appropriate.
- One of the glycoprotein IIb/IIIa receptor blockers as adjunct to acute MI intervention, which usually includes a stent. The bulk of the data and even one head to head comparison favor abciximab (Reopro).
- Clopidogrel 300 mg load and then 75 QD for approximately one month after PCI/stent.
- Lipid panel at time of admission with discharge on dose sufficient to lower LDL < 100 mg.
- If LVEF < 0.40, titration of ACE-I post-procedure to target dose of one of the large RCTs.
- If BP remains > 140/90 after above procedure, then further up-titration of beta blockade or calcium blocker.

(C) Stable angina or asymptomatic ischemia patients should be on following prior to diagnostic catheterization:

- Aspirin or alternative antiplatelet: clopidogrel or ticlopidine.

- Lipid-lowering regimen such that LDL < 130 mg/dl.
- Blood pressure regimen such that resting BP < = 140/90. This should include ACE-I if LVEF < 0.50 or prior MI or should include beta-blocker if prior MI.
- Blood pressure that is refractory to beta-blocker and/or ACE-I, may be treated with titrating calcium blocker.

(D) Patients with left ventricular dysfunction

- Patients should receive dietary counseling with regard to water, and electrolytes and diuretics in an effort to achieve dry weight.
- Digoxin may be used particularly in patients with atrial fibrillation and particularly when beta-blockers are not needed (for example, post-MI patients).
- Symptomatic or asymptomatic patients with LVEF < 0.40 should be titrated to RCT doses (for example captopril 50 mg BID) of ACE-inhibition. If cough or hypersensitivity preclude use, angiotensin receptor blocking agents may be substituted. If rise in creatinine precludes, isordil/hydralazine to RCT dose (i.e. 40 TID/75–100 QD may be substituted.
- In all patients with MI, lipid panel should be checked and statin titrated to LDL < 100.
- After step 3, titrate slowly on beta-blocker, preferably either metoprolol (based on the Metroprolol in Dilated Cardiomyopathy (MDC) trial) or carvedilol.
- Control BP to < 140/90 using first ACE-I (step 3), second either beta (ischemic disease) or hydralazine/isordil and last calcium blocker (unless diastolic dysfunction is primary).

MEDICALLY REFRACTORY AFTER REVASCULARIZATION

Having put a patient through a revascularization procedure, what medicines should they go home on?

(A) Patients who have had either coronary artery bypass graft (CABG) or PCI should go home on following:

- Aspirin and/or clopidogrel.
- Lipid-lowering to have LDL < 100.
- Blood pressure < = 140/90.
- Not smoking or sent to smoking cessation.
- Step 3 should include ACE-I if LVEF < 0.40 or prior MI.
- Step 3 should include beta-blocker if prior MI.
- Diabetes control optimized.

Having established the objectives of therapy, the specific drugs, and the physiologic targets, how long should a patient with persistent symptoms or signs of ischemia receive therapy before he (she) is declared refractory? The implication is that medically refractory patients should go to the catheterization laboratory. It is a reflection of the latitude available in the literature that many similar studies (mostly low-molecular weight heparin and glycoprotein IIb/IIIa receptor blocker trials) were cited for the following five articles, which concluded that the appropriate timing for catheterization was anywhere from immediately to almost never.

- Immediate or 'drive-through'.
- Delay for 24 hours of medical treatment.
- Risk-stratification and ischemia guided.
- Stabilization for 5 days.
- As infrequently as possible [129–132].

REFERENCES

1. Tugwell P. Chapter 7. Deciding on the best therapy. In: Sackett DL, Haynes RB, Guyatt GH, Tugwell P, eds, *Clinical epidemiology: a basic science for clinical medicine*, 2nd edn (Boston: Little Brown, 1991) 187–248.
2. Morrison DA. What constitutes medically refractory? In: Morrison DA, Serruys PW, eds, *Medically refractory rest angina* (New York: Marcel Dekker Inc, 1992) 105–118.
3. Ryan TJ, Antman EM, Brooks NH et al. ACC/AHA guidelines for the management of patients with acute myocardial infarction: 1999 update. A report of the American College of Cardiology/American Heart Association Task Force on Practice Guidelines (committee on the management of acute myocardial infarction), *J Am Coll Cardiol* 1996; **28**:1328–1428.
4. Braunwald E, Antman EM, Beasley JW et al. ACC/AHA guidelines for the management of patients with unstable angina and non-ST-segment elevation myocardial infarction. A report of the American College of Cardiology/American Heart Association Task Force on Practice Guidelines (committee on the management of patients with unstable angina), *J Am Coll Cardiol* 2000; **36**:970–1062.
5. Gibbons RJ, Chatterjee K, Daley J et al. ACC/AHA/ ACP-ASIM guidelines for the management of patients with chronic stable angina. A report of the American College of Cardiology/American Heart Association Task Force on Practice Guidelines (committee on the management of patients with chronic stable angina), *J Am Coll Cardiol* 1999; **33**: 2092–2197.
6. Antiplatelet Trialists Collaboration. Collaborative overview of randomized trials of antiplatelet therapy – I: prevention of death, myocardial infarction and stroke by prolonged antiplatelet therapy in various categories of patients, *BMJ* 1995; **308**:81–106.
7. Lewis RD, Davis JW, Archibald DG et al. Protective effect of aspirin against acute myocardial infarction and death in men with unstable angina. Results of a Veterans Administration cooperative study, *N Engl J Med* 1983; **309**:396–403.
8. Cairns JA, Gent M, Singer J et al. Aspirin, sulfinpyrazone, or both in unstable angina. Results of a Canadian multicenter trial, *N Engl J Med* 1985; **313**:1369–1375.
9. Final report on the aspirin component of the ongoing Physicians' Health Study. Steering Committee of the Physicians' Health Study Research Group, *N Engl J Med* 1989; **321**: 129–135.
10. CAPRIE Steering Committee: a randomized, blinded, trial of clopidogrel versus aspirin in patients at risk of ischemic events (CAPRIE), *Lancet* 1996; **348**:1329–1339.
11. The Clopidogrel in Unstable angina to prevent Recurrent Events trial investigators. Effects of Clopidogrel I addition to aspirin in patients with acute coronary syndromes without ST-segment elevation, *N Engl J Med* 2001; **345**: 494–502.
12. Larosa JC, Hunninghake D, Bush D et al. The cholesterol facts: a summary of the evidence relating dietary fats, serum cholesterol, and coronary heart disease. A joint statement by the American Heart Association and the National Heart, Lung, and Blood Institute. The Task Force on Cholesterol Issues, American Heart Association, *Circulation* 1990; **81**:1721–1733.
13. Gould AL, Rossouw JE, Sanranello NC, Heyse JF, Furberg CD. Cholesterol reduction yields clinical benefit: impact of statin trials, *Circulation* 1998; **97**:946–952.
14. Report from the Committee of Principal Investigators: a cooperative trial in the primary prevention of ischemic heart disease using clofibrate, *Br Heart J* 1978; **40**:1069–1118.
15. Lipid Research Clinics Program Epidemiology Committee: plasma lipid distributions in selected North American populations: the lipid research clinics program prevalence study, *Circulation* 1979; **60**:427–439.
16. Lipid Research Clinics Program: the lipid research clinics coronary primary prevention trial results I. Reduction in incidence of coronary heart disease, *JAMA* 1984; **251**:351–364.
17. Lipid Research Clinics Program: the lipid research clinics coronary primary prevention trial results II. The relationship of reduction in incidence of coronary heart disease to cholesterol lowering, *JAMA* 1984; **251**:365–374.
18. Frick MH, Elo O, Haapa K et al. Helsinki Heart Study: primary-prevention trial with gemfibrozil in middle-age men with dyslipidemia; safety of treatment, changes in risk factors, and

incidence of coronary heart disease, *N Engl J Med* 1987; **317**:1237–1245.

19. Mannihen V, Elo O, Frick MH et al. Lipid alterations and decline in incidence of coronary heart disease in the Helsinki Heart Study, *JAMA* 1988; **260**:641–651.

20. The Coronary Drug Project Research Group. Clofibrate and niacin in coronary heart disease, *JAMA* 1975; **231**:360–381.

21. Canner PL, Berge KG, Wenger NK et al. Fifteen year mortality in coronary drug project patients: long-term benefit with niacin, *J Am Coll Cardiol* 1986; **8**:1245–1255.

22. Rubins HB, Robins SJ, Collins D et al. Distribution of lipids in 8,500 men with coronary artery disease, *Am J Cardiol* 1995; **75**:1196–1201.

23. Rubins HB. High-density lipoprotein and coronary heart disease: lessons from recent intervention trials, *Prev Cardiol* 2000; **3**:33–39.

24. Rubins HB, Robins S, Collins D et al for the Veterans Affairs high-density lipoprotein cholesterol intervention trial study group. Gemfibrozil for the secondary prevention of coronary heart disease in men with low levels of high-density lipoprotein cholesterol, *N Engl J Med* 1999; **341**:410–418.

25. Rubins HB, Robins SJ, Collins D. The Veterans Affairs high-density lipoprotein intervention trial: baseline characteristics of normocholesterolemic men with coronary artery disease and low levels of high-density lipoprotein cholesterol, *Am J Cardiol* 1996; **78**:572–575.

26. Carlson LA, Rosenhamer G. Reduction of mortality in the Stockholm ischemic heart disease secondary prevention study by combined treatment with clofibrate and nicotinic acid, *Acta Med Scand* 1998; **223**:405–418.

27. Shepherd J, Cobbe SM, Ford I et al. Prevention of coronary heart disease with pravastatin in men with hypercholesterolemia, *N Engl J Med* 1995; **333**:1301–1307.

28. Downs JR, Clearfield M, Weis S et al. Primary prevention of acute coronary events with lovastatin in men and women with average cholesterol levels: results of AFCAPS/TEXCAPS, *JAMA* 1998; **279**:1615–1622.

29. Scandinavian Simvastatin Survival Study Group. Randomized trial of cholesterol lowering in 4,444 patients with coronary heart disease: the Scandinavian Simvastatin Survival Study (4S), *Lancet* 1994; **344**:1383–1389.

30. Sacks FM, Pfeffer MA, Moye LA et al. The effect of pravastatin on coronary events after myocardial infarction in patients with average cholesterol levels. Cholesterol and recurrent events trial investigators, *N Engl J Med* 1996; **355**:1001–1009.

31. The Long-term Intervention with Pravastatin in Ischaemic Disease (LIPID) Study Group. Prevention of cardiovascular events and death with pravastatin in patients with coronary heart disease and a broad range of initial cholesterol levels, *N Engl J Med* 1998; **339**:1349–1357.

32. Yusuf S, Peto R, Lewis J, Collins R, Sleight P. Beta-blockade during and after myocardial infarction: an overview of the randomized trials, *Prog in Cardiovasc Dis* 1985; **27**:335–371.

33. Yusuf S, Wittes J, Friedman L. Overview of results of randomized clinical trials in heart disease II. Unstable angina, heart failure, primary prevention with aspirin, and risk factor modification, *JAMA* 1988; **260**:2259–2263.

34. Andersson B, Hjalmarson A, Swedborg K. Adrenergic beta-blockade and heart failure: from endangerment to conquest. Updates, *Textbook of Cardiovascular Medicine* Vol 2, 1999.

35. ISIS-1 (First International Study of Infarct Survival) Collaborative Group: randomized trial of intravenous atenolol among 16,027 cases of suspected acute myocardial infarction: ISIS-1, *Lancet* 1986; July 12:57–65.

36. The MIAMI Research Group. Metoprolol in acute myocardial infarction (MIAMI). A randomized placebo-controlled intervention trial, *Eur Heart J* 1985; **6**:199–226.

37. Roberts R, Rogers WJ, Mueller HS et al for the TIMI Investigators: immediate versus deferred beta-blockade following thrombolytic therapy in patients with acute myocardial infarction. Results of the Thrombolysis in Myocardial Infarction (TIMI) II-B study, *Circulation* 1991; **83**:422–437.

38. Hjalmarson A, Herlitz J, Malek I et al. Effect on mortality of metoprolol in acute myocardial infarction, *Lancet* 1981; Oct 17:823–827.

39. The International Collaborative Study Group. Reduction of infarct size with the early use of timolol in acute myocardial infarction, *N Engl J Med* 1984; **310**:9–15.

40. Norris RM, Sammel NL, Clarke ED, Smith WM, Williams B. Protective effect of propranolol in threatened myocardial infarction, *Lancet* 1978; Oct 28:907–909.

41. Yusuf S, Peto R, Bennett D et al. Early intravenous atenolol treatment in suspected acute myocardial infarction, *Lancet* 1980; Aug 9: **9:** 273–276.

42. Peter T, Norris RM, Clarke ED et al. Reduction of enzyme levels by propranolol after acute myocardial infarction, *Circulation* 1978; **57:** 1091–1095.

43. Yusuf S, Sleight P, Rossi P et al. Reduction in infarct size, arrythmias and chest pain by early intravenous beta-blockade in suspected acute myocardial infarction, *Circulation* 1983; **67:** I32–I41.

44. Ramsdale DR, Faragher EB, Bennett DH et al. Ischemic pain relief in patients with acute myocardial infarction by intravenous atenolol, *Am Heart J* 1982; **103:**459–467.

45. Richterova A, Herlitz J, Holmberg S et al. Goteborg Metoprolol Trial. Effects on chest pain, *Am J Cardiol* 1984; **53:**32D–36D.

46. Waagstein F, Hjalmarson A. Double-blind study of the effect of cardioselective beta-blockade on chest pain in acute myocardial infarction, *Acta Med Scand* 1975 (suppl 587): 201–208.

47. Basu S, Senior R, Raval U et al. Beneficial effect of intravenous and oral carvedilol treatment in acute myocardial infarction. A placebo-controlled randomized trial, *Circulation* 1997; **96:**183–191.

48. Beta-blocker Heart Attack Trial Research Group. A randomized trial of propranolol in patients with acute myocardial infarction I. Mortality results, *JAMA* 1982; **247:**1707–1714.

49. Lopressor Intervention Trial Research Group. The Lopressor Intervention Trial: Multicentre study of metoprolol in survivors of acute myocardial infarction, *Eur Heart J* 1987; **8:** 1056–1064.

50. The Norwegian Multicenter Study Group. Timolol-induced reduction in mortality and reinfarction in patients surviving acute myocardial infarction, *N Engl J Med* 1981; **304:**801–807.

51. Pederson TR for the Norwegian Multicenter Study Group. Six-year follow-up of the Norwegian multicenter study on timolol after acute myocardial infarction, *N Engl J Med* 1985; **313:**1055–1058.

52. Olsson G, Rehnqvist N, Sjogren A, Erhardt L, Lundman T. Long-term treatment with metoprolol after myocardial infarction: effect on 3-year mortality and morbidity, *J Am Coll Cardiol* 1985; **5:**1428–1437.

53. Olsson G, Oden A, Johansson L, Sjogren A, Rehnqvist N. Prognosis after withdrawal of chronic postinfarction metoprolol treatment: a 2–7 year follow-up, *Eur Heart J* 1988; **9:**365–372.

54. MERIT-HF Study Group. Effect of metoprolol CR/XL in chronic heart failure: metoprolol CR/XL randomized intervention trial in congestive heart failure (MERIT-HF), *Lancet* 1999; **353:**2001–2007.

55. Bristow MR, Gilbert EM, Abraham WT et al for the MOCHA Investigators. Carvedilol produces dose-related improvements in left ventricular function and survival in subjects with chronic heart failure, *Circulation* 1996; **94:**2807–2816.

56. Fisher ML, Gottlieb SS, Plotnick GD et al. Beneficial effects of metoprolol in heart failure associated with coronary artery disease: a randomized trial, *J Am Coll Cardiol* 1994; **23:** 943–950.

57. Krum H, Sackner-Bernstein JD, Goldsmith RL et al. Double-blind, placebo-controlled study of the long-term efficacy of carvedilol in patients with severe chronic heart failure, *Circulation* 1995; **92:**1499–1506.

58. Persson H, Eriksson SV, Erhardt L. Effects of beta receptor antagonists on left ventricular function in patients with clinical evidence of heart failure after myocardial infarction. A double-blind comparison of metoprolol and xamoterol, *Eur Heart J* 1996; **17:**741–749.

59. Persson H, Rythe-Alder E, Erhardt L. Effects of beta receptor antagonists in patients with clinical evidence of heart failure after myocardial infarction: double-blind comparison of metoprolol with xamoterol, *Br Heart J* 1995; **74:** 140–148.

60. Waagstein F, Bristow M, Swedborg K et al. Beneficial effects of metoprolol in idiopathic dilated cardiomyopathy, *Lancet* 1993; **342:** 1441–1446.

61. Packer M, Bristow MR, Cohn JN et al for the US Carvedilol Heart Failure Study Group. The effect of carvedilol on morbidity and mortality in patients with chronic heart failure, *N Engl J Med* 1996; **334:**1349–1355.

62. Packer M, Colucci WS, Sackner-Bernstein JD et al for the PRECISE Study Group. Double-blind, placebo-controlled study of the effects of carvedilol in patients with moderate to severe

heart failure (the PRECISE Trial), *Circulation* 1996; **94**:2793–2799.

63. CIBIS Investigators and Committees. A randomized trial of beta-blockade in heart failure the cardiac insufficiency bisoprolol study (CIBIS), *Circulation* 1994; **90**:1765–1773.

64. CIBIS-II Investigators and Committees. The cardiac insufficiency bisoprolol study II (CIBIS II): a randomized trial, *Lancet* 1999; **353**:9–13.

65. The Xamoterol in Severe Heart Failure Study Group. Xamoterol in severe heart failure, *Lancet* 1990; **336**:1–6.

66. Australia–New Zealand Heart Failure Research Collaborative Group. Effects of carvedilol, a vasodilator-beta blocker, in patients with congestive heart failure due to ischemic heart disease, *Circulation* 1995; **92**:212–218.

67. ACE Inhibitor Myocardial Infarction Collaborative Group. Indications for ACE inhibitors in the early treatment of acute myocardial infarction: systemic overview of individual data from 100,000 patients in randomized trials, *Circulation* 1998; **97**:2202.

68. Swedberg K, Held P, Kjekshus J et al for the CONSENSUS II Study Group. Effects of the early administration of enalapril on mortality in patients with acute myocardial infarction, *N Engl J Med* 1992; **327**:678.

69. Gruppo Italiano per lo Studio della Sopravivenza nell' infarto Miocardico: GISSI-3. Effects of lisinopril and transdermal glyceryl trinitrate single and together on 6-weeks mortality and ventricular function after acute myocardial infarction, *Lancet* 1994; **343**:1115.

70. ISIS-4 (Fourth International Study of Infarct Survival) Collaborative Group. ISIS-4: a randomized factorial trial assessing early oral captopril, oral mononitrate, and intravenous magnesium sulfate in 58,050 patients with suspected acute myocardial infarction, *Lancet* 1995; **345**:669.

71. Chinese Cardiac Study Collaboration Group. Oral captopril versus placebo among 13,634 patients with suspect acute myocardial infarction: interim report from the Chinese Cardiac Study (CCS 1), *Lancet* 1995; **345**:686.

72. Latini R. Maggioni AP, Flather M et al. ACE inhibitor use in myocardial infarction. Summary of evidence from clinical trials, *Circulation* 1995; **92**:3132.

73. Gruppo Italiano per lo Studio della Sopravivenza nell' infarto Miocardico. Six-month effects of early treatment with lisinopril and transdermal glyceryl trinitrate singly and together withdrawn six weeks after acute myocardial infarction, *J Am Coll Cardiol* 1996; **27**:337.

74. Zuanetti G, Latini R, Maggioni AP et al for the GISSI-3 Investigators. Effect of the ACE inhibitor lisinopril on mortality in diabetic patients with acute myocardial infarction: Data from the GISSI-3 study, *Circulation* 1997; **96**: 4239.

75. Pfeffer MA, Braunwald E, Moye LA et al for the SAVE Investigators. Effect of captopril on mortality and morbidity in patients with left ventricular dysfunction after myocardial infarction. Results of the survival and ventricular enlargement trial, *N Engl J Med* 1992; **327**:669.

76. Kober L, Torp-Pedersen C, Carlsen JE et al. A clinical trial of the angiotensin converting enzyme inhibitor trandolapril in patients with left ventricular dysfunction after myocardial infarction, *N Engl J Med* 1995; **333**:1670.

77. The Acute Infarction Ramipril Efficacy (AIRE) Study Investigators. Effort of ramipril on mortality and morbidity of survivors of acute myocardial infarction with evidence of clinical heart failure, *Lancet* 1993; **342**:821.

78. Hall AS, Murray GD, Ball SG on behalf of the AIRE Study Investigators. Follow-up study of patients randomly allocated ramipril or placebo for heart failure after myocardial infarction: AIRE Extension (AIREX) Study, *Lancet* 1997; **349**:1493.

79. Cohn JN, Johnson G, Ziesche S et al. A comparison of enalapril with hydralazine-isosorbide dinitrate in the treatment of chronic heart failure, *N Engl J Med* 1991; **325**:303.

80. Budaj A, Cybulski J, Cedro K et al. Effects of captopril on ventricular arrhythmias in the early and late phase of suspected acute myocardial infarction. Randomized, placebo-controlled substudy of ISIS-4, *Eur Heart J* 1996; **17**:1506.

81. Domanski MJ, Exner DV, Borkowf CB et al. Effect of angiotensin-converting enzyme inhibition on sudden cardiac death in patients following acute myocardial infarction, *J Am Coll Cardiol* 1999; **33**:598.

82. Ambrosioni E, Borghi C, Magnani B for the Survival of Myocardial Infarction Long-Term Evaluation (SMILE) Investigators. The effect of

the angiotensin converting enzyme inhibitor zofrenopril on mortality and morbidity after anterior myocardial infarction, *N Engl J Med* 1995; **332**:80.

83. Borghi C, Marino P, Zardini W et al for the FAMIS Working Party. Short and long-term effects of early fosinopril administration in patients with acute anterior myocardial infarction undergoing intravenous thrombolysis: results from the fosinopril in acute myocardial infarction study, *Am Heart J* 1998; **136**:213.

84. Van Gilst WH, Kingma JH, Peels CH et al. Which patient benefits from early angiotensin-converting enzyme inhibition after myocardial infarction? Results of a one-year serial echo-cardiographic follow-up from the Captopril and Thrombolysis study (CATS), *J Am Coll Cardiol* 1996; **28**:114.

85. De Kam DJ, Voors AA, van der Berg MP et al. Effect of very early angiotensin converting enzyme inhibition on left ventricular dilation after myocardial infarction in patients receiving thrombolysis, *J Am Coll Cardiol* 2000; **36**:2047.

86. Flather MD, Lonn EM, Yusuf S. Effects of ACE inhibitors on mortality when started in the early phase of myocardial infarction: evidence from the larger randomized controlled trials, *J Cardiovasc Risk* 1995; **2**:423–428.

87. Curtiss C, Cohn JN, Vrobel T, Franciosa JA. Role of the renin-angiotensin system in the systemic vasoconstriction of chronic congestive heart failure, *Circulation* 1978; **58**:763.

88. Gavras H, Faxon DP, Berkoben J et al. Angiotensin converting enzyme inhibition in patients with congestive heart failure, *Circulation* 1978; **58**:770.

89. Dzau VJ, Colucci WAS, Hollenberg NK, Williams GH. Relation of the renin-angiotensin-aldosterone system to clinical state in congestive heart failure, *Circulation* 1981; **63**:645.

90. The CONSENSUS Trial Study Group. Effects of enalapril on mortality in severe congestive heart failure: results of the Cooperative North Scandinavia Enalapril Survival Study (CONSENSUS), *N Engl J Med* 1987; **316**:1429.

91. The SOLVD Investigators. Effect of enalapril on survival in patients with reduced left ventricular ejection fractions and congestive heart failure, *N Engl J Med* 1991; **325**:293.

92. The SOLVD Investigators. Effect of enalapril on mortality and the development of heart failure in asymptomatic patients with reduced left ventricular ejection fractions, *N Engl J Med* 1992; **327**:685.

93. Kleber F, Niemoller L, Doering W. Impact of converting enzyme inhibition on progression of chronic heart failure: results of the Munich mild heart failure trial, *Br Heart J* 1992; **67**:289.

94. EPIC Investigators. Use of a monoclonal antibody directed against the platelet glycoprotein IIb/IIIa receptor in high-risk coronary angioplasty, *N Engl J Med* 1994; **330**:956–961.

95. EPILOG Investigators. Platelet glycoprotein IIb/IIIa blockade with abciximab with low-dose heparin during percutaneous coronary revascularization, *N Engl J Med* 1997; **336**:1689–1696.

96. EPISTENT Investigators. Randomized placebo-controlled and balloon-angioplasty controlled trial to assess safety of coronary stenting with use of platelet glycoprotein IIb/IIIa blockade, *Lancet* 1998; **352**:87–92.

97. IMPACT II Investigators. Randomized placebo-controlled trial of effect of eptifibatide on complications of percutaneous coronary intervention: IMPACT II, *Lancet* 1997; **349**:1422–1428.

98. RESTORE Investigators. Effects of platelet glycoprotein IIb/IIIa blockade with tirofiban on adverse cardiac events in patients with unstable angina or acute myocardial infarction undergoing coronary angioplasty, *Circulation* 1997; **96**:1445–1453.

99. CAPTURE Investigators. Randomized placebo-controlled trial of abciximab before and during coronary intervention in refractory unstable angina: the CAPTURE study, *Lancet* 1997; **349**:1429–1435.

100. Brener SJ, Barr LA, Burchenal JEB et al. A randomized, placebo-controlled trial of platelet glycoprotein IIb/IIIa blockade with primary angioplasty for acute myocardial infarction, *Circulation* 1998; **98**:734–741.

101. Gibson CM, Goel M, Cohen DJ et al. Six-month angiographic and clinical follow-up of patients prospectively randomized to receive either tirofiban or placebo during angioplasty in the RESTORE trial, *J Am Coll Cardiol* 1998: **32**:28–34.

102. Mark DB, Nelson CU, Califf RM et al. Continuing evolution of therapy for coronary artery disease. Initial results from the era of coronary angioplasty, *Circulation* 1994; **89**:2015–2025.

103. Théroux P, Ouimet H, McCans J et al. Aspirin,

heparin, or both to treat acute unstable angina, *N Engl J Med* 1988; **319**:1105–1111.

104. Théroux P, Waters D, Lam J. Reactivation of unstable angina after the discontinuation of heparin, *N Engl J Med* 1992; **327**:141–145.

105. The RISC Group. Risk of myocardial infarction and death during treatment with low dose aspirin and intravenous heparin in men with unstable coronary artery disease, *Lancet* 1990; **336**:827–830.

106. Oler A, Whooley M, Oler J, Grady D. Adding heparin to aspirin reduces the incidence of myocardial infarction and death in patients with unstable angina. A meta-analysis, *JAMA* 1996; **276**:811–815.

107. Fragmin, and fast revascularization during instability in coronary artery disease investigators. Invasive compared with non-invasive treatment in unstable coronary-artery disease: FRISC II prospective randomized multicentre study, *Lancet* 1999; **354**:708–715.

108. Cannon CP, Weintraub WS, Demopoulos L et al for the TACTICS-TIMI 18 Investigators. Troponin T and I to predict 6-month mortality and relative benefit of invasive vs conservative strategy in patients with unstable angina: primary results of the TACTICS-TIMI 18 troponin substudy, *J Am Coll Cardiol* 2001; **37** (suppl A):325A–326A.

109. Fragmin, and fast revascularization during instability in coronary artery disease investigators. Long-term low-molecular-mass heparin in unstable coronary-artery disease. FRISC II prospective randomised multicentre study, *Lancet* 1999; **354**:701–707.

110. Morrison DA, Sethi G, Sacks J et al for the AWESOME co-investigators. Percutaneous coronary intervention versus bypass graft surgery for patients with medically refractory myocardial ischemia and risk factors for adverse outcomes with bypass; a multicenter, randomized trial, *J Am Coll Cardiol* 2001; **38**:143–149.

111. Morrison DA, Sethi G, Sacks J et al for the AWESOME co-investigators. Percutaneous coronary intervention versus coronary bypass graft surgery for patients with medically refractory myocardial ischemia and risk factors for adverse outcomes with bypass; the VA AWESOME multicenter registry: comparison with the randomized clinical trial, *J Am Coll Cardiol* 2002; **39**:266–273.

112. Falk L, Shah PK, Fuster V. Coronary plaque disruption, *Circulation* 1995; **92**:657–671.

113. Mann JM, Davies MJ. Vulnerable plaque. Relation of characteristics to degree of stenosis in human coronary arteries, *Circulation* 1996; **94**:928–931.

114. Libby P. Molecular bases of the acute coronary syndromes, *Circulation* 1995; **91**:2844–2850.

115. Reimer KA, Lowe JE, Rasmussen MA, Jennings RB. The wavefront phenomenon of ischemic cell death I. Myocardial infarct size vs a duration of coronary occlusion in dogs, *Circulation* 1977; **56**:786–794.

116. Reimer KA, Jennings RB. The 'Wavefront phenomenon' of myocardial ischemic cell death II. Transmural progression of necrosis within the framework of ischemic bed size (myocardium at risk) and collateral flow, *Laboratory Investigation* 1979; **40**:633–644.

117. Glagov S, Weisenberg E, Zarins CK, Stankunavicius R, Kolettis GJ. Compensatory enlargement of human atherosclerotic coronary arteries, *N Engl J Med* 1987; **316**:1371–1375.

118. Ambrose JA, Tannenbaum MA, Alexopoulos D et al. Angiographic progression of coronary artery disease and the development of myocardial infarction, *J Am Coll Cardiol* 1988; **12**:56–62.

119. Ambrose JA, Winters S, Stern A et al. Angiographic morphology and the pathogenesis of unstable angina pectoris, *J Am Coll Cardiol* 1985; **5**:609–616.

120. Zaacks S, Liebson PR, Calvin JE, Parrillo JE, Klein LW. Unstable angina and non-Q myocardial infarction; does the clinical diagnosis have therapeutic implications? *J Am Coll Cardiol* 1999; **33**:107–118.

121. Kono T, Morita H, Nishina T et al. Circadian variations of onset of acute myocardial infarction and efficacy of thrombolytic therapy, *J Am Coll Cardiol* 1996; **27**:774–778.

122. Anderson HV, Cannon CP, Stone PH et al. One-year results of the thrombolysis in myocardial infarction (TIMI) IIIb clinical trial. A randomized comparison of tissue-type plasminogen activator versus placebo and early invasive versus early conservative strategies in unstable angina and non-Q wave myocardial infarction, *J Am Coll Cardiol* 1995; **26**:1643–1650.

123. Anderson TJ. Assessment and treatment of endothelial dysfunction in humans, *J Am Coll Cardiol* 1999; **34**:631–638.

124. Fuster V, Fallon JT, Nemerson Y. Coronary thrombosis, *Lancet* 1996; **348** (suppl 1):S7–S10.

125. Little WC, Constantinescu M, Applegare RJ et al. Can coronary angiography predict the site of subsequent myocardial infarction in patients with mild-to-moderate coronary artery disease? *Circulation* 1988; **78**:1157–1166.

126. Ringqvist I, Fisher LD, Mock M, Davis KB et al. Prognostic value of angiographic indices of coronary artery disease from the Coronary Artery Surgery Study (CASS), *J Clin Invest* 1983; **71**:1854–1866.

127. Califf RM. Evidence to practice in acute coronary syndromes, *Am J Cardiol* 2000; **86** (suppl):1M–3M.

128. Kereiakes DJ, Young J, Broderick TM, Shimshak TM, Abbottsmith CW. Therapeutic adjuncts for immediate transfer to the catheterization laboratory in patients with acute coronary syndromes, *Am J Cardiol* 2000; **82** (suppl):10M–17M.

129. Cohen M. Calming the plaque to delay intervention for 24-hours in acute coronary syndromes, *Am J Cardiol* 2000; **86** (suppl): 18M–26M.

130. Pepine CJ. An ischemia-guided approach for risk stratification in patients with acute coronary syndromes, *Am J Cardiol* 2000; **86** (suppl):27M–35M.

131. Holmes DR. Acute coronary syndromes: extending medical intervention for five days before proceeding to revascularization, *Am J Cardiol* 2000; **86** (suppl):36M–41M.

132. Boden WE. Avoidance of routine revascularization in the management of patients with non-ST-segment elevation acute coronary syndromes, *Am J Cardiol* 2000; **86** (suppl): 42M–47M.

2

Beta-blocking agents

Jason R Wollmuth and Douglass A Morrison

CONTENTS • Biology of the beta-adrenergic system and beta-blockade • Side-effects and contraindications of beta-blockade • Beta-blockade after acute myocardial infarction • Long-term therapy with beta-blockers after myocardial infarction • Beta-blockade for unstable angina • Beta-blockade for stable angina • Beta-blockade for silent ischemia • Beta-blockade for heart failure • Underutilization of beta-blockers in clinical practice • Beta-blockade for hypertension

BIOLOGY OF THE BETA-ADRENERGIC SYSTEM AND BETA-BLOCKADE [1–3]

Beta-receptors have been divided into beta-1, found primarily in heart muscle and involved with heart rate and contractility, and beta-2 found in bronchial and smooth muscle and involved in bronchodilation and vasodilation. Beta-receptors are located on cell membrane and are part of the adenylate cyclase system. The G protein links the adenylate cyclase system to the receptor. Cyclic adenosine monophosphate (AMP) is the intracellular messenger of beta-stimulation. When the system is activated, adenylate cyclase produces cyclic AMP from adenosine triphosphate (ATP), which in turn, opens calcium-channels to promote inotropic (contractility), lusitropic (relaxation), chronotropic (increased heart rate through sinus node stimulation), and dromotropic (conduction through atrioventricular node stimulation) effects [1].

Whereas adrenergic stimulation increases cytosolic calcium in the heart muscle cells, it decreases calcium in vascular smooth muscle, thereby vasodilating the coronary circulation. In this context, beta-blockade might be expected to increase coronary vascular resistance and in selected cases, spasm has been reported. Nevertheless, the beneficial effect of prolonging diastole preferentially often yields a net improvement in coronary perfusion with beta-blockade.

When beta-receptors are chronically blocked the number of beta-receptors increases. Accordingly, if beta-blockade were suddenly stopped, this increase in receptor density could facilitate a hyper-response to adrenergic stimulation, clinically evident as a withdrawal syndrome such as increased risk of infarction after abrupt withdrawal.

Propranolol is considered non-selective, whereas both metoprolol and atenolol are cardioselective, blocking beta-1 but not beta-2 receptors. Some drugs, such as pindolol and timolol, have intrinsic sympathomimetic activity (ISA), meaning they also stimulate adrenergic receptors in addition to their beta-blocking properties. Labetolol has alpha-blocking as well as beta-blocking properties.

Individual beta-blockers have other pharmacologic differences. Water-soluble drugs such as nadolol and atenolol appear to be less able to cross the blood–brain barrier and are therefore less likely to produce central nervous system side-effects such as fatigue and/or depression. The clinical effects of beta-blockade result from the sum of the individual pharmacologic effects.

SIDE-EFFECTS AND CONTRAINDICATIONS OF BETA-BLOCKADE [1–4]

The three major mechanisms for side-effects are:

- Smooth-muscle spasm, producing broncho-spasm or peripheral extremity ischemia.
- Exaggeration of cardioselective blockade, producing bradycardia, heart-block, and heart failure.
- Central nervous involvement, causing fatigue, depression or insomnia.

Accordingly, contraindications to beta-blockade include:

- History of bronchospasm or reversible obstructive airways disease.
- Severe vascular disease, especially if accompanied by Raynaud's phenomenon, brady-cardia, or heart-block (especially advanced degree).
- History of heart failure (clearly this is changing with careful titration after the patient has achieved 'dry' status).
- Severe depression.

Because of the above contraindications, physicians have been reluctant to use beta-blockers in older patients and those with chronic pulmonary disease, diabetes mellitus, or left ventricular dysfunction. However, even among patients with these relative contraindications, there appears to be potential benefits with beta-blockers. Gottlieb et al, reviewed the medical records of over 200,000 patients after myocardial infarction and found that long-term administration of beta-blockers reduced mortality in every subgroup, including patients with COPD, type I diabetes mellitus, low ejection fractions and heart failure [4]. Therefore, despite relative contraindications to beta-blockade, many patients will have significant mortality benefits with long-term beta-blocker administration.

BETA-BLOCKADE AFTER ACUTE MYOCARDIAL INFARCTION [4–18] (TABLE 2.1)

The proposed mechanisms for observed clinical benefit of early intravenous and long-term oral beta-blockade after myocardial infarction include the following:

- Reduction in myocardial oxygen demand by decreased heart rate, systolic blood pressure and double-product.
- Reduction in infarct size secondary to the reduction in myocardial oxygen demand.
- Increased ventricular fibrillation threshold.
- Reduced ischemic ectopy [2, 4, 5].

The largest of the clinical trials examining the effect of beta-blockers in acute myocardial infarction was the ISIS-1 trial [6]. In this trial, 16,027 patients with suspected acute myocardial infarction were randomized to a control group or to a group receiving atenolol (5–10 mg of intravenous (iv) immediately followed by 100 mg orally a day for seven days) [6]. Mortality in the first seven days after myocardial infarction was decreased by 15% and this benefit was maintained over one year. Though there was no decrease in rise of cardiac enzymes, there was a non-significant decrease in reinfarction and non-fatal cardiac arrests. This study suggested that treatment of approximately 200 patients would lead to avoidance of one reinfarction, one cardiac arrest, and one death during the first seven days.

The MIAMI trial continued oral treatment out to 15 days [7]. In this trial 5778 patients were randomized to a control group and a group receiving metoprolol (15 mg iv within 24 hours of onset of pain followed by 200 mg orally for 15 days). There was a 13% decrease in mortality in the metoprolol group though this was non-significant. However, in patients with

Table 2.1 Randomized trials of beta-blockade early after acute MI

Trial name/ first author	References	Subjects	Drug	Endpoints	*p* value statistics
ISIS-1	6	16,027	iv atenolol 5 mg	1 week vascular mortality	$p<0.02$ 15% risk reduction
MIAMI	7	5778	iv metoprolol 5×3	15 day mortality	$p=0.29$ 13% risk reduction
TIMI IIb	8	1434	iv metoprolol 5×3	Mortality Reinfarct	$p=0.98$ $p=0.29$ favors immediate
Hjalmarson	9	1395	iv metoprolol 15	Mortality	$p=0.03$ 36% risk reduction
Sederholm	10	144	Timolol	Infarct size	30% risk reduction
Norris	11	20	iv propranolol 0.1 mg/kg	Infarct size	$p<0.05$
Yusuf	12	214	iv atenolol 5 mg	Infarct size	$2p=0.02$
Peter	13	95	iv propranolol 0.1 mg/kg	Infarct size	27% risk reduction
Yusuf	14	477	iv atenolol 5 mg	Multiple	Significant
Ramsdale	15	18	iv atenolol	Pain relief	$p<0.001$
Goteborg	16, 17	1322	iv metoprolol 15 mg	Infarct size Pain relief	$p=0.05$ $p<0.05$
Basu	18	151	iv carvedilol 12.5	Cardiac events	$p<0.02$

Infarct size estimated by either electrocardiographic Q waves and/or creatinine phosphokinase levels.

three or greater risk predictors (age over 60, abnormal EKG, history of myocardial infarction (MI), angina pectoris, congestive heart failure, hypertension, diabetes, treatment with diuretics, treatment with cardiac glycosides prior to randomization), there was a 29% decrease in mortality. In addition to the decrease in mortality, there was a significant decrease in development of Q waves, need for pain medications, and cardiac enzymes. There were also non-significant decreases in ventricular arrhythmias and reinfarctions in the treatment group.

Two other large randomized trials comparing metoprolol with placebo showed impressive reductions in mortality. In the Goteberg Metoprolol Trial, 1322 patients received either 15 mg of iv metoprolol followed by oral doses or placebo [16, 17]. In this trial there was a 36% decrease in mortality in the group receiving metoprolol. Infarct size, as measured by lactate dehydrogenase (LDH) levels, was 17% less in the metoprolol group. Also, metoprolol decreased the incidence of ventricular fibrillation from 41 episodes in the control group compared with six in the metoprolol group. In a trial by Hjalmarson et al, 1395 patients were randomized to metoprolol or placebo [9]. In the group receiving metoprolol, there was a 36% reduction in mortality at three months.

Finally, in the TIMI II-B study, the effects of immediate beta-blocker therapy was compared with delayed initiation of beta-blockers at six days post-infarction. Though there was no difference in mortality between the two groups, immediate iv therapy resulted in a 50% decrease in reinfarction within six days and a 25% decrease in recurrence of chest pain [8].

It should be noted that the major studies of beta-blockers in early stage acute myocardial infarction were in the pre-thrombolytic era. Thrombolysis reverses some of the clinical complications of acute myocardial infarction, which may, in some cases, make beta-blockers appear less effective. However, adrenergic responses to acute myocardial infarction occur regardless of thrombolysis. Therefore, it would be expected that beta-blockers would decrease fatal ventricular arrhythmias and progression of ischemia to infarction.

LONG-TERM THERAPY WITH BETA-BLOCKERS AFTER MYOCARDIAL INFARCTION [16–27] (TABLE 2.2)

In addition to the improvement in mortality with iv beta-blocker therapy during acute myocardial infarction, there are several clinical trials, which show benefit of beta-blockers in secondary prevention. The major mechanisms for increased cardiovascular mortality during the post-infarction period include persistent myocardial ischemia, cardiac arrhythmias, and left ventricular dysfunction. Elevated levels of circulating catecholamines after myocardial infarction drive increased severity of myocardial ischemia and frequency of ventricular arrhythmias. Beta-blockade can attenuate the undesirable consequences of increased levels of circulating catecholamines. These proposed benefits are reflected in clinical studies, which

Table 2.2 Randomized trials of beta-blockade long-term post myocardial infarct

Trial name/ first author	References	Subjects	Drug	Endpoints	p value statistics
BHAT	19	3837	Propranolol	CV mortality	$p < 0.01$
					26% risk reduction
LIT	20	2395	Metoprolol	All cause mortality	p NS
Norwegian	21	1884	Timolol	Mortality	39% risk reduction
				Reinfarction	28% risk reduction
Olsson	23, 24	301	Metoprolol	Mortality	NS
				Reinfarction	$p < 0.05$
					45% risk reduction
APSI	25	607	Acebutolol	Mortality	$p = 0.019$
					48% risk reduction
				CV mortality	$p = 0.06$
					58% risk reduction
SWORD	26, 27	3121	d-sotalol	Mortality	$p = 0.006$
					65% relative risk increase

Risk reduction is relative risk; NS, not significant

show improved outcome with beta-blockers after myocardial infarction. These trials are listed in Table 2.2 and several will be reviewed here.

The most convincing long-term data for the benefit of beta-blockers after myocardial infarction came from the Norwegian Timolol Trial and the Beta-Blocker Heart Attack Trial (BHAT) [19, 21]. The largest of the long-term beta-blocker trials was the BHAT in which 3837 patients were randomized to receive 60–80 mg of propranolol three times a day or placebo within three weeks of a myocardial infarction. In an average of 25 months of follow-up, there was a decrease in all cause mortality of 28% and a decrease in cardiovascular mortality of 26%. In addition, there was a decrease in sudden death by 28% and a decrease in non-fatal reinfarction by 16% in those receiving propranolol. In the Norwegian timolol trial, 1884 patients were randomized to receive 10 mg of timolol twice a day or placebo [21]. In the initial study, there was a decrease in mortality of 39.4% with timolol as well as a decrease in sudden death of 44.6% and reinfarction of 28.4% at 17 months. A proportion of these patients were followed for an average of 61 months and the decrease in mortality at this time with timolol was 18.3%. In both of these studies, the protective effect of beta-blockers was primarily in the first 12–18 months. The reduction in mortality in the first year was 33% with timolol and 39% with propranolol.

Despite the convincing data seen in the Norwegian timolol trial and BHAT, it should be noted that several trials have failed to show a benefit of beta-blockers in the post-infarct period. In the SWORD trial, 3121 patients were treated with *d*-sotalol and followed for years [26, 27]. The study was stopped early due to a 5% death rate with *d*-sotalol compared to 3.1% with placebo. The increased mortality was accounted for by an increase in arrhythmic deaths. It should be noted however, that *d*-sotalol is primarily a potassium channel blocker with little clinically significant beta-blocking activity, which may explain the results.

Two other studies, the Lopressor Intervention Trial (LIT) and Acebutolol et Prevention Secondaire de L'Infarctus (APSI) trial, were stopped early despite encouraging results [20, 25]. In LIT, 2395 patients were randomized to receive metoprolol or placebo 6–16 days after myocardial infarction [20]. At seven months there was a 22% decrease in mortality though this wasn't maintained at one year. The trial was stopped early secondary to a progressive and marked decline in patient accession. In the APSI trial, 607 high-risk patients were randomized to receive acebutolol or placebo [25]. Despite being stopped early secondary to a lower than expected death rate among the placebo group, there was a 48% reduction in mortality and a 58% reduction in vascular mortality at an average follow-up of 318 days.

A review by Frishman et al, in 1984 examined the overall mortality benefit in 13 major randomized controlled trials which included over 16,000 survivors of acute myocardial infarction. These studies examined total mortality, cardiovascular mortality, sudden death, and non-fatal reinfarction with treatment and mean patient follow-up from nine months to four years. This revealed a 22% reduction in estimated mortality. Despite this, the authors urged caution in interpreting these results because of the significant differences between the trials, including patient populations, type and dosage of beta-blocker used, time of initiation after infarction, and duration of treatment.

BETA-BLOCKADE FOR UNSTABLE ANGINA [29–37] (TABLE 2.3)

The proposed mechanisms for observed clinical benefit of beta-blockade in patients with either stable or unstable myocardial ischemia include the following:

- Reduction in myocardial oxygen demand by decreased heart rate, systolic blood pressure, and double-product.
- Improved myocardial perfusion in patients

Table 2.3 Randomized trials of beta-blockade for unstable angina/non-Q myocardial infarction

Trial name/first author	References	Subjects	Drug
Capucci	29	23	Verapamil/propranolol
HINT	30, 32	338/177	Nifedipine/metoprolol
Fouet	31	70	Diltiazem/propranolol
Hohnloser	33	113	Esmolol 2–24 mg/min
Telford	34	214	Atenolol/heparin
Parodi	35	10	Verapamil/propranolol
Gottlieb	36	81	Propranolol/nifedipine
Theroux	37	100	Propranolol/diltiazem
Smith	101	247	Beta-blocker/diltiazem

with tachycardia by virtue of slowing heart rate preferentially increasing diastole.

- Reduction in ischemia by improved collateral flow.
- Reduction in number and severity of episodes of silent ischemia by any of the above [1–3].

Unlike acute myocardial infarction and congestive heart failure, there is little randomized trial data regarding the use of beta-blockers in unstable angina. Despite their theoretical benefits, clinical benefit hasn't been shown in large placebo-controlled trials. The only major placebo-controlled trial evaluating beta-blockers in unstable angina pectoris is the European Esmolol Study Group trial by Hohnloser et al [33]. In this study 113 patients with unstable angina were randomized to receive esmolol titrated in a step-wise manner at dosages of 2–24 mg/min versus placebo. Clinical events (development of acute MI, the need for urgent revascularization) were decreased from nine in placebo patients to three in patients receiving esmolol. Side-effects from esmolol were generally cardiovascular in origin and improved with decreased dose or discontinuation of the drug. The benefit of esmolol in the setting of unstable angina is the rapidity

with which the drug can be titrated to a desired level of beta-blockade or decreased/discontinued should side-effects develop.

The majority of trials assessing the benefit of beta-blockers in unstable angina have been comparative trials or trials in which beta-blockers are added to another therapy. In a trial by Gottlieb et al, patients with unstable angina on nitrates and nifedipine were randomized to placebo or propranolol [36]. Though the addition of propranolol didn't decrease the incidence of cardiac death, myocardial infarction, and need for revascularization, it was shown to decrease the recurrent resting angina, duration of angina, and nitroglycerin use. In addition, ischemia episodes, based on continuous ECG monitoring, were decreased with propranolol. In the Holland Interuniversity Nifedipine/metoprolol Trial (HINT), 338 patients with unstable angina were treated with nifedipine, metoprolol, or both [30, 32]. Patients were evaluated for recurrent ischemia or myocardial infarction within 48 hours. Approximately half of the patients (177) were treated with beta-blockers prior to enrollment. In these patients, the addition of nifedipine was beneficial. Among patients not on prior beta-blockers, metoprolol improved outcomes, but in these patients, there wasn't any apparent benefit from adding nifedipine. In addition, nifedipine alone may lead to an increased risk of events.

BETA-BLOCKADE FOR STABLE ANGINA [38–68, 79] (TABLE 2.4)

There are very few placebo-controlled trials examining the effects of beta-blockers on patients with stable angina pectoris. Three small, placebo-controlled trials examining the effects of nadolol [39], labetalol [40], and acebutelol [38] on patients with stable angina showed beneficial effects of the beta-blockers such as improvement in frequency of angina attacks, exercise capacity, and nitroglycerin consumption.

The majority of trials with beta-blockers in stable angina are comparative trials with other therapies, primarily calcium-channel antago-

Table 2.4 Randomized trials of beta-blockade for stable angina

Trial name/first author	References	Subjects	Drug
DiBianco	38	44	Acebutolol
Shapiro	39	37	Nadolol
Prida	40	12	Labetalol
DiBianco	41	46	Acebutolol/propranolol
IMAGE	42	288	Metoprolol
TIBET	43, 44	608	Atenolol
FEMINA	45	363	Metoprolol CR
APSIS	46	809	Metoprolol
Carvedilol	47	368	Metoprolol/carvedilol
CIAS	48	140	Celiprolol/propranolol
Betaxolol	49	92	Betaxolol/propranolol
Betaxolol	50	20	Betaxolol/atenolol
Epanolol	51	173	Epanolol/atenolol
Celiprolol	52, 53	92, 55	Celiprolol
MIRSA	54	147	Bisoprolol/atenolol
Epanolol	55	114	Epanolol/metoprolol
Carvedilol	56	248	Carvedilol/verapamil
Atenolol	58	17	Atenolol/nifedipine
Atenolol	59	129	Atenolol/nifedipine
Bisoprolol	60	30	Bisoprolol/nitrates
Atenolol	61	14	Atenolol/isordil
Bupranolol	62	30	Bupranolol/isordil
Propranolol	63	74	Propranolol/nifedipine
Atenolol	64	27	Atenolol/SR nifedipine
Atenolol	65	25	Atenolol/diltiazem
Atenolol	66	30	Atenolol/nicardipine
Atenolol	67	114	Atenolol/nifedipine

nists. In the Total Ischemic Burden European Trial (TIBET), 608 patients with stable angina were randomized to atenolol, nifedipine SR or their combination [43, 44]. Patients underwent maximal exercise testing and 48 hour ambulatory ST segment monitoring outside the hospital prior to initiating therapy and after six weeks of therapy. Both atenolol and nifedipine, as well as their combination, caused significant improvements in exercise parameters and significant reductions in ischemia during daily activity compared with placebo. Withdrawal from the study medication was greatest in the nifedipine group but similar in the atenolol and combination groups. There were no significant differences between the three groups except for a greater fall in systolic and diastolic blood pressure with combination therapy than either treatment alone. In the Angina Prognosis Study in Stockholm (APSIS), 809 patients with stable angina were randomized to metoprolol or verapamil and were followed for an average of 3.4 years [46]. There were no significant differences in death, non-fatal myocardial infarctions, unstable angina, cerebrovascular or peripheral vascular events. In the Felodipine ER and Metoprolol CR in Angina (FEMINA) trial, 363 patients with stable angina, despite optimal beta-blockade, were randomized to three treat-

ment groups: continuation of metoprolol (control), the addition of felodipine to metoprolol, and the replacement of metoprolol with felodipine [45]. Though there were no differences in exercise duration and onset of chest pain with exercise testing, the addition of felodipine increased time to 1 mm ST segment depression and decreased maximal ST segment depression. Replacement of metoprolol with felodipine didn't result in any significant improvement. These studies show benefit of beta-blockers in stable angina, though they don't appear to have any advantage over calcium-channel blockers.

BETA-BLOCKADE FOR SILENT ISCHEMIA [71–78] (TABLE 2.5)

The only major trial comparing a beta-blocker versus placebo in silent myocardial ischemia is the Atenolol Silent Ischemia Study (ASIST) [78]. In this study, 306 patients with mild or no angina (Canadian Cardiovascular Society class I–II), who had an abnormal exercise treadmill test and/or evidence of ischemia on ambulatory monitoring, were randomized to receive atenolol or placebo. The primary outcome was event-free survival with events defined as

Table 2.5 Randomized trials of beta-blockade for silent ischemia

Trial name	References	Subjects	Treatment
ACIP	71–73	558	Revasculation versus atenolol/nifedipine or isordil/diltiazem
TIBBS	74	330	Bisoprolol/nifedipine
TIBBS	75	520	Bisoprolol/nifedipine
TIBET	76	682	Atenolol/nifedipine
CASIS	77	100	Amlodipine/atenolol
ASIST	78	306	Atenolol/placebo

death, resuscitated ventricular tachycardia or fibrillation, myocardial infarction, hospitalization for unstable angina, aggravation of angina, or revascularization. Event-free survival was increased by 58% among patients receiving atenolol. In addition there was a decrease in number and duration of ischemic episodes with atenolol. Finally, atenolol use resulted in fewer first events as well as increased time to first event.

Other trials examining beta-blockers in silent ischemia have been comparative trials with beta-blockers and other anti-anginal medications. The Canadian Amlodipine/Atenolol in Silent Ischemia Study (CASIS) examined the effects of amlodipine, atenolol and their combination on ischemia during treadmill testing and 48 hour ambulatory monitoring [77]. The combination of both atenolol and amlodipine significantly reduced the frequency of ischemic episodes, exercise time to angina, and time to 1 mm ST segment depression over either medication alone. Atenolol was significantly better than amlodipine in decreasing the number of ischemia episodes but less effective in exercise time to angina and time to 1 mm ST segment depression. In the Asymptomatic Cardiac Ischemia Pilot (ACIP) Study, 553 patients were randomized to receive angina-guided medical therapy, ischemia-guided medical therapy, or coronary revascularization [71–73]. Though each treatment strategy resulted in a significant reduction in all exercise-induced variables of myocardial ischemia at 12 weeks, coronary revascularization was significantly better at increasing peak exercise time and decreasing exercise-induced ST segment depression. At one year of follow-up, revascularization resulted in a significant decrease in death, myocardial infarction, non-protocol revascularizations, and hospital admissions over medical therapy.

BETA-BLOCKADE FOR HEART FAILURE [81–95] (TABLE 2.6)

The mechanisms whereby chronic beta-blockade has led to enhanced survival and functional capacity of patients with chronic congestive heart failure are incompletely understood, but include the following:

- Up-regulation of beta-receptors.
- Reduced tachycardia and its consequences.
- Block of the renin-angiotensin system.
- Reduced myocardial oxygen demand leading to improved myocardial energetics [94, 95].

One of the first large studies on the use of beta-blockers in congestive heart failure was the Cardiac Insufficiency Bisoprolol Study (CIBIS) [90]. In this study, 641 patients with New York Heart Association (NYHA) functional class III–IV heart failure and an ejection fraction of less than 40% were randomized to bisoprolol or placebo and followed for an average of 1.9 years. Patients treated with bisoprolol had a significant decrease in hospitalization secondary to cardiac decompensation and a greater improvement in NYHA functional class. There was also a non-significant trend toward a decrease in death and sudden death. The results of this study led to the CIBIS II trial in which 2647 patients with similar characteristics to the first study were randomized to bisoprolol or placebo [91]. In this study, bisoprolol led to a 34% decrease in mortality and a 44% decrease in sudden death. Additionally, bisoprolol use led to significant reductions in the rate of hospital admissions, cardiovascular deaths, and ventricular arrhythmias.

Metoprolol, a cardioselective beta-blocker, has also been shown to be beneficial in congestive heart failure. The Metoprolol in Dilated Cardiomyopathy (MDC) trial, conducted in 383 patients with idiopathic dilated cardiomyopathy, randomized patients to receive metoprolol or placebo [87]. There was a 34% decrease in the primary endpoint (death and need for transplantation) though this did not reach statistical

Table 2.6 Randomized trials of beta-blockade for congestive heart failure

Trial name/ first author	References	Subjects	Drug	Endpoints	RR (95% CI) or risk reduction
MERIT-HF	81	3991	Metoprolol	Mortality	0.66 (0.53–0.81)
				Sudden death	0.59 (0.45–0.78)
				CHF mortality	0.51 (0.33–0.79)
MOCHA	82	345	Carvedilol	Mortality	0.27 (0.12–0.60)
Fisher	83	50	Metoprolol	Multiple	All significant
Krum	84	56	Carvedilol	Multiple	All significant
MEXIS	85, 86	210	Metoprolol/ xamoterol	Multiple	NS difference
MDC	87	383	Metoprolol	Mortality or need for transplant	34% risk reduction $p = 0.058$
US Carvedilol	88	1094	Carvedilol	Mortality	65% risk reduction
				CV admission	24% risk reduction
PRECISE	89	278	Carvedilol	Death or admission	36% risk reduction
CIBIS	90	641	Bisoprolol	Mortality	NS
CIBIS-II	91	2647	Bisoprolol	Mortality	0.66 (0.54–0.81)
				Sudden death	0.56 (0.39–0.80)
Xamoterol	92	516	Xamoterol	Mortality	2.54 x risk increase
ANZ	93	415	Carvedilol	Ejection fraction	Increased
				Exercise time	NS

significance. More recently, the Metoprolol CR/XL Randomized Intervention Trial in Heart Failure (MERIT-HF), examined the use of metoprolol in 3991 patients with NYHA functional class II–IV and an ejection fraction of < 40% [81]. The study was stopped early, secondary to the significant benefit seen among patients receiving metoprolol. In a mean follow-up time of one year, use of metoprolol decreased all-cause mortality by 34%, cardiovascular death by 38%, sudden death by 41%, and deaths from worsening heart failure by 49%.

The most widely studied beta-blocker in the treatment of congestive heart failure has been carvedilol, a non-selective beta-blocker with some alpha-1 blocking properties. The largest of these trials, the US Carvedilol Heart Failure Study Group, randomized 1094 patients to receive carvedilol or placebo [88]. The study was terminated early because of a 65% reduction in mortality as well as a 27% reduction in hospitalizations for cardiovascular causes with carvedilol. In addition, worsening heart failure as an adverse reaction during treatment was less frequent with carvedilol. The PRECISE trial enrolled 278 patients with moderate to severe heart failure and randomized patients to receive carvedilol or placebo [89]. Despite a non-significant trend toward lower mortality, the combined risk of major fatal or non-fatal events was decreased 37% with the use of carvedilol. Patients treated with carvedilol had a greater frequency of symptomatic improvement, a lower risk of clinical deterioration (as assessed by NYHA functional class or by global assessment of progress by the patient or physician), and an increase in ejection fraction. The MOCHA trial, which examined 345 patients with mild to moderate stable heart failure on various doses of carvedilol or placebo, showed similar benefits [82]. In this trial, the all-cause actuarial mortality was decreased 73% in patients receiving carvedilol. In addition, there were dose-related improvements in ejection fraction and survival though there was no improvement in submaximal exercise parameters. As seen in these studies, carvedilol improved survival regardless of NYHA functional class or underlying cause of heart failure.

UNDERUTILIZATION OF BETA-BLOCKERS IN CLINICAL PRACTICE [96–101]

Despite the large volume of data showing clear morbidity and mortality benefits in a variety of cardiovascular diseases, beta-blockers are being underutilized in clinical practice. Several retrospective studies examining utilization rates of beta-blockers in acute myocardial infarction, after myocardial infarction and congestive heart failure have shown this and will be reviewed [96–101].

A large retrospective series by Becker et al, evaluated the utilization of beta-blockers early in acute myocardial infarction in data pooled from the National Registry of Myocardial Infarction (NRMI 2) [96]. The 170,143 patients were classified as high or low risk based on a modified TIMI II risk scale. Only 13.4% of the patients received iv beta-blockers within 72 hours of admission and only 31.5% received oral beta-blockers. High-risk patients were more likely to receive iv beta-blockers (19.7%) versus low-risk patients (10.4%) but both were equally likely to receive oral beta-blockers. Phillips et al, evaluated the pharmacologic profile of 500 patients with acute MI at 12 academic hospitals and found that 61% of patients

received beta-blockers within 72 hours and 51% were discharged on beta-blockers [93]. These usage rates were significantly lower in women. Also, of the 116 with a previous history of myocardial infarction, only 29% were being treated with beta-blockers on admission.

Long-term administration of beta-blockers to patients after myocardial infarction has also been poor. In a large, retrospective review of records of 201,752 patients after myocardial infarction by Gottlieb et al, only 34% of patients received beta-blockers [94]. The utilization rates of beta-blockers were also significantly lower in the very elderly, blacks, and patients with the lowest ejection fractions, heart failure, chronic obstructive pulmonary disease, elevated serum creatinine concentrations, or type I diabetes mellitus. Despite the low utilization rates, there was a 40% reduction in mortality among patients receiving beta-blockers as compared with patients who did not. Soumerai et al, reviewed the medical records of 3737 patients greater than age 65 after myocardial infarction and found only 21% of patients were treated with a beta-blocker [98]. Calcium-channel antagonists were prescribed three times more than beta-blockers. Among the patients who did receive beta-blockers, there was a 43% reduction in mortality and a 22% decrease in rehospitalization. Though there may be some selection bias falsely elevating the mortality reductions in these trials, they do support the data from other randomized, placebo-controlled trials, which demonstrate a mortality benefit with beta-blockade after myocardial infarction.

Beta-blockers are also underutilized in congestive heart failure. Nohria et al, examined 522 patients admitted to academic medical centers with the diagnosis of congestive heart failure and found that only 19% were on beta-blockers at admission [99]. Data from the Systematic Assessment of Geriatric Drug Use via Epidemiology (SAGE) database showed that only 4% of 86,094 patients with congestive heart failure were treated with beta-blockers [100].

From these studies it is clear that beta-blockers are being underutilized in a variety of cardiovascular diseases. Beta-blockers play an important role in the medical management of acute myocardial infarction, stable and unstable angina, silent ischemia, and congestive heart failure.

BETA-BLOCKADE FOR HYPERTENSION [69, 70, 80]

The complex combination of effects that make beta-blockers effective antihypertensive agents is not completely understood. Shortly after initiating beta-blockade, resting cardiac output declines in the order of 20%. This is followed by a reflex rise in resistance, presumably to maintain blood pressure. Then, over several days, resistance and blood pressure decline. Proposed mechanisms for this gradual decline include:

- Inhibition of beta-receptors on terminal neurons that facilitate release of norepinephrine.
- Central nervous reduction in adrenergic outflow.
- Block of the renin-angiotensin.

Beta-blockers are particularly useful antihypertensive agents for patients who have hypertension in addition to angina, heart failure or prior myocardial infarction [101].

REFERENCES

1. Andersson B, Hjalmarson A, Swedborg K. Adrenergic beta-blockade and heart failure: from endangerment to conquest. Updates, *Textbook of Cardiovascular Medicine*, vol 2, 1999.
2. Reeder GS, Gersh BJ. Modern management of acute myocardial infarction, *Current Problems in Cardiology* 2000; **25**:681–782.
3. Cannon CP. Diagnosis and management of patients with unstable angina, *Current Problems in Cardiology* 1999; **24**:681–744.
4. Gottlieb SS, McCarter RJ, Vogel RA. Effect of beta-blockade on mortality among high-risk and low-risk patients after myocardial infarction, *N Engl J Med* 1998; **339**:489–497.
5. Yusuf S, Peto R, Lewis J, Collins R, Sleight P.

Beta-blockade during and after myocardial infarction: an overview of the randomized trials, *Prog in Cardiovasc Dis* 1985; **27**:335–371.
6. ISIS-1 (First International Study of Infarct Survival) Collaborative Group. Randomized trial of intravenous atenolol among 16,027 cases of suspected acute myocardial infarction: ISIS-1, *Lancet* 1986; July 12:57–65.
7. The MIAMI Research Group. Metoprolol in acute myocardial infarction (MIAMI). A randomized placebo-controlled intervention trial, *Eur Heart J* 1985; **6**:199–226.
8. Roberts R, Rogers WJ, Mueller HS et al for the TIMI Investigators. Immediate versus deferred beta-blockade following thrombolytic therapy in patients with acute myocardial infarction. Results of the Thrombolysis in Myocardial Infarction (TIMI) II-B Study, *Circulation* 1991; **83**:422–437.
9. Hjalmarson A, Herlitz J, Malek I et al. Effect on mortality of metoprolol in acute myocardial infarction, *Lancet* 1981; Oct 17: 823–827.
10. The International Collaborative Study Group. Reduction of infarct size with the early use of timolol in acute myocardial infarction, *N Engl J Med* 1984; **310**:9–15.
11. Norris RM, Sammel NL, Clarke ED, Smith WM, Williams B. Protective effect of propranolol in threatened myocardial infarction, *Lancet* 1978; Oct 28:907–909.
12. Yusuf S, Peto R, Bennett D et al. Early intravenous atenolol treatment in suspected acute myocardial infarction, *Lancet* 1980; Aug 9:273–276.
13. Peter T, Norris RM, Clarke ED et al. Reduction of enzyme levels by propranolol after acute myocardial infarction, *Circulation* 1978; **57**: 1091–1095.
14. Yusuf S, Sleight P, Rossi P et al, Reduction in infarct size, arrythmias and chest pain by early intravenous beta-blockade in suspected acute myocardial infarction, *Circulation* 1983; **67**: I32–I41.
15. Ramsdale DR, Faragher EB, Bennett DH et al. Ischemic pain relief in patients with acute myocardial infarction by intravenous atenolol, *Am Heart J* 1982; **103**:459–467.
16. Richterova A, Herlitz J, Holmberg S et al. Goteberg metoprolol trial: effects on chest pain, *Am J Cardiol* 1984; **53**:32D–36D.
17. Waagstein F, Hjalmarson A. Double-blind study

of the effect of cardioselective beta-blockade on chest pain in acute myocardial infarction, *Acta Med Scand* 1975 (suppl 587):201–208.

18. Basu S, Senior R, Raval U et al. Beneficial effects of intravenous and oral carvedilol treatment in acute myocardial infarction. A placebo-controlled randomized trial, *Circulation* 1997; **96**:183–191.

19. Beta-blocker Heart Attack Trial Research Group. A randomized trial of propranolol in patients with acute myocardial infarction I. Mortality results, *JAMA* 1982; **247**:1707–1714.

20. Lopressor Intervention Trial Research Group. The lopressor intervention trial: multicentre study of metoprolol in survivors of acute myocardial infarction, *Eur Heart J* 1987; **8**:1056–1064.

21. The Norwegian Multicenter Study Group. Timolol-induced reduction in mortality and reinfarction in patients surviving acute myocardial infarction, *N Engl J Med* 1981; **304**:801–807.

22. Pederson TR for the Norwegian Multicenter Study Group. Six-year follow-up of the Norwegian multicenter study on timolol after acute myocardial infarction, *N Engl J Med* 1985; **313**:1055–1058.

23. Olsson G, Rehnqvist N, Sjogren A, Erhardt L, Lundman T. Long-term treatment with metoprolol after myocardial infarction: effect on 3-year mortality and morbidity, *J Am Coll Cardiol* 1985; **5**:1428–1437.

24. Olsson G, Oden A, Johansson L, Sjogren A, Rehnqvist N. Prognosis after withdrawal of chronic postinfarction metoprolol treatment: a 2–7 year follow-up, *Eur Heart J* 1988; **9**:365–372.

25. Boissel JP, Leizorovicz A, Picolet H, Peyrieux JC for the APSI Investigators. Secondary prevention after high-risk acute myocardial infarction with low-dose acebutolol, *Am J Cardiol* 1990; **66**:251–260.

26. Waldo AL, Camm AJ, deRuyter H et al for the SWORD Investigators. Effect of *d*-sotalol on mortality in patients with left ventricular dysfunction after recent and remote myocardial infarction, *Lancet* 1996; **348**:7–12.

27. Waldo AL, Camm J, deRuyter H et al for the SWORD Investigators. Survival with oral *d*-sotalol in patients with left ventricular dysfunction: rationale, design, and methods (the SWORD trial), *Am J Cardiol* 1995; **75**:1023–1027.

28. Baber NS, Evans DW, Howitt G et al. Multicentre post-infarction trial of propranolol in 49 hospitals in the United Kingdom, Italy and Yugoslavia, *Br Heart J* 1980; **44**:96–100.

29. Capucci A, Bassein L, Bracchetti D et al. Propranolol versus verapamil in the treatment of unstable angina. A double-blind crossover study, *Eur Heart J* 1983; **4**:148–154.

30. Report of the Holland Interuniversity Nifedipine/metoprolol Trial (HINT) Research Group. Early treatment of unstable angina in the coronary care unit: a randomized, double-blind, placebo controlled comparison of recurrent ischaemia in patients treated with nifedipine or metoprolol or both, *Br Heart J* 1986; **56**:400–413.

31. Fouet A, Usdin JP, Gayet CH et al. Comparison of short-term efficacy of diltiazem and propranolol in unstable angina at rest: a randomized trial in 70 patients, *Br Heart J* 1983; **4**:691–698.

32. Tijssen JGP, Lubsen J. Early treatment of unstable angina with nifedipine and metoprolol—the HINT trial, *J Cardiovas Pharm* 1988 (12 Suppl):S71–S77.

33. Hohnloser SH, Meinertz T, Klingenheben T et al for the European Esmolol Study. Usefulness of esmolol in unstable angina pectoris, *Am J Cardiol* 1991; **67**:1319–1323.

34. Telford AM, Wilson C. Trial of heparin versus atenolol in prevention of myocardial infarction in intermediate coronary syndrome, *Lancet* 1981; **1**:1225–1228.

35. Parodi O, Simonetti I, Michelassi C et al. Comparison of verapamil and propranolol therapy for angina pectoris at rest: a randomized, multiple-crossover, controlled trial in the coronary care unit, *Am J Cardiol* 1986; **57**:899–906.

36. Gottlieb SO, Weisfeldt ML, Ouyang P et al. Effect of the addition of propranolol to therapy with nifedipine for unstable angina pectoris: a randomized, double-blind, placebo-controlled trial, *Circulation* 1986; **73**:231–337.

37. Theroux P, Taemans Y, Morisette D et al. A randomized study comparing propranolol and diltiazem in the treatment of unstable angina, *JACC* 1985; **5**:717–722.

38. DiBianco R, Singh S, Singh J et al. Effects of acebutolol on chronic stable angina pectoris. A placebo-controlled, double-blind, randomized crossover study, *Circulation* 1980; **62** (6):1179–1187.

39. Shapiro W, Park J, DiBianco R et al.

Comparison of nadolol, a new long-acting beta-receptor blocking agent, and placebo in the treatment on stable angina pectoris, *Chest* 1981; **80** (4):425–430.

40. Prida XE, Hill JA, Feldman RL. Systemic and coronary hemodynamic effects of combined alpha and beta-adrenergic blockade (labetolol) in normotensive patients with stable angina pectoris and positive exercise stress test responses, *Am J Cardiol* 1987; **59**:1084–1088.

41. DiBianco R, Singh SN, Shah PM et al. Comparison of the antianginal efficacy of acebutolol and propranolol. A multicenter, randomized, double-blind placebo-controlled trial, *Circulation* 1982; **65** (6):1119–1128.

42. Savonitto S, Ardissiono D, Egstrup K et al. Combination therapy with metoprolol and nifedipine versus monotherapy in patients with stable angina pectoris. Results of the International Multicenter Angina Exercise (IMAGE) Study, *J Am Coll Cardiol* 1996; **27**:311–316.

43. Fox KM, Mulcahy D, Findlay I, Ford I, Dargie RJ. The Total Ischaemic Burden European Trial (TIBET). Effects of atenolol, nifedipine SR and their combination on the exercise test and the total ischaemic burden in 608 patients with stable angina. The TIBET Study Group, *Eur Heart J* 1996; **17**:96–103.

44. Dargie RJ, Ford I, Fox KM. Total Ischaemic Burden European Trial (TIBET). Effects of ischaemia and treatment with atenolol, nifedipine SR and their combination on outcome in patients with chronic stable angina. The TIBET Study Group, *Eur Heart J* 1996; **17**:104–112.

45. Dunselman P, Liem AH, Verdel G et al on behalf of the FEMINA Study Group of the Working Group on Cardiovascular Research. Addition of felodipine to metoprolol versus replacement of metoprolol by felodipine in patients with angina pectoris despite adequate beta-blockade, *Eur Heart J* 1997; **18**:1755–1764.

46. Rehnqvist N, Rjemdahl P, Billing E et al. Treatment of stable angina pectoris with calcium antagonists and beta-blockers. The APSIS study. Angina Prognosis Study in Stockholm, *Cardiologia* 1995; **40** (12 suppl 1):301.

47. Van der Does R, Hauf-Zachariou U, Pfarr E et al. Comparison of safety and efficacy of carvedilol and metoprolol in stable angina pectoris, *Am J Cardiol* 1999; **83**:643–649.

48. Frishman WH, Heiman M, Soberman J, Greenberg S, Eff J. Comparison of celiprolol and propranolol in stable angina pectoris. Celiprolol International Angina Study Group, *Am J Cardiol* 1991; **67**:665–670.

49. Narahara KA. Double-blind comparison of once daily betaxolol versus propranolol four times daily in stable angina pectoris. Betaxolol Investigators Group, *Am J Cardiol* 1990; **65**:577–582.

50. McLenachan JM, Findlay IN, Wilson JT, Dargie HJ. Twenty-four-hour beta-blockade in stable angina pectoris: a study of atenolol and beta-xolol, *J Cardiovasc Pharmacol* 1992; **20**:311–315.

51. Boberg J, Larsen FF, Pehrsson SK. The effects of beta blockade with (epanolol) and without (atenolol) intrinsic sympathomimetic activity in stable angina pectoris. The Visacor Study Group, *Clin Cardiol* 1992; **15**:591–595.

52. Capone P, Mayol R. Celiprolol in the treatment of exercise induced angina pectoris, *J Cardiovasc Pharmacol* 1986; **8** (suppl 4):S135–S137.

53. Eff J, Godfrey J, Garutti R, Capone P. Celiprolol in angina pectoris: a controlled study, *J Card Pharm* 1986; **8**:S132–S134.

54. Muinck ED, Buchner-Moell D, van de Ven LLM, Lie KI on behalf of MIRSA Study Group. Comparison of the safety and efficacy of biso-prolol versus atenolol in stable exercise-induced angina pectoris: a Multicenter International Randomized Study of Angina Pectoris (MIRSA), *J Cardiovasc Pharm* 1992; **19**:870–875.

55. Ryden U. Efficacy of epanolol versus metoprolol in angina pectoris: report from a Swedish multicentre study of exercise tolerance, *J Intern Med* 1992; **231**:7–11.

56. Hauf-Zachariou U, Blackwood RA, Gunawardena KA et al. Carvedilol versus verapamil in chronic stable angina: a multicentre trial, *Eur J Clin Pharmacol* 1997; **52**:95–100.

57. Raftery EB. The preventative effects of vasodilating beta-blockers in cardiovascular disease, *Eur Heart J* 1996; **17** (suppl B):30–38.

58. Wallace WA, Weilington KU, Chess MA, Uiang CS. Comparison of nifedipine gastrointestinal therapeutic system and atenolol on antianginal efficacies and exercise hemodynamic responses in stable angina pectoris, *Am J Cardiol* 1994; **73**:23–28.

59. de Vries RJ, van den Reuvel AF, Uok DJ et al.

Nifedipine gastrointestinal therapeutic system versus atenolol in stable angina pectoris. The Netherlands Working Group on Cardiovascular Research (WCN), *Int J Cardiol* 1996; **57**:143–150.

60. van den Ven UU, Vermeulen A, Tans JG et al. Which drug to choose for stable angina pectoris: a comparative study between bisoprolol and nitrates, *Int J Cardiol* 1995; **47**:217–223.

61. Waysbort J, Meshulam N, Brunner D. Isosorbide-5-mononitrate and atenolol in the treatment of stable exertional angina, *Cardiology* 1991; **79** (suppl 2):19–26.

62. Krepp HP. Evaluation of the antianginal and anti-ischemic efficacy of slow-release isosorbide-5-mononitrate capsules, bupranolol and their combination, in patients with chronic stable angina pectoris, *Cardiology* 1991; **79** (suppl 2):14–18.

63. Kawanishi DT, Reid CU, Morrison EC, Rahimtoola SH. Response of angina and ischemia to long-term treatment in patients with chronic stable angina: a double-blind randomized individualized dosing trial of nifedipine, propranolol and their combination, *J Am Coll Cardiol* 1992; **19**:409–417.

64. Meyer TE, Adnams C, Commerford P. Comparison of the efficacy of atenolol and its combination with slow-release nifedipine in chronic stable angina, *Cardiovasc Drugs Ther* 1993; **7**:909–913.

65. Steffensen R, Grande P, Pedersen F, Raunso S. Effects of atenolol and diltiazem on exercise tolerance and ambulatory ischaemia, *Lot J Cardiol* 1993; **40**:143–153.

66. Parameshwar J, Keegan J, Mulcahy D et al. Atenolol or nicardipine alone is as efficacious in stable angina as their combination: a double blind randomized trial, *Int J Cardiol* 1993; **40**:135–141.

67. Foale RA. Atenolol versus the fixed combination of atenolol and nifedipine in stable angina pectoris, *Eur Heart J* 1993; **14**:1369–1374.

68. Tilmant PY, Lablanche JM, Thieuleux FA, Dupuis BA, Bertrand ME. Detrimental effect of propranolol in patients with coronary arterial spasm countered by combination with diltiazem, *Am J Cardiol* 1983; **52**:230–233.

69. Messerli FR, Grossman E, Goldbourt U. Are beta-blockers efficacious as first-line therapy for hypertension in the elderly? A systematic review, *JAMA* 1998; **279**:1903–1907.

70. Psaty BM, Smith NL, Siscovick DS et al. Health outcomes associated with antihypertensive therapies used as first-line agents: a systematic review and meta-analysis, *JAMA* 1997; **277**:739–745.

71. Pepine CJ, Geller NL, Knatterud GL et al for the ACIP Investigators. The Asymptomatic Cardiac Ischemia Pilot (ACIP): design of a randomized clinical trial, baseline data and implications for a long-term outcome trial, *J Am Coll Cardiol* 1994; **24**:1–10.

72. Chaitman BR, Stone PH, Knatterud GL et al for the ACIP Investigators. The Asymptomatic Cardiac Ischemia Pilot (ACIP) Study: Impact of anti-ischemia therapy on 12-week rest electrocardiogram and exercise test outcomes, *J Am Coll Cardiol* 1995; **26**:585–593.

73. Rogers WJ, Bourassa MG, Andrews TC et al for the ACIP Investigators. Asymptomatic Cardiac Ischemia Pilot (ACIP) Study: outcome at 1-year for patients with asymptomatic cardiac ischemia randomized to medical therapy or revascularization, *J Am Coll Cardiol* 1995; **26**:594–605.

74. von Arnim T. Medical treatment to reduce total ischemic burden. Total Ischemic Burden Bisoprolol Study (TIBBS): a multicenter trial comparing bisoprolol and nifedipine. The TIBBS Investigators, *J Am Coll Cardiol* 1995; **25**:231–238.

75. von Arnim T for the TIBBS Investigators. Prognostic significance of transient ischemic episodes: response to treatment shows improved prognosis, *J Am Coll Cardiol* 1996; **28**:20–24.

76. Dargie HJ, Ford I, Fox KM on behalf of the TIBET study group. Total Ischemic Burden European Trial (TIBET). Effects of ischaemia and treatment with atenolol, nifedipine SR and their combination on outcome in patients with chronic stable angina, *Eur Heart J* 1996; **17**:104–112.

77. Davies FR, Habibi H, Klinke WP et al for the Canadian Amlodipine/Atenolol in Silent Ischemia Study (CASIS) Investigators: Effect of amlodipine, atenolol and their combination on myocardial ischemia during treadmill exercise and ambulatory monitoring, *J Am Coll Cardiol* 1995; **25**:619–625.

78. Pepine CJ, Cohn PF, Deedwania PC et al for the

ASIST Study Group. Effects of treatment on outcome in mildly symptomatic patients with ischemia during daily life. The Atenolol Silent Ischemia Study (ASIST), *Circulation* 1994; **90**:762–768.

79. Bassan MM, Weiler-Ravell D, Shalev O. Comparison of the antianginal effectiveness of nifedipine, verapamil, and isosorbide dinitrate in patients receiving propranolol: a double-blind study, *Circulation* 1983; **68**: 568–575.

80. Wassertheil-Smoller S, Oberman A, Blaufox MD, Davis B, Langford H. The Trial of Antihypertensive Interventions and Management (TAIM) Study: final results with regard to blood pressure, cardiovascular risk, and quality of life, *Am J Hypertens* 1992; **5**:37–44.

81. MERIT-HF Study Group. Effect of metoprolol CR/CL in chronic heart failure: metoprolol CR/XL randomized intervention trial in congestive heart failure (MERIT-HF), *Lancet* 1999; **353**:2001–2007.

82. Bristow MR, Gilbert EM, Abraham WT et al for the MOCHA Investigators. Carvedilol produces dose-related improvements in left ventricular function and survival in subjects with chronic heart failure, *Circulation* 1996; **94**:2807–2816.

83. Fisher ML, Gottlieb SS, Plotnick GD et al. Beneficial effects of metoprolol in heart failure associated with coronary artery disease: a randomized trial, *J Am Coll Cardiol* 1994; **23**: 943–950.

84. Krum H, Sackner-Bernstein JD, Goldsmith RL et al. Double-blind, placebo-controlled study of the long-term efficacy of carvedilol in patients with severe chronic heart failure, *Circulation* 1995; **92**:1499–1506.

85. Persson H, Eriksson SV, Erhardt L. Effects of beta receptor antagonists on left ventricular function in patients with clinical evidence of heart failure after myocardial infarction. A double-blind comparison of metoprolol and xamoterol, *Eur Heart J* 1996; **17**:741–749.

86. Persson H, Rythe-Adler E, Erhardt L. Effects of beta receptor antagonists in patients with clinical evidence of heart failure after myocardial infarction: double-blind comparison of metoprolol with xamoterol, *Br Heart J* 1995; **74**:140–148.

87. Waagstein F, Bristow M, Swedborg K et al. Beneficial effects of metoprolol in idiopathic dilated cardiomyopathy, *Lancet* 1993; **342**: 1441–1446.

88. Packer M, Bristow MR, Cohn JN et al for the US Carvedilol Heart Failure Study Group: The effect of carvedilol on morbidity and mortality in patients with chronic heart failure, *N Engl J Med* 1996; **334**:1349–1355.

89. Packer M, Colucci WS, Sackner-Bernstein JD et al for the PRECISE Study Group. Double-blind, placebo-controlled study of the effects of carvedilol in patients with moderate to severe heart failure the PRECISE trial, *Circulation* 1996; **94**:2793–2799.

90. CIBIS Investigators and Committees. A randomized trial of beta-blockade in heart failure the Cardiac Insufficiency Bisoprolol Study (CIBIS), *Circulation* 1994; **90**:1765–1773.

91. CIBIS-II Investigators and Committees. The Cardiac Insufficiency Bisoprolol Study II (CIBIS II): a randomized trial, *Lancet* 1999; **353**:9–13.

92. The Xamoterol in Severe Heart Failure Study Group. Xamoterol in severe heart failure, *Lancet* 1990; **336**:1–6.

93. Australia–New Zealand Heart Failure Research Collaborative Group. Effects of carvedilol, a vasodilator-beta blocker, in patients with congestive heart failure due to ischemic heart disease, *Circulation* 1995; **92**:212–218.

94. Carson PE. Beta-blocker therapy in heart failure: pathophysiology and clinical results, *Current Problems in Cardiology* 1999; **24**:421–460.

95. Yusuf S, Wittes J, Friedman L. Overview of results of randomized clinical trials in heart disease II. Unstable angina, heart failure, primary prevention with aspirin, and risk factor modification, *JAMA* 1988; **260**:2259–2263.

96. Becker RC, Burns M, Gore JM et al. Early assessment and in-hospital management of patients with acute myocardial infarction at increased risk for adverse outcomes: a nationwide perspective of current clinical practice, *Am Heart J* 1998; May 153 (5 pt 1):786–796.

97. Phillips BJ, Yim JM, Brown EJ et al. Pharmacologic profile of survivors of acute myocardial infarction at US academic hospitals, *Am Heart J* 1996; May 131 (5):872–878.

98. Soumerai SB, McLaughlin TJ, Spiegelman D et al. Adverse outcomes of underuse of beta-blockers in elderly survivors of acute myocardial infarction, *JAMA* 1997; **277**:115–121.

99. Nohria A, Chen YT, Morton DJ et al. Quality of

care for patients hospitalized with heart failure at academic medical centers, *Am Heart J* 1998; June 137 (6):1028–1034.

100. Gambassi G, Forman DE, Lapane KL et al. Management of heart failure among very old persons living in long-term care: has the voice of trials spread? *Am Heart J* 2000; June 139 (1 pt 1):85–93.

101. Smith NL, Reiber GE, Psaty BM et al. Health outcomes associated with beta-blocker and diltiazem treatment of unstable angina, *JACC* 1998; **32** (5):1305–1311.

3

Statins and other lipid-lowering agents

Douglass A Morrison and Stephen P Thomson

CONTENTS • Lipid and lipoprotein biology • The 'cholesterol hypothesis' or the 'classic diet-heart' hypothesis • Applying the cholesterol hypothesis to the primary and secondary prevention of coronary artery disease • Summary: lessons from the trials • We can do better

LIPID AND LIPOPROTEIN BIOLOGY [1, 2]

Lipids are an important source of metabolic energy and are required for the formation of cellular membranes, steroid hormones, and vitamin D. Lipids are insoluble in water and for that reason, move together, as macromolecular complexes of lipids (cholesterol, esterfied cholesterol, triglycerides and phospholipids) and proteins, called lipoproteins. The protein components are apolipoproteins or enzymes. The apolipoproteins are structural proteins, which often direct lipoproteins to particular tissues, by means of receptors and receptor binding sites. Lipoproteins are structured with the most hydrophobic components, triglycerides and cholesteryl esters, as a central droplet, which is surrounded by more polar components, free cholesterol, proteins, and phospholipids. Because of the presence of the phosphate group, phospholipids are the most highly charged of the lipids. The most frequently measured lipids, in clinical practice, are cholesterol and triglycerides.

Cholesterol is both absorbed in the gut, and secreted back into the gut, in the form of bile. In addition, the body synthesizes as much cholesterol as it absorbs, primarily in the gut, liver, and central nervous system. An intermediate step in the synthesis of cholesterol is the conversion of 3-hydroxy-3-methylglutaryl CoA (HMG-CoA) to mevalonic acid by HMG-CoA reductase. This step is important because it is the site of down regulation in response to a variety of physiologic functions, the most important of which is a high intracellular level of cholesterol. It is also the site of action of the statin drugs or HMG-CoA reductase inhibitors. Measured cholesterol includes both free cholesterol, which has no fatty acyl group attached to its OH group, and esterified cholesterol, which has a fatty acyl group bound by an ester link. Free cholesterol has a slight electrical charge and can interact with water, but esterified cholesterol has little interaction with water.

Triglycerides are the major energy store. Triglycerides in the gut undergo digestion to fatty acids and monoglycerides. They are absorbed and transformed into chylomicrons for transport. The liver can also synthesize triglycerides, which are then assembled into lipoprotein particles, the very low-density lipoproteins (VLDL), for transport. Following absorption of the products of fat digestion, chylomicrons are formed. Chylomicrons are secreted into intestinal lymphatics and via the thoracic duct, enter the bloodstream accounting for the postprandial rise in triglycerides. The

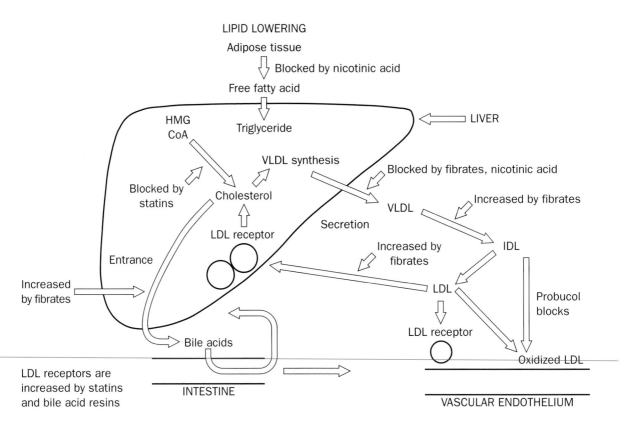

Figure 3.1 Schema of cholesterol metabolism and site of action of enzymes and selected lipid-lowering agents at sites in adipose tissue, liver, intestine, and vascular endothelium.

triglyceride component of chylomicrons is removed by lipoprotein lipase. Lipoprotein lipase also removes triglycerides from VLDL. Low-density lipoprotein (LDL) is formed after the triglycerides have been removed from VLDL. Low-density lipoproteins is small enough to cross capillary endothelium and enter tissue fluid; it supplies cholesterol to tissues. When intracellular cholesterol pools are depleted, the cells can synthesize an LDL receptor, which migrates to the cell surface where it can combine with LDL in the tissue fluid. LDL particles are heterogeneous: some are small and dense, whereas other particles are larger and less cholesterol depleted. About 2/3

to 4/5 of serum cholesterol is present in LDL; most of the remainder is high-density lipo-protein (HDL) with a small amount being VLDL. Low levels of HDL are associated with higher risk of coronary artery disease, and small, dense LDL.

Low-density lipoproteins, VLDL, and lipoprotein (a) are the three major apolipoprotein-B containing lipoproteins found in blood. Elevated levels of LDL, VLDL, intermediate-density lipoprotein (IDL) and lipoprotein (a) can all promote atherosclerosis. High-density lipoproteins appears to be protec-tive against atherosclerosis.

There are three interconnected pathways of

lipoprotein metabolism: (a) transport of dietary or exogenous fat, (b) transport of hepatic or endogenous fat, and (c) reverse cholesterol transport [2].

- Exogenous fat transport. The secretion of dietary fat as chylomicrons requires apolipoprotein B-48. The triglycerides within the chylomicrons are hydrolyzed by lipoprotein lipase with apolipoprotein C-II as a co-factor. The liver removes the chylomicron remnant.
- Endogenous fat transport. The liver synthesizes and secretes triglyceride-rich VLDL using apolipoprotein B-100. In the blood, VLDL is broken down into free fatty acids and glycerol by lipoprotein lipase and apolipoprotein C-2. VLDL and intermediate-density lipoprotein (IDL) is produced. Some of the IDL is removed via LDL receptors. Alternatively, the triglycerides in IDL can be further hydrolyzed to LDL, which is removed by apolipoprotein B-100 via the LDL receptor.
- Reverse cholesterol transport. Free cholesterol is removed from peripheral cells, such as macrophages, through the transfer of cholesterol across the cell membrane by the ABC1 transporter. Nascent HDL, consisting of phospholipid and apolipoprotein A-1, picks up the free cholesterol from the transporter. A spherical or mature HDL molecule is formed by the action of lecithin-cholesterol acyl transferase. Approximately half of this mature HDL will be removed by the HDL (SR-B1) receptor and the other half by transfer to apolipoprotein-B-containing lipoproteins, VLDL, IDL, and LDL.

There are at least four mechanisms by which HDL may be protective against atherosclerosis: reverse cholesterol transport, inhibition of LDL oxidation, reduction in levels of adhesion proteins and increased fibrinolysis.

THE 'CHOLESTEROL HYPOTHESIS' OR THE 'CLASSIC DIET-HEART' HYPOTHESIS [1–12]

Population studies, epidemiologic studies, and clinical trials have demonstrated that serum cholesterol and LDL concentrations are positively associated with the risk of atherosclerotic coronary artery disease (CAD) [3–11]. Conversely, HDL cholesterol appears to be inversely related to risk of CAD. Although there are age and gender differences for cholesterol and LDL levels, risk for CAD is related to elevations of these lipids in all categories. Risk appears to be continuous but a major therapeutic dilemma is whether there is a 'threshold' or level below which risk or cost is no longer justified by gain from treatment.

Epidemiological studies consistently support the cholesterol hypothesis, particularly robust data sets from the Framingham study and the Multiple Risk Factor Intervention Trial (MR FIT) database, which link high LDL and low HDL with increased risk for CAD [3–10]. Supportive evidence has been derived from primary prevention (prior to the development of either a myocardial infarction or symptoms of CAD) and secondary prevention (after symptoms, myocardial infarction, or the development of angiographic coronary artery disease) trials. Reducing LDL and increasing HDL have been associated with decreases in CAD event rates.

APPLYING THE CHOLESTEROL HYPOTHESIS TO THE PRIMARY AND SECONDARY PREVENTION OF CORONARY ARTERY DISEASE [13–47]

Primary prevention trials using bile acid binding resins, fibrates and niacin, include the World Health Organization Trial, the Lipid Research Clinics Coronary Primary Prevention Trial and the Helsinki Heart Study [13–18] (see Table 3.1).

The WHO trial randomized 15,745 healthy men in three centers: Edinburgh, Prague, and

Table 3.1 Randomized trials of primary prevention using lipid-lowering agents			
Trial name	**Reference**	**Subjects**	**Intervention**
WHO	13	15,745	Clofibrate 1.6 gm
LRC-CPPT	14–16	3806	Cholestyramine 24 gm
Helsinki Heart	17, 18, 101	4081	Gemfibrozil 600 BID
WOSCOPS	26, 89	6595	Pravastatin 40 mg QHS
AFCAP/TexCAPS	27	5608/997	Lovastatin 20–40 mg/day
Upjohn	103	2278	Colestipol

Budapest. Patients were randomized to receive either clofibrate 1.6 gm/day or an olive oil placebo (!) if they were among the upper third of the distribution of serum cholesterol (groups 1 and 2); the third group, which also received the placebo, was among the lower third of the cholesterol distribution. Over an average of 5.3 years, 83,534 persons-years of observational experience was accumulated. The trial showed lower rates of non-fatal infarction among the group 3 subjects with lower cholesterol, supporting the cholesterol hypothesis. Additionally, among the two groups with high cholesterol, clofibrate was associated with a significant reduction in non-fatal myocardial infarction (MI), thereby supporting the concept of cholesterol lowering for primary prevention. However, overall mortality was not reduced because of a disconcerting increase in liver and biliary deaths among the clofibrate cohort.

The Lipid Research Clinics Coronary Primary Prevention Trial evaluated 3806 male volunteers between the ages of 35 and 59 who were randomly assigned to either 24 gm of cholestyramine or placebo. The cholestyramine was associated with average reductions of total and LDL cholesterol of 8.5% and 12.6% respectively. The trial demonstrated significant reductions in coronary death, non-fatal MI, positive exercise tests, and coronary bypass graft surgery, in association with the cholesterol reductions. However, there was a disconcerting increase in deaths by accident or violence, which counterbalanced the reductions in coronary death leading to a slight and insignificant reduction in overall mortality among the cholestyramine group.

The Helsinki Heart Study was a five-year double-blind randomized trial comparing gemfibrozil 600 mg twice daily (BID) versus placebo in 4081 middle-aged, healthy men who had elevated cholesterol. Over the course of the study, plasma lipids changed very little in the placebo group whereas gemfibrozil was associated with an 11% decline in total cholesterol, a 10% decline in LDL cholesterol and 10% increase in HDL cholesterol. These favorable changes in lipid profile were associated with an overall 34% (95% confidence interval 8.2–52.6%) reduction in cardiac endpoints (fatal and non-fatal MIs and cardiac death).

Primary prevention trials using the statin drugs include the West of Scotland Primary Prevention Study (WOSCOPS) and the Air Force/Texas Coronary Artery Prevention Study (AFCAPS/TexCAPS) [26, 27] (see Table 3.1).

The West of Scotland study was a landmark in the history of primary prevention. A total of 6595 men ages 45 to 64 years of age, who had average serum cholesterol of 272 ± 23 mg/dl, were randomly allocated between placebo and 40 mg pravastatin. Placebo was associated with no change in lipids, whereas, the pravastatin group had an average reduction of cholesterol of 20% and LDL cholesterol of 26%. These lipid changes were associated with a 22% reduction in overall mortality (95% CI 0–40%). Looking further, there was a 32% reduction in cardiovascular deaths; a 33% reduction in coronary heart disease deaths; a 31% reduction in non-fatal MI; and a 31% reduction in definite coronary events.

AFCAPS/TexCAPS carried the primary prevention concept further by evaluating 6605 men and women, who had normal to mildly elevated cholesterol levels (180–264 mg/dl). Lovastatin 20–40 mg/day was given to lower LDL < 110 mg/dl. After an average of 5.2 years, lovastatin was associated with a significant reduction in incidence of first major cardiac event (sudden cardiac death, fatal and non-fatal myocardial infarction, and unstable angina) (RR = 0.63%; 95% CI 0.5–0.79). Lovastatin was also associated with a 25% reduction in LDL and a 6% increase in HDL cholesterol. The results were comparable for women as well as men.

Secondary prevention trials using bile acid binding resins, fibrates or niacin include the Coronary Drug Project (CDP), the Stockholm Ischemic Heart Disease Trial, Scottish and Newcastle upon Tyne studies of clofibrate, and the Veterans Affairs High-Density Lipoprotein Cholesterol Intervention Trial (VA-HIT) [19–25] (see Table 3.2).

The Coronary Drug Project was an ambitious undertaking involving 8341 patients randomized to one of six different groups at 53 centers in the US. The six arms of the trial were: 2.5 mg conjugated estrogens; 5.0 mg conjugated estrogen; 1.8 gm clofibrate; 6.0 mg dextrothyroxine; 3.0 gm niacin; or lactose placebo. There were more than 1000 subjects in each active treatment arm and 2789 subjects in the placebo arm. All subjects were males age 30–64 years, and all had at least one prior MI, at least three months previously. The primary endpoint was all-cause mortality. The results were disappointing; specifically, none of the treatments was associated with significant mortality reduction. However, niacin was associated with a significant mortality reduction at 15 years [20].

The Stockholm Ischaemic Heart Disease Study was a smaller trial (276 in one group and 279 in the other) of post-MI survivors, which used both clofibrate and nicotinic acid in the

Table 3.2 Randomized trials of secondary prevention using lipid-lowering agents

Trial name	Reference	Subjects	Intervention
4S	28	4444	Simvastatin 20–40 mg
LIPID	30, 90	9014	Pravastatin 40 mg/day
CARE	29, 87, 91	4159	Pravastatin 40 mg/day
MIRACL	48	3086	Atorvastatin 80 mg/day
CDP	19, 20	2789	Niacin, gemfibrozil
Scottish	109	717	Clofibrate
Newcastle	110	497	Clofibrate 1500 mg
VAHIT	23, 24, 93, 94	2531	Gemfibrozil 1200 mg/day
Stockholm	25	555	Clofibrate, niacin
BIP	82	3090	Bezafibrate 400 mg

active treatment group. Despite its smaller size, this trial reported significant decreases in all-cause mortality (26%) and ischemic heart disease mortality (36%). Similarly, a Scottish study, which included infarct survivors, who also had angina, randomized between clofibrate and placebo, reported statistically significant differences. Clofibrate was associated with a 62% lower mortality than placebo. A study from Newcastle randomized 497 patients, who had angina, a prior MI or both, between clofibrate and placebo. The investigators found significant reduction in the combined rate of death and non-fatal MI. Several intriguing findings were reported: (a) the protection afforded by clofibrate appeared to be limited to patients with angina; (b) the reduction in death appeared to be limited to sudden death; and (c) there appeared to be a similar degree of protection regardless of patient's initial cholesterol levels.

The VA-HIT study was another landmark in the evolution of the cholesterol hypothesis because it showed a reduction in CAD events by means of increasing HDL rather than decreasing LDL cholesterol. In this trial, 2531 men with known coronary disease (defined as either documented MI; angina with objective evidence of ischemia; prior coronary revascularization; or coronary angiographically documented narrowing) were randomized between 1200 mg gemfibrozil/day and placebo. The primary endpoint was non-fatal MI or death from coronary cause. The overall result was a 22% risk reduction (95% CI 7–35%). Importantly, although LDL cholesterol was not changed by gemfibrozil versus placebo, HDL cholesterol was increased by 6% and triglycerides reduced by 31%. These data have been interpreted as providing confirmation of the clinical importance of reverse cholesterol transport and HDL cholesterol as a protective factor.

The Bezfibrate Infarction Prevention (BIP) study used bezafibrate to examine similar issues, but their population was younger and had fewer diabetic patients than VA-HIT. They had similar changes in triglycerides and HDL, albeit in a population with lower event rates.

Accordingly the event rate differences between their control and active intervention arms did not achieve significance.

Secondary prevention trials with statins include the Scandinavian Simvastatin Survival Study (4S), the Cholesterol and Recurrent Events Trial (CARE), the Long-Term Intervention with Pravastatin in Ischemic Disease (LIPID) trial, and the Myocardial Ischemia Reduction with Aggressive Cholesterol Lowering (MIRACL) trial [28–31, 48] (see Table 3.2).

The Scandinavian Simvastatin Survival Study randomized 4444 patients with angina or prior MI and serum cholesterol 213–310 mg/dl to placebo or up to 40 mg/day of simvastatin (treatment goal < 213 mg/dl). Over 5.4 years of median follow-up, simvastatin was associated with 25% and 35% reductions in total and LDL cholesterol and 8% increase in HDL cholesterol. These favorable changes in lipid profile were accompanied by a significant reduction in overall mortality (relative risk of death for simvastatin versus placebo = 0.7; 95% CI 0.58–0.85). There were also significant reductions in coronary death, fatal and non-fatal cerebrovascular events, and myocardial revascularization procedures. Importantly, simvastatin was associated with comparable reductions in event rates across all quartiles of baseline lipids.

The CARE trial was a secondary prevention trial of men and women with closer to average cholesterol levels. Men and postmenopausal women who had had a prior MI and whose total cholesterol was < 240 mg/dl and LDLs were between 115–174 mg/dl, were eligible. In a five-year trial, 4159 subjects were randomly allocated to placebo or 40 mg pravastatin. The primary endpoint was a composite of fatal cardiac event or non-fatal MI. There was a significant 24% reduction in the primary endpoint (95% CI 9–36%). Significant reductions in percutaneous intervention (PCI), coronary artery bypass graft (CABG) and stroke were also observed in association with pravastatin therapy. A source of continued controversy is whether favorable clinical events accrue from LDL reduction across the spectrum of levels versus some sort of threshold or target. The CARE investigators came down on the side of a target, specifically ~ 125 mg/dl of LDL. A major contribution of the CARE trial was the clear demonstration of efficacy among women.

LIPID enrolled patients with prior MI or unstable angina and total cholesterol between 155–270 mg/dl. A total of 9014 patients were randomized between placebo and 40 mg pravastatin, and followed for a mean of 6.1 years. A reduction in overall mortality of 22% (95% CI 13–31%) was seen with pravastatin. Significant reductions were observed in MI, death from coronary causes, stroke and myocardial revascularization. As such, there is a remarkable consistency in the relative rate reductions between the results of 4S, CARE, and LIPID.

Recently the MIRACL study reported on relatively acute secondary prevention with high dose (80 mg/day) atorvastatin. A total of 3086 patients with unstable angina and/or non-Q MI were randomized between placebo and atorvastatin and followed for 16 weeks. A composite of death, non-fatal MI, cardiac arrest, or objectively documented myocardial ischemia, which necessitated hospitalization, constituted the primary endpoint. Atorvastatin was associated with a 16% reduction (95% CI 0–0.3) in the primary endpoint.

Quantitative angiographic regression studies have included FATS, MAAS, LCAS, MARS, REGRESS, HARP, BECAIT, POSCH, CLAS, PLAC I, NHLBI-II, and SCAT and STARS [31–45] (see Table 3.3). FATS demonstrated reduced incidence of coronary events and angiographic reduced rate of progression of atherosclerosis in association with lipid-lowering using lovastatin, colestipol or niacin. MAAS reported fewer new lesions and total occlusion and less progression among subjects taking simvastatin as opposed to placebo. In LCAS, fluvastatin use was associated with less angiographic progression over 2.5 years. CCAIT was a Canadian trial of lovastatin 40–80 mg, which demonstrated reduced angiographic progression of coronary

Table 3.3 Randomized trials of angiographic regression with lipid-lowering agents			
Trial name	**Reference**	**Subjects**	**Intervention Results**
FATS	32	146 men	Lovastatin/niacin/colestipol
MAAS	33	381	Simvastatin 20 mg
LCAS	34	340	Fluvastatin 20 mg BID
CCAIT	106	331	Lovastatin 40–80 mg
MARS	35	270	Lovastatin 80 mg
REGRESS	36, 100	885	Pravastatin 40 mg
HARP	37	79	Pravastatin, niacin, cholestyramine
BECAIT	38, 39	92	Bezafibrate 200 TID
POSCH	39	838	Ileal bypass
CLAS	49, 111	188	Colestipol, niacin
PLAC I	44	559	Pravastatin 40 mg
NHLBI II	40, 104	143	Cholestyramine 24 gm
SCAT	95	460	Simvastatin 40 mg
STARS	105	90	Cholestyramine 16 gm

artery disease at two years. MARS demonstrated slower progression and some evidence for regression with lovastatin. REGRESS was a large (885 patients) Dutch study that demonstrated both angiographic and clinical event reductions with pravastatin. By demonstrating decreased angina, REGRESS also contributed to the speculation that statins may have anti-ischemic properties (part of the rationale for the cited MIRACL study). HARP was a relatively small study of patients with normal cholesterol levels, which failed to demonstrate angiographic regression or slowed progression. BECAIT included angiography two and five years after randomization between placebo and bezafibrate; improvements in serum lipids and fibrinogen were associated with slowed angiographic progression and reduced clinical events. POSCH was a surgical (ileal bypass) trial which is included as 'proof of concept' namely that lipid lowering, regardless of how it is achieved, appears to be associated with less angiographic progression (all the way

to 10 years). CLAS (I and II) demonstrated regression in CAD out to four years with a combination of colestipol and niacin. Cholestyramine was associated with angiographic improvement in the NHLBI type II study. Pravastatin was associated with reduction in angiographic progression of CAD and clinical events, as well as cerebrovascular events in PLAC I. Both clinical and angiographic benefits were observed with simvastatin among initially normocholesterolemic subjects in SCAT. The STARS demonstrated efficacy of both diet and 16 gm of cholestyramine on angiographic CAD progression.

Secondary prevention among patients who have had a revascularization or transplant (Table 3.4) [49–61]

Among the subset of CLAS patients who had prior CABG, colestipol was associated with significantly fewer new lesions and significantly

Table 3.4 Trials of lipid-lowering agents in patients who have undergone revascularization or transplant

Trial	Reference	Subjects	Intervention	Outcome
Post-CABG				
CLAS	49, 111	162	Colestipol/niacin	Graft patency
Post-CABG trial	58	1351	Lovastatin/cholesty	Graft disease
Post-PCI				
Weintraub et al	112	404	Lovastatin 40 mg	Restenosis
APPLE	113	239	Lovastatin 40 mg	Restenosis
PREDICT	114	695	Pravastatin 40 mg	Restenosis
FLARE	115	1054	Pravastatin 40 mg	Restenosis
PTCA versus medical therapy				
Pitt et al	57	341	Atorvastatin 80 mg	Ischemic events
Endothelial function				
Treasure et al	61	23	Lovastatin 40 BID	Vasodilatation
Post-transplant				
Wenke	59	72	Simvastatin	Transplant survival
Kobashigawa	60	97	Pravastatin	Transplant survival

less progression than placebo. In the post CABG trial, 1351 patients were randomized in a 2×2 factorial design between lovastatin and coumadin after CABG. Both angiographic measures of progression and repeat vascularization were reduced by effective cholesterol lowering but not by coumadin. Taken together, these two studies support lipid-lowering as a means of reducing repeat vascularization after CABG.

The experience with statins, used in an attempt to reduce restenosis, after PCI, have been disappointing. Weintraub and coworkers from Emory University randomized 404 patients between 80 mg of lovastatin and placebo, beginning fully 7–10 days before elective PCI. They found no difference in angiographic restenosis. In PREDICT, 695 patients were randomized between pravastatin 40 mg and placebo; no difference in clinical events or angiographic restenosis was detected. In APPLE, a total of 239 patients were randomized between placebo and a combination of probucol and lovastatin 20 mg. Again, no differences in clinical or angiographic restenosis were observed. In the FLARE trial, 1054 patients were randomized between fluvastatin 80 mg and placebo with repeat angiography at approximately two years. There was no reduction in angiographic restenosis with fluvastatin. These disappointing results all suggest that statins are not associated with a significant improvement in restenosis.

Other trials have documented prolonged survival and reduced rate of rejection among transplant patients treated with statins [59, 60]. There are some mechanistic studies suggesting improved endothelial function with statin use among CAD patients [61].

Dietary management (Table 3.5) [49, 52–55; 62–79]

In much the same way that between and within population comparisons of cholesterol have been associated with CAD risk, similar comparisons have supported the link between diets high in saturated fats and cholesterol, and CAD incidence. Dietary intervention trials have demonstrated that reducing the amount of cholesterol and saturated fat in the diet can lead to reduced serum levels of both total and LDL cholesterol. Showing that dietary reductions in serum lipids are accompanied by reductions in CAD events has strengthened the link.

The Leiden Intervention Trial examined coronary angiography after two years on a vegetarian diet and reported no progression of CAD among subjects with a favorable total/HDL cholesterol ratio (< 6.9 median value). Although the Oslo intervention study included smoking cessation, it was a practical 'real-world' look at the potential effectiveness of risk factor counseling. A total of 1232 subjects were randomly allocated to an intervention group (which included a 45% reduction in smoking in the intervention group; extraordinary by anyone's standards!). After five years, the diet and smoking intervention group had 47% fewer myocardial infarctions. The intervention group had significant improvements in total cholesterol and total/HDL ratios.

The Lyon Diet Heart Study used an alphalinolenic acid-rich Mediterranean diet and was stopped early by its safety committee after 2.5 years because there was a 73% reduction in cardiac deaths and non-fatal MIs [80]. A total of

Table 3.5 Dietary intervention trials			
Trial	Reference	Subjects	Outcomes
Leiden	68	39	Angiographic
Oslo	70	1232	Clinical
Lyon	80	605	Clinical

605 patients were randomized after their first MI to either the Mediterranean diet or a prudent post-MI diet. The intervention diet was adapted from that associated with low cardiac and overall mortality in the seven-country study. The cohort ingesting the Mediterranean diet were found to have increased serum levels of alpha-linolenic acid, vitamins A and C without change in LDL cholesterol, weight or blood pressure.

The National Cholesterol Education Program, the Secondary Prevention Panel, AHA panel, and the 27th Bethesda Conference: Matching the Intensity of Risk Factor Management with the Hazard for Coronary Disease Events, are all in agreement that dietary modification of elevated lipids is an important first step. Dietary measures should include weight loss for the obese, and reduction in total fat to < 30% of calories,

saturated fat to < 7% of total calories, and cholesterol to < 200 mg/day. Even more recent evidence has raised the possibility that having less saturated and more mono and polyunsaturated fats may be more important than either total fat or proportion of fat in the diet. Such a program can reasonably be expected to reduce serum LDL by 15–25 mg/dl. All these recommendations deserve emphasis for patients coming to revascularization, all the more so for high-risk revascularization, the topic of this book.

Pharmacological management (Tables 3.1–3.4) (Figs 3.2 and 3.3)

The entire field of lipid lowering was revolutionized by the introduction of 3-hydroxy-3-methylglutaryl-CoA reductase inhibitors

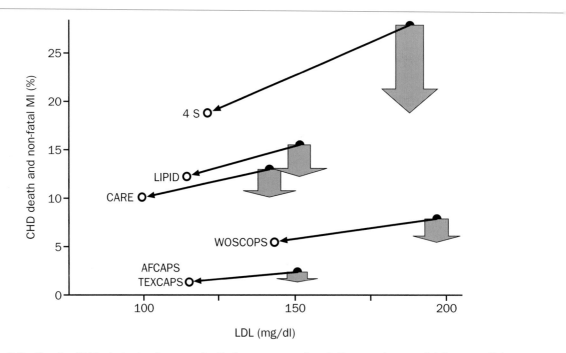

Figure 3.2 Graph of LDL cholesterol versus death from coronary heart disease plus non-fatal myocardial infarction, in several large statin intervention trials. Subject's LDL are shown on x-axis with thin arrows from pre- to post-intervention LDL levels. Death from coronary heart disease plus non-fatal-myocardial infarction is graphed on y-axis with large arrows showing reductions in events with therapy. Large reductions in events only occur among patients with high-risk before intervention.

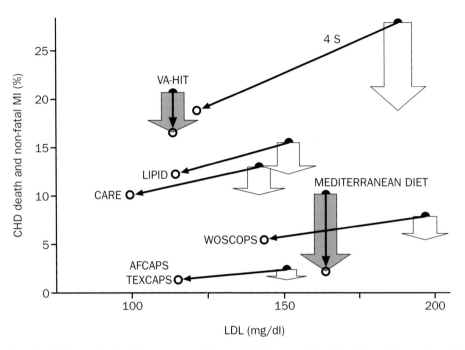

Figure 3.3 Graph of LDL cholesterol versus death from CAD plus non-fatal MI with addition of two trials, VAHIT and Mediterranean diet, which effected cardiac events through HDL and triglycerides, rather than through LDL reduction which appears to be primary mechanism of statins.

(statins). Statins lower LDL to a far greater extent than any of the other agents (20–60%), have far fewer side-effects and are thus much better tolerated by patients. These two characteristics made possible the large-scale primary and secondary prevention trials which have demonstrated not only reduction in coronary events and coronary death, but also overall mortality. All of these agents (lovastatin [Mevacor], pravastatin [Pravachol], simvastatin [Zocor], atorvastatin [Lipitor], fluvastatin [Lescol], and cerivastatin [Baycol]) work by competitive inhibition of HMG-CoA reductase, an important enzyme in hepatic cholesterol synthesis. All of them reproducibly lower total and LDL cholesterol. Major side-effects include mild elevations in serum transaminases and a

less frequent and less severe myopathy than has been seen with the fibrates.

Significant reductions in clinical event rates have been observed in statin primary prevention studies such as WOSCOPS and AFCAP/TexCAPS [26, 27]. Secondary prevention trials with statins that demonstrated significant improvements in clinical event rates include 4S, CARE, and LIPID [28–30]. Overall survival was significantly improved in 4S, and in LIPID and demonstrated borderline significance in WOSCOPS [26, 28, 30].

The bile acid binding resins, cholestyramine (Questran) and colestipol (Colestid), bind bile acids in the gut, thereby interrupting the enterohepatic recirculation. They also increase the conversion of cholesterol into bile acids in the liver. As a consequence, the hepatic LDL receptor population is increased and LDL is cleared more rapidly from the blood. In clinical trials, such as the Lipid Research Clinics Coronary Primary Prevention Trial, decreases in LDL on the order of 10–30% have been observed. Major side-effects are gastrointestinal including bloating, flatulence, and constipation. Additionally, these drugs may interfere with the absorption of fat-soluble drugs such as thiazides, warfarin, digoxin, thyroxine and even the statins.

Nicotinic acid was the first lipid-lowering drug for which mortality reduction was demonstrated. Nicotinic acid leads to decreased mobilization of free fatty acids from peripheral adipose so there is less substrate for hepatic synthesis of lipoprotein lipid. Reduced hepatic secretion of lipoproteins results in decreases in LDL by 10–25%, and reduced very low-density lipoproteins (VLDL). High-density lipoproteins may be seen to increase by 5–35% with niacin, which is a greater increase in this cardioprotective moiety than with any other agent. Triglycerides are also reduced with niacin, often by as much as 25–50%. Niacin is relatively cheap and is available over the counter. The primary limitation in niacin use is that large doses are required (1–2 gm), and these are usually accompanied by prostaglandin-mediated side-effects, such as flushing, dizziness, and palpitations which are often poorly tolerated. One approach to enhance patient compliance is titration of the dose gradually; another is aspirin pre-treatment. Niacin is relatively contraindicated in patients with diabetes and gout because of dose-dependent increases in glucose and uric acid. Major clinical trials testing the effectiveness of niacin include the Coronary Drug Project, the Stockholm Ischemic Heart Disease Secondary Prevention Trial, CLAS, FATS, UCSF-SCOR and HARP [19, 20, 25, 32, 37, 81].

The fibrates, gemfibrozil (Lopid), clofibrate, bezafibrate, and fenofibrate, increase fatty acid oxidation in the liver and skeletal muscle and decrease secretion of triglyceride rich lipoproteins. They are the most effective triglyceride lowering agents with 20–50% reductions having been reported. They have much less effect on LDL (5–15%) but are also associated with some increase in HDL (10–20%). The most important side-effect is myopathy but abdominal pain, rash, increased incidence of gallstones and erectile dysfunction have all been reported.

The World Health Organization (WHO) trial of clofibrate was particularly disappointing because of an unexplained increased incidence of non-cardiac deaths. Both the Helsinki Heart Trial and the Veterans Affairs High-density lipoprotein Intervention Trial (VA-HIT) strongly support the use of gemfibrozil. The Coronary Drug Project, the Stockholm Ischemic study, and BIP have also looked at event rates with fibrate intervention [19, 20, 25, 82].

SUMMARY: LESSONS FROM THE TRIALS [13–47; 49–79; 81–108]

As summarized in the accompanying tables, the prospective randomized clinical trials demonstrate the following:

- Primary prevention of cardiac events (reduced frequency of fatal and non-fatal myocardial infarction and in some cases, overall mortality) is feasible with available agents (Table 3.1). The decision-making factors are level of LDL and HDL cholesterol and presence of other risk factors which determine overall risk (Fig. 3.2).
- Secondary prevention of cardiac events (myocardial infarction and all cause mortality) is a safe and practical reality for most patients (Table 3.2). The decision-making factors are level of LDL cholesterol and presence of other risk factors which determine overall risk (Fig. 3.2).
- Coronary angiographic regression or modified progression of angiographic disease can be accomplished with lipid lowering in many patients (Table 3.3).
- Improved outcomes (either clinical or

angiographic or both) among patients who have already undergone CABG, PCI, or transplantation can be derived from safe lipid-lowering therapies (Table 3.4).

- Prevention of cardiac events and/or slowed angiographic progression can be achieved with dietary interventions, which lower serum lipids or in the case of the Mediterranean diet, change specific lipids and/or micronutrients (Table 3.5).

WE CAN DO BETTER [116, 117]

For patients who have had a documented MI, a PCI, or a CABG, there is no good reason not to check a lipid panel and commence lipid lowering for all patients with an LDL cholesterol > 130 mg/dl. More often than not, statins are the safest and cheapest place to start, but especially among subgroups with low HDL, elevated triglycerides, and diabetes, gemfibrozil, niacin, and other fibrates are among the alternatives and dietary intervention should be attempted. High-risk intervention should be considered only after medical therapy has been exhausted and that should now include lipid lowering, which is aimed at preventing events rather than simply relieving symptoms (like some antianginals). Furthermore, data support life-long lipid lowering post PCI or post CABG [96, 97]. The continued use of optimal medical therapy and risk factor modification should be a mandatory goal to improve quality of life and longevity [57–61].

REFERENCES

1. Willet W. Diet and coronary heart disease. In: Willet W, ed, *Nutritional Epidemiology* (New York: Oxford University Press, 1998), 414–466.
2. Kwiterovich PO Jr. The metabolic pathways of high-density lipoprotein, low-density lipoprotein and triglycerides: a current review, *Am J Card* 2000; **86** (suppl):5L–10L.
3. Larosa JC, Hunninghake D, Bush D et al. The cholesterol facts: a summary of the evidence relating dietary fats, serum cholesterol, and coronary heart disease. A joint statement by the American Heart Association and the National Heart, Lung, and Blood Institute. The Task Force on Cholesterol Issues, American Heart Association, *Circulation* 1998; **97**:946–952.
4. Verschuren WM, Jacobs DR, Bloemberg BP et al. Serum total cholesterol and long-term coronary heart disease mortality in different cultures, *JAMA* 1995; **274**:131–135.
5. Kannel WB, Castelli WP, Gordon T. Cholesterol in the prediction of atherosclerotic disease: new perspectives based on the Framingham Study, *Ann Intern Med* 1979; **90**:85–91.
6. Gordon T, Castelli WP, Hjortland MC, Kannel WB, Dawber TR. High density lipoprotein as a protective factor against coronary heart disease, *Am J Med* 1977; **62**:707–714.
7. Kannel WB, Castelli WP, Gordon T, McNamara PM. Serum cholesterol, lipoproteins, and the risk of coronary heart disease. The Framingham Study, *Ann Intern Med* 1971; **74**:1–12.
8. Gordon DJ, Probstfield JL, Garrison RJ et al. High-density lipoprotein cholesterol and cardiovascular disease: four prospective American studies, *Circulation* 1989; **79**:8–15.
9. Martin MJ, Hulley SB, Browner WS, Kuller LH, Wentworth D. Serum cholesterol, blood pressure, and mortality: implications from a cohort of 361,662 men, *Lancet* 1986; **ii**:933–939.
10. Neaton JD, Blackburn H, Jacobs D et al. Multiple Risk Factor Intervention Trial Research Group: serum cholesterol and mortality findings for men screened in the Multiple Risk Factor Intervention Trial, *Arch Int Med* 1992; **152**:1490–1500.
11. Multiple Risk Factor Intervention Trial Research Group. Multiple Risk Factor Intervention Trial, *JAMA* 1982; **248**:1465–1477.
12. Maron DJ. The epidemiology of low levels of high-density lipoprotein cholesterol in patients with and without coronary artery disease, *Am J Card* 2000; **86** (suppl):11L–14L.
13. Report from the Committee of Principal Investigators. A cooperative trial in the primary prevention of ischemic heart disease using clofibrate, *Br Heart J* 1978; **40**:1069–1118.
14. Lipid Research Clinics Program Epidemiology Committee. Plasma lipid distributions in selected North American populations: the lipid

research clinics program prevalence study, *Circulation* 1979; **60**:427–439.

15. Lipid Research Clinics Program. The lipid research clinics coronary primary prevention trial results I. Reduction in incidence of coronary heart disease, *JAMA* 1984; **251**:351–364.

16. Lipid Research Clinics Program. The lipid research clinics coronary primary prevention trial results II. The relationship of reduction in incidence of coronary heart disease to cholesterol lowering, *JAMA* 1984; **251**:365–374.

17. Frick MH, Elo O, Haapa K et al. Helsinki Heart Study: primary-prevention trial with gemfibrozil in middle-age men with dyslipidemia; safety of treatment, changes in risk factors, and incidence of coronary heart disease, *N Engl J Med* 1987; **317**:1237–1245.

18. Mannihen V, Elo O, Frick MH et al. Lipid alterations and decline in incidence of coronary heart disease in the Helsinki Heart Study, *JAMA* 1988; **260**:641–651.

19. The Coronary Drug Project Research Group. Clofibrate and niacin in coronary heart disease, *JAMA* 1975; **231**:360–381.

20. Canner PL, Berge KG, Wenger NK et al. Fifteen year mortality in coronary drug project patients: long-term benefit with niacin, *J Am Coll Cardiol* 1986; **8**:1245–1255.

21. Rubins HB, Robins SJ, Collins D et al. Distribution of lipids in 8500 men with coronary artery disease, *Am J Cardiol* 1995; **75**:1196–1201.

22. Rubins HB. High-density lipoprotein and coronary heart disease: lessons from recent intervention trials, *Prev Cardiol* 2000; **3**:33–39.

23. Rubins HB, Robins S, Collins D et al for the Veterans Affairs High-density Lipoprotein Cholesterol Intervention Trial Study Group. Gemfibrozil for the secondary prevention of coronary heart disease in men with low levels of high-density lipoprotein cholesterol, *N Engl J Med* 1999; **341**:410–418.

24. Rubins HB, Robins SJ, Collins D. The Veterans Affairs High-density Lipoprotein Intervention Trial: baseline characteristics of normocholesterolemic men with coronary artery disease and low levels of high-density lipoprotein cholesterol, *Am J Card* 1996; **78**:572–575.

25. Carlson LA, Rosenhamer G. Reduction of mortality in the Stockholm ischemic heart disease secondary prevention study by combined treatment with clofibrate and nicotinic acid, *Acta Med Scand* 1988; **223**:405–418.

26. Shepherd J, Cobbe SM, Ford I et al. Prevention of coronary heart disease with pravastatin in men with hypercholesterolemia, *N Engl J Med* 1995; **333**:1301–1307.

27. Downs JR, Clearfield M, Weis S et al. Primary prevention of acute coronary events with lovastatin in men and women with average cholesterol levels: results of AFCAPS/TEXCAPS, *JAMA* 1998; **279**:1615–1622.

28. Scandinavian Simvastatin Survival Study Group. Randomized trial of cholesterol lowering in 4444 patients with coronary heart disease: the Scandinavian Simvastatin Survival Study (4S), *Lancet* 1994; **344**:1383–1389.

29. Sacks FM, Pfeffer MA, Moye LA et al. The effect of pravastatin on coronary events after myocardial infarction in patients with average cholesterol levels. Cholesterol and recurrent events trial investigators, *N Engl J Med* 1996; **335**: 1001–1009.

30. The Long-Term Intervention with Pravastatin in Ischaemic Disease (LIPID) Study Group. Prevention of cardiovascular events and death with pravastatin in patients with coronary heart disease and a broad range of initial cholesterol levels, *N Engl J Med* 1998; **339**:1349–1357.

31. Rossouw JE. Lipid-lowering interventions in angiographic trials, *Am J Cardiol* 1995; **76**: 86C–92C.

32. Brown G, Albers JJ, Fisher LD et al. Regression of coronary artery disease as a result of intensive lipid-lowering therapy in men with high levels of apoliprotein B, *N Engl J Med* 1990; **323**:1289–1298.

33. MAAS Investigators. Effect of simvastatin on coronary atheroma: the Multicentre Anti-Atheroma Study (MAAS), *Lancet* 1994; **344**: 633–638.

34. Herd JA, Ballantyne CM, Farmer JA et al. Effects of fluvastatin on coronary atherosclerosis in patients with mild to moderate cholesterol elevations (Lipoprotein and Coronary Atherosclerosis Study (LCAS)), *Am J Card* 1997; **80**:278–286.

35. Blankenhorn DA, Azen SP, Kramsch DM et al. Coronary angiographic changes with lovastatin therapy. The Monitored Atherosclerosis Regression Study (MARS), *Ann Int Med* 1993; **119**:969–976.

36. Jukema JW, Bruschke AVG, van Boven AJ et al. Effects of lipid lowering by pravastatin on progression and regression of coronary artery disease in symptomatic men with normal to moderately elevated serum cholesterol levels. The Regression Growth Evaluation Statin Study (REGRESS), *Circulation* 1995; **91**:2528–2540.

37. Sacks FM, Pasternack RC, Gibson CM et al for the Harvard Atherosclerosis Reversibility Project (HARP) group. Effect on coronary atherosclerosis of decrease in plasma cholesterol concentrations in normocholesterolaemic patients, *Lancet* 1994; **344**:1182–1186.

38. Ericsson CG, Hamsten A, Nilsson J et al. Angiographic assessment of effects of bezafibrate on progression of coronary artery disease in young male postinfarction patients, *Lancet* 1996; **347**:849–853.

39. Buchwald H, Varco RL, Matts JP et al and the POSCH group. Effect of partial ileal bypass surgery on mortality and morbidity from coronary heart disease in patients with hypercholesterolemia, *N Engl J Med* 1990; **323**:946–955.

40. Levy RI, Breniske JF, Epstein SE et al. The influence of changes in lipid values induced by cholestyramine and diet on progression of coronary artery disease: results of the NHLBI type II coronary intervention study, *Circulation* 1984; **69**:325–337.

41. Gotto AM. Assessing the benefits of lipid-lowering therapy, *Am J Card* 1998; **82**:2M–4M.

42. Roussow JE, Lewis B, Rifkind BM. The value of lowering cholesterol after myocardial infarction, *N Engl J Med* 1990; **323**:1112–1119.

43. Ballantyne CM. Clinical trial endpoints: angiograms, events, and plaque instability, *Am J Cardiol* 1998; **82**:5M–11M.

44. Pitt B, Mancini GBJ, Ellis SG et al for the PLAC I Investigators. Pravastatin Limitation of Atherosclerosis in the Coronary Arteries (PLAC-I): reduction in atherosclerosis progression and clinical events, *J Am Coll Cardiol* 1995; **26**:1133–1139.

45. K Lance Gould. Coronary arteriography and lipid lowering: limitations, new concepts, and new paradigms in cardiovascular medicine, *Am J Cardiol* 1998; **82**:12M–21M.

46. Herd JA. Relation of clinical benefit to metabolic effects in lipid-lowering therapy, *Am J Cardiol* 1998; **82**:22M–25M.

47. Jones PH. Future of lipid-lowering trials: what else do we need to know? *Am J Cardiol* 1998; **82**:32M–38M.

48. Schwartz GG, Olsson AG, Ezekowitz MD et al for the MIRACL study investigators. Effects of atorvastatin on early recurrent ischemic events in acute coronary syndromes. The MIRACL study: a randomized clinical trial, *JAMA* 2001; **285**:1711–1718.

49. Blankenhorn DH, Nessim SA, Johnson RL et al. Beneficial effects of combined colestipol niacin therapy on coronary atherosclerosis and coronary venous bypass grafts, *JAMA* 1987; **257**:3233–3240.

50. Eritsland J, Arnesen H, Seljefiot I et al. Influence of serum lipoprotein (a) and homocysteine levels on graft patency after coronary artery bypass grafting, *Am J Cardiol* 1994; **74**:1099–1102.

51. Bates ER. Raising high-density lipoprotein cholesterol and lowering low-density lipoprotein cholesterol as adjunctive therapy to coronary revascularization, *Am J Cardiol* 2000; **86** (suppl):28L–34L.

52. Rhodes KS, Bookstein UC, Aaronson US, Mercer NM, Orringer CE. Intensive nutrition counseling enhances outcomes of National Cholesterol Education Program dietary therapy, *J Am Diet Assoc* 1996; **96**:1003–1010.

53. Singh RB, Rasrogi SS, Verma R et al. Randomized controlled trial of cardioprotective diet in patients with recent acute myocardial infarction: results of one year follow up, *BMJ* 1992; **304**:1015–1019.

54. Schuler G, Rambrecht R, Schlierf G et al. Regular physical exercise and low-fat diet. Effects on progression of coronary artery disease, *Circulation* 1992; **86**:1–11.

55. Superko HR, Krauss RM. Coronary artery disease regression: convincing evidence for the benefit of aggressive lipoprotein management, *Circulation* 1994; **90**:1056–1069.

56. Gould AL, Rossouw JE, Sanranello NC, Heyse JF, Furberg CD. Cholesterol reduction yields clinical benefit: impact of statin trials, *Circulation* 1998; **97**:946–952.

57. Pitt B, Waters D, Brown WV et al for the Atorvastatin versus Revascularization Treatment Investigators. Aggressive lipid-lowering therapy compared with angioplasty in stable coronary disease, *N Engl J Med* 1999; **341**:70–76.

58. The Post Coronary Artery Bypass Graft Trial

Investigators: The effect of aggressive lowering of low-density lipoprotein cholesterol levels and low-dose anticoagulation on obstructive change in saphenous-vein coronary-artery bypass grafts, *N Engl J Med* 1997; **336**:153–162.

59. Wenke K, Meiser B, Thiery J et al. Simvastatin reduces graft vessel disease and mortality after transplantation, *Circulation* 1997; **96**:1398–1402.

60. Kobashigawa JA, Katznelson S, Laks H et al. Effect of pravastatin on outcomes after cardiac transplantation, *N Engl J Med* 1995; **333**:621–627.

61. Treasure CB, Klein JL, Weintraub WS et al. Beneficial effects of cholesterol-lowering therapy on the coronary endothelium in patients with coronary artery disease, *N Engl J Med* 1995; **332**:481–487.

62. Keys A. *Seven countries: a multivariate analysis of death and coronary heart disease* (Cambridge: Harvard University Press, 1980).

63. Shekelle RB, Shryock AM, Paul O et al. Diet, serum cholesterol, and death from coronary heart disease. The Western Electric Study, *N Engl J Med* 1981; **304**:65–70.

64. Gordon T, Kagan A, Garcia-Palmieri M et al. Diet and its relation to coronary heart disease and death in three populations, *Circulation* 1981; **63**:500–515.

65. Scott DW, Gorry GA, Gotto AM. Editorial. Diet and coronary heart disease: the statistical analysis of risk, *Circulation* 1981; **63**:516–518.

66. Enholm C, Huttunen JK, Pietinen P et al. Effect of diet on serum lipoproteins in a population with a high risk of coronary heart disease, *N Engl J Med* 1982; **307**:850–855.

67. Kushi LH, Lew RA, Stare FJ et al. Diet and 20-year mortality from coronary heart disease, *N Engl J Med* 1985; **312**:811–818.

68. Arntzenius AC, Kromhout D, Barth JD et al. Diet, lipoproteins, and the progression of coronary atherosclerosis. The Leiden Intervention Trial, *N Engl J Med* 1985; **312**:805–811.

69. Blankenhorn DH. Editorial. Two new diet-heart studies, *N Engl J Med* 1985; **312**:851–853.

70. Hjermann I, Velve Byre K, Holme I, Leren P. Effect of diet and smoking intervention on the incidence of coronary heart disease. Report from the Oslo Study Group of a Randomized Trial in Healthy Men, *Lancet* 1981; Dec 12:1303–1310.

71. National Cholesterol Education Program. Second report of the expert panel on detection, evaluation, and treatment of high blood cholesterol in adults, *Circulation* 1994; **89**:1333–1445.

72. Smith SC Jr, Blair SN, Criqui MH et al. The secondary prevention panel. Preventing heart attack and death in patients with coronary disease, *Circulation* 1995; **92**:2–4.

73. The 27th Bethesda Conference. Matching the intensity of risk factor management with the hazard for coronary disease events. September 14–15, 1995, *J Am Coll Cardiol* 1996; **27**:957–1047.

74. Pearson T, Rapaport E, Criqui M et al. Optimal risk factor management in the patient after coronary revascularization. AHA Medical/ Scientific Statement, *Circulation* 1994; **90**:3125–3133.

75. Sacks FM. Why cholesterol as a central theme in coronary artery disease? *Am J Cardiol* 1988; **82**:14T–17T.

76. Summary of the second report of the National Cholesterol Education Program (NCEP) Expert Panel on Detection, Evaluation, and Treatment of High Blood Cholesterol in Adults (Adult Treatment Panel II), *JAMA* 1993; **269**:3015–3023.

77. Miller M. Differentiating the effects of raising low levels of high-density lipoprotein cholesterol versus lowering normal triglycerides: further insights from the Veterans Affairs high-density lipoprotein intervention trial, *Am J Card* 2000; **86** (suppl):23L–27L.

78. Piepho RW. The pharmacokinetics and pharmacodynamics of agents proven to raise high-density lipoprotein cholesterol, *Am J Cardiol* 2000; **86** (suppl): 35L–40L.

79. Ginsburg HN. Non-pharmacologic management of low levels of high-density lipoprotein cholesterol, *Am J Cardiol* 2000: **86** (suppl): 41L–45L.

80. De Logeril M, Renaud S, Mamelle N et al. Mediterranean alpha-linoleic acid-rich diet in secondary prevention of coronary heart disease, *Lancet* 1994; **343**:1454–1459.

81. Kane JP, Malloy MJ, Ports TA et al. Regression of coronary atherosclerosis during treatment of familial hypercholesterolemia with combined drug regimens, *JAMA* 1990; **264**:3007–3012.

82. The BIP Study Group. Secondary prevention by raising HDL cholesterol and reducing triglycerides in patients with coronary artery disease. The Bezafibrate Infarction Prevention Study, *Circulation* 2000; **102**:21–27.

83. Sprecher DL. Raising high-density lipoprotein cholesterol with niacin and fibrates: a compara-

tive review, *Am J Cardiol* 2000: **86** (suppl): 46L–50L.

84. Pearson TA. Divergent approaches to the treatment of dyslipidemia with low levels of high-density lipoprotein cholesterol, *Am J Cardiol* 2000: **86** (suppl):57L–61L.

85. Smith SC Jr. Clinical treatment of dyslipidemia: practice patterns and missed opportunities, *Am J Cardiol* 2000: **86** (suppl):62L–65L.

86. Sacks FM, Tonkin AM, Shepherd J et al for the Prospective Pravastatin Pooling Project Investigators Group. Effect of pravastatin on coronary disease events in subgroups defined by coronary risk factors. The Prospective Pravastatin Pooling Project, *Circulation* 2000; **102**:1893–1900.

87. Sacks FM, Alaupovic P, Moye LA et al. VLDL, apolipoproteins B, CIII, and E, and risk of recurrent coronary events in the Cholesterol And Recurrent Events (CARE) Trial, *Circulation* 2000; **102**:1886–1892.

88. Holme I. An analysis of randomized trials evaluating the effect of cholesterol reduction on total mortality and coronary heart disease incidence, *Circulation* 990; **82**:1916–1924.

89. Shepherd J for the West of Scotland Coronary Prevention Study Group. The West of Scotland Coronary Prevention Study. A trial of cholesterol reduction in Scottish men, *Am J Cardiol* 1995; **76**:113C–117C.

90. Tonkin AM for the LIPID Study Group. Management of the long-term Intervention with Pravastatin in Ischaemic Disease (LIPID) Study after the Scandinavian Simvastatin Survival Study (4S), *Am J Cardiol* 1995; **76**:107C–112C.

91. Pfeffer MA, Sacks FM, Moye LA et al for the CARE Investigators. Cholesterol and recurrent events: a secondary prevention trial for normolipemic patients, *Am J Cardiol* 1995; **76**:98C–106C.

92. De Faire U, Ericsson CG, Grip L et al. Secondary preventive potential of lipid-lowering drugs. The Bezafibrate Coronary Atherosclerosis Intervention Trial (BECAIT), *Eur Heart J* 1996; **17** (suppl):37–42.

93. Coronary Drug Project Research Group. National history of myocardial infarction in the coronary drug project: long-term prognostic importance of serum lipid levels, *Am J Cardiol* 1978; **42**:489–498.

94. The Coronary Drug Project Research Group. Implications of findings in the coronary drug project for secondary prevention trials in coronary heart disease, *Circulation* 1981; **63**:1342–1350.

95. Teo KK, Burton JR, Buller CE et al for the SCAT Investigators. Long-term effects of cholesterol lowering and angiotensin-converting enzyme inhibition on coronary atherosclerosis. The Simvastatin/Enalapril Coronary Atherosclerosis Trial (SCAT), *Circulation* 2000; **102**:1748–1754.

96. Bradford RH, Shear CL, Chremos AN et al. Expanded Clinical Evaluation of Lovastatin (EXCEL) Study Results. Two-year efficacy and safety follow-up, *Am J Cardiol* 1994; **74**:667–673.

97. Kannel WB. The worth of controlling plasma lipids, *Am J Cardiol* 1998; **81**:1047–1049.

98. Cohen MV, Byrne MJ, Levine B, Gutowski T, Adelson R. Low rate of treatment of hypercholesterolemia by cardiologist in patients with suspected and proven coronary artery disease, *Circulation* 1991; **83**:1294–1304.

99. Pearson TA, Laurora I, Chu H, Kafonek S. The Lipid Treatment Assessment Project (L-TAP), *Arch Intern Med* 2000; **160**:459–467.

100. Kastelein JJP, Jukema JW, Zwinderman AH et al for the REGRESS Study Group. Lipoprotein lipase activity is associated with severity of angina pectoris, *Circulation* 2000; **102**:1629–1633.

101. Manninen V, Tenkanen L, Koskinen P et al. Joint effects of serum triglyceride and LDL cholesterol concentrations in coronary heart disease risk in the Helsinki heart study, *Circulation* 1992; **85**:37–45.

102. Kwiterovich PO. State-of-the-art update and review: clinical trials of lipid-lowering agents, *Am J Cardiol* 1998; **82** (12A):3U–17U.

103. Dorr AE, Gunderson KK, Schneider JC Jr, Spencer TW, Martin WB. Colestipol hydrochloride in hypercholesterolemic patients: effect on serum cholesterol and mortality, *J Chron Dis* 1978; **31**:5–14.

104. Breniske JF, Levy RI, Kelsey SF et al. Effects of therapy with cholestyramine on progression of coronary atherosclerosis: results of the NHLBI Type II coronary intervention study, *Circulation* 1984; **69**:313–324.

105. Watts GF, Lewis B, Brunt JN et al. Effects on coronary artery disease of lipid-lowering diet or diet plus cholestyramine, in the St Thomas Atherosclerosis Regression Study (STARS), *Lancet* 1992; **339**:563–569.

106. Waters D, Higginson L, Gladstone P et al. Effect of monotherapy with HMG-CoA reductase inhibitor on the progression of coronary atherosclerosis as assessed by serial quantitative arteriography: the Canadian Coronary Atherosclerosis Intervention Trial, *Circulation* 1994; **89**:959–968.

107. Shah PK, Amin J. Low high-density lipoprotein level is associated with increased restenosis rate after coronary angioplasty, *Circulation* 1992; **85**:1279–1285.

108. Guyton JR. Effect of niacin on atherosclerotic cardiovascular disease, *Am J Cardiol* 1998; **82**:18U–23U.

109. Scottish Society of Physicians. Ischaemic heart disease: a secondary prevention trial using clofibrate, *BMJ* 1971; **4**:775–784.

110. Newcastle-upon-Tyne Physicians group. Trial of clofibrate in the treatment of ischaemic heart disease, *BMJ* 1971; **4**:767–775.

111. Cashin-Hemphill L, Mack WJ, Pogoda JM et al. Beneficial effects of colestipol-niacin on coronary atherosclerosis: a 4-year follow-up, *JAMA* 1990; **264**:3013–3017.

112. Weintraub WS, Boccuzzi SJ, Klein JL et al for the Lovastatin Restenosis Trial Study Group. Lack of effect of lovastatin on restenosis after coronary angioplasty, *N Engl J Med* 1994; **331**:1331–1337.

113. O'Keefe JH, Stone GW, McCallister BD et al. Lovastatin plus probucol for prevention of restenosis after percutaneous transluminal coronary angioplasty, *Am J Cardiol* 1996; **77**:649–652.

114. Bertrand ME, McFadden EP, Fruchart JC et al. Effect of pravastatin on angiographic restenosis after coronary balloon angioplasty. The PREDICT Trial Investigators, *J Am Coll Cardiol* 1997; **30**:863–869.

115. Serruys PW, Foley DP, Jackson G et al. A randomized placebo-controlled trial of fluvastatin for prevention of restenosis after successful coronary balloon angioplasty. Final results of the fluvastatin angiographic restenosis (FLARE) trial, *Eur Heart J* 1999; **20**:58–69.

116. Executive Summary of the third report of the National Cholesterol Education Program (NCEP) Expert Panel on Detection, Evaluation, and Treatment of High Blood Pressure, and Cholesterol in Adults (Adult Treatment Panel III), *JAMA* 2001; **285**:2486–2497.

117. Taubes G. The soft science of dietary fat, *Science* 2001; **291**:2536–2545.

4

Angiotensin-converting enzyme inhibitors

Hoang M Thai and Douglass A Morrison

CONTENTS • Introduction • ACE inhibition in the early post myocardial infarction setting • ACE inhibition in the long-term post myocardial infarction setting • ACE inhibition in the congestive heart failure setting • The role of ACE inhibition in cardiovascular protection and hypertension • The role of ACE inhibition as adjunctive therapy following revascularization • Conclusion

INTRODUCTION

The beneficial effects of attenuating the conversion of angiotensin I to angiotensin II (AII) through the use of angiotensin-converting enzyme (ACE) inhibitors have been firmly established in the therapy of heart failure from various causes. It is believed that these pharmacologic agents are effective in the treatment of heart failure and even of asymptomatic patients with left ventricular (LV) dysfunction, because they decrease the formation of AII. It is generally agreed that the most important effects of ACE inhibition in the treatment of heart failure include the improvement of abnormal ventricular loading conditions and the attenuation of ventricular remodeling. However, since ACE inhibitors can also promote the effects of other important neurohormones, such as bradykinin and prostaglandins, and because AII may be produced by alternate pathways, the specificity and magnitude of the contribution of AII blockade to the prevention and evolution of heart failure has not been determined precisely.

It is clear that an important clinical setting in which the use of ACE inhibitors has demonstrated an unquestioned survival benefit is in the setting of heart failure following acute myocardial infarction (MI). With over 100,000 patients enrolled in a combination of trials that initiated ACE inhibition from within 24 hours of an acute MI to days later, the reduction in mortality seen in this setting is established [1–21]. In the review that follows, the effects of ACE inhibition on major clinical parameters following myocardial infarction will be discussed, both in an acute and chronic setting [22–34]. The long-term benefits of ACE inhibition in the treatment of chronic heart failure will be evaluated [22–34], along with the role of ACE inhibition in cardiovascular protection including the role of ACE inhibitors as anti-hypertensive agents [35–55]. Finally, the role of ACE inhibition as an adjunctive therapy along with coronary revascularization, both surgical and percutaneous interventions, will be examined [56–62].

ACE INHIBITION IN THE EARLY POST MYOCARDIAL INFARCTION SETTING [1–2]

Over 98,000 patients were studied in five major clinical trials (CONSENSUS-II, GISSI-3, ISIS-4, SMILE and CCS-1) evaluating the effectiveness of ACE inhibition within 24 hours of an acute MI [2–5, 17]. Three of these five studies showed

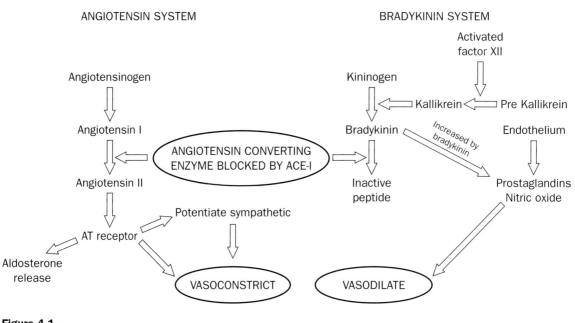

Figure 4.1
Pathophysiologic/pharmacologic scheme of action. Shown are the bradykinin and angiotensin systems and where angiotensin-converting enzyme inhibition works on each.

significant mortality reductions with the use of ACE inhibitors in the early post MI period. The failure to show a significant mortality benefit in CONSENSUS II, has been attributed to small sample size and the possibility of a significant increase in hypotension with a trend towards increasing mortality among patients enrolled with systolic blood pressure < 90 mmHg (approximately 10%) [2]. Patients with a systolic below 90 mmHg were excluded from ISIS-4 and below 100 mmHg were excluded from GISSI-3. Similarly, the failure to observe a survival benefit in SMILE was likely a function of inadequate sample size. A more recent meta-analysis of these five studies reports an overall risk reduction of 6.7% with 4.9 fewer deaths per 1000 treated [22].

In the studies showing survival benefit, most of the benefits were seen within the first week of therapy, with GISSI-3 and ISIS-4 showing nearly

a third of the total mortality reduction occurring within the first day of treatment [1, 6]. This early survival benefit persisted for the length of the follow-up period, from six months to one year, despite early discontinuation of therapy as early as six weeks after MI [4, 7]. This result was not surprising since the mortality rate of a myocardial infarction tends to be the highest in the period immediately following the clinical event. The total reduction in mortality ranged from 6–7% in CCS-1 and the ISIS-4 trials respectively, to as high as 11% in GISSI-3. As a whole this translates into approximately five lives saved per 1000 treated. The subgroup analyses revealed that the greatest proportional improvement in mortality was among patients with the highest risk profiles, mainly those with anterior wall myocardial infarctions, diabetes, previous MI and heart failure [4, 8]. In these high-risk patients, the lives saved per 1000 treated increased 10-fold to 50 per 1000 treated. In particular, among patients with electrocardiographic (ECG) evidence of an anterior wall MI there was a 12.7% reduction in mortality compared to only a 2% reduction in patients with ECG changes elsewhere. In terms of lives saved, in the anterior wall MI subgroup 11 lives were saved per 1000 treated, compared to only one saved per 1000 treated in the non-anterior MI subgroup. These findings reinforce the axiom in clinical medicine that any beneficial effects that result from a particular intervention will usually be the most pronounced among subjects with the highest risks and during the time period that is associated with the highest mortality. Although there was no subgroup among which the use of an ACE inhibitor proved harmful, patients with hypotension (systolic blood pressure < 100) and cardiogenic shock were excluded from these studies. Additionally, the use of an intravenous ACE inhibitor did not demonstrate a survival

benefit among patients with heart failure following a myocardial infarction (Table 4.1). As a result of these clinical studies, the use of an oral ACE inhibitor early in the post MI period, especially in patients with depressed LV function and/or anterior wall myocardial infarction, has been given a class I indication by the joint 1996 American College of Cardiology/American Heart Association (ACC/AHA) 'Guidelines for the management of patients with acute myocardial infarction' task force [9].

ACE INHIBITION IN THE LONG-TERM POST MYOCARDIAL INFARCTION SETTING

The Survival and Ventricular Enlargement (SAVE) trial remains the seminal study that evaluated the long-term benefits of ACE inhibition in patients with depressed LV function (ejection fraction < 40%) following myocardial

Table 4.1 Major randomized trials of angiotensin-converting enzyme inhibitors (ACE-I) in the early post myocardial infarction period

Trial name	Ref	ACE-I (dose)	n	Endpoint	RR (CI)	p
GISSI-3	3	Lisinopril (10 QD)	18,895	Mortality	0.88 (0.79–0.99)	0.03
ISIS-4	4	Captopril (50 TID)	58,050	Mortality	0.93 (0.87–0.99)	0.02
CCS-1	5	Captopril (12.5 TID)	14,962	Mortality	0.94 (0.84–1.05)	0.03
(CONSENSUS II)	2	Enalaprilat iv (1 mg over 2 hours, then enalapril (20 QD)	6090	Mortality	1.10 (0.93–1.29)	0.26
SMILE	17	Zofenopril 7.5 mg to 30 mg BID	1556	Mortality	0.75 (0.4–1.11)	0.19

RR, risk ratio; CI, 95% confidence interval.

infarction. The uniqueness of this trial was that the study cohort was essentially asymptomatic and not in overt heart failure at the time of enrolment [10]. There were a total of 2231 patients with an LV ejection fraction (EF) of less than 40% randomized to captopril (50 mg TID) or placebo, 3–16 days after an acute myocardial infarction. After a follow-up period that lasted an average of 3.5 years, the results showed a 19% reduction in overall mortality and a 21% reduction in cardiovascular mortality with captopril treatment. The need for re-hospitalization was reduced by 22% along with a 37% reduction in the future development of heart failure. Interestingly, recurrent MI was reduced by 25%, raising the possibility that ACE inhibition may reduce ischemia. A similar study to the SAVE trial was the Trandolapril Cardiac Evaluation (TRACE) trial [11]. A total of 6676 patients, within 3–7 days after an MI, were screened to find 2606 patients without overt heart failure but with echocardiographic wall motion scores that denoted an LV ejection fraction of less than 35%. Of those, 1749 patients were randomized to the ACE inhibitor trandolapril or placebo. After a follow-up period ranging from 2–4 years, the results were consistent with the SAVE study. There was a reduction of overall mortality by 22% with a reduction of progression to severe heart failure by 29% in those patients treated with trandolapril. However, unlike the SAVE study there was not an appreciable reduction in the rate of recurrent MI among the ACE inhibitor treated group. This finding was repeated in the Acute Infarction Ramipril Efficacy (AIRE) trial [12], in which investigators identified 2006 high-risk patients with overt failure after myocardial infarction. Randomization to ramipril or placebo among these patients took place between days 3 and 10 post MI. Despite the disappointing lack of reduction in recurrent ischemia, ramipril therapy reduced overall mortality in this high-risk cohort by 26% (17% ramipril versus 23% placebo) and progression to severe heart failure by 23% (Table 4.2). A follow-up study from the AIRE investigators

reported sustained survival benefits at five years, with a 28% reduction in mortality (28% ramipril versus 39% placebo) [13]. While ACE inhibitors are not known to have anti-arrhythmic effects, ramipril was associated with a reduced incidence of sudden death by 30% in the AIRE trial. A similar finding was noted with trandolapril in the TRACE study. It is speculated that reduction in the progression to severe heart failure that is seen among these studies, may account for the decline in sudden cardiac death. Several studies provide further insights into this observation. In the Vasodilator Heart Failure Trial II (VHeFT II) study, 804 men, age 18–75 years, with chronic clinical heart failure (CHF) and left ventricular ejection fraction (LVEF) < 45% were randomized to enalapril (10 mg twice daily (BID)) or a hydralazine/isosorbide dinitrate combination. After a two-year follow-up period there was a 28% reduction in mortality in the ACE inhibitor group. This result was attributed to a reduction of sudden death among patients with less severe CHF symptoms, New York Heart Association (NYHA) class I or II [14]. A possible anti-arrhythmic effect of ACE inhibition was demonstrated in a sub-study from the ISIS-4 trial. In ISIS, captopril treatment reduced was accompanied by reduced frequency of premature ventricular beats (PVB) at days 3 and 14 post MI compared to placebo; this included the number of patients with more than 10 PVB per hour. However, the number of patients with ventricular tachycardia and complex ventricular rhythms were similar in both groups [15]. While it is not yet clear that ACE inhibitors deserve to be classified as an anti-arrhythmic agent, the role of ACE inhibition in reducing sudden death is convincing. In a recent meta-analysis of 15,104 patients, it was found that ACE inhibitor therapy reduced the risk of sudden death by 20% (odds ratio 0.80) [16]. Despite many possible theories, ranging from prohibition of ventricular remodeling to prevention of recurrent ischemic events, the actual mechanism, by which ACE inhibition affects sudden death in a post-myocardial infarct setting, remains unknown.

Table 4.2 Major randomized trials of angiotensin-converting enzyme inhibitors (ACE-I) in the late post myocardial infarction period

Trial name	Ref	ACE-I (dose)	n	Endpoint	RR (CI)	p
SAVE	10	Captopril (50 TID)	2231	Mortality	0.81 (0.68–0.97)	0.019
AIRE	12	Ramipril (10 QD)	1986	Mortality	0.73 (0.6–0.89)	0.002
TRACE	11	Trandolapril (4 QD)	1749	Mortality	0.78 (0.67–0.91)	0.001
SMILE	17	Zofrenopril (30 BID)	1556	1 yr mortality	0.75 (0.4–1.11)	0.19

RR, risk ratio; CI, 95% confidence interval; QD, once daily; BID, twice daily; TID, three times daily.

The long-term benefit of ACE inhibitors in high-risk patients following a myocardial infarction was again demonstrated in the Survival of Myocardial Infarction Long-Term Evaluation (SMILE) trial [17]. In SMILE, patients with an anterior wall MI, who did not receive thrombolytic therapy, were randomized to the ACE inhibitor zofrenopril or placebo, within 24 hours of their infarct, and continued for a total of six weeks. A total of 1556 patients were enrolled, zofrenopril was initially started at a dose of 7.5 mg BID; this was progressively titrated up until the target dose of 30 mg BID was reached. The clinical primary endpoint of mortality and severe heart failure was reduced by 33%, with an absolute reduction of 3.5% (7.1% zofrenopril versus 10.6% placebo) at six weeks. At 12 months the absolute benefit was 4% (10% zofrenopril versus 14% placebo), with a 29% relative reduction in the primary endpoint. Since such dramatic results were seen with ACE inhibitor use in an acute MI setting without the benefit of thrombolytic therapy, several trials designed to study the efficacy of combined ACE inhibition and thrombolytic therapy were initi-

ated. The Fosinopril in Acute Myocardial Infarction Study (FAMIS) studied 285 patients with anterior wall MI treated with a thrombolytic agent and randomized to fosinopril (10 or 20 mg QD) or placebo within nine hours of presentation. Therapy was continued for at least three months and the patients followed for another two years. The primary endpoint of mortality and progression to severe heart failure (NYHA III or IV) was significantly reduced with ACE inhibition/thrombolytic combination compared to placebo/thrombolytic therapy (18% versus 27%) [18]. This reduction in mortality was not observed in the Captopril and Thrombolysis Study (CATS), in which captopril was used within six hours of thrombolytic therapy in 298 patients [19]. The small size of these studies may play a role in the inconsistencies of the findings. A common result among these trials was the attenuation of LV dilation with early ACE inhibition, and a separate meta-analysis of 845 patients revealed that this was particularly significant among patients that did not achieve reperfusion [20]. This finding suggests that ACE inhibitors provide a protective anti-ischemic benefit in the post MI period. Similar findings were demonstrated in the SAVE study with a 25% reduction in recurrent ischemia and the CATS trial, in which there was a 37% reduction in ischemic related events three months to 12 months post infarct.

ACE INHIBITION IN THE CONGESTIVE HEART FAILURE (CHF) SETTING [22–34]

The use of ACE inhibitors in the treatment of chronic heart failure represents one of the most effective therapeutic interventions in modern medicine. The initial role of ACE inhibitors as afterload-reducing agents came about from the observation that chronic compensated heart failure is often accompanied by neurohormonal activation of the renin angiotensin system [22]. These observations led to initial studies that measured hemodynamic changes in heart failure patients treated acutely with ACE inhibitors [23, 24]. As it became apparent that the patients treated in these studies achieved favorable reductions in pulmonary capillary wedge pressure, systemic resistance and clinical symptoms of heart failure, there was an increased interest in expanding these hemodynamic studies to include other more tangible clinical results. The first major study to address the question of whether ACE inhibitors improve survival in symptomatic heart failure patients was the Cooperative North Scandinavian Enalapril Survival Study (CONSENSUS); in this trial 253 patients with symptomatic, severe heart failure (NYHA class III–IV) were randomized to enalapril or placebo. The follow-up period lasted 10 years, with the greatest reduction in mortality occurring in the first six months of the study, in which there was a 40% reduction in overall mortality. The overall mortality at one year was reduced by 31%, and the relative risk reduction was sustained over the duration of the study [25]. The Survival of Left Ventricular Dysfunction (SOLVD) investigators attempted to clarify whether ACE inhibitors improve the survival of patients without symptoms of heart failure as well as patients with mild–moderate symptoms of heart failure; in effect incorporating a preventive strategy in the treatment of left ventricular (LV) dysfunction. Two parallel studies in the SOLVD trial were designed to answer these questions. Over 2500 patients with mild–moderate (New York Heart Association (NYHA) class II–III) heart failure were randomized to enalapril (10 mg BID) and placebo. The length of follow-up averaged 41 months; enalapril was associated with an overall mortality reduction of 16%, beginning at six months and continuing for four years. The major difference was a reduction in death by progressive heart failure [26]. In the preventive strategy, the SOLVD investigators randomized 4228 patients, all of whom are asymptomatic with a LVEF < 35%, the use of enalapril resulted in a 29% reduction in the combined endpoint of progression to symptomatic heart failure and cardiovascular mortality at a follow-up of three years [27]. Other studies, such as VHeFT II [14] and the Munich Mild Heart Failure (MHFT) [28] trial confirmed the earlier trials, and expanded the use of ACE inhibitors to mildly symptomatic and asymptomatic patients with LV dysfunction. Although it appears that the greatest survival benefit with ACE inhibitors are seen among patients with the most severe form of LV dysfunction, it is clear that the use of ACE inhibitors also confer a preventive benefit to those patients within the milder spectrum of this disease (Table 4.3). Despite the proven benefit, the utilization of ACE inhibitors remains low. In addition, when ACE inhibitors are used, they are frequently not used at adequate (based on randomized clinical trials) doses. Accordingly, the effectiveness of ACE inhibitors are attenuated, especially among the elderly [29–32]. The current recommendation for the use of ACE inhibitors essentially follows the available clinical evidence. All patients with symptomatic or asymptomatic LV dysfunction (LVEF < 40%) should be started on an ACE inhibitor, beginning with low doses to reduce the likelihood of hypotension or azotemia [33, 34]. Doses should be gradually

Table 4.3 Major randomized trials of angiotensin-converting enzyme inhibitors (ACE-I) in chronic heart failure

Trial name	Ref	ACE-I (dose)	n	Endpoint	RR (CI)	p
CONSENSUS	25	Enalapril (20 QD)	253	10 yr mortality	0.56 (0.34–0.91)	0.003
SOLVD	26	Enalapril (20 QD)	2569	1 yr mortality	0.82 (0.7–0.97)	0.004
SOLVD (Prevention)	27	Enalapril (20 QD)	4228	CHF	0.63 (0.56–0.72)	0.001
V-HeFT II	14	Enalapril (20 QD)	804	2 yr mortality	0.72	0.016

RR, risk ratio; CI, 95% confidence interval.

titrated to maintenance doses equivalent to enalapril 10 mg BID or captopril 50 mg TID, doses used in the clinical trials.

THE ROLE OF ACE INHIBITION IN CARDIOVASCULAR PROTECTION AND HYPERTENSION [35–55]

Depressed LV function after myocardial infarction is associated with the development of ventricular remodeling, beginning with ventricular dilation, then with progression to the formation of fibrotic scar, and subsequently followed by infarcted segment elongation, all of which can occur within hours of myocardial necrosis [35–37]. ACE inhibitors attenuate LV remodeling after MI in the animal model of ischemic heart failure [38]. This seminal observation led to the many clinical trials that evaluated the role of ACE inhibition early in the post MI setting. From these studies it is clear that ACE inhibitors limit the increase in ventricular volumes and infarct size. Possible explanations for these unique properties may lie in ACE inhibitors' anti-ischemic activity, since AII can

increase myocardial oxygen demand via vasoconstriction, as well as other protective effects such as limiting the myocardial degradation of high-energy phosphate stores after myocardial ischemia and restoration of impaired endothelial dependent vasorelaxation [39, 40]. Clinical evidence of anti-ischemic activity of ACE inhibitors come from the SAVE trial in which recurrent ischemia after an acute MI was decreased with captopril, and the HOPE study, in which major adverse cardiac events such as unstable angina, acute MI, cardiovascular death and stroke were reduced by ramipril. Other investigators have demonstrated improved ventricular systolic and diastolic function during exercise [41] and an increase in myocardial blood flow to ischemic regions with intravenous quinaprilat [42]. This data is intriguing since there is no evidence that ACE inhibitors stabilize or promote regression of atherosclerosis [43–45]. Ordinarily, progression of atherosclerosis precedes ischemia, either through plaque rupture in acute ischemia or through limitation of flow reserves in chronic ischemia. In the Simvastatin/Enalapril Coronary Atherosclerosis Trial (SCAT) 460 patients, with normal serum cholesterol, were randomized to simvastatin/placebo and/or enalapril/placebo and followed for two years. There was no difference between enalapril and placebo in preventing the progression of coronary atherosclerosis. Simvastatin alone slowed the progression of coronary disease, but there was no additive benefit with enalapril [43]. It is conceivable that the preservation of endothelial function by ACE inhibitors during ischemic stress alone may play a major role in the cardioprotective, anti-ischemic effects of ACE inhibition. Several trials have evaluated the role that ACE inhibitors have on impaired endothelial function in patients with coronary artery disease. The Trial on Reversing Endothelial Dysfunction (TREND) study randomized patients with coronary artery disease to quinapril or placebo; patients with heart failure, hypertension and hyperlipidemia were excluded. The primary endpoint was coronary vessel response to acetylcholine infusion at six months. Quinapril, which has a high tissue ACE specificity, improved coronary endothelial function [46]. Increased nitric oxide release due to direct preservation of bradykinin and inhibition of AII's vasoconstrictive effects on the coronary vasculature appear to have major roles in the improvement of coronary endothelial function with ACE inhibition [47]. Other factors that may contribute to anti-ischemic, cardio-protective effects of ACE inhibitors include:

- Enhanced endogenous fibrinolytic activity via decreased tissue plasminogen activator (t-PA) antigen levels and plasminogen activator inhibitor type 1 activity.
- Inhibition of procoagulant activity post MI through the reduction of tissue factor levels.
- Inactivation of macrophages and monocytes by decreasing chemoattractant protein-I [48, 49].

It is important to note that while these findings contribute greatly to our understanding of ACE inhibitors, they as yet have not achieved any significant relevance in the clinical spectrum. In light of ACE inhibitors' cardiovascular protective effects, the remaining issue is whether this translates to a much greater range of clinical settings in which ACE inhibition will provide similar benefits as in the post MI heart failure milieu. The use of ACE inhibitors as antihypertensive agents has yielded mixed results in clinical studies. Over 9500 high-risk patients were randomized in the HOPE study [50]. To qualify patients had to be either diabetic with at least one coronary risk factor or have had evidence of prior vascular disease, including coronary heart disease, stroke or vascular disease. After randomization to ramipril (5–10 mg QD) or placebo the patients were then followed until a predetermined number had reached the primary endpoint of any cardiovascular event (cardiovascular death, myocardial infarction, or stroke). The study was stopped prematurely after 54 months because patients randomized in the ramipril group had a 22% reduction in the relative risk of reaching the primary endpoint. In addition, several of the secondary endpoints were also significantly reduced by ramipril, including: unstable angina, heart failure, and subsequent revascularization. The uniqueness of this study was that these benefits were achieved by ramipril independent of blood pressure lowering [50]. Especially dramatic was the effect that ACE inhibition had on myocardial infarction, stroke and mortality in diabetics with reductions in each subset ranging from 22–33% [51]. These significant results were not seen in the CAPP, STOP Hypertension-2 and UKPDS studies in which ACE inhibitors were compared to other anti-hypertensive agents including: beta-blockers, calcium-channel blockers and diuretics. Perhaps the major difference among these trials was that the study cohort in the HOPE trial consisted of patients who are at a much higher risk of developing macrovascular and microvascular events [52–54].

THE ROLE OF ACE INHIBITION AS ADJUNCTIVE THERAPY FOLLOWING REVASCULARIZATION [56–62]

While it is clear that revascularization of viable myocardium in patients with depressed ventricular function improves their overall prognosis, the role of ACE inhibitors as adjunctive therapy in these patients was only recently examined in the APRES study [55]. In this trial 159 patients with stable angina, no overt heart failure and LVEF ranging from 30–50% were randomized to ramipril or placebo. These patients subsequently underwent revascularization, either percutaneous coronary intervention (PCI) or via coronary artery bypass grafting (CABG). After a three year follow-up ramipril reduced the composite primary endpoint of cardiac death, acute MI, and progression to clinical heart failure by 58% (10% ramipril versus 23% placebo). This effect was independent of LVEF and method of revascularization [55].

The use of ACE inhibitors as adjunctive therapy along with PCI gained popularity after several small studies suggested that restenosis rate correlated with serum ACE level, particularly in patients with the D/D angiotensin I-converting enzyme genotype [56]. In addition, neo-intimal hyperplasia following intracoronary stenting was attenuated with quinapril in these patients [57]. However, despite promising results that demonstrated ACE inhibitor's suppression of neointimal proliferation in an animal model of coronary injury [58, 59], two large clinical studies, MERCATOR and MARCATOR, using cilazapril following percutaneous coronary angioplasty failed to demonstrate any significant benefit in preventing restenosis [60, 61]. This issue is far from settled, however. In the recently completed ValPREST study, 250 patients undergoing coronary stenting were randomized to the angiotensin receptor blocker, valsartan (80 mg QD), or placebo (patients were allowed to take ACE inhibitors at unspecified dosages for other reasons). After six months the valsartan treated patients had a 50% reduction in the rate of in-stent restenosis (19.2% valsartan versus 38.6% placebo) along with a 58% reduction in the re-intervention rate. Even more intriguing was that the valsartan group included twice as many diabetic patients than the placebo group [62].

CONCLUSION

Over the last 20 years, ACE inhibition has become standard therapy for patients with congestive heart failure and myocardial infarction, following several large clinical trials that demonstrated significant reductions in mortality and morbidity. Based on the evidence available, the clinical indication for ACE inhibition has expanded to include asymptomatic patients with depressed LV function. The HOPE trial has begun the transition from secondary to primary prevention. Because the effects of angiotensin II receptor stimulation are believed to contribute significantly to the pathophysiology of heart failure, and given the success of ACE inhibitors, future clinical and basic investigations will focus on alternative modalities designed to manipulate the renin-angiotensin system.

REFERENCES

1. ACE Inhibitor Myocardial Infarction Collaborative Group. Indications for ACE inhibitors in the early treatment of acute myocardial infarction: systematic overview of individual data from 100,000 patients in randomized trials, *Circulation* 1998; **97**:2202–2212.
2. Swedberg K, Held P, Kjekshus J et al for the CONSENSUS II Study Group. Effects of the early administration of enalapril on mortality in patients with acute myocardial infarction, *N Engl J Med* 1992; **327**:678–684.
3. Gruppo Italiano per lo Studio della Sopravivenza nell' infarto Miocardico: GISSI-3. Effects of lisinopril and transdermal glyceryl trinitrate singly and together on six weeks mortality and ventricular function after acute

myocardial infarction, *Lancet* 1994; **343**:1115–1122.

4. ISIS-4 (Fourth International Study of Infarct Survival) Collaborative Group. ISIS-4: a randomized factorial trial assessing early oral captopril, oral mononitrate, and intravenous magnesium sulfate in 58,050 patients with suspected acute myocardial infarction, *Lancet* 1995; **345**:669–685.

5. Chinese Cardiac Study Collaboration Group. Oral captopril versus placebo among 13,634 patients with suspect acute myocardial infarction: interim report from the Chinese Cardiac Study (CCS 1), *Lancet* 1995; **345**:686–687.

6. Latini R, Maggioni AP, Flather M et al. ACE inhibitor use in myocardial infarction. Summary of evidence from clinical trials, *Circulation* 1995; **92**:3132–3137.

7. Gruppo Italiano per lo Studio della Sopravivenza nell' infarto Miocardico. Six month effects of early treatment with lisinopril and transdermal glyceryl trinitrate singly and together withdrawn six weeks after acute myocardial infarction, *J Am Coll Cardiol* 1996; **27**:337.

8. Zuanetti G, Latini R, Maggioni AP et al for the GISSI-3 Investigators. Effect of the ACE inhibitor lisinopril on mortality in diabetic patients with acute myocardial infarction: data from the GISSI-3 study, *Circulation* 1997; **96**:4239–4245.

9. Ryan TJ, Anderson JL, Antman EM et al. ACC/AHA guidelines for the management of patients with acute myocardial infarction. A report of the American College of Cardiology and the American Heart Association Task Force on Practice Guidelines (Committee on Management of Acute Myocardial Infarctions), *J Am Coll Cardiol* 1996; **28**:1328–1428.

10. Pfeffer MA, Braunwald E, Moye LA et al for the SAVE Investigators. Effect of captopril on mortality and morbidity in patients with left ventricular dysfunction after myocardial infarction. Results of the Survival and Ventricular Enlargement Trial, *N Engl J Med* 1992; **327**:669–677.

11. Kober L, Torp-Pedersen C, Carlsen JE et al. A clinical trial of the angiotensin converting enzyme inhibitor trandolapril in patients with left ventricular dysfunction after myocardial infarction, *N Engl J Med* 1995; **333**:1670–1676.

12. The Acute Infarction Ramipril Efficacy (AIRE) Study Investigators. Effect of ramipril on mortality and morbidity of survivors of acute myocardial infarction with evidence of clinical heart failure, *Lancet* 1993; **342**:821–828.

13. Hall AS, Murray GD, Ball SG, on behalf of the AIRE Study Investigators. Follow-up study of patients randomly allocated ramipril or placebo for heart failure after myocardial infarction: AIRE Extension (AIREX) Study, *Lancet* 1997; **349**:1493–1497.

14. Cohn JN, Johnson G, Ziesche S et al. A comparison of enalapril with hydralazine-isosorbide dinitrate in the treatment of chronic congestive heart failure, *N Engl J Med* 1991; **325**:303–310.

15. Budaj A, Cybulski J, Cedro K et al. Effects of captopril on ventricular arrhythmias in the early and late phase of suspected acute myocardial infarction. Randomized, placebo-controlled substudy of ISIS-4, *Eur Heart J* 1996; **17**:1506–1510.

16. Domanski MJ, Exner DV, Borkowf CB et al. Effect of angiotensin converting enzyme inhibition on sudden cardiac death in patients following acute myocardial infarction, *J Am Coll Cardiol* 1999; **33**:598–604.

17. Ambrosioni E, Borghi C, Magnani B, for the Survival of Myocardial Infarction Long-Term Evaluation (SMILE) Investigators. The effect of the angiotensin converting enzyme inhibitor zofrenopril on mortality and morbidity after anterior myocardial infarction, *N Engl J Med* 1995; **332**:80–85.

18. Borghi C, Marino P, Zardini W et al for the FAMIS Working Party. Short and long term effects of early fosinopril administration in patients with acute anterior myocardial infarction undergoing intravenous thrombolysis: results from the Fosinopril in Acute Myocardial Infarction Study, *Am Heart J* 1998; **136**:213–225.

19. Van Gilst WH, Kingma JH, Peels CH et al. Which patient benefits from early angiotensin-converting-enzyme inhibition after myocardial infarction? Results of a one-year serial echocardiographic follow-up from the Captopril and Thrombolysis Study (CATS), *J Am Coll Cardiol* 1996; **28**:114–121.

20. De Kam DJ, Voors AA, van der Berg MP et al. Effect of very early angiotensin converting enzyme inhibition on left ventricular dilation after myocardial infarction in patients receiving thrombolysis, *J Am Coll Cardiol* 2000; **36**: 2047–2053.

21. Flather MD, Lonn EM, Yusuf S. Effects of ACE inhibitors on mortality when started in the early phase of myocardial infarction: evidence from the larger randomized controlled trials, *J Cardiovasc Risk* 1995; **2**:423–428.

22. Curtiss C, Cohn JN, Vrobel T, Franciosa JA. Role of the renin-angiotensin system in the systemic vasoconstriction of chronic congestive heart failure, *Circulation* 1978; **58**:763–770.

23. Gavras H, Faxon DP, Berkoben J et al. Angiotensin converting enzyme inhibition in patients with congestive heart failure, *Circulation* 1978; **58**:770–776.

24. Dzau VJ, Colucci WAS, Hollenberg NK, Williams GH. Relation of the renin-angiotensin-aldosterone system to clinical state in congestive heart failure, *Circulation* 1981; **63**:645–651.

25. The CONSENSUS Trial Study Group. Effects of enalapril on mortality in severe congestive heart failure: results of the Cooperative North Scandinavian Enalapril Survival Study (CONSENSUS), *N Engl J Med* 1987; **316**:1429–1435.

26. The SOLVD Investigators. Effect of enalapril on survival in patients with reduced left ventricular ejection fractions and congestive heart failure, *N Engl J Med* 1991; **325**:293–302.

27. The SOLVD Investigators. Effect of enalapril on mortality and the development of heart failure in asymptomatic patients with reduced left ventricular ejection fraction, *N Engl J Med* 1992; **327**:685–691.

28. Kleber F, Niemoller L, Doering W. Impact of converting enzyme inhibition on progression of chronic heart failure: results of the Munich Mild Heart Failure Trial, *Br Heart J* 1992; **67**:289.

29. Smith NL, Psaty BM, Pitt B et al. Temporal patterns in the medical treatment of congestive heart failure with angiotensin-converting enzyme inhibitors in older adults, 1989 through 1995, *Arch Intern Med* 1998; **158**:1074–1080.

30. McDermott MM, Feinglass J, Lee P et al. Heart failure between 1986 and 1994: temporal trends in drug-prescribing practices, hospital readmissions, and survival at an academic medical center, *Am Heart J* 1997; **134**:901–909.

31. Havranek EP, Abrams F, Stevens E et al. Determinants of mortality in elderly patients with heart failure: the role of angiotensin-converting enzyme inhibitors, *Arch Intern Med* 1998; **158**:2024–2028.

32. Luzier AB, Forrest A, Adelman M et al. Impact of angiotensin-converting enzyme inhibitor under-dosing on rehospitalization rates in congestive heart failure, *Am J Cardiol* 1998; **82**:465–469.

33. Lang RM, Di Bianco R, Broderick GT et al. First dose effects of enalapril 2.5 mg and captopril 6.25 mg in patients with heart failure: a double blind, randomized, multicenter study, *Am Heart J* 1994; **128**:551–556.

34. ACC/AHA Task Force Report. Guidelines for the evaluation and management of heart failure, *Circulation* 2001; **104**:2996–3007.

35. Gaudron P, Eilles C, Kugler I, Ertl G. Progressive left ventricular function and remodeling after myocardial infarction. Potential mechanisms and early predictors, *Circulation* 1993; **87**:755–763.

36. Pfeffer MA, Braunwald E. Ventricular remodeling after myocardial infarction: Experimental observations and clinical implications, *Circulation* 1990; **81**:1161–1172.

37. Pfeffer MA, Pfeffer JM, Lamas GA. Development and prevention of congestive heart failure following myocardial infarction, *Circulation* 1993; **87**:IV120–IV125.

38. Pfeffer JM, Pfeffer MA, Fletcher PJ et al. Progressive ventricular remodeling in rat with myocardial infarction, *Am J Physiol* 1991; **260**:H1406–H1414.

39. Li K, Chen X. Protective effects of captopril and enalapril on myocardial ischemia and reperfusion damage of rat, *J Mol Cell Cardiol* 1987; **19**:909–912.

40. Piana RN, Wang SY, Friedman M et al. Angiotensin-converting enzyme inhibition preserves endothelium-dependent coronary microvascular responses during short-term ischemia-reperfusion, *Circulation* 1996; **93**:544–551.

41. Willenheimer R, Rydberg E, Oberg L et al. ACE inhibition with ramipril improves left ventricular function at rest and post exercise in patients with ischaemic heart disease and preserved left ventricular systolic function, *Eur Heart J* 1999; **20**:1647–1656.

42. Schneider CA, Voth E, Moka D et al. Improvement of myocardial blood flow to ischemic regions by angiotensin-converting enzyme inhibition with quinaprilat IV: a study using 15O water dobutamine stress positron emission tomography, *J Am Coll Cardiol* 1999; **34**:1005–1011.

43. Teo KK, Burton JR, Butler CE et al. Long-term effects of cholesterol lowering and angiotensin-converting enzyme inhibition on coronary atherosclerosis: the Simvistatin/Enalapril coronary atherosclerosis trial (SCAT), *Circulation* 2000; **102**:1748–1754.

44. MacMahon S, Sharpe N, Gamble G et al.

Randomized, placebo-controlled trial of the angiotensin-converting enzyme inhibitor, ramipril, in patients with coronary or other occlusive arterial disease, *J Am Coll Cardiol* 2000; **36**:438–443.

45. Cashin-Hemphill L, Holmvang G, Chang RC et al. Angiotensin-converting enzyme inhibitor as antiatherosclerotic therapy: no answer yet. The QUIET Investigators, QUinapril Ischemic Event Trial, *Am J Cardiol* 1999; **83**:43–47.

46. Mancini GBJ, Henry GC, Macaya C et al. Angiotensin-converting enzyme inhibition with quinapril improves endothelial vasomotor dysfunction in patients with coronary artery disease. The TREND (Trial on Reversing Endothelial Dysfunction) Study, *Circulation* 1996; **94**:258–265.

47. Prasad A, Husain S, Quyyumi AA. Effect of enalaprilat on nitric oxide activity in coronary artery disease, *Am J Cardiol* 1999; **84**:1–6.

48. Wright RA, Flapan AD, Alberti KG et al. Effects of captopril therapy on endogenous fibrinolysis in men with recent, uncomplicated myocardial infarction, *J Am Coll Cardiol* 1994; **24**:67–73.

49. Soejima H, Ogawa H, Yasue H et al. Angiotensin-converting enzyme inhibition reduces monocyte chemoattractant protein-1 and tissue factor levels in patients with myocardial infarction, *J Am Coll Cardiol* 1999; **34**:983–988.

50. Heart Outcomes Prevention Evaluation (HOPE) Study Investigators. Effects of an angiotensin-converting enzyme inhibitor, ramipril, on cardiovascular events in high-risk patients, *N Engl J Med* 2000; **342**:145–153.

51. Heart Outcomes Prevention Evaluation (HOPE) Study Investigators. Effects of ramipril on cardiovascular and microvascular outcomes in people with diabetes mellitus: Results of the HOPE study and MICRO-HOPE substudy, *Lancet* 2000; **355**:253–259.

52. Hansson L, Lindholm LH, Niskanen L et al for the Captopril Prevention Project (CAPP) study group. Effect of angiotensin-converting enzyme inhibition compared with conventional therapy on cardiovascular morbidity and mortality in hypertension: the Captopril Prevention Project (CAPP) randomised trial, *Lancet* 1999; **353**: 611–616.

53. Hansson L, Lindholm LH, Ekbom T et al. Randomized trial of old and new antihypertensive drugs in elderly patients: cardiovascular mortality and morbidity in the Swedish Trial in Old Patients with Hypertension-2 study, *Lancet* 1999; **354**:1755–1762.

54. Efficacy of atenolol and captopril in reducing risk of macrovascular and microvascular complications in type 2 diabetes: UKPDS 39, UK Prospective Diabetes Study Group, *BMJ* 1998; **317**:713–720.

55. Kjoller-Hansen L, Steffensen R, Grande P. The Angiotensin-converting Enzyme Inhibition Post Revascularization Study (APRES), *J Am Coll Cardiol* 2000; **35**:881–888.

56. Ribichini F, Steffenino G, Dellavalle A et al. Plasma activity and insertion/deletion polymorphism in the angiotensin I-converting enzyme: a major risk factor and marker of risk for coronary stent restenosis, *Circulation* 1998; **97**:147–154.

57. Kondo J, Sone T, Tsuboi H et al. Effect of quinapril on intimal hyperplasia after coronary stenting as assessed by intravascular ultrasound, *Am J Cardiol* 2001; **87**:443–445.

58. Powell JS, Clozel JP, Muller RK et al. Inhibitors of angiotensin-converting enzyme prevent myointimal proliferation after vascular injury, *Science* 1989; **245**:186–188.

59. Huber KC, Schwartz RS, Edwards WD et al. Effects of angiotensin-converting enzyme inhibition on neointimal proliferation in a porcine coronary injury model, *Am J Heart* 1993; **125**:695–701.

60. Multicenter European Research Trial with Cilazapril after Angioplasty to Prevent Transluminal Coronary Obstruction and Restenosis (MERCATOR) Study Group. Does the new angiotensin converting enzyme inhibitor cilazapril prevent restenosis after percutaneous transluminal coronary angioplasty? Results of the MERCATOR study: a multicenter, randomized, double-blind, placebo controlled trial, *Circulation* 1992; **86**:100–110.

61. Faxon DP for the Multicenter American Research Trial with Cilazapril After Angioplasty to Prevent Transluminal Coronary Obstruction and Restenosis (MARCATOR) Study Group. Effect of high dose angiotensin-converting enzyme inhibition on restenosis: final results of the MARCATOR study, a multicenter, randomized, double-blind, placebo controlled trial of cilazapril, *J Am Coll Cardiol* 1995; **25**:362–369.

62. Peters S, Gotting B, Trummel M et al. Valsartan for Prevention of Restenosis After Stenting of Type B2/C Lesions: The Val-PREST Trial, *J Invas Cardiol* 2001; **13**:93–97.

5

Anticoagulants in unstable angina and acute myocardial infarction

Kodangudi B Ramanathan

CONTENTS • Introduction • Anticoagulation for unstable angina • Anticoagulation in acute myocardial infarction

INTRODUCTION [1–11]

In 1912 Dr Herrick in his initial description of an acute myocardial infarction (MI) recognized the role of coronary thrombosis in its causation [1]. However, the role of anticoagulants in treating this condition has always remained controversial. Early studies favored the use of anticoagulants in the treatment of acute myocardial infarction and in 1948 the American Heart Association recommended the use of anticoagulants in acute myocardial infarction unless any definite contraindications existed [2]. However, in the 1960s the role of thrombosis itself in the causation of acute coronary syndromes came into question [3]. Confirmation was provided by the demonstration of an occlusive coronary thrombus in greater than 80% of patients with acute myocardial infarction by De Wood et al in 1980 [4].

The past decade has witnessed significant progress in our understanding of the pathogenesis of acute coronary syndrome and its relation to coronary thrombosis. The basic underlying pathology in the majority of instances is coronary atherosclerosis. Coronary atherosclerosis leads to formation of atherosclerotic plaques. The rupture of these plaques triggers coronary thrombosis and hence the development of coronary occlusion culminating in an acute myocardial infarction [5, 6]. Although plaque development leads to coronary stenosis, the relationship between the severity of stenosis and occlusive thrombus formation leading to acute myocardial infarction is not always predictable. While the development of angina appears to be related to the severity of stenosis, plaque rupture leading to acute myocardial infarction takes place among patients with only moderate coronary obstruction [7, 8].

Among the acute coronary syndromes, unstable angina represents one end of the spectrum. In this instance, a significant obstruction to coronary blood flow leads to angina at rest but without demonstrable evidence for myocardial necrosis. Q wave myocardial infarction or what used to be called transmural myocardial infarction represents the other end of the spectrum where a completed obstruction to coronary flow results in myocardial necrosis. The myocardial necrosis in most instances proceeds in a wave front pattern from the endocardium to the epicardium [9]. The non-Q wave infarct or what used to be called subendocardial infarction represents a pattern midway between these two conditions. In this situation, there is some myocardial necrosis and typically an incomplete obstruction to coronary blood flow or complete obstruction with partial protection of the myocardium by coronary collaterals [10, 11]. The role of thrombus formation varies in these three conditions but these three conditions are interchangeable and can progress from one to the other. The atherosclerotic plaque that leads to unstable angina with minimal thrombus formation and absence of myocardial necrosis can lead to either a non-Q or a Q wave myocardial infarction over time as thrombus formation stimulates further thrombus formation and progression of coronary occlusion. Since these three conditions are so closely related and distinctions are sometimes difficult to make between them, the term acute coronary syndrome has become more commonplace. However, in this chapter we will continue to maintain the traditional names since the use of anticoagulants has preceded the evolution in terminology.

ANTICOAGULATION FOR UNSTABLE ANGINA [12–37]

Unstable angina could represent varying forms of angina. It could be rest angina, post-infarction angina or it could simply be a form of angina on exertion that has changed from a stable pattern with predictable exertion to one that is no longer predictable. Irrespective of the nature of presentation, it always represents either an increase in myocardial oxygen demand and/or a decrease in supply in someone with critical coronary artery disease [12]. Although in the short-term, progression to myocardial infarction is rather uncommon, over the subsequent eight months, 57% of patients progress to either an acute coronary syndrome or angiographic total coronary occlusion [13, 14]. Since unstable angina can lead to an acute coronary syndrome with platelet aggregation and thrombus formation in a patient with atherosclerotic heart disease, the goal of treatment will be to prevent vascular occlusion. Besides

antianginal agents that either decrease myocardial oxygen demand or increase supply or both, the main focus of treatment will be to prevent platelet aggregation and clot formation. Antiplatelet agents, including the newer forms of adenosine diphosphate (ADP) antagonists and glycoprotein IIb/IIIa antagonists, are discussed elsewhere in this book. Coumarin derivatives have a limited role in the treatment of unstable angina since the syndrome has a limited time course. The syndrome either resolves with treatment or progresses to myocardial infarction with or without Q waves.

Among the antithrombin agents are heparin and direct thrombin inhibitors. For many years we have used unfractionated heparin in the treatment of various medical conditions to prevent clotting. The last few years have witnessed the development of low molecular weight heparins that require little monitoring and offer better treatment benefit in comparison to the unfractionated form. This chapter will discuss the present day use of low molecular weight heparins. Direct thrombin inhibitors include hirudin, hirulog and the newly introduced argotroban. These agents have a limited but important role in the treatment of unstable angina. Although studies have been conducted comparing antiplatelet agents such as aspirin to heparin, it is now recognized that the combination works better than either alone [15]. Heparin is useful in the first 48–72 hours. Aspirin that is started simultaneously with heparin maintains such benefit beyond that early period in all forms of acute coronary syndromes. Beyond historical reasons, further discussion on the relative superiority is not warranted and use of heparin will be assumed to be in conjunction with aspirin administration.

However, not all glycoprotein (GP) IIb/IIIa agents are used in combination with heparin. These agents are far more potent than aspirin and the benefit of their combination has to be weighed against the possibility of increased bleeding complications. The individual trials with each of the GP IIb/IIIa agents utilized a distinct schedule for heparin usage. These will be alluded to in the chapter dealing with their use. As a final note, although use of warfarin has little benefit in the acute phase of unstable angina, its use to prevent unstable angina after resolution to a stable pattern has been studied and will be alluded to. Thrombolytics have no place in the treatment of unstable angina. The trials conducted so far have yielded either a neutral or a negative advantage to patients.

Unfractionated heparin in unstable angina

Historically, earlier trials were either conducted in an unblinded fashion or using clinical trial techniques that would not stand up to the scrutiny of modern clinical trials. Paul Wood from England was one of the earliest to report the benefit of anticoagulation in unstable angina. In 1961, he reported a marked difference in morbidity as measured by the development of myocardial infarction or mortality, with the use of anticoagulants compared to placebo [16]. Similar benefits were reported by Vakil from India in 1964 [17]. Telford and Wilson reported the first randomized double-blind control trial of anticoagulants in unstable angina in 1981. They reported an 80% reduction in the incidence of myocardial infarction with the use of heparin in unstable angina [18].

Among the trials that compared the use of aspirin to heparin, Theroux et al found that the addition of aspirin to heparin conferred only a minimal benefit [19]. In the RISC trial, the investigators found that the combination of aspirin and heparin provided the greatest benefit with reduction in the event rate from 5.1 to 1.4% [20]. In comparison, use of heparin alone did not show any benefit in this study. Similarly, in the ATACS trial the most benefit was derived from the combined use of heparin and aspirin compared to aspirin alone [21]. A meta-analysis of the various trials clearly demonstrated a 56% reduction in fatal and non-fatal myocardial infarction with combined heparin and aspirin therapy [22].

Low molecular weight heparin in unstable angina

Low molecular weight heparins (LMWHs) are derived from unfractionated heparin (UFH) using chemical and enzymatic depolymerization. Compared to UFH, the LMWHs have the following beneficial features: they have greater anti-Xa to anti-IIa ratios; are less likely to be inactivated by platelet factor 4; have less non-specific binding; have greater inhibition of thrombin generation and have longer half-lives. All these features lead to more reliable anticoagulation without frequent monitoring of activated partial thromboplastin time (APPT) as with UFH [23]. Heparin-induced thrombocytopenia (HIT), a potentially lethal syndrome that leads to arterial and venous thrombosis occurs in up to 5% of patients receiving UFH. This syndrome occurs only very rarely among those on LMWH. However, the latter cannot be used as an alternative for patients developing this syndrome with UFH since LMWH cross reacts with UFH. Although many LMWH agents have been developed or are in the process of development, only a few have been tested in the acute coronary syndromes by controlled clinical trials. These agents share many common features but differ in their molecular weights and anti-Xa to anti-IIa ratios [24].

Gurfinkel and colleagues conducted the earliest trial using LMWH [25]. They used nadroparin and found this agent to be superior to aspirin alone or aspirin and UFH. This was a small trial with only 219 patients and the agents were used in an open labeled fashion. However, a larger subsequent trial (FRAXIS) using the same agent failed to show any benefit over UFH [26]. Similarly, in the FRISC trial (Fragmin during Instability in Coronary Artery Disease), dalteparin was compared to placebo in a large clinical trial of 2357 patients. There was an early reduction in death and recurrent myocardial infarction with dalteparin compared to aspirin in acute coronary syndrome (1.8% vs 4.8%) [27]. A subsequent trial comparing dalteparin and UFH (FRIC) however, failed to show any benefit for dalteparin over UFH. Death or MI occurred among 9.3% of patients treated with dalteparin compared to 7.6% of patients treated with UFH (p = ns) [28].

Although neither nadroparin nor dalteparin demonstrated greater benefit over UFH in acute coronary syndromes, enoxaparin, another LMWH, showed consistent superiority over UFH in two well-conducted large clinical trials. The ESSENCE study (Enoxaparin in Non-Q Wave Coronary Events Study) was undertaken in 3171 patients with acute coronary syndrome and enoxaparin was administered at a dose of 1 mg/kg body weight given subcutaneously twice daily [29]. The TIMI 11B trial was similarly undertaken in 3910 patients and in this study, 30 mg of enoxaparin was administered intravenously as a bolus followed by subcutaneous administration of 1 mg/kg twice daily [30]. In both studies enoxaparin was superior to UFH. In ESSENCE the combined mortality/morbidity end-point (death, MI and recurrent angina) was reduced to 16.6% by enoxaparin compared to 19.8% with UFH (p = 0.02). In TIMI 11B the combined end-point of death, MI or urgent revascularization was statistically less frequent with enoxaparin compared to UFH (14.2% vs 16.7% p = 0.03). A meta-analysis of the combined end-point in the two studies showed a statistically significant 20% reduction in any ischemic event early and late after the advent of the acute coronary syndrome [31].

The rationale for the differences between the various kinds of LMWH is unclear. It is apparent that these agents have different molecular weights and also have differing ratios of inhibition of Xa versus thrombin. However, these trials have been conducted in such a varied fashion such that it would be unfair to suggest superiority of one agent over the other without a head-to-head comparison in large clinical trials [24]. The only conclusion that could be drawn at present would be that the LWMHs are equally efficacious as UFH in the early stages of acute coronary syndrome. The choice between the two agents has to be made based upon the ease of usage of the former without frequent

laboratory tests along with a relative safety from heparin-induced thrombocytopenia. On the other hand, LMWHs are more expensive, are not beneficial long-term after discharge from the hospital and may pose a problem when administered prior to surgery since the effect cannot easily be reversed with protamine. Finally, all the above-mentioned studies were conducted under the rubric of acute coronary syndrome that includes not only unstable angina but also non-Q or non-ST elevation MI.

Direct thrombin inhibitors in unstable angina

These agents inhibit thrombin directly without requiring antithrombin III for their effect. They are not inactivated by platelet factor 4 and were expected to provide a better alternative to unfractionated heparin [23]. Unfortunately, the theoretical advantages did not translate into clinical practice. The only approved use for hirudin analogues has been to provide anticoagulation in the presence of heparin-induced thrombocytopenia [32]. Bivalirudin has also been approved as an alternative to heparin in percutaneous interventions, a situation that will be alluded to later.

Studies in acute coronary syndromes have always combined unstable angina and non-ST elevation myocardial infarctions similar to the reports with LMWHs. In GUSTO IIb, hirudin did not demonstrate any superiority over UFH. Death or MI following the use of UFH was 9.1% and with hirudin there was a non-significant reduction to 8.3%. The investigators in the Organization to Assess Strategies for Ischemic Syndromes (OASIS) conducted two trials. In the OASIS-1 pilot study the combined end-point of death, MI or refractory angina was reduced among patients receiving hirudin compared to those given UFH [34]. The second trial that included greater than 10,000 patients, however, failed to demonstrate statistically significant superiority of hirudin over UFH for the chosen end-point of death or MI. However, as in the pilot study, when refractory angina was added to the composite end-point, there was significant improvement with hirudin over UFH (5.6% vs 6.7%, $p = 0.01$) [35]. A meta-analysis of OASIS-1, OASIS-2 and GUSTO-IIb did demonstrate significant reduction in mortality risk from MI of 28% among patients treated with hirudin. Unfortunately this mortality advantage was not maintained for more than 35 days. Further, major bleeding was more common with hirudin in comparison to UFH especially among the OASIS-2 study patients [35].

The interest in hirudin, originally derived from the saliva of the medicinal leech and its analogues hirulog (bivalirudin), argatroban and inagotran peaked at a time when alternatives were being pursued for UFH because of its inconsistent effect in acute coronary syndromes. With the advent of LMWHs and IIb-IIIa platelet antagonists such enthusiasm appears to have lessened. However, trials using these agents as adjuncts to thrombolysis in ST elevation myocardial infarctions are continuing and will be discussed later.

Oral anticoagulants in unstable angina

While short-term administration of heparin (fractionated or unfractionated) or antithrombins has been useful in unstable angina and acute myocardial infarction, long-term use of these parenteral agents is neither practical nor useful in most circumstances. Further, following discontinuation of these agents, reactivation of the underlying disease process may occur [36]. Long-term anticoagulation with warfarin has been shown in some studies to be of benefit in preventing recurrences of the anginal syndrome. Williams et al have shown a 65% ($p < 0.05$) reduction in total ischemic recurrence rate following six months of treatment with oral anticoagulants [37]. In the ATACS (Antithrombotic Therapy in Acute Coronary Syndromes) trial there was a significant reduction in the composite end-point of death, MI and recurrent ischemia with oral anticoagulants. Moderate intensity prolongation of international normalized ratio (INR) between 2.0 and 2.5

resulted in the reduction of the composite end-point from 27.5 to 10.5% ($p = 0.004$) [21]. The OASIS pilot study (hirudin vs UFH) was conducted with two doses of warfarin. A small fixed dose of 3 mg of warfarin conferred no benefit but moderate prolongation of INR from 2.0 to 2.5 led to significant reduction in the need for re-hospitalization (58%, $p = 0.03$) [34]. The large subsequent OASIS-2 trial failed to show benefit among all the patients but among the centers in countries with strict adherence to protocol and maintenance of INR between 2.0 and 2.5, there appeared to be a significant benefit [32, 35].

The need for anticoagulation assumes that the unstable anginal syndrome will be treated long-term by medical therapy alone. While this might indeed have been the norm in days prior to the evolution of interventional therapy, at present, there is considerable controversy regarding the need for interventions in such patients. The role of anticoagulation, as a prelude to percutaneous intervention will be addressed later.

ANTICOAGULATION IN ACUTE MYOCARDIAL INFARCTION [38–56]

The primary role of anticoagulation in unstable angina is to prevent its progression to an acute myocardial infarction. In the completed acute myocardial infarction anticoagulation has three major goals. Although the occurrence of thrombus has been demonstrated in greater than 80% of patients with an acute transmural or Q wave myocardial infarction, existing anticoagulants cannot dissolve the preformed thrombus [4]. However, anticoagulants can prevent extension of the infarct by curtailing further thrombus formation. This will be the first or primary goal for anticoagulation.

Besides preventing extension of thrombus in the coronary artery, anticoagulants also prevent thrombus formation at the site of myocardial infarct that can lead to arterial thromboembolism. Prevention of arterial thromboembolism will be the second goal. On the venous side, immobilization imposed as a treatment for

Table 5.1 Guidelines for the use of anticoagulants in unstable angina and acute myocardial infarction

Clinical diagnosis	Agent	Recommendation
Unstable angina	Unfractionated heparin for 48 hours	Grade 1A
Unstable angina	Low molecular weight heparin for 48 hours	Grade 1A
Unstable angina	Hirudin over heparin for heparin-induced thrombocytopenia	Grade 1C
Unstable angina	Long-term warfarin therapy for intolerance to aspirin	Grade 2C
Acute myocardial infarction with ST elevation with thrombolytic therapy, rtPA, rPA, or TNK-PA	Unfractionated heparin	Grade 2A
Post-MI with high risk for systemic embolism	Warfarin therapy for 3 months	Grade 2A
Post-MI with atrial fibrillation	Long-term warfarin therapy	Grade 1A
Acute myocardial infarction: All	Low dose unfractionated heparin or low molecular weight heparin until ambulation	Grade 1A

patients with an acute MI often leads to formation of deep venous thrombosis that can lead to pulmonary emboli with attendant mortality and morbidity. Prevention of venous thrombosis will be the third goal.

Both the terminology of acute myocardial infarction and its treatment have been in a perpetual state of evolution. While discussing unstable angina, numerous studies discussed were conducted in acute coronary syndromes. Acute coronary syndrome included unstable angina and non-ST elevation myocardial infarction and these studies will not be discussed again. The role of anticoagulation has also changed with the availability of thrombolytics in ST elevation myocardial infarctions. Until recently the only widely used antiplatelet agent was aspirin. The availability of more potent agents that target the final glycoprotein IIb/IIIa pathway on the platelet has also made changes in the way that we use parenteral and oral anticoagulants. Instead of dwelling on the historical past, the focus of the discussion will be limited to what is being done at present with some pointers to what

may be happening in the near future. Table 5.1 provides general guidelines, along with the strength of evidence, for the use of anticoagulants in unstable angina and acute myocardial infarction as derived from the sixth ACCP consensus conference on antithrombotic therapy in coronary artery disease [32].

Prevention of morbidity and mortality

Most studies with anticoagulants were not large enough to make definitive statements regarding their usefulness in the treatment of acute myocardial infarction. Chalmers et al did an overview of anticoagulant trials in the pre-thrombolytic era and Collins et al did an excellent review of the anticoagulant trials in the post-thrombolytic era [38, 39]. Chalmers et al in their pooled analysis demonstrated a 21% risk reduction ($p < 0.05$) with the use of anticoagulants. Collins et al performed a more detailed analysis of various trials and their conclusion was that in the absence of aspirin and fibrinolytic therapy, heparin reduced mortality by 3.5% that was statistically significant ($p = 0.002$).

In the post-thrombolytic era, while the use of aspirin and fibrinolysis are mandated, especially in the ST elevation myocardial infarction, the role for heparin use has remained controversial. Both GISSI-2 and ISIS-3 trials failed to demonstrate survival benefit among patients receiving subcutaneous heparin post-thrombolysis [40, 41]. The GUSTO-1 trial on the other hand clearly demonstrated the superiority of alteplase and intravenous heparin over streptokinase and subcutaneous or intravenous heparin [42]. This led the ACC/AHA committee to recommend the routine use of intravenous heparin with the initiation of thrombolysis by alteplase [43]. The recommendation for alteplase is being followed when reteplase or tenecteplase (TNK/t-PA) is used as well [44]. Although streptokinase use has declined in the US, the agent is still used widely in other countries where adjunctive use of intravenous heparin may not be advantageous.

The use of LMWH has been less studied in combination with thrombolytics. Among the recent trials, the Biochemical Markers In Acute Coronary Syndrome (BIOMACS) trial studied patients receiving streptokinase. They were randomized to receive either dalteparin or placebo. Dalteparin use in comparison to placebo resulted in a non-significant increase in TIMI grade 3 flow (68% vs 52%; $p < 0.10$) [45]. In the Heparin Aspirin Reperfusion Trial (HART-2), patients receiving tissue plasminogen activator (t-PA) were randomized to receive either enoxaparin or UFH. In this study again there was a trend towards better TIMI grade 3 flow among patients receiving enoxaparin [46]. Finally, in the Assessment of the Safety and Efficacy of a New Thrombolytic agent trial (ASSENT PLUS) dalteparin is being compared to UFH among patients receiving recombinant tissue-plasminogen activator (rt-PA). Preliminary results seem to indicate greater TIMI 3 flow with dalteparin [47]. In spite of all these preliminary data, there is at present no consensus on the use of LMWH in combination with fibrinolytic agents in the treatment of acute myocardial infarction.

The antithrombins have had a checkered history in the treatment of ST elevation MI in combination with thrombolytics. The earlier trials TIMI-9A, HIT-3 and GUSTO-IIA were abandoned due to excessive bleeding caused by the high dose of hirudin used [24]. Even with reduction in the dose of hirudin, the TIMI-9B trial failed to show any significant benefit for hirudin over heparin in ST elevation MI treated with thrombolysis [48]. GUSTO-IIB and HIT-4 similarly failed to demonstrate significant reduction in 30-day mortality with hirudin compared to heparin among patients treated with thrombolytics [33, 49].

Bivalirudin is being compared to heparin in a large trial of 17,000 patients with ST elevation myocardial infarction receiving streptokinase for thrombolysis. The result of this HERO-2 trial is awaited [24].

Prevention of systemic embolization

Systemic embolization especially in acute myocardial infarction leads to a stroke that can be catastrophic. The thrombus tends to form at the infarct site in the left ventricle and is more common in an anterior infarct than in an inferior infarct. The risk factors include the size of infarction, nature of wall motion abnormality, the presence of congestive heart failure and occurrence of atrial fibrillation. The presence of akinesis or dyskinesis favors thrombus formation and a large dyskinetic area in the anterior wall leads to formation of thrombus in up to 40% of patients [32].

The risk of stroke is between 1–3% following all myocardial infarctions and this almost doubles among patients with anterior myocardial infarction (2–6%). Most systemic emboli occur within a few days following myocardial infarction. However, in the presence of poor left ventricular function, systemic emboli can occur much later [32].

Randomized and non-randomized trials, both

large and small have demonstrated reduction in systemic embolization and thrombus formation with anticoagulation. An overview of four relatively major trials demonstrated a marked reduction in mural thrombus formation with an odds ratio of 0.32 [50].

Thrombolytics may have decreased the incidence of systemic embolization by reducing the incidence of atrial fibrillation that is one of the major risk factors for thrombus formation in the left atrium. Konty et al evaluated the low molecular weight heparin, dalteparin, in a study of prevention of arterial thromboembolism following acute myocardial infarction. The use of dalteparin along with aspirin and thrombolytics was associated with less thrombus formation but hemorrhagic complications were more frequent among those that received the LMWH [51].

Finally, left ventricular aneurysm formation is frequently associated with clot formation but embolic complication in this condition is infrequent. At present even in the presence of a clot in a chronic LV aneurysm, anticoagulation cannot be routinely recommended.

Anticoagulation for venous thromboembolism

In the past when patients with myocardial infarction were immobilized for a long period of time, the occurrence of venous thrombosis leading to pulmonary embolization was a dreaded complication. With the advent of thrombolytics along with routine use of aspirin, the incidence of venous thrombosis and pulmonary embolus formation has become less frequent. In the pre-thrombolytic era, use of heparin was associated with a 50% reduction in the incidence of pulmonary emboli post-MI. However, in the present thrombolytic era, the beneficial effects of heparin, either low dose or high dose, for prevention of pulmonary embolism is debatable. Some of the changes such as earlier mobilization, percutaneous intervention and use of IIb/IIIa agents ought to have had some role in the prevention of venous

thrombosis that leads to pulmonary embolization [32].

Anticoagulation for percutaneous intervention during acute myocardial infarction

Anticoagulation has always remained an integral part of any percutaneous intervention (PCI) since its original description by Gruntzig in 1977 [52]. However, the role of PCI in the treatment of acute myocardial infarction has been controversial. In the ST elevation myocardial infarction, its role as an adjunctive modality to thrombolysis was abandoned after some major trials showed increased mortality with that approach [53]. However, primary angioplasty as an alternative to thrombolysis is becoming increasingly popular among major institutions that are geared to reperfuse acutely ischemic and infracting myocardium rapidly and adequately [54]. It does appear that this approach might be associated with a superior outcome in these institutions. The use of heparin in these instances is mandated both for the treatment of myocardial infarction and to assist in the performance of percutaneous intervention. Unfractionated heparin has in general been used in these instances to maintain an activated clotting time (ACT) of around 300.

The use of low molecular weight heparin as an alternative to UFH in percutaneous intervention in acute myocardial infarction has been less well studied. Part of the problem is that activated clotting time that determines the level of anticoagulation during PCI can no longer be used with LMWH. The only reliable way to measure the level of anticoagulation is to perform anti-Xa levels. The methodology is not available in all the laboratories and may be time consuming and expensive. Furthermore, the reference levels for adequate anticoagulation are unclear.

ACUTE II investigators studied the use of enoxaparin among 525 patients with acute coronary syndrome. They continued enoxaparin until the time for percutaneous intervention and switched to UFH at the time of intervention. They reported slight reduction in rehospitalization and revascularization with the use of LMWH [46]. The FRISC-2 study was undertaken with the use of dalteparin in patients with acute coronary syndrome. Patients were given dalteparin for 5–6 days and randomized to either conservative management or interventional therapy, surgical or percutaneous. This study demonstrated superior benefit with intervention compared to conservative management. From the anticoagulation standpoint it might be that therapy with LMWH provided the necessary cooling off period required before intervention, surgical or percutaneous, could be safely carried out in patients with unstable coronary syndromes [55].

Among antithrombins, Bittl et al studied bivalirudin in patients with unstable angina undergoing angioplasty. They demonstrated decreased bleeding complications with bivalirudin compared to heparin but there was no significant difference in the composite endpoint of death, myocardial infarction or abrupt vessel closure when compared to heparin [56].

REFERENCES

1. Herrick JB. Clinical features of sudden obstruction of the coronary arteries, *JAMA* 1912; **59**:2015–2020.
2. Wright IS, Marple CD, Beck DF. Report of the committee for the evaluation of anticoagulants in the treatment of coronary thrombosis with myocardial infarction, *Am Heart J* 1948; **36**: 801–815.
3. Chapman I. The cause-effect relationship between recent coronary artery occlusion and acute myocardial infarction, *Am Heart J* 1974; **87**:267–271.
4. DeWood MA, Spores J, Notske R et al. Prevalence of total coronary occlusion during the early hours of transmural myocardial infarction, *N Engl J Med* 1980;**303**:897–902.
5. Davies MJ, Thomas AC. Plaque fissuring—the cause of acute myocardial infarction, sudden ischemic death and crescendo angina, *Br Heart J* 1985; **53**:363.
6. Davies MJ, Bland MJ, Hangartner WR et al. Factors influencing the presence or absence of acute coronary thrombi in sudden ischemic death, *Eur Heart J* 1989; **2**:941–944.
7. Ambrose J, Tannenbaum M, Alexopoulos D et al. Angiographic progression of coronary artery disease and the development of myocardial infarction, *J Am Coll Cardiol* 1988; **12**:56–62.
8. Little WC, Constantinescu M, Applegate RJ et al. Can coronary angiography predict the site of a subsequent myocardial infarction in patients with mild-to-moderate coronary artery disease, *Circulation* 1988; **78**:1157–1166.
9. Reimer KA, Jennings RB. The 'wavefront phenomenon' of myocardial ischemic cell death. II. Transmural progression of necrosis within the framework of ischemic bed size (myocardium at risk) and collateral flow, *Lab Invest* 1979; **40**:633.
10. Keen WD, Savage MP, Fischman DL et al. Comparison of coronary angiographic findings during the first 6 hours non-Q wave and Q wave myocardial infarction, *Am J Cardiol* 1994; **74**:324.
11. Christian TF, Gibbons RJ, Clements IP et al. Estimates of myocardium at risk and collateral flow in acute myocardial infarction using electrocardiographic indexes with comparison to radionuclide and angiographic measures, *J Am Coll Cardiol* 1995; **26**:388.
12. Moise A, Theroux P, Taeymans Y et al. Unstable angina and progression of coronary atherosclerosis, *N Engl J Med* 1983; **309**:685.
13. Kaski JC, Chester MR, Chen L et al. Progression of coronary disease in patients with unstable angina pectoris. The role of complex stenosis morphology, *Circulation* 1995; **92**:2058.
14. Chester M, Chen L, Kaski JC. Identification of patients at high risk for adverse coronary events while awaiting routine coronary angioplasty, *Br Heart J* 1995; **73**:216–222.
15. Holdright D, Patel D, Cunningham D et al. Comparison of the effect of heparin and aspirin versus aspirin alone on transient myocardial ischemia and in-hospital prognosis in patients with unstable angina, *J Am Coll Cardiol* 1994; **24**:39.
16. Wood P. Acute and sub-acute coronary insufficiency, *BMJ* 1961; **1**:1779–1782.
17. Vakil RJ. Preinfarction syndrome-management and follow-up, *Am J Cardiol* 1964; **14**:55–63.
18. Telford AM, Wilson C. Trial of heparin versus

atenolol in prevention of myocardial infarction in intermediate coronary syndrome, *Lancet* 1981; **1**:1225–1228.

19. Theroux P, Ouimet H, McCans J et al. Aspirin, heparin or both to treat acute unstable angina, *N Engl J Med* 1988; **319**:1105–1111.

20. The RISC group. Risk of myocardial infarction and death during treatment with low-dose aspirin and intravenous heparin in men with unstable coronary artery disease, *Lancet* 1990; **336**:827–830.

21. Cohen M, Adams PC, Parry G et al. Combination antithrombotic therapy in unstable rest angina and non-Q wave infarction in nonoption aspirin users: primary end point analysis from the ATACS trial, *Circulation* 1994; **89**:81–88.

22. Cairns JA, Lewis HD Jr, Meade TW et al. Antithrombotic agents in coronary artery disease, *Chest* 1995; **108**:380S–400S.

23. Miller WL, Reeder GS. Adjunctive therapies in the treatment of acute coronary syndromes, *Mayo Clin Proc* 2001; **76**:391–405.

24. Antman EM. The search for replacements for unfractionated heparin, *Circulation* 2001; **103**:2310–2314.

25. Gurfinkel EP, Eustaquio EJ, Mejail RI et al. Low molecular weight heparin vs regular heparin or aspirin in the treatment of unstable angina and silent ischemia, *J Am Coll Cardiol* 1995; **26**: 313–318.

26. The FRAXIS study group. Comparison of two treatment durations (6 days and 14 days) of a low molecular weight heparin in the initial management of unstable angina or non-Q wave myocardial infarction: FRAXIX (FRAxiparine in ischemic syndrome), *Eur Heart J* 1999; **20**: 1553–1562.

27. FRISC study group. Low molecular weight heparin (Fragmin) during instability in coronary artery disease (FRISC), *Lancet* 1996; **347**:561–568.

28. Klein W, Buchwald A, Hillis WS et al. Comparison of low molecular weight heparin with unfractionated heparin acutely and with placebo for six weeks in the management of unstable coronary artery disease. Fragmin in Unstable Coronary Artery Disease Study (FRIC), *Circulation* 1997; **97**:61–68.

29. Cohen M, Demers C, Gurfinkel EP et al. A comparison of low molecular weight heparin with unfractionated heparin for unstable coronary artery disease. Efficacy and Safety of Subcutaneous Enoxaparin in Non-Q Wave Coronary Events Study Group, *N Engl J Med* 1997; **337**:447–452.

30. Antman EM, McCabe CH, Gurfinkel EP et al. Enoxaparin prevents death and cardiac ischemic events in unstable angina/non-Q wave myocardial infarction: results of the Thrombolysis in Myocardial Infarction (TIMI) 11B trial, *Circulation* 1999; **100**:1593–1601.

31. Antman EM, Cohen M, Radley D et al. Assessment of the treatment effect of enoxaparin for unstable angina/non-Q wave myocardial infarction. TIMI 11B-ESSENCE meta-analysis, *Circulation* 1999; **100**:1602–1608.

32. Cairns JA, Theroux P, Lewis JD et al. Antithrombotic agents in coronary artery disease, *Chest* 2001; **119**:228S–252S.

33. Global Use of Strategies to Open Occluded Coronary Arteries (GUSTO) IIb investigators. A comparison of recombinant hirudin with heparin for the treatment of acute coronary syndromes, *N Engl J Med* 1996; **335**:775–782.

34. Organization to Assess Strategies for Ischemic Syndromes (OASIS) Investigators. Comparison of the effects of two doses of recombinant hirudin compared with heparin in patients with acute myocardial ischemia without ST elevation: a randomized trial, *Circulation* 1997; **96**:769–777.

35. Organization to Assess Strategies for Ischemic Syndromes (OASIS-2) Investigators. Effects of recombinant hirudin (lepirudin) compared with heparin of death, myocardial infarction, refractory angina, and revascularisation procedures in patients with acute myocardial ischemia without ST elevation: a randomized trial, *Lancet* 1999; **353**:429–438.

36. Theroux P, Waters D, Lam J et al. Reactivation of unstable angina following discontinuation of heparin, *N Engl J Med* 1992; **327**:141–145.

37. Williams DO, Kirby MG, McPherson K et al. Anticoagulant treatment in unstable angina, *Br J Clin Pract* 1986; **40**:114–116.

38. Chalmers TC, Matta RJ, Smith J Jr et al. Evidence favoring the use of anticoagulants in the hospital phase of acute myocardial infarction, *N Engl J Med* 1977; **297**:1091–1096.

39. Collins R, MacMahon S, Flather M et al. Clinical effects of anticoagulant therapy in suspected acute myocardial infarction: systematic overview of randomized trials, *BMJ* 1996; **313**:652–659.

40. The International Study Group. In-hospital mor-

tality and clinical course of 20,891 patients with suspected acute myocardial infarction randomized between alteplase and streptokinase with or without heparin, *Lancet* 1990; **336**:71–73.

41. ISIS-3 Collaborative Group. ISIS-3: a randomized comparison streptokinase vs tissue plasminogen activator vs anistreplase and of aspirin plus heparin vs aspirin alone among 41,299 cases of suspected acute myocardial infarction, *Lancet* 1992; **339**:753–770.

42. GUSTO investigators. An international randomized trial comparing four thrombolytic strategies for acute myocardial infarction, *N Engl J Med* 1993; **329**:673–682.

43. Ryan TJ, Antman EM, Brooks NH et al. 1999 update: ACC/AHA guidelines for the management of patients with acute myocardial infarction: a report of the American College of Cardiology/American Heart Association Task Force on Practice Guidelines (Committee on Management of Acute Myocardial Infarction), *J Am Coll Cardiol* 1999; **34**:890–911.

44. Levine GN, Ali MN, Schafer AI. Antithrombotic therapy in patients with acute coronary syndromes, *Arch Intern Med* 2001; **161**:937–948.

45. Frostfeldt G, Ahlberg G, Gustafsson G et al. Low molecular weight heparin (dalteparin) as adjuvant treatment of thrombolysis in acute myocardial infarction: a pilot study. Biochemical markers in acute coronary syndromes (BIO-MACS II), *J Am Coll Cardiol* 1999; **33**: 627–633.

46. Aguilar OM, Kleiman NS. Low molecular-weight heparins, *J Inv Cardiol* 2001; **13**:3A–7A.

47. Chesebro JH, Verheugt FW. Introduction. Expanding the horizon in unstable coronary artery disease, *Clin Cardiol* 2000; **23** (suppl 1): I1–I3.

48. Antman EM for the TIMI 9B investigators. Hirudin in acute myocardial infarction: Thrombolysis and Thrombin Inhibition in Myocardial Infarction (TIMI) 9B trial, *Circulation* 1996; **94**:911–921.

49. Neuhaus KL, Molhoek GP, Zeymer U et al. Recombinant hirudin (lepirudin) for the improvement of thrombolysis with streptokinase in patients with acute myocardial infarction: results of the HIT-4 trial, *J Am Coll Cardiol* 1999; **34**:966–973.

50. Vaitkus PT, Barnathau ES. Embolic potential prevention and management of mural thrombus complicating anterior myocardial infarction: a meta-analysis, *J Am Coll Cardiol* 1993; **22**:100–109.

51. Kontny F, Dale J, Abildgaard U et al. Randomized trial of low molecular weight heparin (dalteparin) in prevention of left ventricular thrombus formation and arterial embolism after acute anterior myocardial infarction. The Fragmin in Acute Myocardial Infarction (FRAMI) study, *J Am Coll Cardiol* 1997; **30**: 962–969.

52. Hurst JW. The first coronary angioplasty as described by Andreas Gruentzig, *Am J Cardiol* 1986; **57**:185–186.

53. Simoons ML, Betriu A, Col J et al. Thrombolysis with tissue plasminogen activator in acute myocardial infarction: no additional benefit from immediate percutaneous coronary angioplasty, *Lancet* 1988; **1**:197.

54. Grines CL, Browne KF, Marco J et al. A comparison of immediate angioplasty with thrombolytic therapy for acute myocardial infarction, *N Engl J Med* 1993; **328**:673.

55. Long-term low molecular mass heparin in unstable coronary artery disease: FRISC II prospective randomized multicentre study. FRagmin and Fast Revascularization during InStability in Coronary artery disease. Investigators, *Lancet* 1999; **354**:701–707.

56. Bittl JA, Strony J, Brinker JA et al. Treatment with bivalirudin (hirulog) as compared with heparin during coronary angioplasty for unstable or post-infarction angina: Hirulog Angioplasty Study Investigators, *N Engl J Med* 1995; **333**:764–769.

6

Antiplatelet therapy

H Daniel Lewis Jr

CONTENTS • Introduction • Aspirin therapy • Thienpyridine therapy • Glycoprotein IIb/IIIa antagonist therapy • Risk factors • Summary

INTRODUCTION [1–14]

Approximately 2.5 million patients with acute coronary syndrome (ACS) are admitted to hospitals in the US each year. This includes about 1.5 million patients with unstable angina and about one million with acute ST-segment elevation myocardial infarction (MI) and acute non ST-segment elevation myocardial infarction (NSTEMI) [1].

Management of unstable angina (UA) is based on the principle of more aggressive therapy for the patients at higher risk. Therapy associated with greater adverse effects is weighed against greater benefit in the higher risk patient. Greater benefit for the higher risk patient has been shown for surgical, percutaneous interventional, and medical therapy. Therefore risk assessment is fundamental in the management of medical therapy. Unstable angina cannot be distinguished from NSTEMI initially. Since early therapy is critical, these two entities are considered together as acute coronary syndrome (ACS), and risk is assessed based on clinical, electrocardiographic (ECG), and enzymatic features [2]. Troponin positivity [3], even at low levels, and TIMI-risk score [4], incorporating ST-segment deviations, recent or prolonged chest pain, age, and other independent risk factors, as well as enzyme elevations,

have been shown to be predictive of better outcome with more aggressive therapy: early invasive strategy [5, 6], low molecular weight heparin (LMWH) [7], and glycoprotein (GP) IIb/IIIa receptor inhibitors [8, 9]. Troponin positivity cannot be taken out of context; it is valuable only in the setting of an acute ischemic event. The features most predictive of higher risk are prolonged or recurrent chest pain, ST-segment deviation, and positive troponin. Higher troponin is more predictive, as is greater ST-segment deviation. New data suggests that C-reactive protein is another important risk factor [10, 11].

All of the acute coronary events: unstable angina, NSTEMI, ST-segment elevation myocardial infarction, and sudden death, are characteristically caused by a ruptured atherosclerotic plaque leading to platelet aggregation and subsequent fibrin thrombus formation, and/or platelet emboli to distal arterioles [12–14]. The specific clinical event is related to the degree and duration of obstruction of coronary arterial flow. Hence, antiplatelet therapy is the cornerstone of medical therapy for unstable angina and the other acute coronary events. Anti-ischemic therapy with beta blockers, nitrates, blood pressure control, statin therapy, and avoidance of smoking are of great importance as well.

ASPIRIN THERAPY [15–22]

Aspirin has been the mainstay of antiplatelet therapy for unstable angina since the Veterans Administration Cooperative Study in 1983 first proved that aspirin can prevent myocardial infarction [15]. That randomized clinical trial showed that 324 mg per day of aspirin for 12 weeks in patients with unstable angina was associated with a 51% reduction in MI ($p = 0.001$), and suggested a 51% reduction in mortality ($p = 0.054$). The Canadian Cooperative Study in 1985 showed very similar results with aspirin 300 mg four times a day in patients with unstable angina [16]. It confirmed increased survival, showed the benefit in women as well as men, and showed that sulfinpyrazone was not effective.

Théroux in 1988 and 1992 confirmed the benefit of aspirin in patients with unstable angina, demonstrated that heparin was even more effective than aspirin, and that the effects are additive to those of aspirin [17, 18]. Théroux also showed that aspirin is required to prevent rebound myocardial infarction when heparin is discontinued. In 1990 RISC demonstrated the benefit of aspirin in even lower dosage, 75 mg daily [19]. A meta-analysis of all the randomized trials of heparin plus aspirin compared to aspirin alone showed a relative risk reduction of 52%, and when the low molecular weight heparin trials are included a risk reduction of 62% [20].

The randomized clinical trial is the most reliable (unbiased) method of determining the value of a therapy. In the case of aspirin therapy in coronary artery disease a vast amount of evidence has been collected. The Antiplatelet Trialists Collaboration was a meta-analysis of 145 randomized trials of prolonged antiplatelet therapy vs control in 70,000 high-risk patients with primary occlusive disease and 30,000 subjects from the general population [21]. It showed no differences in effectiveness of aspirin therapy with increasing dosage from 75 to 3000 mg per day. It did show proportionately increased adverse events, particularly gastrointestinal bleeding, with higher dosages. The meta-analysis also showed the benefit of chronic aspirin therapy in high-risk patients reducing vascular events by about one fourth, non-fatal MI by one third, non-fatal stroke by one third, and vascular death by one sixth ($2p < 0.0001$).

ISIS-2 showed decreased mortality and decreased recurrent myocardial infarction with acute aspirin therapy, 160 mg per day, in patients with acute myocardial infarction [22]. It showed the benefit, a 21% decrease in myocardial infarction, to be of similar magnitude to that of fibrinolytic therapy, and it showed aspirin to have additive benefit in combination therapy. It also showed that aspirin is necessary to prevent a rebound increase in recurrent myocardial infarction with streptokinase therapy.

Since the aspirin preparation in ISIS-2 was enteric coated, the initial dose was taken immediately and chewed. We also know that chewed aspirin is more rapidly absorbed buccally (P. Sleight, personal communication). Although 80 mg is adequate for a daily dose, 160 to 325 mg is preferable for the first dose to assure reaching an adequate initial serum level plateau.

Aspirin causes irreversible inhibition of platelet cyclooxygenase by acetylation suppressing the synthesis of thromboxane A_2, a platelet aggregant and potent vasoconstrictor. Platelet aggregation inhibition is therefore related to the life of the platelet and lasts 3–7 days. Aspirin does not inhibit platelet aggregation by any other pathway. Because an antiplatelet drug that works by a different mechanism, blocking a different pathway, may have more potent or additive effects, a search for new antiplatelet agents has been a priority. Sulfinpyrazone was shown by the Canadian Cooperative Study not to be effective in unstable angina [16] and dipyridamole has never demonstrated a clear beneficial effect greater than aspirin, or in addition to aspirin, in clinical trials involving patients with coronary artery disease.

THIENPYRIDINE THERAPY [23–29]

Ticlopidine, a thienpyridine, inhibits adenosine diphosphate (ADP)-induced platelet aggregation. A randomized, placebo-controlled clinical trial in patients with unstable angina showed ticlopidine to reduce death or non-fatal MI by 46.3% [23]. It is associated with less gastrointestinal bleeding than aspirin. The disadvantages are several days' delay in optimal beneficial clinical effect, higher cost, frequent gastrointestinal side-effects, occasional rash, and rare neutropenia, thrombocytopenia, and liver function abnormalities. Ticlopidine has not been shown to have clinical benefits in addition to aspirin in patients with coronary artery disease except in association with percutaneous intervention [24].

Because of the infrequent, but serious adverse effects of ticlopidine, another thienpyridine, clopidogrel, was evaluated in 19,185 patients with recent ischemic stroke, recent MI, or symptomatic peripheral vascular disease in the Clopidogrel versus Aspirin in Patients at Risk of Ischemic Events (CAPRIE) trial [25]. The composite end-point of vascular death, MI, or ischemic stroke was 5.32% with clopidogrel and 5.83% with aspirin, a relative risk reduction of 8.7% ($p = 0.043$) in favor of clopidogrel. There was slightly more bleeding in the aspirin-treated patients, slightly more rash and diarrhea in the clopidogrel-treated patients, and no excess of neutropenia or thrombocytopenia. Consequently, clopidogrel is recommended for patients with unstable angina who have contraindications for aspirin therapy.

Studies have also compared clopidogrel with ticlopidine for percutaneous coronary intervention (PCI) with stent placement. Comparable efficacy and a better safety profile have led to utilization of clopidogrel in addition to aspirin for coronary stent procedures [26, 27].

The Clopidogrel in Unstable angina to prevent Recurrent ischemic Events: CURE (OASIS-4) trial was reported at the 50th Annual Scientific Session of the American College of Cardiology March 19, 2001 [28, 29]. It evaluated 12,562 patients with ACS (75% unstable angina and 25% NSTEMI) randomly assigned to clopidogrel 300 mg oral load and 75 mg oral daily vs placebo in addition to usual therapy. Approximately 99% of the patients received aspirin, 46% iv heparin, and 56% LMWH. There were 3737 primary coronary events (cardiovascular death, MI, or stroke), 11.47% in placebo-treated and 9.28% in clopidogrel-treated patients, relative risk (RR), 0.80, $p = 0.00005$. Cardiovascular death RR was 0.92 and MI RR 0.73. Major, non-life-threatening bleeding was increased from 2.7% to 3.6%, RR 1.36, $p = 0.003$. Refractory ischemia was reduced by about a sixth. The effect of clopidogrel was additive to the effect of aspirin. If 1000 patients with non ST-segment elevation acute coronary syndrome are treated with clopidogrel for nine months you could expect to prevent 28 major events in 23 patients at a cost of three major non-life-threatening bleeds. After peer review and publication of CURE, clopidogrel in addition to aspirin may become the standard treatment for patients with non ST-segment elevation acute coronary syndrome.

GLYCOPROTEIN IIB/IIIA ANTAGONIST THERAPY [30–46]

Glycoprotein IIb/IIIa receptor activation on the surface of platelets increases its affinity for binding to fibrinogen and von Willebrand factor resulting in cross-linking and platelet aggregation [30]. This is the final common pathway for platelet aggregation regardless of the stimulus or pathway. Consequently the GP IIb/IIIa receptor antagonists are the most potent platelet aggregation inhibitors. Various GP IIb/IIIa antagonists have different pharmacokinetic and pharmacodynamic properties that significantly affect their clinical features and usefulness.

Abciximab (Reopro) is a large Fab fragment of murine-human chimeric antibody that has a short plasma half-life but a strong affinity for the receptor thereby affecting platelet aggregation for 24–48 hours. It is not specific for the receptor, and can affect other receptors on other cells. The small synthetic molecules, eptifibatide (Integrilin), a peptide, and tirofiban (Aggrastat), a non-peptide, are both highly specific GP IIb/IIIa receptor blockers in equilibrium with plasma levels and having a half-life of 2–3 hours. Platelet aggregation is inhibited for 4–8 hours. All three drugs are given by intravenous infusion.

Abciximab has been evaluated in a number of trials involving percutaneous coronary intervention. Many of the patients had unstable angina. Abciximab has been very effective in preventing the complications of the interventions, and in reducing death or MI in several of the trials. The combined results of EPIC, EPISTENT and EPILOG showed a 20% reduction in mortality over the long-term in the patients randomly assigned to abciximab [31–34]. The CAPTURE trial entered patients with refractory unstable angina scheduled for angioplasty in 20–24 hours with abciximab continued for one hour after the procedure [35]. Death, MI, or urgent revascularization at 30 days was reduced from 15.9% to 11.3% with abciximab (RR 0.71, $p = 0.012$). Death or MI was reduced 47%, $p = 0.003$. Abciximab is approved by the FDA for the treatment of UA/NSTEMI with PCI or when PCI is planned within 24 hours. Because of its longer duration of action, abciximab is less desirable in patients who may need coronary artery bypass grafts (CABG).

Tirofiban was evaluated in patients with UA/NSTEMI in the PRISM and PRISM-PLUS trials [36, 37]. In PRISM at the end of the 48-hour infusion, death, MI, or refractory ischemia was reduced from 5.6% with unfractionated heparin to 3.8% with tirofiban (RR 0.67, $p = 0.01$). At 30 days there was a trend in favor of tirofiban. In PRISM-PLUS the tirofiban alone arm was dropped because of excess mortality. Death, MI or refractory ischemia at seven days was reduced from 17.9% in the unfractionated heparin group to 12.9% in the tirofiban plus unfractionated heparin (RR 0.68, $p = 0.004$), and was still significantly reduced at

30 days and six months. Death or MI at 30 days was reduced by 30%, $p = 0.03$. Tirofiban has been approved for the treatment of ACS managed medically as well as with percutaneous coronary intervention (PCI). It is usually administered with aspirin and heparin.

Eptifibatide was evaluated in UA/NSTEMI patients in the PURSUIT trial [38]. The infusion would last for 72 hours or up to 96 hours if PCI was performed. Death or MI at 96 hours was reduced from 9.1% to 7.6% by eptifibatide (RR 0.84, $p = 0.01$), and from 15.7% to 14.2% (RR 0.91, $p = 0.042$) at 30 days. Eptifibatide is also approved for ACS (UA/NSTEMI) with or without PCI.

Boersma and colleagues analyzed data from the CAPTURE, PURSUIT, and PRISM-PLUS randomized trials of abciximab, eptifibatide, and tirofiban therapy, respectively, in ACS patients before a possible PCI [39]. During the infusions and before PCI the three trials showed a 2.5% rate of death or non-fatal MI in the GP IIb/IIIa inhibitor group ($N = 6125$) vs 3.8% in the placebo group ($N = 6171$), a 34% relative reduction ($p < 0.001$). In the 48 hours after a PCI was performed in 1358 patients assigned GP IIb/IIIa inhibition, the event rate was 4.9% vs 8.0% in the 1396 placebo patients, a 41% reduction, $p < 0.001$). There was no further benefit or worsening subsequent to 48 hours after PCI. This was considered conclusive evidence of the benefits of GP IIb/IIIa inhibitors for patients with ACS, as well as for adjunctive therapy with PCI.

The GUSTO-IV ACS trial of 7600 patients with ACS presented at the European Cardiology Society meeting in September 2000 cast doubt on the validity of the above data [40, 41]. There was no improvement in MI, death, or revascularization with abciximab 24-hour or 48-hour infusions over placebo in relatively low-risk patients with ACS who did not have PCI. This data does not support the use of abciximab in patients with ACS if they do not have percutaneous intervention.

The reason for the disparity from earlier data is not known. Possibilities include: (1) that these lower-risk patients do not derive benefit; (2) that the results are drug specific and that abciximab does not keep adequate levels of inhibition of platelet aggregation during infusion and may even stimulate platelet aggregation; (3) that prior studies were misleading; and (4) that the present study is flawed. GUSTO-IV ACS awaits peer review and publication. At present it is not clear that abciximab, or perhaps GP IIb/IIIa inhibitors, are indicated in patients with ACS, unless they are having PCI.

The TARGET trial, the first direct comparison of two GP IIb/IIIa inhibitors, was presented at the 73rd Scientific Sessions of the American Heart Association in November 2000 [42]. The 4812 patients undergoing primary coronary stenting, and pretreated with clopidogrel and heparin, were randomly assigned to abciximab or tirofiban. The combined incidence of death, non-fatal MI, or urgent repeat cardiac procedures at 30 days was 20% lower in the abciximab-treated patients compared with the tirofiban-treated patients (6.01% vs 7.55%, $p = 0.037$). Although the reason for the difference in beneficial effects is not known, abciximab's non-specificity for the receptor, allowing additional effects such as binding to the Mac1 receptor on monocytes, has been suggested. There was a higher rate of minor bleeding with abciximab (5.6% vs 3.5%, $p = 0.008$), but no significant difference in major bleeding.

The oral IIb/IIIa inhibitors have been evaluated in several clinical trials for longer duration therapy after acute coronary syndrome with or without percutaneous coronary intervention. They have not been shown to be beneficial in these clinical trials [43–45] and although the reason for the disappointing results is not yet known, inadequate maintenance of plasma levels has been suggested.

TACTICS-TIMI 18, presented at the 73rd Scientific Sessions of the American Heart Association in November 2000, was a trial of early invasive versus early conservative strategy [46]. Patients with ACS (UA/NSTEMI) ($N = 2220$) were randomly assigned to cardiac catheterization and usually PCI in 4–48 hours vs only medical treatment unless they met pre-specified clinical criteria that would lead to intervention. All patients received aspirin, heparin, and tirofiban. The early invasive strategy led to decreased incidence of death, MI, or re-hospitalization for worsening chest pain at six months (15.9% vs 19.4% OR 0.78, $p = 0.025$) and decreased rate of death or MI at 6 months (7.3% vs 9.5%, OR 0.74, $p < 0.05$). The use of the GP IIb/IIIa inhibitors is thought to have improved the success of the procedures, making the invasive strategy better.

RISK FACTORS [4, 6, 47–49]

The TACTICS-TIMI 18 troponin sub-study showed even greater benefit of the early invasive strategy in patients with positive troponin at 0.1 mg/dl and at 0.01 mg/dl [6]. Death as well as MI were statistically significantly reduced at 30 days in these patients, but there was no clear benefit in patients with negative troponin. The conclusion from evaluation of 7600 patients from the GUSTO-IV study was that with the third generation improved precision troponin T-test 0.03 mg/L is the most appropriate cut-off level for high and low risk ACS patients [47]. In PARAGON B the treatment effects of GP IIb/IIIa inhibitors were most pronounced in, and limited to, the troponin positive patients [48].

The TIMI risk score was developed from patients in TIMI IIb [4]. When applied to 1915 patients with UA/NSTEMI in PRISM-PLUS there was increased benefit with tirofiban reducing the composite end-point of death, MI, or refractory ischemia at 30 days in patients with increased risk score 4–7 and particularly 5–7 [9]. In OPUS/TIMI 16 the TIMI risk score showed additional predictive power over troponin alone [49]. In TIMI 18, the TIMI risk score predicted the patients who would benefit from LMWH.

SUMMARY

Because the distinction cannot be made initially, patients with unstable angina should be grouped together with NSTEMI as ACS. Risk assessment is fundamental in the management of these patients because higher risk is associated with greater improvement with more aggressive treatments. This is true not only for early invasive strategy, but also with addition of LMWH and with addition of GP IIb/IIIa inhibitors. The best prognostic indicators are troponin positivity even at a low level, dynamic ST-segment deviations, and clinical characteristics including recent prolonged or recurrent chest pain, age, and left ventricular dysfunction, which are independent prognostic indicators.

All patients with unstable angina and NSTEMI should be treated immediately with aspirin and heparin, which have been shown clearly to reduce MI and death rates. After appropriate peer review of the CURE trial it may be that all patients with ACS should be treated with clopidogrel in addition. However, because of increased bleeding risk the question regarding duration of treatment remains. Long-term combination antiplatelet therapy may be most beneficial in patients at high risk, including those with end-stage coronary artery disease, diffuse disease in more than one vascular bed, or poor left ventricular function.

All patients with ACS who are having PCI should be treated with clopidogrel in addition to aspirin, and with a GP IIb/IIIa inhibitor. After the TARGET trial has been reviewed and been published, abciximab may be preferable. When PCI is not planned the data does not clearly support the use of abciximab. The small molecule GP IIb/IIIa inhibitors tirofiban and eptifibatide are the only ones approved for ACS without PCI. They should probably be used only with high-risk patients, perhaps only if ischemia is refractory and intervention is not an option. The oral GP IIb/IIIa inhibitors have not been shown to be efficacious for longer-term therapy.

Patients with possible ACS should be risk assessed in the emergency department with low-risk patients having stress tests before discharge, or being sent home on aspirin for further non-invasive testing to confirm the diagnosis and for risk factor and anti-ischemic management. High-risk patients should be admitted to the hospital on aggressive antithrombotic therapy (aspirin, heparin, clopidogrel, and a GP IIb/IIIa inhibitor) and anti-ischemic therapy for early invasive management. The use of LMWH depends on the comfort of the operator with management in the catheterization laboratory with intervention. Intermediate-risk patients should be admitted to the hospital on moderately aggressive antithrombotic therapy (aspirin, heparin, and probably clopidogrel) to be monitored. If subsequent developments indicate high risk (enzymes, ECG, or clinical changes), the patient is switched to the high risk track. If the ischemia stabilizes, the patient becomes low risk and undergoes non-invasive testing while still in the hospital.

REFERENCES

1. Cohen M, Ferguson JJ III, Harrington RA. Trials of glycoprotein IIb-IIIa inhibitors in non-ST-segment elevation acute coronary syndromes: applicability to the practice of medicine in the US, *Clin Cardiol* 1999; **22** (suppl VI):2–12.
2. Braunwald E, Antman EM, Beasley JW et al. ACC/AHA guidelines for the management of patients with unstable angina and non-ST-segment elevation MI. Executive summary and recommendations: a report of the American College of Cardiology/American Heart Association Task Force on Practice Guidelines (Committee on the Management of Patients with Unstable Angina), *J Am Coll Cardiol* 2000; **36**:970–1062.
3. Hamm CW, Ravkilde J, Gerhardt W et al. The prognostic value of serum troponin T in unstable angina, *N Engl J Med* 1992; **327**:146–150.
4. Antman EM, Cohen M, Bernink PJLM et al. The TIMI risk score for unstable angina/non-ST-elevation MI: a method for prognostication and

therapeutic decision making, *JAMA* 2000; **284**: 835–842.

5. FRagmin, and Fast Revascularization during InStability in Coronary artery disease (FRISC II) Investigators. Invasive compared with non-invasive treatment in unstable coronary-artery disease: FRISC II prospective randomised multi-centre study, *Lancet* 1999; **354**:708–715.

6. Cannon CP, Weintraub WS, Demopoulos L et al for the TACTICS-TIMI 18 Investigators. Troponin T and I to predict 6 month mortality and relative benefit of invasive vs conservative strategy in patients with unstable angina: primary results of the TACTICS-TIMI 18 Troponin Substudy, *J Am Coll Cardiol* 2001; **37** (suppl A):325A–326A.

7. FRagmin, and Fast Revascularization during InStability in Coronary artery disease (FRISC II) Investigators. Long-term low molecular mass heparin in unstable coronary-artery disease. FRISC II prospective randomised multicentre study, *Lancet* 1999; **354**:701–707.

8. Hamm CW, Heeschen C, Goldman B et al for the c7E3 Fab Antiplatelet Therapy in Unstable Refractory Angina (CAPTURE) Study Investigators. Benefit of abciximab in patients with refractory unstable angina in relation to serum troponin T levels, *N Engl J Med* 1999; **340**:1623–1629.

9. Morrow DA, Antman EM, McCabe CH et al. An integrated clinical approach to predicting the benefit of tirofiban: application of the TIMI risk score for unstable angina/non-ST elevation MI in PRISM-PLUS, *J Am Coll Cardiol* 2001; **37** (suppl A):344A.

10. Morrow DA, Rifai N, Antman EM et al. C-reactive protein is a potent predictor of mortality independently of and in combination with troponin T in acute coronary syndromes: a TIMI 11A substudy, *J Am Coll Cardiol* 1998; **31**: 1460–1465.

11. Cannon CP, Weintraub WS, Demopoulos L et al for the TACTICS-TIMI 18 Investigators. High sensitivity C-reactive protein (hs-CRP) 6 month mortality and relative benefit of invasive vs conservative strategy in patients with unstable angina: primary results of the TACTICS-TIMI 18 C-Reactive Protein Substudy. Presented at the American College of Cardiology 50th Annual Scientific Session, March 2001.

12. Fuster V, Badimon A, Badimon L, Chesebro JH. The pathogenesis of coronary artery disease and the acute coronary syndromes, *N Engl J Med* 1992; **326**:242–250; 310–318.

13. Davies M, Thomas A, Knapman P et al. Intramyocardial platelet aggregation in patients with unstable angina suffering sudden ischemic cardiac death, *Circulation* 1986; **73**: 418–427.

14. Falk E. Unstable angina with fatal outcome: dynamic coronary thrombosis leading to infarction and/or sudden death, *Circulation* 1985; **71**:699–708.

15. Lewis HD Jr, Davis JW, Archibald DG et al. Protective effects of aspirin against acute myocardial infarction and death in men with unstable angina: results of a Veterans Administration Cooperative Study, *N Engl J Med* 1983; **309**:396–403.

16. Cairns JA, Gent M, Singer J et al. Aspirin, sulfin-pyrazone, or both in unstable angina: results of a Canadian multicenter trial, *N Engl J Med* 1985; **313**:1396–1375.

17. Théroux P, Ouimet H, McCans J et al. Aspirin, heparin, or both to treat acute unstable angina, *N Engl J Med* 1988; **319**:1105–1111.

18. Théroux P, Waters D, Lam J. Reactivation of unstable angina after the discontinuation of heparin, *N Engl J Med* 1992; **327**:141–145.

19. The RISC Group. Risk of myocardial infarction and death during treatment with low-dose aspirin and intravenous heparin in men with unstable coronary artery disease, *Lancet* 1990; **336**:827–830.

20. Oler A, Whooley M, Oler J, Grady D. Adding heparin to aspirin reduces the incidence of myocardial infarction and death in patients with unstable angina. A meta-analysis, *JAMA* 1996; **276**:811–815.

21. Antiplatelet Trialists' Collaboration. Collaborative overview of randomised trials of antiplatelet therapy, I: prevention of death, myocardial infarction, and stroke by prolonged antiplatelet therapy in various categories of patients [erratum appears in *BMJ* 1994; **308**:1540]. *BMJ* 1994; **308**:81–106.

22. ISIS-2 (Second International Study of Infarct Survival) Collaborative Group. Randomised trial of intravenous streptokinase, oral aspirin, both, or neither among 17,187 cases of suspected acute myocardial infarction: ISIS-2, *Lancet* 1988; **2**: 349–360.

23. Balsano F, Rizzon P, Violi F et al. Antiplatelet

treatment with ticlopidine in unstable angina: a controlled multicenter clinical trial. The Studio della Ticlopidina nell'Angina Instabile Group, *Circulation* 1990; **82**:17–26.

24. Leon MB, Baim DS, Popma JJ et al. A clinical trial comparing three antithrombotic drug regimens after coronary artery stenting, *N Engl J Med* 1998; **339**:1665–1671.

25. CAPRIE Steering Committee. A randomised, blinded, trial of Clopidogrel versus Aspirin in Patients at Risk of Ischaemic Events (CAPRIE), *Lancet* 1996; **348**:1329–1339.

26. Bertrand ME, Rupprecht HJ, Urban P et al for the CLASSICS Investigators. Double-blind study of the safety of clopidogrel with and without a loading dose in combination with aspirin compared with ticlopidine in combination with aspirin after coronary stenting: the Clopidogrel Aspirin Stent International Cooperative Study (CLASSICS), *Circulation* 2000; **102**:624–629.

27. Moussa I, Oetgen M, Roubin G et al. Effectiveness of clopidogrel and aspirin versus ticlopidine and aspirin in preventing stent thrombosis after coronary stent implantation, *Circulation* 1999; **99**:2364–2366.

28. CURE Study Investigators. The Clopidogrel in Unstable angina to prevent Recurrent Events (CURE) trial programme. Rationale, design and baseline characteristics including a meta-analysis of the effects of thienopyridines in vascular disease, *Eur Heart J* 2000; **21**:2033–2041.

29. The Clopidogrel in Unstable angina to prevent Recurrent Events (CURE) trial investigators. Effects of clopidogrel in addition to aspirin in patients with acute coronary syndromes without ST-segment elevation, *N Engl J Med* 2001; **345**: 494–502.

30. Lefkovist J, Plow EF, Topol EJ. Platelet glycoprotein IIb/IIIa receptors in cardiovascular medicine, *N Engl J Med* 1995; **332**:1553–1559.

31. The EPIC Investigators. Use of a monoclonal antibody directed against the platelet glycoprotein IIb/IIIa receptor in high-risk coronary angioplasty, *N Engl J Med* 1994; **330**:956–961.

32. The EPISTENT Investigators. Randomised placebo-controlled and balloon-angioplasty-controlled trial to assess safety of coronary stenting with use of platelet glycoprotein-IIb/IIIa blockade. Evaluation of Platelet IIb/IIIa Inhibitor for Stenting, *Lancet* 1998; **352**:87–92.

33. The EPILOG Investigators. Platelet glycoprotein

IIb/IIIa receptor blockade and low-dose heparin during percutaneous coronary revascularization, *N Engl J Med* 1997; **336**:1689–1696.

34. Lincoff AM, Califf RM, Topol EJ. Platelet Glycoprotein IIb/IIIa receptor blockade in coronary artery disease, *J Am Coll Cardiol* 2000; **35**:1103–1115.

35. The CAPTURE Investigators. Randomized placebo-controlled trial of abciximab before and during coronary intervention in refractory unstable angina: The CAPTURE study, *Lancet* 1997; **349**:1429–1435.

36. Platelet Receptor Inhibition in Ischemic Syndrome Management (PRISM) Study Investigators: a comparison of aspirin plus tirofiban with aspirin plus heparin for unstable angina, *N Engl J Med* 1998; **338**:1498–1505.

37. The PRISM-PLUS Study Investigators. Inhibition of the platelet glycoprotein IIb/IIIa receptor with tirofiban in unstable angina and non-Q wave myocardial infarction, *N Engl J Med* 1998; **338**:1488–1497.

38. The PURSUIT Trial Investigators. Inhibition of platelet glycoprotein IIb/IIIa with eptifibatide in patients with acute coronary syndromes, *N Engl J Med* 1998; **339**:436–443.

39. Boersma E, Akkerhuis KM, Théroux P et al. Platelet glycoprotein IIb/IIIa receptor inhibition in non-ST-elevation acute coronary syndromes: early benefit during medical treatment only, with additional protection during percutaneous coronary intervention, *Circulation* 1999; **100**:2045–2048.

40. The GUSTO IV-ACS investigators. Effect of glycoprotein. IIb/IIIa receptor blocker abciximab on outcome in patients with acute coronary syndromes without early coronary revascularization: the GUSTO IV-ACS randomized trial, *Lancet* 2001; **357**:1915–1924.

41. James S, Lindahl B, Venge P et al. No beneficial effect of 24–48 hours abciximab infusion in aspirin and heparin treated acute coronary syndrome patients with elevated troponin without early revascularization procedures: A GUSTO-IV ACS Substudy, *J Am Coll Cardiol* 2001; **37** (suppl A):326A.

42. Topol EJ, Moliterno DJ, Hermann HC et al for the TARGET investigators. Comparison of two platelet glycoprotein IIb/IIIa inhibitors, tirofiban and abciximab for the prevention of ischemic events with percutaneous coronary revascularizatin, *N Engl J Med* 2001; **344**:1888–1894.

43. Cannon CP, McCabe CH, Wilcox RG et al. Oral glycoprotein IIb/IIIa inhibition with orofiban in patients with unstable coronary syndromes (OPUS/TIMI 16) Trial. *Circulation* 2000; **102**: 149–156.

44. The SYMPHONY Investigators. Comparison of sibrafiban with aspirin for prevention of cardio-vascular events after acute coronary syndromes: a randomised trial. Sibrafiban versus Aspirin to Yield Maximum Protection from Ischemic Heart Events Post-acute Coronary Syndromes, *Lancet* 2000; **355**:337–345.

45. Second SYMPHONY Investigators. Randomized trial of aspirin, sibrafiban, or both for secondary prevention after acute coronary syndromes, *Circulation* 2000; **103**:1727–1733.

46. Cannon CP, Weintraub WS, Demopoulos LA et al for the TACTICS-TIMI 18 investigators. Comparison of early invasive and conservative strategies in patients with unstable coronary syndromes treated with glycoprotein IIb/IIIa inhibitor tirofiban, *N Engl J Med* 2001; **344**: 1879–1887.

47. Lindahl B, Venge P, Armstrong E et al. Troponin-T 0.03 µg/L is the most appropriate cut-off level between high and low risk acute coronary syndrome patients: prospective verification in a large cohort of placebo patients from the GUSTO-IV ACS Study, *J Am Coll Cardiol* 2001; **37** (suppl A):326A.

48. Newby LK, Ohman EM, Christenson RH et al for the PARAGON-B investigators. Benefit of glyco-protein IIb/IIIa inhibition in patients with acute coronary syndromes and troponin T-positive status. The PARAGON-B troponin T substudy, *Circulation* 2001; **103**:2891–2896.

49. Cannon CP, McCabe CH, Antman EM et al. Are there high-risk patients who are troponin negative? Further risk stratification with the TIMI risk score in patients with acute coronary syndrome: results from OPUS-TIMI 16, *J Am Coll Cardiol* 2001; **37** (suppl A):326A.

Section II: The benefits of revascularization

To prolong a life: summary of the coronary bypass trials

Robert C Brooks and Katherine M Detre

In 1967, Rene Favaloro and his colleagues at the Cleveland Clinic demonstrated the feasibility of surgical coronary revascularization using an aortocoronary saphenous vein graft (SVG) [1]. This technique was enthusiastically adopted, modified, and applied for the treatment of chronic coronary artery occlusive disease and acute coronary syndromes. The number of coronary artery bypass graft (CABG) surgeries exploded over the next decade, prompting a growing concern over the appropriate application of the procedure and raising important questions. Does CABG revascularization improve patient survival, particularly in patients who do not require it for control of refractory symptoms? Which patients benefit from the surgery?

Several large randomized controlled trials were undertaken to examine the outcomes of CABG surgery compared with medical therapy for the treatment of patients with chronic stable angina. These trials, which enrolled patients from 1972–1984, were conducted predominantly on men 65 years of age or younger. They excluded patients with acute myocardial infarctions (MI), unstable angina, or severe angina requiring urgent surgery. Medical therapy was not tightly controlled, nor even necessarily similar, between the two treatment groups. Risk factor interventions, such as smoking cessation

and lipid-lowering therapy, were not standard at the time. Because crossovers between the treatment arms were very common, particularly from the medical to the surgical groups, these were trials of early revascularization compared to initial medical therapy with later revascularization if needed for refractory or progressive symptoms.

The first randomized controlled trial was the Veterans Administration Cooperative Study of Coronary Artery Bypass Surgery (VA Study). Six hundred and eighty-six patients were enrolled at 13 sites from 1972–1974. Patients were excluded for recent MI within six months or for uncompensated heart failure, but a large number of patients with systolic dysfunction were included. Impaired left ventricular (LV) function, defined as either a left ventricular ejection fraction (LVEF) less than 50% or hypokinesis/akinesis of more than 25% of the heart border on left ventriculograms, was present in 55% of the patients. A category of 'high angiographic risk' patients was specified *a priori*, which included patients with three-vessel coronary disease and impaired LV function. The primary end-point of the study was total mortality, with secondary end-points of non-fatal MI and angina.

Saphenous vein grafts were used almost exclusively in this study, with only 3% of the grafts from the internal mammary artery (IMA). Perioperative (30-day) mortality was 5.8% in the surgical arm. Using an intention-to-treat analysis for the study population as a whole, a trend toward improved survival was seen with initial CABG therapy after five years. This benefit became statistically significant by seven years (77% survival in the early surgery group versus 70% in the medical group, $p = 0.043$), but was lost again by 11 years (58% versus 57% survival) [2].

When survival was compared in angiographically and clinically defined subgroups of patients, early CABG appeared beneficial compared to initial medical therapy only in certain groups. A clear survival advantage was seen for patients with left main coronary artery stenosis $\geqslant 50\%$ who were assigned to initial revascularization compared to those assigned to initial medical therapy (survival at 42 months was 88% in the surgical group compared to 65% in the medical group, $p = 0.016$) [3]. At seven years, a significant improvement in survival was seen for patients with impaired LV function (74% in the surgical group versus 63% in the medical group, $p = 0.049$), and a non-significant trend toward improved survival was seen among patients with three-vessel disease (75% survival with surgery compared to 63% survival with the medical group, $p = 0.061$) [2]. Both of these differences diminished at 11 years of follow-up. In other groups, including all patients without left main disease taken together, patients with one- and two-vessel disease, and patients with normal LV function, no mortality advantage was seen for initial surgery at any time. In the subset of patients with two-vessel disease, decreased survival was seen by 11 years with initial surgical treatment (55% survival versus 69% in the medical group, $p = 0.045$).

According to these results, only patients with more severe disease, and thus a poorer short-term prognosis, were likely to have a survival benefit from initial surgery. Two pre-specified subgroup analyses conducted on patients at higher risk for cardiovascular mortality were consistent with this hypothesis. Patients in the *a priori* high angiographic risk category due to the presence of three-vessel disease and concomitant impaired LV function demonstrated improved survival at seven years with surgery (76% survival in CABG group versus 52% in medical group, $p = 0.002$) [2]. This difference diminished but remained significant at 11 years. No significant mortality difference was seen for all other (low angiographic risk) patients as a group at any time point.

A regression model was used, as well, to develop a clinical risk score for estimating the probability of dying in the medically treated patients. Twenty non-invasive risk factors that were present in at least 20% of the patients were evaluated, and four variables were found that best fit the model: history of MI, history of hypertension, resting ST-segment depression on ECG, and NYHA functional class III/IV. (A history of heart failure was not considered for inclusion because it was present in only 8% of the study population). The risk prediction model was cross-validated with an independent sample of 535 patients from the University of Alabama, and then used to divide patients into high-, middle-, and low-risk tertiles. The high-risk tertile of patients (approximately 25% or higher predicted five year mortality) showed a survival benefit with initial CABG, with 86% survival at five years compared to 63% in the medical therapy group, $p = 0.0006$) [2]. The middle-risk tertile showed no difference in mortality with the two treatment arms, while the low-risk tertile (approximately 15% or less predicted five year mortality) showed a survival benefit with medical treatment at five years (93% survival versus 82% with initial CABG, $p = 0.012$) that diminished and became non-significant by seven years. These findings indicate that two-thirds of the patients who fit the VA Study eligibility criteria could have been risk-stratified and managed medically, without the need for diagnostic angiography or early surgery.

Applying the clinical risk score to the high angiographic risk subgroup further reinforced the relationship between patient risk and the benefit of surgery. When the high angiographic risk group was subdivided into clinical risk tertiles, the mortality rate with medical treatment rose dramatically with increasing clinical risk score, while the surgical mortality remained similar. As a result, a marked mortality improvement was seen with CABG in the high clinical risk subgroup (76% survival at seven years with surgery versus 36% with initial medical treatment, $p = 0.002$), while only a trend was observed in the middle risk tertile (79% survival versus 50%, $p = 0.069$) and no difference was seen in the low clinical risk subgroup (77 versus 79% survival at seven years, $p = 0.8$).

The overall conclusion of the study was that stable patients with coronary artery disease at highest risk of death have a survival advantage with a strategy of initial surgery, while lower risk patients do not. Depending on known prognostic indicators, the cumulative seven year mortality in surgical patients ranged only from 12–30%, while that of medically treated patients ranged from 10–64% [2]. Initial CABG treatment helped by improving the prognosis of the highest risk patients. Left main disease, decreased LV function, three-vessel disease, and clinical risk scores all appeared useful in defining the high-risk patient who would benefit from initial surgery.

While this analysis concentrated on long-term cardiovascular risk, differences in surgical risk also would be expected to effect the benefit of early surgery. A wide institutional variation was seen in perioperative mortality in this study. When only the 10 sites with lower surgical mortality rates (average perioperative mortality 3.4%) were included, for example, survival of patients with three-vessel disease was better with initial CABG than with medical treatment ($p = 0.014$ at seven years) [4]. This difference was not statistically significant when all hospitals were included. Thus, institutional and individual surgical risks appeared to be meaningful considerations, along with overall cardiovascular risk, when assessing the likely benefit of early revascularization.

The European Coronary Surgery Study was the second large multicenter randomized controlled trial of CABG versus medical therapy. The 768 patients enrolled from 1973–1976 were required to have stable angina, multivessel disease (with > 50% stenosis of two or more vessels), and normal ventricular function (LVEF > 50%). The majority of grafts used were SVGs, with 54 patients receiving IMA grafts [5]. Perioperative mortality was lower in this trial, at 3.2%, as was the long-term mortality in the population as a whole. Overall results showed a more impressive benefit for initial CABG treatment compared with the strategy of initial medical treatment and delayed revascularization if needed. Total population survival after five years was 92.4% in the surgery group compared to 83.1% in the medical treatment group, $p = 0.0001$) [6]. This difference was still significant at 12 years of follow-up (70.6% survival in the surgery arm versus 66.7% in the medical group, $p = 0.04$).

In subgroup analyses, the extent of disease by angiography again appeared important. Patients with three-vessel disease had improved survival in the surgery group compared to the medical group at five years (94% versus 82%, $p = 0.0002$) and 10 years (78% versus 68%, $p = 0.01$) [6]. Patients with two-vessel disease, on the other hand, showed no mortality difference. The investigators also noted that proximal left anterior descending (LAD) artery stenosis was a predictor of poorer prognosis with medical treatment and benefit from initial CABG. Patients with proximal LAD stenosis as a component of their multivessel disease had improved survival with initial surgical treatment compared to medical therapy (76% versus 65% survival at 10 years, $p = 0.007$). Patients without proximal LAD stenosis did not (81% surgery group survival at 10 years compared to 83% in the medical group, $p > 0.2$). Proximal LAD stenosis was common in the study, being present in 78% of the patients with three-vessel disease and 61% of patients with two-vessel disease.

These investigators also used a regression

model to identify non-invasive clinical risk factors which were predictive of survival in their cohort. Older age, abnormal resting ECG, a markedly positive (versus positive or normal-to-slightly-positive) exercise ECG, and the presence of peripheral arterial disease were all associated with poorer survival in the medical treatment group [6]. Two of these factors, older age and a markedly positive stress test, were also associated with mortality benefit from early surgery. The oldest tertile of patients (over age 53) showed a 10-year survival of 72% with initial CABG compared to 56% with medical therapy ($p = 0.007$), while younger patients showed no survival difference between treatment groups. The study excluded patients 65 years of age and older, however. Patients with markedly positive exercise ECG (non-imaging) stress test results had 75% survival at 10 years with initial surgery versus 62% survival with medical therapy ($p = 0.007$), while patients with other stress test results showed no mortality difference by treatment assignment. Resting ECG abnormalities and peripheral arterial disease had little effect on the benefit from surgery. The absence of treated hypertension was associated with a mortality benefit from surgery, interestingly, while patients with a history of hypertension showed no difference in survival between the two treatment groups.

Overall, the European study results thus supported the idea that higher risk patients benefit from initial surgical therapy, while lower risk patients do not. Besides three-vessel disease, the study suggested that the presence of a proximal LAD stenosis or a markedly abnormal exercise test may be useful for identifying higher risk patients among a population with multivessel disease and normal ventricular function.

The last large randomized trial of CABG versus medical therapy was the Coronary Artery Surgery Study (CASS), which enrolled 780 patients in the US and Canada from 1975–1979. The study required patients to have mild–moderate stable exertional angina or prior MI, and bypassable stenosis of at least 70% in two

vessels, or in the proximal LAD, or the proximal right coronary artery (RCA) in a right-dominant circulation, or the proximal circumflex artery in left dominant circulation, or a 50–70% left main artery stenosis. Patients were excluded if they had more than 70% stenosis of the left main artery, severe (class III or IV) angina, recent MI (within three weeks), uncompensated heart failure or a primary clinical problem of heart failure. Randomization was stratified by the number of diseased vessels and the presence or absence of LV dysfunction. About 10% of the patients were female.

Of the 390 patients randomized to and receiving initial surgical therapy, 96% had SVGs and 16% had IMA grafts. A much lower 1.4% perioperative mortality rate was observed in this trial compared to the prior studies, likely due to improving operative techniques as well as patient characteristics. For the overall population, no significant difference in survival was seen between the medical and surgical groups out to 10 years of follow-up (82% survival in surgical group at 10 years versus 79% in the medical group, $p = 0.25$).

In subgroup analyses, no difference in survival between treatment arms was seen by number of diseased vessels. Survival in patients with three-vessel disease, for example, was 75% with medical therapy versus 76% with surgical therapy at 10 years ($p = 0.7$) [7]. Similarly, no differences in mortality were observed between treatments by location of disease, including patient subgroups with proximal LAD stenosis or LAD stenosis along with two- or three-vessel disease. Patients with left main disease also did not benefit statistically from early CABG, but this result was likely due to having too few patients in this subgroup. Only 14 patients with left main disease were enrolled, with 100% survival at 10 years in the surgical group compared to 50% survival with medical therapy.

As with the VA trial, however, patients with impaired left ventricular function did appear to benefit in CASS from early surgical revascularization. Patients with LVEF less than 50% showed a survival advantage with initial CABG compared to medical therapy which was detectable by seven years and persisted at 10 years (79% survival at 10 years with surgery versus 61% with medical therapy, $p < 0.01$) [7]. Patients with normal EF (> 50%) had no difference in survival with different initial therapies and, in fact, were more likely to be alive and free of MI with initial medical treatment (75% versus 68% at 10 years, $p = 0.04$). The long-term prognosis was good and quite similar for patients with normal EF randomized to initial medical therapy whether they had one-, two-, or three-vessel disease (85% survival at 10 years). The presence or absence of clinical heart failure was not associated with a benefit for surgery compared to medical treatment, but patients with overt heart failure were excluded from the trial, and very few patients with EF < 35% were included.

The overall results of the CASS study were similar to the VA study, with no mortality benefit for early surgery in the population as a whole, but subgroup analyses showing a benefit with early CABG for higher risk patients. Impaired LV function was the major determinant of poor prognosis with medical therapy and of survival benefit with initial surgery in this trial.

In 1994, the Coronary Artery Bypass Graft Surgery Trialists Collaboration published a meta-analysis of the randomized studies on CABG versus medical therapy for stable angina [8]. Individual patient data from the three large trials and four other smaller trials was included, using a stenosis cut-off of 50% for defining a diseased vessel. An intention to treat analysis was used again, ignoring the effect of crossovers. The vast majority of grafts used were SVGs, with only 9.9% of patients receiving left IMA grafts. Most of the patients had normal LV function, with only 19.7% having an EF less than 50%.

The perioperative (30-day) mortality rate in patients randomized to initial surgery was 3.2% for all studies combined, with a combined rate of death and MI of 10.3%. Crossover rates from the medical group to later CABG were similar in the trials, with 25% of patients at five years and 41% at 10 years receiving surgery. Survival in the overall population was improved with initial surgical therapy at five years (89.8% with CABG versus 84.2% with medical therapy, $p < 0.0001$), and this effect persisted at 10 years of follow-up (73.6% survival with CABG versus 69.5% with medical therapy, $p = 0.03$). The combined end-point of death and MI was higher with initial surgery treatment after one year (11.6% with CABG versus 8.0% with medical therapy, OR 1.55, $p < 0.001$), but this effect was no longer significant after five years.

In subgroup analyses defined by extent of angiographic disease, patients with left main disease demonstrated improved survival after five years with initial surgical treatment (odds ratio (OR) for death 0.32 with surgery versus medical therapy, 95% CI 0.15–0.70) [8]. This benefit was no longer significant at 10 years of follow-up, but was likely attenuated by the high crossover rate from medical to surgical therapy in this group (65% at 10 years in patients with left main disease). Patients with three-vessel disease also showed improved survival at five and 10 years with initial CABG therapy (odds ratio for death 0.58, 95% CI 0.42–0.80 at five years; OR 0.76, 95% CI 0.60–0.97 at 10 years). No difference between the treatment groups was seen for patients with one- or two-vessel disease. The presence or absence of proximal LAD lesions did not change the conclusions about surgical benefit based on the number of diseased vessels. Patients with three-vessel disease without proximal LAD stenosis retained a mortality advantage with early CABG (OR 0.47 at five years, 95% CI 0.25–0.89), while patients with one- or two-vessel disease including proximal LAD stenosis did not (OR 0.58, 95% CI 0.34–1.01).

Left ventricular dysfunction appeared less important as a determinant of short-term mortality benefit with surgery in the meta-analysis than it had in the individual studies, probably because the largest (European) study excluded patients with abnormal LVEF. However, LV function remained important as a predictor of prognosis and long-term benefit. Patients with normal and abnormal LV function had similar significant relative risk reductions for death at five years with CABG versus medical therapy (OR 0.39 and 0.41, respectively). The magnitude of the absolute survival benefit was much larger in patients with LV dysfunction, however, since the mortality rate with medical treatment was roughly twice as high (25.2% versus 13.3% at five years). At 10 years of follow-up, the odds ratio for death remained significantly improved with early surgery in patients with LV dysfunction (OR 0.65, 95% CI 0.45–0.92), but were no longer significant in patients with normal LV function (OR 0.89, 95% CI 0.73–1.10). The mean survival time at 10 years for patients with abnormal LV function increased 10.6 months with surgery compared to medical therapy.

Two different risk scores, the VA study non-invasive clinical risk score and a multivariate risk score developed by the meta-analysis authors, were used to look at higher versus lower risk patient subgroups. The Collaborative Group risk score was based on a step-wise logistic regression analysis of 10-year mortality data of the two treatment arms combined. Included variables were age, class III or IV angina, history of MI, abnormal EF, proximal LAD stenosis, RCA stenosis, history of diabetes, and history of hypertension. When the overall study population was separated into three risk strata using the VA risk score, only the highest risk tertile showed significantly improved mortality at five years with initial surgery compared to medical therapy (OR 0.50, 95% CI 0.35–0.72) [8]. The middle tertile risk group showed a trend toward benefit with surgery (OR 0.63, 95% CI 0.39–1.01). Similar results were seen using the Collaborative Group risk score, except that the benefit with surgery reached significance with both the highest and middle risk tertiles (OR 0.54 and 0.55). The middle tertile group using the Collaborative Group score, which included invasive variables, had a higher mortality rate with medical treatment than the middle VA score tertile (13.9% versus

11.5% at five years), suggesting that the improved benefit from early surgery was due to it being a higher risk group. The lowest risk tertiles by either risk score index showed trends toward increased mortality with initial surgical treatment (OR 1.17 and 1.18), which did not reach statistical significance.

A number of concerns exist regarding the meta-analysis and interpretation of the results. Significant heterogeneity of trial methods existed, including the methodology for inter-pretation of angiograms and the presence of a core lab for such interpretations. There was no standardization of medical therapy, which lead to significant differences in the treatment arms, such as more beta-blocker use and less aspirin use in the medical treatment group at one year versus the surgical group [8]. The crossover rate from the medical group to CABG was increased with more angiographically severe disease, which could tend to underestimate the benefit of initial surgical revascularization in patients with three-vessel disease or left main disease. However, the conclusion of the meta-analysis is similar to the conclusions of the individual large trials: initial CABG therapy improved survival over the first 5–10 years compared to initial medical therapy in higher-risk patients.

What happens, then, after the first 10 years? Twenty-two year follow-up data from the VA Study [9] provide insight into the natural history of disease in these patients, who received little routine risk factor intervention. Many of the medically treated patients eventually required CABG. Crossover from the medical group to surgery slowed after the first decade, but 66% of the medical patients received CABG by 22 years. Graft lifetimes were limited. In this study popu-lation with SVGs, mortality rates in patients initially treated with surgery accelerated after seven years, and remained higher than medical patients thereafter. At 22 years, 48% of surgical patients had required re-operation, at much higher perioperative mortality rates (10.3% com-pared to 5.8% for the initial bypass). Crossover and re-operation were not predictable from base-line clinical or angiographic risk factors.

Survival rates were not significantly different at 22 years for the study population overall (25% medical group survival versus 20% surgical, $p = 0.24$), and the early benefit in high-risk patients disappeared over time. High angiographic risk patients (with three-vessel disease and impaired LV function) had a 20% survival at 22 years with initial medical therapy compared to 15% survival with initial CABG. Survival figures for the high clinical risk score tertile were also statistically similar at 11% for the medical group versus 12% for the surgical group. Long-term data also suggested that some patients may benefit from the delayed use of surgical revascularization. Low-risk patients had improved survival at 22 years with initial medical therapy, similar to the trend seen in the meta-analysis at 10 years. For patients without the combination of three-vessel disease and LV dysfunction (low angiographic risk), 22-year survival was 31% with medical therapy versus 24% with surgery ($p < 0.05$). Low and middle tertile clinical risk patients together had improved survival, as well, with initial medical therapy compared to surgery (35% versus 26%, $p < 0.05$). Overall, study patients randomized to initial medical therapy were more likely to be alive and free of MI at 22 years than surgical patients (18% versus 11%, $p = 0.0031$).

Thus, early bypass therapy improved survival in high-risk patients with stable angina for the first decade, but the benefit was limited by the life span of the grafts and progression of native vessel atherosclerosis. Higher mortality with re-operation made survival after two decades similar. In lower risk patients, early bypass therapy did not improve survival at any time, and may decrease very long-term survival.

Since patients with unstable angina constitute a higher risk population for cardiovascular events and death than stable angina patients, does early bypass improve mortality in unstable angina patients? Two randomized controlled trials compared treatment with CABG versus medical therapy for patients with progressive or rest angina and ST-T wave changes. The National Heart, Lung, and Blood Institute sponsored a study that enrolled 288 patients from 1972–1976 [10]. Mortality in the hospital was similar, and no overall survival difference was observed between medical and surgical groups at a mean 30 months of follow-up. The second and larger trial was a VA Cooperative Study that enrolled 468 men less than 70 years old from 1976–1982 [11]. Patients with left main disease or severe LV dysfunction (LVEF < 30%) were excluded. Similar to the stable angina trials of that time, medical therapy was not standardized. An intention-to-treat analysis was used, ignoring the 43% crossover from medical to surgical therapy by five years. Operative mortality was 4.1%.

Study results were notably similar to trials of stable angina patients. No significant overall survival difference was seen between the medical and surgical treatment groups at five years (84% survival in the surgical group versus 81% in the medical group, $p = 0.45$) [11]. Subgroup analyses showed that patients with three-vessel disease had improved survival at 60 months with surgery compared to medical therapy (89% versus 75%, $p < 0.02$), while no differences in survival between treatment groups was seen for patients with one- or two-vessel disease. The results suggested that patients with decreased LV function (defined as LVEF < 50% or LVEDP $\geq$ 16 mmHg) might benefit, as well, from early surgery. There was a trend towards improved survival in patients with abnormal LV function (79% survival at 60 months with surgery versus 67% with medical treatment, $p = 0.22$). When patients were separated into tertiles by LVEF, the patients with the poorest LV function (EF 30–58%) demonstrated a survival advantage with initial CABG therapy (86% survival at 60 months with surgery versus 73% with medical therapy, $p = 0.03$). Regression analysis showed that mortality of medical patients over five years was significantly dependent on LVEF ($p = 0.004$), while mortality of surgical patients was not ($p = 0.76$).

High risk subgroups, again, seemed to benefit from initial surgical revascularization. Patients with three-vessel disease and impaired

LV function had improved five year survival with initial surgery compared to medical treatment (91% survival with surgery versus 71% medical, $p < 0.05$). A high risk *a priori* subgroup was defined by the presence of prolonged chest pain not easily relieved by nitrates and accompanied by ST-T wave changes. No survival difference by treatment group was found for these patients in the presence of normal LV function, while a significant survival benefit was seen in such patients who also had abnormal LV function (eight year survival 87% with surgery versus 54% with medical therapy, $p < 0.04$) [12]. The results of the unstable angina trials thus supported the conclusions from the studies on stable angina: higher risk patients, most easily defined by three-vessel disease and impaired LV function, derive a mortality benefit from early CABG, while lower risk patients survive just as readily with initial trials of medical therapy.

Unfortunately, it is difficult to know the true relevance of such older trial data to current medical practice. Many dramatic improvements have occurred in both surgical and medical treatments over the last 25 years that have improved patient survival. Internal mammary artery grafts have been shown to maintain patency longer and improve long-term patient survival compared with SVGs [13, 14], and are now the conduit of choice for initial surgery. Other surgical factors, such as improvements in anesthesia techniques, cardio-pulmonary bypass technology, and methods of myocardial protection have also improved surgical outcomes. Most of the current medical therapies and risk factor interventions that are used for patients with coronary artery disease (CAD) and systolic heart failure were not in uniform use at the time of these prior studies [15, 16]. Antiplatelet agents are now standard, with aspirin having been shown to reduce all-cause mortality, as well as cardiovascular mortality and cardiovascular events, in people with prior MI. Lipid-lowering therapy has been shown to improve mortality in primary and secondary prevention of CAD, as well as decreasing mor-

tality after revascularization. Smoking cessation has been shown to improve overall survival in patients with CAD and survival after CABG. Beta-blockers and angiotensin-converting enzyme inhibitors have become standard therapy to improve mortality after MI and with systolic heart failure.

An additional level of complexity was added by the development of various methods of percutaneous revascularization over the last 15 years. Coronary angioplasty has been shown to produce similar clinical outcomes when compared to CABG for all but the highest risk patients (such as left main disease) and certain subgroups (such as treated diabetics) [17]. Coronary artery bypass grafting itself can now be performed less invasively, using a limited thoracotomy incision rather than median sternotomy. Thus, major changes and improvements in all treatments for patients with CAD make it difficult or impossible to know whether similar results would be obtained today if older trials of medical therapy versus CABG were repeated.

As these treatments have evolved, more recent randomized controlled trials in specific patient populations have compared early routine revascularization to medical therapy, with mixed results. These trials have used both surgical and percutaneous revascularization methods. The Medicine, Angioplasty, or Surgery Study (MASS) randomized 214 patients from 1988–1991 with severe (> 80%) proximal LAD stenosis, stable angina and normal LVEF to medical therapy, CABG using the left IMA graft, or percutaneous transluminal coronary angioplasty (PTCA) (without stent) [18]. No difference in survival was seen over five years between the three groups. The excellent prognosis of such patients with current treatment, however, makes it difficult to see treatment differences. Five year survival in the medical group was 97.1%.

The Asymptomatic Cardiac Ischemia Pilot Study evaluated 558 patients with stable coronary disease, ischemia on exercise testing, and asymptomatic ischemia on ambulatory ECG monitoring. Patients were randomized from 1991–1993 to angina-guided medical treatment, ischemia-guided medical treatment, or revascularization with PTCA or CABG. Two-year mortality was significantly lower in the revascularization group (1.1%) compared to the angina-guided (6.6%, $p < 0.005$) or ischemia-guided (4.4%, $p < 0.05$) groups. Not all studies support a benefit from early invasive interventions, however. The Veterans Affairs Non-Q Wave Infarction Strategies in Hospital (VAN-QWISH) Trial randomized 920 patients with acute non-Q wave MI from 1993–1995 to early invasive testing and revascularization versus a 'conservative' strategy of routine stress testing with invasive management for recurrent symptoms or objective signs of ischemia [19]. Survival was significantly worse at hospital discharge, one month, and one year in the invasive-strategy group compared to the conservative-strategy group, although longer-term follow-up showed no significant differences.

As the prognosis of CAD patients improves with medical management advances, invasive intervention becomes a more relevant alternative for patients with known poor prognosis. The BARI 2D Study will examine the issue of early revascularization versus medical therapy in the high-risk subgroup of diabetics. Patients with stable angina or documented ischemia will be randomized to revascularization plus aggressive medical therapy versus aggressive medical therapy alone, with end-points of five year mortality, MI, angina, and quality of life.

It does not appear likely, however, that the large randomized controlled trials of the 1970s comparing CABG with medical therapy will be redone using current standards of care. Given the lack of data on survival benefit with current revascularization techniques versus current medical therapy, decisions regarding revascularization can be based on: (1) non-mortality benefits, such as symptomatic improvement or quality of life issues (see Chapters 8 and 9), or (2) the assumption that the major lesson of earlier trials is still valid: the higher risk the patient,

the more likely the patient is to have a mortality benefit from early revascularization.

If one assumes that the 'high-risk' patient will still have a survival benefit from early revascularization, what should be incorporated into the determination of risk? The trial evidence suggests that a combination of clinical and angiographic risk factors for long-term cardiovascular death can be used to define patients who are more likely to benefit from early surgery. Clinical risk factors that have been associated with a poorer prognosis in patients with CAD include poor functional status (often manifested as markedly abnormal stress test results or more severe angina); ventricular dysfunction; older age; history of MI, diabetes or hypertension; resting ST-segment depression; and history of arrhythmias. Angiographic risk factors clearly include left main and three-vessel disease, and may include proximal occlusions of major vessels, such as the LAD, which put large areas of myocardium at risk. The evidence suggests that combinations of these risk factors are additive with regard to risk and with regard to likely benefit from early surgery. In addition, risk factors for perioperative morbidity and mortality with CABG have been well delineated over the last 20 years, so that individual surgical risk can be calculated and added to the analysis [20]. Many of the major surgical risk factors effect patients who were largely excluded from the randomized trials, including patients over age 65, women, and people with prior CABG.

REFERENCES

1. Favoloro RG. Saphenous vein autograft replacement of severe segmental coronary artery occlusion: operative technique, *Ann Thorac Surg* 1968; **5**:334–339.
2. Veterans Administration Coronary Artery Bypass Surgery Cooperative Study Group. Eleven-year survival in the Veterans Administration randomized trial of coronary bypass surgery for stable angina, *N Engl J Med* 1984; **311**:1333–1339.

3. Takaro T, Peduzzi P, Detre KM et al. Survival in subgroups of patients with left main coronary artery disease. Veterans Administration Co-operative Study of Surgery for Coronary Arterial Occlusive Disease, *Circulation* 1982; **66**:14–22.

4. Takaro T, Hultgren HH, Detre KM et al. Results of the VA randomized study of medical and surgical management of angina pectoris. In: Hammermeister KE, ed, *Coronary Bypass Surgery: the late results*, (New York: Praeger Publishers, 1983), 17–42.

5. European Coronary Surgery Study Group. Coronary-artery bypass surgery in stable angina pectoris: survival at two years, *Lancet* 1979; **i**:889–893.

6. Varnauskas E and the European Coronary Surgery Study Group. Twelve-year follow-up of survival in the randomized European Coronary Surgery Study, *N Engl J Med* 1988; **319**:332–337.

7. Alderman EL, Bourassa MG, Cohen LS et al. Ten-year follow-up of survival and myocardial infarction in the randomized coronary artery surgery study, *Circulation* 1990; **82**:1629–1646.

8. Yusuf S, Zucker D, Peduzzi P et al. Effect of coronary artery bypass graft surgery on survival: overview of 10-year results from randomised trials by the Coronary Artery Bypass Graft Surgery Trialists Collaboration, *Lancet* 1994; **344**:563–570.

9. Peduzzi P, Kamina A, Detre K for the VA Coronary Artery Bypass Surgery Cooperative Study Group. Twenty-two-year follow-up in the VA Cooperative Study of Coronary Artery Bypass Surgery for Stable Angina, *Am J Cardiol* 1998; **81**:1393–1399.

10. Russell RO Jr, Moraski RE, Kouchoukos N et al. Unstable angina pectoris: national cooperative study group to compare surgical and medical therapy: II. In-hospital experience and initial follow-up results in patients with one, two and three vessel disease, *Am J Cardiol* 1978; **42**:839–848.

11. Parisi AF, Khuri S, Deupree RH et al. Medical compared with surgical management of unstable angina: five-year mortality and morbidity in the Veterans Administration Study, *Circulation* 1989; **80**:1176–1189.

12. Sharma GVRK, Deupree RH, Khuri SF et al. Coronary bypass surgery improves survival in high-risk unstable angina: results of a Veterans Administration Cooperative Study with an eight-year follow-up, *Circulation* 1991; **84** (suppl III):III260–III267.

13. Loop FD, Lytle BW, Cosgrove DM et al. Influence of the internal mammary artery graft on 10-year survival and other cardiac events, *N Engl J Med* 1986; **314**:1–6.

14. Cameron A, Davis KB, Green G, Schaff HV. Coronary artery bypass surgery with internal thoracic artery grafts: effects on survival over a 15-year period, *N Engl J Med* 1996; **334**:216–219.

15. Gibbons RJ, Chatterjee K, Daley J et al. ACC/AHA/ACP-ISM guidelines for the management of patients with chronic stable angina. A report of the American College of Cardiology/American Heart Association Task Force on Practice Guidelines (Committee on Management of Patients with Chronic Stable Angina), *J Am Coll Cardiol* 1999; **33**:2092–2197.

16. Ryan TJ, Antman EM, Brooks NH et al. 1999 update: ACC/AHA guidelines for the management of patients with acute myocardial infarction. A report of the American College of Cardiology/American Heart Association Task Force on Practice Guidelines (Committee on Management of Acute Myocardial Infarction), *J Am Coll Cardiol* 1999; **34**:890–911.

17. The Bypass Angioplasty Revascularization Investigation (BARI) Investigators. Comparison of coronary bypass surgery with angioplasty in patients with multivessel disease, *N Engl J Med* 1996; **335**:217–225.

18. Hueb WA, Soares PR, Almeida de Oliveira S et al. Five-year follow-up of the Medicine, Angioplasty, or Surgery Study (MASS): a prospective, randomized trial of medical therapy, balloon angioplasty, or bypass surgery for single proximal left anterior descending coronary artery stenosis, *Circulation* 1999; **100** (suppl II):II107–II113.

19. Boden WE, O'Rourke RA, Crawford MH et al. Outcomes in patients with acute non-Q wave myocardial infarction randomly assigned to an invasive as compared with a conservative management strategy, *N Engl J Med* 1998; **338**:1785–1792.

20. Eagle KA, Guyton RA, Davidoff R et al. ACC/AHA guidelines for coronary artery bypass graft surgery: a report of the American College of Cardiology/American Heart Association Task Force on Practice Guidelines (Committee to Revise the 1991 Guidelines for Coronary Artery Bypass Graft Surgery), *J Am Coll Cardiol* 1999; **34**:1262–1346.

8

To improve a life: relief of symptoms, exercise tolerance, ACME and RITA-2

Edward D Folland

CONTENTS • The relationship between degree of coronary artery stenosis, severity of symptoms, and exercise tolerance • The importance of randomized clinical trials in evaluating symptom relief • The effect of revascularization on symptoms • The effect of revascularization on exercise performance • Summary

The purpose of coronary revascularization is to improve the length and/or quality of life for patients afflicted with coronary artery disease. Issues of survival are addressed elsewhere in this text. This chapter focuses on the effect of coronary revascularization on symptoms and exercise tolerance, which are both important and interrelated elements of quality of life.

The cardinal symptom of myocardial ischemia is angina or its equivalent, which occurs whenever myocardial oxygen demand exceeds the ability of the coronary circulation to supply sufficient oxygen to meet that demand. Angina and exercise tolerance are related, because it is often the onset of angina which limits exercise tolerance for patients with coronary artery disease. Since exercise tolerance is easily quantified, it can be used as an objective surrogate to measure inherently subjective symptoms.

THE RELATIONSHIP BETWEEN DEGREE OF CORONARY ARTERY STENOSIS, SEVERITY OF SYMPTOMS, AND EXERCISE TOLERANCE

Both coronary stenosis and exercise tolerance are readily quantified, enabling the investiga-

tion of their relationship. But first a distinction needs to be made between chronic stable angina, in which coronary stenosis is relatively constant, and acute coronary syndromes in which coronary stenosis is dynamic and unpredictable. Although unstable coronary syndromes (unstable angina and acute myocardial infarction) account for a large part of the disability of coronary artery disease, they do not lend themselves readily to this kind of study. Therefore, this chapter will focus on the effects of revascularization on symptoms and exercise tolerance for patients with chronic stable angina.

It has long been assumed that a direct linkage exists between the angiographic severity of coronary artery stenosis, the work threshold for myocardial ischemia and maximum tolerance of treadmill exercise for patients with stable angina pectoris [1]. This linkage was tested by the ACME Study, a Veterans Affairs Cooperative Study comparing angioplasty to medical therapy for patients having single and double vessel coronary artery disease, stable angina pectoris and inducible ischemia on treadmill exercise testing [2]. The study afforded an ideal opportunity to correlate quantitatively measured coronary artery stenosis with exercise tolerance in a well-defined population of 227 patients having single vessel coronary artery disease. In addition, these patients were randomly assigned to medical or interventional treatment and re-studied six months later by angiography and exercise testing. Coronary artery stenoses were measured by quantitative methods using hand-held calipers and computer-based analysis, and also by qualitative estimate by the physician investigators. The results supported the conventional wisdom that coronary stenosis limits exercise tolerance. There was, however, rather poor statistical correlation between coronary stenosis and maximal duration of exercise tolerance due to several factors. One factor identified from the study was the technical variability of coronary stenosis measurement. The standard deviation of the mean variability of percent diameter stenosis between two independent measurements of the same stenosis by the same observer was 9.4% and 7.3% for caliper and computer-based methods, respectively. Improvements of coronary stenosis outside the range of technical variability of the method predicted statistically significant improvements of exercise tolerance. Furthermore, visual estimation of percent diameter stenosis, the crudest of the three methods employed, was most effective in relating degree of stenosis to exercise performance. Patients having a visual estimate of 90% or more diameter stenosis had significantly lower exercise tolerance than patients whose visual stenosis estimate was less than 90%. This probably underscores the limitations of quantitative methods in making small measurements.

THE IMPORTANCE OF RANDOMIZED CLINICAL TRIALS IN EVALUATING SYMPTOM RELIEF

Coronary artery bypass surgery and randomized clinical trials developed simultaneously during the decades of the 1970s and 1980s. Perhaps no other operation has been subjected to such rigorous scientific scrutiny, and for

good reason. Most prior surgical treatments for angina pectoris, no matter how illogically conceived, appeared to have some beneficial effect on symptoms. Most notable of these was the internal mammary ligation procedure. In 1959, Leonard Cobb and Robert A Bruce subjected this procedure to a randomized clinical trial where eight of 17 subjects underwent the mammary ligation and the other nine underwent a sham procedure [3]. Both patients and physicians who assessed the outcome were blinded to the choice of treatment. Symptoms improved in 32% of the ligated patients and in 43% of the sham patients, supporting the hypothesis that the benefit of the operation was a placebo effect. By the time direct coronary bypass surgery was introduced in 1968, the importance of the placebo effect was fully recognized and it was clear that the new operation should be evaluated by a randomized therapeutic trial. Since a sham procedure was neither feasible nor ethical, the operation was compared to the only alternative treatment, anti-anginal drug therapy. Three landmark trials were undertaken: The Veterans Administration Cooperative Study of Medical versus Surgical Treatment for Stable Angina [4], The European Coronary Surgery Study Group [5], and The Coronary Artery Surgery Study (CASS) [6]. When percutaneous intervention became available it was likewise subjected to the same kind of scientific scrutiny, both in comparison with medical therapy and with bypass surgery. The results of these clinical trials form the basis of this chapter.

THE EFFECT OF REVASCULARIZATION ON SYMPTOMS

Coronary artery bypass versus medicine

The primary end-point of most studies comparing bypass surgery and medical therapy is survival; however, symptom relief was included as a secondary end-point in most trials. In all cases, symptom relief was significantly greater with surgery than with medical treatment. The response of patients in the Veterans Administration study is typical. Figure 8.1 displays the symptom response of 354 medically-treated and 332 surgically-treated patients at one and five year follow-up [7]. The angina status of half the patients was unknown at baseline. Of those for whom this information is available, twice as many surgically-treated patients (approximately 60%) report mild or no angina at one year compared to medically-treated patients. Although the difference narrows somewhat at five years, there remains a statistically significant advantage favoring surgical therapy.

Percutaneous intervention versus medicine

The first published comparison of angioplasty and medical therapy was accomplished by the Veterans Administration Angioplasty

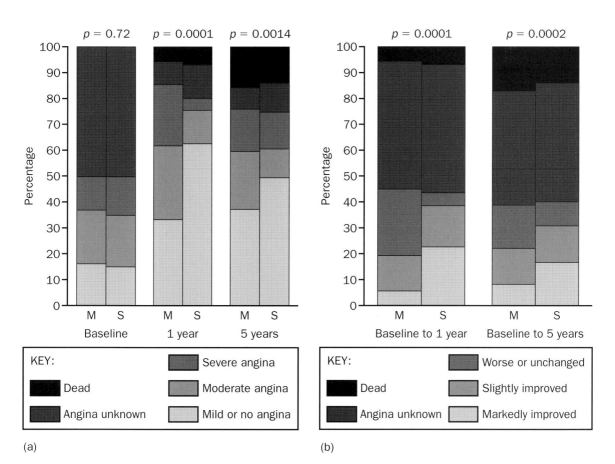

Figure 8.1
Severity (left panel) and change (right panel) of angina in 354 medically (M) and 332 surgically (S) treated patients. Surgically treated patients had less angina and greater improvement at both one and five years follow-up than patients randomized to medical treatment. (From reference 7, with permission.)

Compared to Medicine (ACME) study [8]. This trial randomly assigned 212 patients with stable single vessel coronary artery disease with objective evidence of ischemia on treadmill thallium stress testing to either an initial strategy of percutaneous transluminal coronary angioplasty (PTCA) or to a progressive program of anti-anginal drug therapy. Patients treated by PTCA were re-dilated if needed because of symptomatic re-stenosis. Patients treated medically underwent aggressive, step-wise treatment with beta-blockers, nitrates and calcium-channel blockers to either complete symptom suppression or maximal side-effect tolerance. All patients were interviewed monthly to assess angina status and returned at six months for repeat thallium stress testing and coronary angiography. Figure 8.2 shows the monthly percentage of the two treatment groups reporting *no* angina. At baseline only 8% of 107 medically-treated and 9% of 105 PTCA-treated patients reported no angina during the preceding 30 days. At six months 64% of PTCA-treated patients reported no angina during the preceding 30 days, compared to 46% of medically-treated patients ($p = 0.01$). For the PTCA group this improvement was most evident at the first month following randomization, while the medically-treated group improved gradually over the follow-up period. This advantage of PTCA over medical treatment appears to persist at 2.4 years mean follow-up when 63% of PTCA-treated patients and 49% of medically-treated patients were

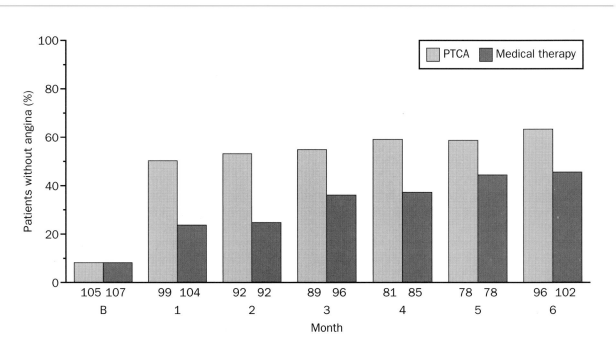

Figure 8.2
Patients who were free from angina at baseline (B) and at each month after random assignment to interventional (PTCA) or medical therapy. The numbers below the bars indicate how many patients from each treatment group were evaluated at each month. Interventionally treated patients had earlier and more complete relief than medically treated patients ($p = 0.01$ at six months). (From reference 8, with permission.)

angina-free. The statistical significance of this difference is borderline, however ($p = 0.08$). Underlying this difference in symptoms is a contrast in change in percent stenosis of index lesions for the two treatment groups at baseline compared to six months (Fig. 8.3). When the percent diameter stenosis of the medically-treated patients is virtually unchanged from baseline to six months, the stenosis of PTCA-treated patients falls from 79.2% to 53.8%. These differences in symptoms and stenosis might be even greater using current interventional methods employing stents.

The ACME trial also included a pilot study of 101 patients with double vessel coronary artery disease [9]. This group demonstrated a smaller difference in symptom relief compared to medical therapy, presumably due to greater restenosis and less complete revascularization engendered by multiple vessel interventions. A more definitive comparison of PTCA and medical therapy for patients with multivessel disease comes from the British Randomized Interventional Treatment of Angina group (RITA-2) who randomly assigned 1018 stable patients to PTCA or medical treatment [10]. Of these patients, 60% had single, 33% double and

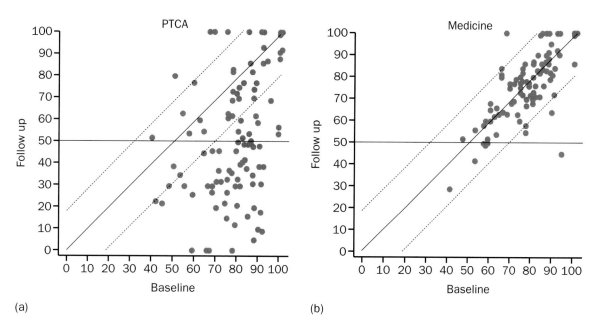

(a)　　　　　　　　　　　　　　　　　　(b)

Figure 8.3

Scatterplots representing the change in diameter stenosis from baseline to six months for 108 coronary artery lesions in 91 interventionally treated patients (PTCA) and for 103 lesions in 94 medically treated patients. The dotted lines on either side of the line of identity represent ±2 standard deviations (18.8%) of the technical variability of the caliper method. The mean percent diameter stenosis of the lesions in PTCA treated patients is reduced from 79.2 to 53.8 from baseline to follow-up. The mean diameter stenosis of medically treated patients remains unchanged. (From reference 2, with permission.)

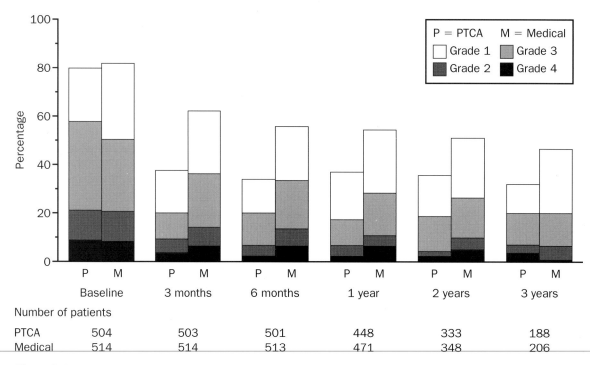

Figure 8.4
Severity of angina in 1018 patients randomized to medical (M) or interventional (PTCA) therapy in the RITA 2 Trial. Angina grades are those of the Canadian Cardiovascular Society classification. PTCA patients experience substantially greater relief from angina at three months which is sustained at three years. (From reference 10, with permission.)

7% triple vessel coronary artery disease. The angina status of the RITA-2 patients at baseline, three months, six months, one year, two years and three years follow-up is shown in Fig. 8.4. Again, RITA-2 shows the same advantage of coronary revascularization over medical treatment seen in the ACME trial and the VA surgical versus medical therapy trial. Roughly twice as many patients are rendered free from angina by revascularization during the first year, and this advantage persists three years later.

The symptom relief of coronary intervention comes with a cost, which must be factored into the treatment decision. While none of 107 medically-treated patients having single vessel

disease in the ACME study underwent coronary bypass surgery in the first six months, seven of 105 PTCA-treated patients required bypass [8], however, this difference disappeared by 2.4 years follow-up [11]. In RITA-2 the risk of death or non-fatal myocardial infarction was higher at 2.7 years follow-up for PTCA-treated patients (6.3%) compared to medically-treated patients (3.3%) [10]. Most of this difference was procedure-related, occurring in the first three months following randomization. Again, current techniques employing stents and glycoprotein IIb/IIIa inhibitors might be expected to reduce this difference.

Percutaneous intervention versus bypass surgery

PTCA and coronary bypass surgery have been compared in several major trials, including the Bypass Angioplasty Revascularization Investigation (BARI) [12], the Randomized Intervention Treatment of Angina (RITA) trial [13], the Coronary Angioplasty versus Bypass Revascularization Investigation (CABRI) [14], the Emory Angioplasty versus Surgery Trial (EAST) [15], the German Angioplasty Bypass Surgery Investigation (GABI) [16] and others. In BARI, 1829 patients judged suitable for either PTCA or bypass surgery were randomized to the two treatments. As demonstrated in Fig. 8.5,

patients assigned to bypass surgery had significantly less angina at six months, one and three years follow-up compared to angioplasty-treated patients. At five years the difference was less, but still statistically significant (20.3% PTCA versus 15.6% bypass, $p = 0.015$). Mortality was significantly better at seven years follow-up for surgical compared to PTCA treatment (survival = 84.4% versus 80.9%) [12]. This difference is virtually entirely due to a subgroup of 353 patients with treated diabetes mellitus for whom surgery conferred a particularly large survival advantage (76.4% versus 55.7%). Furthermore, the likelihood of repeat revascularization is much higher for PTCA patients at seven years than for surgically-treated patients

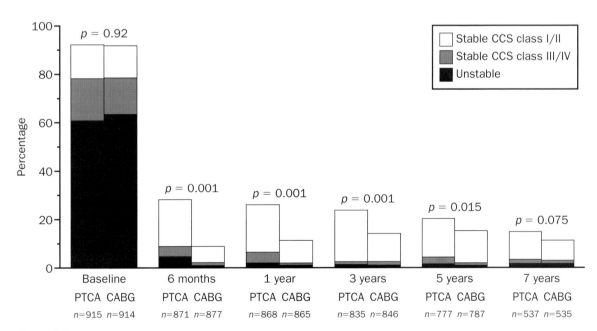

Figure 8.5
Severity of angina in 1829 patients having multivessel coronary artery disease who were randomized to angioplasty (PTCA) and coronary bypass surgery (CABG) in the BARI Trial. Severity is graded by the Canadian Cardiovascular Society (CCS) classification. Surgically treated patients experienced significantly greater relief from angina compared to those treated by angioplasty. (From reference 12, with permission.)

(59.7% versus 13.1%, $p < 0.001$). Once more, the BARI patients were studied prior to current methods of intervention and should be viewed in that light.

THE EFFECT OF REVASCULARIZATION ON EXERCISE PERFORMANCE

Coronary artery bypass versus medicine

Both the VA and CASS randomized studies compared exercise performance among patients randomized to medical and surgical treatment strategies. Approximately 55% of patients in the VA study underwent stress testing. A variety of protocols were employed; therefore, maximum oxygen consumption was utilized as a measure of exercise performance which is independent of the testing protocol. A highly significant advantage was seen for the surgically-treated patients for whom maximum oxygen consumption rose by 24% at both one and five years follow-up, in contrast to the medically-treated patients whose maximum oxygen consumption rose by 5% and 15%, respectively [17]. In CASS, treadmill exercise tests were performed at six, 18 and 60 months post-randomization. At all three follow-up points surgically assigned patients experienced significantly longer exercise time, less exercise-induced angina and less ST-segment depression (Fig. 8.6) [18].

Percutaneous intervention versus medicine

In the VA ACME trial of patients having stable single-vessel coronary artery disease, treadmill exercise time was a primary end-point. A highly significant advantage ($p < 0.0001$) was seen at six months among patients randomized to PTCA treatment for whom time on the modified Bruce protocol test increased by 2.1 minutes, in contrast to the patients randomized to medical treatment for whom treadmill time increased by 0.5 minutes [8]. Figure 8.7 demonstrates angina-free treadmill time for ACME patients at baseline and six months follow-up. The shift of the curves upward and to the right at six months indicates that both treatments are effective in reducing exercise-induced angina and prolonging treadmill time. The cohort randomized to PTCA demonstrates significantly better ($p < 0.01$) improvement in angina-free exercise time compared to medically treated patients.

In the RITA-2 trial, which included patients having multivessel as well as single vessel coronary artery disease, approximately 90% of patients had Bruce treadmill exercise tests at three, six, 12 and 36 month follow-up. Once again, patients randomized to PTCA demonstrated significantly greater improvement of exercise time when compared to the medically-treated cohort (Fig. 8.8) [10]. Furthermore, subgroup analysis in RITA-2 showed the greatest improvement among patients randomized to PTCA who had severe symptoms or limited exercise tolerance at the time of the baseline evaluation.

Percutaneous intervention versus bypass surgery

The RITA trial reports results of treadmill testing for 67% of 1011 patients having multivessel coronary artery disease who were technically suitable for PTCA or bypass surgery and were randomly assigned to the two treatment strategies [13]. As seen in Fig. 8.9, there is a significant initial advantage for PTCA-treated cohort in terms of improvement of exercise tolerance. However, at six, 12 and 24 month follow-up both groups were equally improved, increasing exercise duration on the Bruce protocol by approximately three minutes. The advantage for PTCA at one month is almost surely related to the fact that the surgical patients hadn't yet fully recovered from their operation.

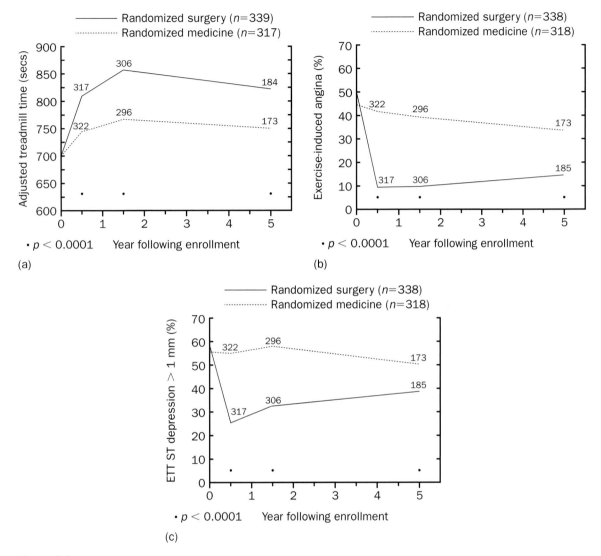

Figure 8.6
Treadmill exercise test results of 780 patients randomized to surgical or medical therapy in the Coronary Artery Surgery Study (CASS). (a) represents adjusted treadmill time, (b) exercise-induced angina and (c) ST segment depression of 1 mm or more. Surgically treated patients demonstrated advantages in all three categories. (From reference 18, with permission.)

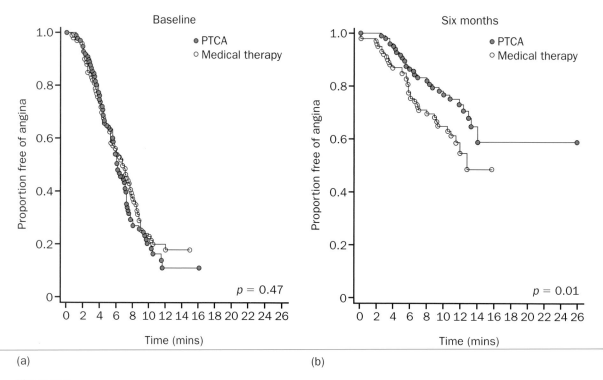

Figure 8.7
Duration of angina-free exercise on the treadmill for 212 patients randomized to angioplasty (PTCA) or medical therapy in the ACME Study. The proportion of patients who were free from angina is plotted on the vertical axis, and the length of time to onset of angina on the horizontal axis. Data were censored at the patients' total exercise time if they did not have angina during the test. (a) shows the treatment groups at baseline, and (b) shows the groups six months after randomization. Patients assigned to the PTCA treatment group increase their angina-free exercise time significantly more than those assigned to medical treatment. (From reference 8, with permission.)

SUMMARY

Both surgical and catheter-based approaches to coronary revascularization have been proven to be more effective than medical therapy in relieving ischemic symptoms and improving exercise performance. In general, both methods of revascularization are approximately twice as effective as drug therapy. Sixty to seventy percent of patients are rendered virtually free from symptoms by revascularization versus 30–40% by medical treatment after 6–12 months of therapy. Both methods also can be expected to improve average exercise tolerance measured by the Bruce treadmill protocol by 2–3 minutes, which is significantly greater than improvements observed with medical treatment. Patients demonstrating particular benefit compared to medical treatment are those who are most symptomatic and who have most limited treadmill performance prior to treatment. When bypass surgery and percutaneous intervention

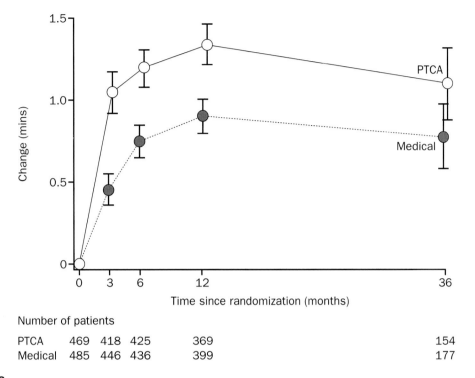

Number of patients

PTCA	469	418	425	369	154
Medical	485	446	436	399	177

Figure 8.8
Change in exercise time (mean minutes with standard error) at 3, 6, 12 and 36 months compared to baseline (0) for patients randomized to medical treatment and PTCA in the RITA-2 Trial. Patients assigned to PTCA demonstrated significantly greater improvement in treadmill exercise time compared to those assigned to medical therapy. (From reference 10, with permission.)

are compared against each other comparable benefits are seen, although symptom relief appears to be somewhat more complete with surgery, and treadmill performance improves more rapidly with percutaneous intervention. The benefits of surgery are more durable as evidenced by the greater likelihood of percutaneously-treated patients to return for repeat revascularization during the first year. This discrepancy is likely to diminish as further progress is achieved in prevention of recurrent stenosis following percutaneous intervention. Choice of treatment in any individual case requires integration of this information with other aspects of the patient's clinical situation, including co-morbidity such as diabetes mellitus, the particular coronary anatomy, the quality of left ventricular function and the nature of clinical presentation.

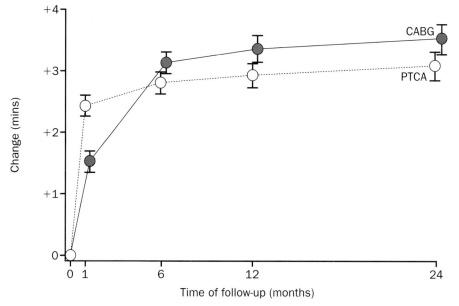

Number of patients and *p*-value for treatment difference were:

Group	1	6	12	24
			Time (mo)	
CABG	291	309	247	171
PTCA	318	322	276	191
p	0.0002	0.20	0.14	0.19

Figure 8.9
Change in exercise time (mean minutes with standard error) at 1, 6, 12 and 24 months compared to baseline (0) for patients randomized to PTCA and coronary bypass (CABG) in the RITA Trial. Both treatment groups experienced similar improvement except at one month when the surgically treated patients probably hadn't recovered fully from their operations. (From reference 13, with permission.)

REFERENCES

1. Bruce RA, Hornsten TR. Exercise stress testing in evaluation of patients with ischemic heart disease, *Prog Cardiovasc Dis* 1969; **11**:371–390.
2. Folland ED, Vogel RA, Hartigan P et al and the Veterans Affairs ACME Investigators. Relation between coronary artery stenosis assessed by visual, caliper, and computer methods and exercise capacity in patients with single-vessel coronary artery disease, *Circulation* 1994; **89**: 2005–2014.
3. Cobb LA, Thomas GI, Dillard DH, Merendino KA, Bruce RA. An evaluation of internal-mammary-artery ligation by a double-blind technic, *N Engl J Med* 1959; **260**:1115–1118.
4. The Veterans Administration Coronary Artery Bypass Surgery Cooperative Study Group. Eleven-year survival in the Veterans Administration randomized trial of coronary bypass surgery for stable angina, *N Engl J Med* 1984; **311**:1333–1339.
5. Varnauskas E and the European Coronary Surgery Study Group. Twelve-year follow-up of

survival in the Randomized European Coronary Surgery Study, *N Engl J Med* 1988; **319**:332–337.

6. CASS Principal Investigators and their associates. Myocardial infarction and mortality in the Coronary Artery Surgery Study (CASS) Randomized Trial, *N Engl J Med* 1984; **310**: 750–758.

7. Peduzzi P, Hultgren H, Miller C, Pfeifer J. The five-year effect of coronary artery bypass surgery on relief of angina, *Prog Cardiovasc Dis* 1986; **38**:267–272.

8. Parisi AF, Folland ED, Hartigan P on behalf of the Veterans Affairs ACME Investigators. A comparison of angioplasty with medical therapy in the treatment of single-vessel coronary artery disease, *N Engl J Med* 1992; **326**:10–16.

9. Folland ED, Hartigan PM, Parisi AF for the Veterans Affairs ACME Investigators. Percutaneous transluminal coronary angioplasty versus medical therapy for stable angina pectoris: outcomes for patients with double-vessel versus single-vessel coronary artery disease in a Veterans Affairs Cooperative randomized trial, *J Am Coll Cardiol* 1997; **29**:1505–1511.

10. RITA-2 Trial Participants. Coronary angioplasty versus medical therapy for angina: the Second Randomised Intervention Treatment of Angina (RITA-2) trial, *Lancet* 1997; **350**:461–468.

11. Hartigan PM, Giacomini JC, Folland ED, Parisi AF on behalf of the Veterans Affairs Cooperative Studies Program ACME Investigators. Two to three-year follow-up of patients with single-vessel coronary artery disease randomized to PTCA or medical therapy (results of a VA Cooperative Study), *Am J Cardiol* 1998; **82**: 1445–1450.

12. The BARI Investigators. Seven-year outcome in the Bypass Angioplasty Revascularization Investigation (BARI) by treatment and diabetic status, *J Am Coll Cardiol* 2000; **35**:1122–1129.

13. RITA Trial Participants. Coronary angioplasty versus coronary artery bypass surgery: the Randomised Intervention Treatment of Angina (RITA) trial, *Lancet* 1993; **341**:573–580.

14. CABRI trial participants. First year results of CABRI (Coronary Angioplasty versus Bypass Revascularization Investigation), *Lancet* 1995; **346**:1179–1184.

15. King SB III, Lembo NJ, Weintraub WS et al for the Emory Angioplasty versus Surgery Trial (EAST). A randomized trial comparing coronary angioplasty with coronary bypass surgery, *N Engl J Med* 1994; **331**:1044–1050.

16. Hamm CW, Reimers J, Ischinger T et al for the German Angioplasty Bypass Surgery Investigation (GABI). A randomized study of coronary angioplasty compared with bypass surgery in patients with symptomatic multivessel coronary disease, *N Engl J Med* 1994; **331**:1037–1043.

17. Hultgren H, Peduzzi P, Shapiro W, van Heeckeren D. Effect of medical versus surgical treatment on exercise performance at five years, *Prog Cardiovasc Dis* 1986; **38**:279–284.

18. CASS Principal Investigators and their associates. Coronary Artery Surgery Study (CASS): a randomized trial of coronary artery bypass surgery. Quality of life in patients randomly assigned to treatment groups, *Circulation* 1983; **68**:951–960.

9

Rationale and design for the Clinical Outcomes Utilizing Revascularization and Aggressive druG Evaluation (COURAGE) trial

William E Boden

CONTENTS • Introduction • Review of previous trials • Objectives of the COURAGE trial • Hypothesis • Design overview • Pre-randomization testing • Risk factor intervention • Intensive medical therapy: guidelines and management • Percutaneous coronary revascularization • Post-randomization management guidelines • Discussion

INTRODUCTION

Continued evolutions in medical therapy and percutaneous coronary interventions (PCI) have improved the outcomes associated with coronary heart disease (CHD). Previous clinical trials have compared these two therapeutic strategies in a randomized fashion, but have not been suitably powered to assess the combined benefit of these treatments on 'hard' prognostically important end-points (death, recurrent myocardial infarction (MI), re-hospitalization of biomarker-positive acute coronary syndrome (ACS)). These trials also predated the use of coronary stents and glycoprotein IIb/IIIa inhibitors and have not employed aggressive lipid-lowering as standardized therapy. These limitations affect the applicability of prior trial results to contemporary practice. This report describes the rationale and design for Clinical Outcomes Utilizing Revascularization and Aggressive druG Evaluation (COURAGE), a multicenter prospective, randomized trial comparing morbidity, mortality and resource utilization in patients with symptomatic CHD and objective evidence of myocardial ischemia following randomization to a strategy of PCI and intensive medical therapy versus intensive medical therapy alone. Patients with symptomatic CHD (CCS Class I–III) exhibiting objective signs of myocardial ischemia on stress testing with either single or multivessel CHD will be included, as well as patients with prior CABG surgery. Major exclusions are persistent CCS Class IV angina, angiographic left main stenosis > 50%, left ventricular ejection fraction (LVEF) < 30% or severe three-vessel CHD with proximal left anterior descending (LAD) disease > 70% and LVEF < 35%. The trial hypothesis is that the combination of PCI and aggressive, multifaceted medical therapy will be superior to intensive medical therapy alone. By combining these two therapeutic strategies, the results of COURAGE promises to advance a new treatment paradigm in the management of CHD, namely that the best clinical outcomes in symptomatic CHD patients can be achieved by a combination of catheterized revascularization coupled with aggressive medical therapy. As of April 2002, 1680 patients have been randomized.

Despite significant improvements in the management of coronary heart disease (CHD) in the last three decades, CHD remains the single most important cause of morbidity and mortality in the western world. Since the early 1970s, numerous large-scale clinical trials have established the respective roles of medical therapy, percutaneous coronary intervention (PCI) and coronary artery bypass grafting (CABG) in patients with stable and unstable CHD. Coronary artery bypass grafting surgery is considered the treatment of choice for patients with significant obstruction of the left main coronary artery, as well as for those with triple vessel disease and left ventricular systolic dysfunction. Percutaneous coronary intervention is recommended for a proximal coronary artery stenosis jeopardizing a large area of myocardium, stenosis producing severe inducible ischemia and for treatment of angina refractory to medical therapy [1]. Catheter-based techniques utilizing coronary stents have also improved the procedural success rate of coronary interventions and reduced complications such as restenosis.

Concurrent with the evolution of PCI and CABG surgery, there has been a revolution in the medical therapeutics of CHD. Aspirin has been proven to be of benefit in both primary and secondary prevention of coronary events [2]. Beta-blockers have been demonstrated conclusively to prolong life after myocardial infarction [3]. ACE inhibitors have been shown to favorably affect survival in a number of ways including the modulation of the renin angiotensin system and beneficial effects on

vascular remodeling [4, 5]. Numerous clinical trials have confirmed the important role of aggressive lipid-lowering and antiplatelet therapy along with optimal blood pressure control to reduce the progression of CHD [6–11]. To date however, no randomized trial has attempted to incorporate all of these proven therapeutic modalities in the setting of catheter-based revascularization for the management of patients with CHD.

REVIEW OF PREVIOUS TRIALS

The first randomized trial evaluating standard balloon PCI versus medical management was the Angioplasty Compared to Medicine study (ACME) trial. The ACME randomized 212 patients with stable angina or a recent MI (within three months) with angiographic evidence of 70% to 99% stenosis of one major coronary artery, and a positive exercise-tolerance test [12]. Exclusion criteria included previous CABG or PCI, or ongoing unstable angina. The primary end-points in this study were changes in exercise tolerance between baseline and follow-up exercise test, frequency of angina attacks, and the use of nitroglycerin between baseline and the final month of study. By six months, each group showed improvement in exercise capacity, although the PCI group had more improvement than the medical therapy group ($p = 0.01$). More PCI patients were angina-free ($p = 0.01$), but there was a higher incidence of subsequent CABG surgery in the PCI group [12]. The ACME trial also randomized a small number of patients with two-vessel coronary artery disease. This study suggested that the symptomatic improvement and increase of exercise tolerance associated with balloon PCI compared to medical therapy (principally aspirin, beta-blockers and nitrates) might be diminished for patients with two-vessel disease compared to patients with single-vessel disease [13].

The second trial comparing PCI to medical therapy was the recently completed RITA-2

(Randomized Intervention Treatment of Angina) trial conducted in the UK and Ireland [14]. A total of 1018 patients at 20 centers (40% with multi-vessel coronary artery disease), were randomized to PCI or medical therapy and were followed for a median of 2.7 years. Patients in the medical arm were treated with anti-anginal medications as in the ACME trial; lipid-lowering was left at the discretion of the supervising physician. The primary end-point was the composite of death and 'definite' myocardial infarction. At the trial conclusion, 32 PCI patients versus 17 patients managed medically suffered death or non-fatal MI (6.3% versus 3.3% $p = 0.02$). There were 21 (4.2%) non-fatal MIs in the PCI group versus 10 (2.0%) in the medically-treated group. This difference can be likely explained by the seven procedure-related infarcts in the PCI group. However, PCI patients with class II angina or poor exercise tolerance at baseline appeared to benefit with a 20% lower frequency of angina and better exercise performance. This benefit diminished, however, over the course of the following two years. The PCI group reported improved quality of life as compared with the medical group [15].

The MASS (The Medical Angioplasty and Surgery Study) trial, a single center randomized three-arm trial compared PCI, medical treatment and CABG (left internal mammary artery (LIMA) to the left anterior descending coronary artery) for the treatment of isolated severe proximal LAD stenosis in patients with a lesion ideal for treatment with PCI [16]. A total of 214 patients were randomized and followed for three years. The primary end-point of the study was the combined incidence of cardiac death, MI or refractory angina requiring revascularization. There was no difference in mortality or MI rate among the three groups. However, the combined end-point occurred more frequently in patients who received PCI (24%) and medical therapy (17%), compared to those assigned to CABG surgery (3% $p < 0.006$).

The Atorvastatin Versus Revascularization Treatment (AVERT) trial was an open-label, randomized, multicenter trial of patients with stable, minimally symptomatic coronary artery disease [17]. Patients with a serum LDL of > 115 mg/dl and a stenosis of 50% or more in at least one coronary artery were included in the study. The patients were randomized to receive treatment with 80 mg of atorvastatin per day or to undergo PCI (principally balloon angioplasty) followed by usual care. 'Usual Care' was not protocol-driven, did not mandate lipid-lowering and was left to the discretion of the treating physician. The patients were followed for 18 months. The primary end-point of the study was the between-group difference in a composite ischemic event (cardiovascular death, cardiac arrest, non-fatal myocardial infarction, the need for coronary bypass grafting or angioplasty, cerebrovascular accident, or worsening angina). Thirteen percent of patients in the atorvastatin arm versus 21% of patients in the PCI/usual care arm had an ischemic event, a difference of 36% ($p = 0.048$). Twelve percent of patients in the atorvastatin arm underwent a revascularization procedure, either CABG or PCI. Sixteen percent of patients in the PCI arm underwent a repeat revascularization procedure. Treatment with atorvastatin, as compared to PCI, was associated with a significantly longer time to a first ischemic event ($p < 0.03$), with a risk reduction of 36%.

There are shortcomings in the above-mentioned trials. In the ACME trial, only 4% of 9500 patients met eligibility criteria. This fact raises obvious concerns about the generalizability of this study to clinical practice. The trial was not powered to address the 'hard' clinical end-points of death or non-fatal MI. The ACME, RITA-2 and the MASS trials did not use aggressive lipid-lowering in any of the treatment arms. In addition, all the trials predated the use of glycoprotein IIb/IIIa inhibitors and the use of coronary stents. In AVERT, relatively simple medical therapy was used to compare one drug versus the usual care. None of the trials was configured to measure the combined benefit from all the therapies at the same time. All the trials were designed to establish the superiority of either PCI without concomitant medical treatment compared to medical therapy alone in the management of CHD (see Table 9.5).

OBJECTIVES OF THE COURAGE TRIAL

The principal objectives of the COURAGE trial are to assess prospectively both 'hard' end-point outcomes (death, non-fatal MI, re-hospitalization for biomarker-positive acute coronary syndrome), and other health care outcomes (resource utilization, quality of life measures, cost effectiveness and cost utility measures) during long-term (1.5–6 years) follow-up after randomization to PCI, plus intensive medical therapy versus intensive medical therapy alone in all but the very highest risk CHD patients who meet one or more ACC/AHA Joint Task Force Class I (definite) or II (probable) indication for PCI [1].

HYPOTHESIS

The hypothesis of the COURAGE trial is that clinically meaningful long-term outcomes (death, non-fatal MI, resource utilization and quality of life) in all but the very highest risk CHD patients will be superior in patients randomized to a strategy of optimal catheter-based PCI and intensive medical therapy compared to those who are randomized to a strategy of intensive medical therapy alone during a minimum three year follow-up, when outcomes are compared using the intention-to-treat principle.

We project a cumulative three-year event rate of 19% in the medical therapy only arm and 15% in the PCI plus medical therapy arm (absolute difference of 4%; relative difference of 21%). A sample size of 2964 patients will be needed to test the hypothesis with a power of 80%. If a cumulative loss to follow-up rate of 10% is factored in for the duration of the trial, an adjusted sample size of 3120 is necessary to achieve the required number of end-points.

Randomization will take place over a period of four years and all patients will be followed for a minimum of one and a half years. All statistical analyses will be performed using two-sided tests with a level of significance at 0.05.

DESIGN OVERVIEW

The COURAGE trial is a large-scale multicenter, randomized controlled trial that is powered for a composite trial primary end-point of all-cause mortality, non-fatal MI, and hospitalized ACS with biomarker (troponin) positivity. Secondary trial end-points include quality of life assessment, resource utilization, and hospitalization for unstable angina with negative biomarkers. Major trial end-points are listed in Table 9.1.

Patients eligible for inclusion will consist of those with chronic angina pectoris (CCS Class I–III), stable post-MI patients and asymptomatic myocardial ischemia who have either single or multi-vessel CAD (Table 9.2). The only major exclusions to patient enrollment will be persistent CCS Class IV angina status refractory to medical therapy, angiographic unprotected left main stenosis > 50%, left ventricular ejection fraction < 30% in patients with multi-vessel CAD, and a markedly-positive (e.g., Bruce Stage I) exercise stress test. Exclusion criteria are listed in Table 9.3.

PRE-RANDOMIZATION TESTING

Patients who are protocol-eligible based on the clinical inclusion/exclusion criteria will first undergo non-invasive diagnostic testing including an assessment of LV ejection fraction (radionuclide ventriculography, 2-D echocardiography or left ventricular contrast angiography) and a stress test (exercise treadmill, pharmacologic and exercise myocardial perfusion scintigraphy, exercise or pharmacologic wall motion analysis) to verify and quantify objective evidence of inducible myocardial ischemia or regional wall motion abnormality, unless there are new, resting ischemic electrocardiographic (ECG) changes, or if the patient presents with ACS with symptoms of definite or classic angina and has a caliper-measured lesion ≥ 80%, or if the patient has definite or classic angina with one lesion at least 70% stenosed and another coronary artery at least 50% stenosed.

Table 9.1 Trial end-points

1. Primary
   - All-cause mortality
   - Non-fatal MI*
   - Hospitalized ACS with biomarker positivity
2. Secondary
   - Quality of life measures
   - Resource utilization, cost, cost effectiveness analysis
   - Hospitalization for unstable angina with negative biomarkers
3. Tertiary
   - Death
   - MI
   - Stroke
   - Cardiac mortality
   - Myocardial revascularization (PCI or CABG)
   - Death, MI or hospitalization for unstable angina
   - Hospitalization for CHF
   - Hospitalization for other cardiac events
   - Repeat cardiac catheterization
   - Angina status (Canadian Cardiovascular Society Class)
   - Exercise treadmill test (ETT) duration

---

*MI: (a) Spontaneous: Total CK ≥ 1.5 × UNL with ≥ 5% MB fraction. (b) Peri PCI: Total CK ≥ 3.0 × UNL with ≥ 5% MB fraction. (c) Peri CABG: Total CK ≥ 5.0 × UNL with ≥ 5% MB fraction.

The two therapeutic strategies, which will be compared randomly, are PCI (balloon PTCA, directional coronary atherectomy, rotoblator or coronary stents, alone or in combination) in addition to intensive medical therapy, versus a strategy of intensive medical therapy alone (defined below). Within each medical center, patients will be randomized into two strata based on the history of prior CABG surgery. Other subgroups of particular interest include extent of CAD (single versus multi-vessel), history of prior MI, diabetes, LV function (EF > 50% versus EF 30–50%), demographic variables, and various risk categories.

In patients who are randomized to the PCI and intensive medical therapy arm, PCI should be performed within 105 days of the diagnostic catheterization. If coronary anatomy is suitable for myocardial revascularization, potential study subjects will be randomized to either arm and treated. Procedure and catheterization films will be forwarded to the Angiographic Core Laboratory for assessment and coding.

RISK FACTOR INTERVENTION

The COURAGE trial site clinical coordinator will perform a comprehensive risk factor assessment, including fasting blood tests. Patients will be counseled prior to discharge and an individualized risk intervention program will be devised for each patient regarding diet, weight loss, smoking cessation/relapse prevention and the role of regular aerobic exercise. The intervention and goals are based largely on AHA guidelines and are summarized in Tables 9.4–9.7 [18].

INTENSIVE MEDICAL THERAPY: GUIDELINES AND MANAGEMENT

Medical therapy in COURAGE will conform to current updated AHA treatment guidelines [19]. It is aggressive and multifaceted, targeted for the dual purpose of achieving athero-

Table 9.2 Inclusion criteria

1. CCS class I–III CHD patients, including patients with:
   - Prior PCI or CABG with objective evidence of ischemia.
   - Chronic stable angina.
   - Post-MI patients without Class IV angina, severe LV dysfunction or arrhythmia.
   - Asymptomatic ischemia detected by exercise or perfusion scintigraphy or 24 hour ambulatory ECG monitoring.
   - Patients with an 80% or greater lesion in one or more vessels subtending a 'large area' of myocardium even in the absence of objective evidence for ischemia.
2. Patients who meet an existing ACC/AHA Joint Task Force Class I or II indications for PCI. These indications are:
   - Single vessel CAD patients who are asymptomatic to severely symptomatic and who have a 'large area' of ischemic myocardium subtending a significant (> 50% diameter reduction) coronary stenosis (ACC/AHA Class I indication) or a 'moderate area' of ischemia (ACC/AHA Class II indication).
   - Multi-vessel CAD patients who are asymptomatic or mildly symptomatic who have a 'large ischemic area' or 'moderate ischemic area' (ACC/AHA Class II indication) for asymptomatic or minimally symptomatic patients.
3. Has at least one vessel for angioplasty meeting one of the following criteria:
   - RCA: proximal to the PDA in a right dominant vessel.
   - LCX: proximal to two or more OM branches or proximal to the PDA and PL branches in a left dominant vessel.
   - LAD: proximal or mid vessel.
   - SVG or LIMA: graft must supply the same regions as outlined above or in the opinion of the interventionalist the coronary stenosis subtends a major mass of myocardium.
4. Has objective evidence of myocardial ischemia including one of the following:
   - Spontaneous new ST-T changes on resting ECG defined as either $\geq$ 1.0 mm ST-segment deviation from the baseline (80 mm from J point) or > 2.0 mm T wave inversion (or pseudonormalizations if the T waves were previously inverted) in a minimum of two contiguous leads within one of three ECG lead groups (anterior = V1–4; inferior = II, III, aVF; lateral = I, aVL, V5–6).
   - Objective evidence of stress induced myocardial ischemia as detected by standard 12 lead exercise stress test; exercise or pharmacological stress (adenosine or dipyridamole) coupled with perfusion scintigraphy (technetium sestamibi or thallium-based isotopes); exercise or pharmacological stress (dobutamine) coupled with 2-D echocardiography or exercise radionuclide ventriculography, based on one of the following:
     (a) Less than 1.0 mm ST-segment deviation from baseline on standard treadmill exercise using 12 lead ECG.
     (b) One or more scintigraphic perfusion defects (reversible or partial reversible) during exercise technetium sestamibi or thallium-based isotope imaging.
     (c) One or more scintigraphic perfusion defects (reversible or partial reversible) with pharmacological stress (dipyridamole, adenosine) during technetium sestamibi or thallium imaging.
     (d) One or more wall motion abnormalities during exercise radionuclide ventriculography or 2-dimension echocardiography (exercise or dobutamine).

Table 9.3 Exclusion criteria

1. CHD associated with unstable angina and symptoms refractory to maximal oral and intravenous medical therapy (persistent CCS Class IV).
2. Post-MI course complicated by persistent rest angina, shock, and persistent CHF, etc., for which the need or likelihood of urgent myocardial revascularization is high.
3. Coronary angiographic exclusions:
   - Patients with no prior CABG and left main coronary disease ≥ 50%.
   - Coronary arteries technically unsuitable or hazardous for PCI.
   - Patients with non-significant coronary artery disease in whom PCI would not be considered appropriate or indicated.
4. Ejection fraction < 30%, except < 35% if patients have three-vessel disease including > 70% LAD proximal stenosis.
5. Cardiogenic shock.
6. Pulmonary edema or CHF unresponsive to standard medical therapy.
7. CABG or PCI within the last 6 months.
8. Concomitant valvular heart disease likely to require surgery or affect prognosis during follow-up period.
9. Congenital or primary cardiac muscle disease likely to affect prognosis during follow-up period.
10. Resuscitated out of hospital, sudden death or symptomatic sustained or non-sustained ventricular tachycardia.
11. Significant systemic hypertension (BP > 200/100 mmHg) unresponsive to medical therapy.
12. Lipid exclusion criteria: fasting TG > 400 mg/dl, LDL > 250 mg/dl, LDL > 200 if already on a HMG COA reductase inhibitor.
13. Pregnant or women likely to become pregnant.
14. Significant co-morbidity likely to cause death in the 1.5–6 year follow-up period.
15. Significant active history of substance abuse.
16. Refusal to give informed consent or follow study protocol.
17. Participation in another long-term clinical trial.
18. Refusal of patient's physician to allow participation in the study.

---

sclerotic plaque stabilization (or regression), and reducing subsequent ischemic events. The guidelines are provided to ensure a consistent therapeutic approach with the understanding that a particular drug may be administered for more than one purpose. The goals of therapy are to keep COURAGE patients as symptom-free as possible within their individual tolerance for medication, and to configure prophylactic therapy targeted to abolish ischemia and treat aggressively all abnormal cardiac risk factors.

All patients will receive antithrombotic therapy with aspirin (enteric coated) 80–325 mg/day. In case of aspirin allergy, clopidogrel 75 mg/day will be prescribed. For patients with stable CCS class I–III angina, the post-randomization anti-ischemic therapy is outlined in Table 9.5. Patients with unstable angina will be characterized as low- to high-risk

Table 9.4 Risk factor goals

1. Smoking	Cessation	
2. Total dietary fat	< 30% Calories	
3. Saturated fat	< 7% Calories	
4. Dietary cholesterol	< 200 mg/day	
5. LDL cholesterol	60–85 mg/dl (1.56–2.21 mmol/L)	
6. HDL cholesterol (Secondary goal)	> 40 mg/dl (1.04 mmol/L)	
7. Triglycerides (TG) (Secondary goal)	< 150 mg/dl (1.69 mmol/L)	
8. Physical activity	30–45 minutes of moderate intensity activity five times/week supplemented by an increase in daily lifestyle activities.	
9. Body weight by Body Mass Index (BMI)	Initial BMI	Weight loss goal
• Desirable < 25	25–27.5	BMI < 25
• Overweight 25.0–29.0	> 27.5	10% relative weight loss
• Obese > 30.0	> 27.5	10% relative weight loss
10. Blood pressure	< 130/85 mmHg	
11. Diabetes	HbA1c < 7.0%	

by the criteria indicated in Table 9.6 and therapy will be initiated according to Table 9.7. If an unstable angina patient is randomized to PCI plus aggressive medical therapy, unfractionated heparin and tirofiban will be continued for a minimum of 12 hours post-PCI with a total duration of therapy of at least 48 hours. If an acute coronary syndrome patient is randomized to aggressive medical therapy only, tirofiban and heparin will be continued for 48 hours. The stabilized patient will then undergo non-invasive stress testing to assess the severity of the residual ischemia. Coronary angiography followed by myocardial revascularization will be considered for those patients with severe residual ischemia.

In keeping with published therapeutic guidelines, the goal of antihypertensive therapy will be to achieve and maintain a target blood pressure (BP) of 130/85 mmHg or below [20]. All patients with BP exceeding 130/85 mmHg will be prescribed antihypertensive therapy. If therapy is needed ACE inhibitor (lisinopril), beta-blocker without ISA, amlodipine, angiotensin II receptor blocker (losartan) or a diuretic may be used. Within each treatment class, an attempt will be made to maximize the dosage, as tolerated clinically, to achieve and maintain the desired treatment targets. If the blood pressure remains elevated a second drug from a different class may be added to achieve the target goal.

The centerpiece of medical therapy in each arm of the COURAGE trial is aggressive low-density lipoprotein (LDL) reduction (cholesterol range of 60–85 mg/dl). Secondary goals include achieving and maintaining high-density lipoprotein cholesterol levels > 40 mg/dl and triglyceride levels < 150 mg/dl. Fasting lipid profiles will be analyzed at the

Table 9.5 Anti-ischemic therapy for patients with stable CHD

		LVEF > 40%	LVEF < 40%
Recommendation	Secondary prevention	Q wave MI	
		Long-acting metoprolol	ACE inhibitor (lisinopril)
		Non-Q wave MI	
		Diltiazem or long acting metoprolol	Long acting metoprolol (if tolerated)
		+/− ACE inhibitor	
Guidelines	Symptomatic ischemia	Maximize-existing drug therapy	Maximize existing drug therapy
		Amlodipine	Amlodipine
		Long-acting metoprolol	Long-acting metoprolol
		Isosorbide 5-mononitrate	Isosorbide 5-mononitrate
	Silent ischemia		
		Amlodipine	Amlodipine
		Long-acting metoprolol	Long-acting metoprolol
		Isosorbide 5-mononitrate	Isosorbide 5-mononitrate
	Diabetics		
		ACE inhibitor	
		recommended for all	
		diabetics	

core laboratory at baseline, six months and annually, until the end of the trial. Simvastatin will be used as the first line of therapy to achieve and maintain the aggressive LDL-cholesterol goal. If additional LDL reduction is required on maximum-dose simvastatin (80 mg QD), a bile acid sequestrant will be added. A lipid management algorithm for initiating and titrating simvastatin therapy is listed in Table 9.8. Patients with HDL < 40 mg/dl will be treated with extended release niacin (Niaspan).

The goal for diabetes management in COURAGE patients is to maintain fasting blood glucose levels between 80–126 mg/dl and HBA$_{1C}$ levels at < 7.0%. These guidelines are in accord with published recommendations of the American Diabetes Association and the DCCT Consensus Report [21, 22]. As new therapies become available during the course of the trial, and their safety and efficacy are demonstrated,

they will be incorporated as part of the therapeutic and risk intervention program.

PERCUTANEOUS CORONARY REVASCULARIZATION

In patients randomized to PCI plus medical therapy, the intent will be to perform as complete a myocardial revascularization as possible, while minimizing the possibility of procedure-related complications. In all patients, procedural strategy will be predetermined.

Revascularization of the culprit stenosis will be undertaken, as guided by the previously obtained non-invasive testing. In patients with multi-vessel disease, complete myocardial revascularization will not be mandated by protocol if, in the judgement of the operator, this poses undue risk to the patient. Complete myocardial

Table 9.6 Risk categorization for patients with unstable angina/non-ST segment elevation

Patient characteristics	High risk	Intermediate risk	Low risk
Angina	Rest angina with at least one of the following:	Current or recent rest angina without high risk criteria but with at least one of the following:	No CCS III or IV angina but angina with at least one of the following:
Other criteria	• Prolonged ongoing course (> 20 min) • ST segment depression > 1 mm during pain in multiple leads • Elevated serum level of cardiac markers of ischemic injury (Troponin I or T) • Clinical or laboratory evidence of LV systolic dysfunction	• Deep T wave inversions (> 3 mm) in multiple leads • Age > 65 years • Diabetes mellitus • New CCS Class III or IV angina within the past two weeks • Prior myocardial infarction by history or ECG evidence	• Increased angina frequency, severity, or duration with activity • Angina provoked at a lower threshold • New onset angina within two weeks or two months of presentation • Any of the above with normal or unchanged ECG

Table 9.7 Therapy according to risk stratification for patients with unstable angina

High risk	Intermediate risk	Low risk
Aspirin, beta-blockers, nitrates, unfractionated heparin, low molecular weight heparin and glycoprotein IIb/IIIa inhibitors	Aspirin, beta-blockers, nitrates, unfractionated heparin, low molecular weight heparin and glycoprotein IIb/IIIa inhibitors	Aspirin, beta-blockers, amlodipine, and nitrates as needed

Table 9.8 Lipid algorithm for COURAGE

Primary goal	LDL 60–85 mg/dl	

1. Initiating therapy
   - For subjects on statins other than simvastatin:

LDL (mg/dl)	Initial therapy
< 60	Back titrate to simvastatin at equivalent half dose
50–85	Simvastatin at equivalent dose
> 85	Simvastatin dose at one step higher than current equivalent

   - For subjects not on any lipid medication at baseline:

LDL (mg/dl)	Initial therapy
< 100	Simvastatin 10 mg qhs
100–129	Simvastatin 20 mg qhs
> 130	Simvastatin 40 mg qhs

2. Titrating therapy

• LDL > 85 mg/dl	Double dose every 4–6 weeks until LDL < 85 mg/dl
• LDL < 50 mg/dl	Back titrate to previous dose
• LDL > 85 mg/dl Simvastatin 80 mg	Add bile acid binding resin and titrate, as necessary

Secondary goals	HDL	> 40 mg/dl
	Triglycerides	< 150 mg/dl

qhs, at bedtime.

revascularization will also not be undertaken if incomplete revascularization is thought to be adequate, based upon regional left ventricular function, collateral flow to the chronic total occlusion, or nuclear perfusion imaging.

Prior to the procedure, patients will receive aspirin (> 160 mg/dl) for at least one day and one dose of a calcium-channel blocker. Heparin will be administered and activated clotted time will be maintained at a level dependent on the use of glycoprotein IIb/IIIa inhibitors. Twelve lead ECGs will be obtained before and within 24 hours after the procedure. Creatine kinase levels with myocardial isoenzymes will be measured at eight and 16 hours after the procedure or before discharge. Following the procedure, calcium-channel blockers will be continued for at least one month and aspirin (325 mg) will be continued indefinitely. In patients with stent placements, clopidogrel treatment will be used for a period of 2–4 weeks after the procedure.

Angiographic success will be defined as a reduction in the stenosis to less than 50% or a 20% reduction in the stenosis. When a stent is placed, angiographic success will be defined as a residual stenosis of less than 10% and normal TIMI grade 3 flow. Clinical success will be defined as angiographic success plus the absence of in-hospital MI, emergency CABG or death.

Medical therapy will be initiated as soon as possible after randomization. Except for beta-blocker or calcium-channel blocker for post-MI secondary prevention, an attempt will be made to discontinue all routine anti-ischemic medical therapy within 3–6 months after randomization to PCI in patients who remain asymptomatic after a successful PCI procedure. If symptoms persist or recur, medical therapy will be maintained or reinitiated, respectively.

POST-RANDOMIZATION MANAGEMENT GUIDELINES

Regular protocol-mandated assessments (clinic visits) and procedures (ECG, stress testing, lipid profiles, quality of life assessments) will be performed at specified intervals after discharge. If a patient develops worsening or persistent angina after randomization to intensive medical therapy, the following management guidelines will be used:

- In all patients with CCS Class I–III angina, intensify medical therapy; if the patient stabilizes to CCS Class I–II, continue medical therapy indefinitely.
- If symptoms do not stabilize, or progress after 6–8 weeks of maximum medical therapy, patients should undergo stress testing with ECG-gated sestamibi SPECT imaging. If there is a high-risk result (EF < 35% or severe reversible ischemia) the patient should undergo catheterization and revascularization, as indicated clinically.

If a patient destabilizes after being randomized to PCI plus medical therapy, the following guidelines are recommended:

- For patients with CCS Class I–II, and no evidence of spontaneous ischemic ECG changes at rest, a repeat stress test (exercise or pharmacological) with ECG-gated sestamibi imaging will be obtained. If this is positive for severe inducible ischemia or EF < 35%, the patient should be considered for re-catheterization.
- If the patient is CCS Class III–IV after maximizing medical therapy, repeat cardiac catheterization and/or PCI should be performed.

DISCUSSION

Evidence-based medicine has evolved to include a multitude of pharmacologic interventions, which have been demonstrated conclusively to reduce long-term cardiac events. The roles of aspirin, beta-blockers and ACE inhibitors have been elucidated in multiple well-designed and conducted randomized trials. Although the individual roles of these interventions have been established, no study has examined clinical outcomes utilizing the combination of all proven therapies to assess their impact on reducing the clinical event rates due to CHD.

The COURAGE trial is the first randomized controlled trial whose central goal is to utilize multifaceted, aggressive guideline-driven medical therapy with or without PCI. Equal importance will be given to the preventive aspect of CHD treatment and an organized effort will be made to modify risk factors and co-morbid conditions.

Another important trial end-point is to analyze the health economics associated with the two therapeutic approaches. The literature reveals only a modest amount of descriptive data or methodological approaches that are useful in evaluating cost and outcomes associated with PCI. The vast majority of published literature has limited generalizability or comparability. Moreover, there is virtually no economic data that can be used for medical decision-making regarding the choice between medical therapy and medical therapy in combination with PCI. In the COURAGE trial, we will determine the cost and effectiveness of PCI in the setting of optimal medical therapy. Comprehensive information regarding in-hospital costs of PCI and cumulative health costs will be gathered over a period of three years.

Improvements in the quality of life (QOL) are also considered a significant end-point in the medical care of patients with CHD [23, 24]. Health-related QOL is characterized by its application to well-being and satisfaction associated with how an individual is affected by disease, accidents and treatment [25]. The assessment of health economics and QOL outcomes are moving into a new era as clinical trials attempt to intertwine these two domains in analyzing the effectiveness and utility of interventions. Two major approaches have emerged, including psychometric methods and utility assessment [26]. In the COURAGE trial, prospective QOL assessment is embedded in the trial proper, along with economic measures to determine overall cost quality outcomes. This approach will also enhance the interpretation of the trial outcomes and increase the value of the data for health policy implementation.

Despite the wide applicability of PCI in the management of CHD, no long-term, prospective randomized trial has been designed and powered to compare its effect coupled with contemporary multifaceted aggressive medical therapy, on incident CHD morbidity and mortality. The COURAGE trial seeks to advance a new treatment paradigm in the management of symptomatic CHD. It emphasizes the role of PCI with an equal emphasis on the role of intensive medical therapy in the management of patients with CHD. This management strategy has not been tested in a large-scale multicenter, randomized clinical trial to date.

REFERENCES

1. Ryan TJ, Bauman WB, Kennedy JW et al. Guidelines for percutaneous transluminal coronary angioplasty: a report of the American Heart Association/American College of Cardiology Task Force on Assessment of Diagnostic and Therapeutic Cardiovascular Procedures (Committee on Percutaneous Transluminal Coronary Angioplasty), *Circulation* 1993; **88**:2987–3007.
2. Yusuf S, Wittes J, Friedman L. Overview of results of randomized clinical trials in heart disease 1. Treatments following myocardial infarction, *JAMA* 1988; **260**:2088.
3. Beta Blocker Heart Attack Trial Research Group. A randomized trial of propranolol in patients with acute myocardial infarction, *JAMA* 1982; **247**:1707–1714.
4. Pfeiffer MA, Braunwald E, Moye LA et al. Effect of captopril on mortality and morbidity in patients with left ventricular dysfunction after myocardial infarction: results of the survival and ventricular enlargement trial, *N Engl J Med* 1992; **327**:669.
5. The SOLVD investigators. Effect of angiotensin converting enzyme inhibitor enalapril on survival in patients with reduced left ventricular ejection fraction and congestive heart failure, *N Engl J Med* 1991; **325**:293.
6. Brown BG, Zhao X-Q, Sacco DE et al. Lipid lowering and plaque regression: new insights into prevention of plaque disruption and clinical events in coronary disease, *Circulation* 1993; **87**:1781–1791.
7. Blankenhom DH, Azen SP, Dramsch D et al. Coronary angiographic changes with lovastatin therapy: the Monitored Atherosclerosis Regression Study (MARS), *Ann Int Med* 1993; **119**:969–976.
8. Waters D, Higginson L, Gladstone P et al. Effect of monotherapy with an HMG CoA reductase inhibitor on the progression of coronary atherosclerosis as assessed by serial quantitative arteriography: the Canadian Coronary Atherosclerosis Intervention Trial, *Circulation* 1994; **89**:959–968.
9. Waters D, Craven TE, Lesperance J. Prognostic significance of progression of coronary atherosclerosis, *Circulation* 1993; **87**:1067–1075.
10. Scandinavian Simvastatin Survival Study Group. Randomized trial of cholesterol lowering in 4444 patients with coronary heart disease: the Scandinavian Simvastatin Survival Study (4S), *Lancet* 1994; **344**:1383.
11. Shepherd J, Cobbe SM, Ford I et al. Prevention of coronary heart disease with pravastatin in men with hypercholesterolemia, *N Engl J Med* 1995; **333**:1301–1307.
12. Parisi AF, Folland ED, Hartigan P et al. A comparison of angioplasty with medical therapy in the treatment of single-vessel coronary artery disease, *N Engl J Med* 1992; **326**:10–16.
13. Folland ED, Hartigan PM, Parisi AF. Percutaneous; transluminal coronary angioplasty (PTCA) compared to medical therapy for stable angina pectoris. Outcomes for patients with double-vessel compared to single-vessel coronary artery disease in a randomized VA Cooperative study, *J Am Coll Cardiol* 1997; **29**:1505–1511.

14. RITA-2 Trial Participants. Coronary angioplasty versus medical therapy for angina: the second Randomized Intervention Treatment of Angina (RITA-2) trial, *Lancet* 1997; **350**:461–469.

15. Pocock SJ, Henderson RA, Rickards AF et al. Meta-analysis of randomised trials comparing coronary angioplasty with bypass surgery, *Lancet* 1995; **346**:1184–1189.

16. Hueb WA, Bellotti G, De Oliveira SA et al. The Medicine, Angioplasty or Surgery Study (MASS): a prospective, randomized trial of medical therapy, balloon angioplasty or bypass surgery for single proximal left anterior descending artery stenosis. *J Am Coll Cardiol* 1995; **26**:1600–2605.

17. Pitt B, Waters D, Brown WV, van Boeven AJ, Schwartz L, Title LM. Aggressive lipid-lowering therapy compared with angioplasty in stable coronary artery disease (for the Atorvastatin Versus Revascularization Treatment Investigators), *N Engl J Med* 1999; **341**:70–76.

18. Grundy SM, Balady GJ, Criqui MH et al. Guide to primary prevention of cardiovascular diseases. A statement for healthcare professionals from the Task Force on Risk Reduction. American Heart Association Science Advisory and Coordinating Committee, *Circulation* 1997; **95:** 2329–2331.

19. Smith SC, Blair SN, Criqui MH et al. Preventing heart attack and death in patients with coronary disease, *Circulation* 1995; **92**:2–4.

20. Report of the Joint National Committee on Detection, Evaluation and Treatment of High Blood Pressure. A cooperative study, *JAMA* 1997; **237**:255–261.

21. American Diabetes Association. Standards of medical care for patients with diabetes mellitus (position statement), *Diabetes Care* 1997; **20** (suppl 1):S5–S13.

22. DCCT Research Group. The effect of intensive diabetes treatment on the development and progression of long-term complications in insulin-dependent diabetes mellitus. The Diabetes Control and Complications Trial, *N Engl J Med* 1993; **329**:977.

23. Wenger N, Furberg C. Cardiovascular disorders. In: Spilker B, ed. *Quality of Life Assessments in Clinical Trials* (New York: Raven Press, 1990) 335–345.

24. Stewart A. Conceptual and methodological issues in defining quality of life: state of the art, *Prog in Cardiovasc Nursing* 1992; **7**:3–11.

25. Grant M, Padilla GV, Ferrell BR et al. Assessment of quality of life with a single instrument, *Sem Oncol Nurs* 1990; **6**:260–270.

26. Dedhiya S, Kong SX. Quality of life: an overview of the concept and measures, *Pharm World Sci* 1995; **17**:114–118.

10

Results of randomized controlled trials in patients with non-ST segment elevation acute coronary syndromes (TIMI-IIIB, VANQWISH, FRISC-II, TACTICS TIMI-18)

William E Boden

CONTENTS • Use of non-invasive and invasive testing in risk stratification • Medical management versus coronary intervention in patients with stable coronary artery disease • Trials of non-ST segment elevation acute coronary syndromes (non-Q wave MI or unstable angina) • Differential rates of revascularization among trials and use of adjunctive therapies • Tailored therapeutic modalities and intensity to risk profile

USE OF NON-INVASIVE AND INVASIVE TESTING IN RISK STRATIFICATION

The management of acute coronary syndromes has been largely predicated on the performance of routine, diagnostic coronary angiography to define abnormal coronary anatomy. Such an approach seeks to identify the so-called culprit stenosis, or stenoses, for which the goal is to perform myocardial revascularization with either coronary bypass surgery or percutaneous coronary intervention (PCI). Presumably, the purpose of performing early coronary angiography and myocardial revascularization is to improve both short-term and long-term clinical outcomes. Unquestionably, this management approach is associated with improved symptoms and quality of life short term, but it remains unclear whether such a strategy favorably alters clinical outcomes such as death or recurrent non-fatal myocardial infarction.

Prior to undertaking an invasive evaluation, it seems most appropriate to achieve control of symptoms and objective findings of myocardial ischemia in patients who present at hospital with unstable angina. In the majority of patients, bed rest and intensification of antithrombotic (IV heparin and aspirin), anti-ischemic (IV nitroglycerin plus calcium-channel blocker and/or beta-blocker) and/or platelet glycoprotein IIb/IIIa receptor antagonist therapy will be effective pharmacotherapy.

In patients who have persistent or refractory symptoms of angina, or recurrent ECG findings of myocardial ischemia, despite maximal medical therapy, or if patients demonstrate hemodynamic instability, use of intra-aortic balloon counterpulsation may be extremely effective, until cardiac catheterization and myocardial revascularization can be safely performed.

If coronary angiography cannot be deferred as an elective procedure because the patient exhibits persistent, or recurrent, ischemia despite intensification of medical therapy, prompt coronary angiography must be undertaken, followed by myocardial revascularization, if possible. Clearly, the risk of undertaking PCI or coronary artery bypass graft (CABG) surgery is higher in such patients, compared to the morbidity associated with performing such revascularization procedures on stable elective coronary artery disease (CAD) patients. Nevertheless, myocardial revascularization may be the most appropriate strategy to undertake in those patients with unstable angina whose myocardium is at risk for infarction, and should be reserved for those patients who do not adequately respond to medical therapy.

The approach to the 'stabilized' unstable angina patient is somewhat more controversial. One approach would be to subject *all* unstable angina patients to diagnostic coronary angiography, irrespective of their initial response to medical therapy in the CCU. The rationale for this approach is that the acute coronary syndrome was likely presaged by accelerated coronary atherosclerosis, and the 'stabilization' achieved with medical therapy is likely only to be temporary, and is not likely to affect the underlying coronary stenosis or stenoses.

However, studies have indicated that most coronary lesions that presage plaque rupture in unstable angina are minor (< 50% stenosis), and that high-grade CAD is not invariably the angiographic finding in patients who present with acute coronary syndromes [1, 2]. Thus, it remains unproven that *all* patients with unstable angina should undergo *routine* coronary angiography prior to hospital discharge. We believe that such a decision must be individualized, taking into account several factors (patient's age, physical activity level, ECG findings of ischemia, other medical conditions, etc) which may influence diagnostic and therapeutic decision-making.

An alternative strategy may be employed. According to this approach, intensive medical therapy (antithrombotic, antiplatelet and anti-ischemic), as previously described, should be initiated as soon as the patient has been admitted to a monitored care facility. If the patient stabilizes on maximal medical therapy in the CCU or telemetry unit, these intravenous medications can be changed to equivalent oral therapy. If the patient does not develop spontaneous angina or ECG findings of recurrent ischemia as his/her physical activity is advanced, urgent coronary angiography can be deferred, and myocardial perfusion imaging with sestamibi or thallium can be performed.

If the patient objective findings of a 'high-risk' scan (multiple perfusion defects; an extensive anteroseptal perfusion defect; increased lung uptake; increased left ventricular (LV) cavity dilatation [increased cardiac blood pool]), he/she should undergo prompt diagnostic coronary angiography followed by myocardial revascularization, as outlined above. On the other hand, if the patient exhibits a normal, or low-risk, myocardial perfusion scan, it would be appropriate to continue antithrombotic and anti-ischemic therapy, and to follow the patient's clinical course closely post-discharge.

MEDICAL MANAGEMENT VERSUS CORONARY INTERVENTION IN PATIENTS WITH STABLE CORONARY ARTERY DISEASE

In an effort to define better therapeutic modalities, intervention therapy has been compared with medical therapy. The two main trials that have compared bypass surgery with medical therapy, the National Cooperative Study [3] and the Veterans Administration Cooperative Study [4], have shown similar survival rates with the two therapeutic modalities. In the former study, mortality at one year was 8% in surgical patients and 6% in medical patients. In the latter, the rates of myocardial infarction (MI) after two years were 11.7% and 12.2%, respectively. Rates of crossover to surgery were 19% at one year in the National Cooperative Study and 34% at two years in the Veterans

Administration Study. Importantly, subsets of patients in the Veterans Administration Study benefited in the long term from surgery. Thus, the five-year survival rate in patients with three-vessel disease was 89% with surgery compared with 75% with medical treatment ($p = 0.02$), and the mortality in patients with an ejection fraction between 30% and 49% was reduced from 27% to 14%.

TRIALS OF NON-ST SEGMENT ELEVATION ACUTE CORONARY SYNDROMES (NON-Q WAVE MI OR UNSTABLE ANGINA)

Thrombolysis in Myocardial Infarction (TIMI) III-B trial

With the development of percutaneous procedures for myocardial revascularization, trials have been reoriented to conservative strategy. The TIMI III-B trial was the prototype of these trials [5]. By study design, patients in the early invasive strategy arm had coronary angiography within 24–48 hours after randomization, followed by coronary angioplasty or bypass surgery in the presence of suitable anatomy. These procedures were performed in the conservative strategy arm with failure of medical therapy, defined by recurrent chest pain with ST-T changes, a ≥ 20 minute period of ischemic ST-segment shifts on a 24-hour Holter monitor, a predischarge positive stress thallium exercise test before completion of stage 2 of the Bruce protocol, re-hospitalization for unstable angina, or angina class III or IV with a positive exercise test during follow-up. A total of 1473 patients with unstable angina or non-Q wave MI were randomized. The primary end point included death, MI, or positive treadmill test at six weeks; it occurred in 18.1% of patients assigned to the conservative strategy and in 16% of patients assigned to invasive strategy ($p = $ NS). Death or MI occurred in 7.8% and 7.2% of patients at six weeks ($p = $ NS) and in 12.2% and 10.8% at one year ($p = $ NS). A large proportion (64%) of patients assigned to medical treatment crossed over to invasive treatment because of recurrent angina or an early positive test for ischemia. Also, the average length of initial hospital stay, the incidence of re-hospitalization within six weeks, and the number of days of re-hospitalization were all decreased with invasive treatment. Another important subset of acute coronary syndromes includes patients with non-Q wave MI.

It is generally agreed that patients recovering from acute non-Q wave MI sustain less myocardial necrosis and have a lower in-hospital mortality, whereas most (but not all) studies indicate that such patients have the same or higher long-term mortality than do patients recovering from acute Q wave MI. Moreover, the majority of published studies indicate that both early and late ischemic complications (reinfarction; post-infarction angina) are consistently higher in non-Q wave MI patients compared to Q wave MI patients, presumably due to the large degree of residually ischemic, jeopardized myocardium that remains at risk within the perfusion zone of the infarct-related coronary artery. Accordingly, the management of acute non-Q wave MI patients has become increasingly aggressive during the last decade, although the hypothesis (that an invasive approach would be superior to a conservative approach) has never been adequately tested prospectively in a large group of such patients with this type of acute coronary syndrome.

Most data in the management of non-Q wave MI have been retrospectively acquired, and certain clinical variables have emerged as powerful predictors of adverse one-year outcome. These include recurrent infarct extension (reinfarction), post-infarction angina associated with transient electrocardiographic changes (early recurrent ischemia), followed by persistent ST-segment depression on serial post-non-Q wave MI electrocardiograms (ECGs), congestive heart failure (CHF), and left ventricular hypertrophy.

Such data support a balanced diagnostic approach to identify high-risk subsets of post-non-Q wave MI management. Approximately

30–35% of non-Q wave MI patients comprise this high-risk subset, defined as those with rein-farction, post-infarction angina, CHF, or persistent ST-segment depression. Invasive testing and interventional maneuvers should be reserved for patients considered at high-risk according to the presence of two or more of the above covariates of risk. Alternatively, the remaining asymptomatic, or low-risk patients, appear to be appropriate candidates for conservative management, which would include a functional assessment of risk (stress test, preferably with sestamibi or thallium) followed by diagnostic coronary angiography only for clinical need or for objective evidence of inducible ischemia.

VA Non-Q wave Infarction Strategies in-Hospital (VANQWISH) trial [6]

This multicenter randomized trial was designed to compare long-term clinical events, resource utilization and other health care outcomes in non-Q wave acute myocardial infarct (AMI) patients who were randomized prospectively to an early 'invasive' strategy (routine coronary angiography followed by myocardial revascularization, if feasible) versus an early 'conservative' strategy (medical therapy and non-invasive, pre-discharge stress testing with planar thallium perfusion scintigraphy), where the selective use of coronary angiography and myocardial revascularization was guided by the outcomes of the non-invasive tests using protocol guidelines, or by clinical course.

The VANQWISH trial was initiated in April 1993, at 15 Department of Veterans Affairs medical centers. The trial primary end-point was to assess the effect of these two randomized management strategies on all-cause mortality and recurrent non-fatal infarction in patients with creatine kinase isoenzyme containing M and B subunits (MB-CK) confirmed non-Q wave MI during long-term follow-up which ranged from 12–44 months (mean 2.5 years). Secondary trial objectives included a comprehensive analysis of risk stratification covariates, and detailed cost-effectiveness comparisons between diagnostic arms, including functional status and quality of life assessments. Enrollment was completed on December 31, 1995, and the uniform one-year follow-up concluded on December 31, 1996.

A total of 920 patients were randomized within 1–3 days of acute non-Q wave MI to either an invasive ($n = 462$) or a conservative ($n = 458$) strategy. An equivalence design was used and death or non-fatal infarction was the combined trial primary end-point during a 12–44 month (mean 2.5 year) follow-up. Baseline clinical characteristics were well-balanced between the two randomized groups, and revealed a moderate–high risk profile of non-Q wave infarction patients: 30% had anterior infarction, 54% were hypertensive, 26% had diabetes, 43% were current smokers, 43% had prior infarction, and 45% had angina within three weeks of the index non-Q wave infarction.

There were 152 events (80 deaths; 72 non-fatal myocardial infarctions) in the 'invasive' arm and 140 events (59 deaths; 80 non-fatal myocardial infarctions) in the 'conservative' arm during cumulative follow-up ($p = 0.35$). Non-Q wave myocardial infarction patients randomized to the invasive strategy had a significantly higher mortality (21 versus six deaths, two-sided; $p = 0.007$) at hospital discharge (mean = 8.8 days), at one month (23 versus nine deaths, respectively; $p = 0.021$), and at one year (58 versus 36 deaths, respectively; $p = 0.025$). The cumulative occurrence of death or non-fatal infarction in the conservative and invasive strategies did not differ during long-term follow-up (hazard ratio, 0.87; 95% confidence interval, 0.68–1.10). However, all-cause mortality was significantly lower in non-Q wave infarction patients randomized to the conservative strategy compared to the invasive strategy (hazard ratio, 0.72; 95% confidence interval, 0.51–1.01).

These data indicate that non-Q wave myocardial infarction patients do not benefit from early aggressive management, and may be harmed. A conservative, ischemia-guided approach to management was both safe and effective in the majority of patients with uncomplicated non-Q wave myocardial infarction.

Fragmin and Fast Revascularization during Instability in Coronary Artery Disease (FRISC-II) trial

The FRISC-II trial enrolled 2457 patients with unstable coronary artery disease from among 61 enrolling sites in Scandinavia between 1996–1998. All patients underwent routine ECG and biomarker testing and were subsequently treated with multifaceted medical therapy, consisting of aspirin, IV heparin, IV nitroglycerin, beta-blockers and low molecular weight heparin (dalteparin) for 4–6 days prior to catheterization and revascularization. Patients were randomized to a routine invasive strategy where coronary angiography was undertaken followed by myocardial revascularization (PCI or CABG surgery) or a non-invasive strategy, where bicycle exercise testing was performed without perfusion imaging. Patients in the non-invasive strategy could cross over to the invasive strategy only if they developed recurrent infarction, CCS Class III–IV angina, or a markedly positive exercise test, defined as: exercise-induced hypotension or ST-segment elevation, > 3 mm ST-segment depression, or a markedly positive exercise test during the first stage of exercise.

In contrast to the VANQWISH trial, patients in the FRISC-II trial had much less clinical co-morbidity; only 13% were diabetic (26% in VANQWISH), 30% were hypertensive (54% in VANQWISH), 23% had prior MI (45% in VANQWISH) and only 57% had abnormal cardiac enzymes or elevated troponins (100% in VANQWISH).

In FRISC-II, 78% of patients in the invasive strategy underwent myocardial revascularization and approximately 30% in the non-invasive strategy underwent subsequent revascularization. For the trial primary composite end-point of death or MI at six months of follow-up, there were 12.1% events in the non-invasive strategy and 9.4% events in the routine invasive strategy; RR (95% CI) = 0.78 (0.62–0.98), p = 0.031. The rate of six-month death was low, with a rate of 1.9% in the invasive arm and 2.9% in the non-invasive arm; RR (95% CI) = 0.65 (0.39–1.09), p = 0.10.

However, in FRISC-II, it was observed that all of the benefit of the routine invasive strategy was restricted to those patients with positive biomarkers (abnormal troponins), which occurred in 57% of patients, and in those with initial ECG ST-segment depression, which occurred in 45% of patients. There was no significant advantage of the routine invasive strategy for the trial primary end-point among patients without ST-segment depression or in patients who were biomarker (troponin) negative.

Thus, while FRISC-II was the first trial to demonstrate improved clinical outcomes in patients with non-ST-segment elevation acute coronary syndrome (ACS) who underwent a routine invasive strategy with a high rate of myocardial revascularization, this effect was not observed in all subsets of patients, underscoring the need to risk stratify patients into low, intermediate and high-risk subsets.

Importantly, FRISC-II also emphasized the critical importance of aggressive, multifaceted medical therapy, since all patients received the benefits of antiplatelet and antithrombin therapy, coupled with anti-ischemic therapy, which may have induced 'plaque passivation' and optimized the benefits of subsequent myocardial revascularization.

Treat Angina with Aggrastat and Determine Cost of Therapy with an Invasive or Conservative Strategy. Thrombolysis in Myocardial Infarction 18 (TACTICS TIMI-18)

Since there is continued debate as to whether a routine, early invasive versus a conservative approach is optimal for the management of patients with unstable angina and non ST-segment elevation MI, the international TACTICS TIMI-18 trial was undertaken in 2200 patients with this syndrome who had either ECG changes, elevated cardiac markers and/or a prior history of coronary artery disease, all of whom were treated with aspirin, heparin and the glycoprotein (GP) IIb/IIIa inhibitor tirofiban. Patients were randomized to an early invasive strategy with routine catheterization within 4–48 hours of randomization and revascularization as appropriate, or to a more conservative ('selective invasive') strategy, with catheterization performed only if the patient had objective evidence of recurrent ischemia or a positive stress test. The primary end-point was a composite of death, myocardial infarction or re-hospitalization for an acute coronary syndrome (ACS) at six months.

The results of TACTICS showed that the rate of the primary end-point was reduced with the early invasive strategy as compared with the conservative strategy, 15.9% versus 19.4%, with an odds ratio (OR) of 0.78 and 95% CI of 0.62–0.97, $p = 0.025$). The rate of death or MI at six months was similarly reduced (7.3% versus 9.5%, respectively). With an OR = 0.74, and 95% CI of 0.54–1.00, $p = 0.0498$. These beneficial effects were also observed at 30 days, and there was no early hazard associated with the routine invasive strategy, as has been reported in other trials such as TIMI-IIIB and VANQWISH.

While the TACTICS trial supports the early 'upstream' use of tirofiban in patients with non-ST segment elevation ACS, it is important to emphasize that the results parallel those of the FRISC-II trial closely, namely that all of the benefit of the routine invasive strategy was observed in the subset on TACTICS patients who were biomarker (troponin) positive (41% of patients) and in those who had ST-segment depression (38%); in the other patients (those who were biomarker-negative and those without ECG ST-segment depression) there was a neutral effect, that is to say, the results were similar regardless of whether the routine inva-

sive or conservative strategies were employed.

Thus TACTICS, like FRISC-II and VANQWISH, supports the fundamental role of risk stratification. It appeared that the 15% of the highest risk patients in TACTICS (with TIMI risk scores > 5) benefited from the invasive strategy, the 25% of low-risk patients with a TIMI risk score of < 3 benefited from a conservative strategy, and the 60% of patients with an intermediate risk (TIMI risk score between 3–5) trended toward improved outcomes with the invasive strategy, although this was of borderline significance.

DIFFERENTIAL RATES OF REVASCULARIZATION AMONG TRIALS AND USE OF ADJUNCTIVE THERAPIES

It is clear that there are significant differences among the published trials in the rates of revascularization and the use of antiplatelet and antithrombin therapy. For example, in the TIMI-IIB trial, cardiac catheterization was performed in 98% of patients in the invasive arm and in 65% of the conservative arm patients; angioplasty was performed in 38% and 26% of patients, respectively; and surgery in 25% and 24%, respectively. By contrast, in the VANQWISH trial, revascularization rates at 1.5 years were 44% with early aggressive management and 33% with early medical treatment (p = NS). In the FRISC-II trial, 78% of the patients in the routine invasive arm underwent myocardial revascularization, and in TACTICS, 61% of patients in the invasive strategy underwent revascularization. These differences could explain some of the differences in outcomes among the various published trials.

Similarly, stents were not available during the era of the TIMI-IIIB and VANQWISH trials, and were not widely employed in the FRISC-II trial, although stenting was widely available during the conduct of the TACTICS trial.

Regarding antiplatelet and antithrombin therapy, standard aspirin and heparin were used in TIMI-IIB and VANQWISH, aspirin and dalteparin were used in FRISC-II (only 10% of

FRISC-II patients received abciximab) and in TACTICS, all patients received aspirin, unfractionated heparin and tirofiban. These differences in pharmacotherapy could likewise explain the differences in clinical outcomes among the various trials.

Currently available data suggest that medical management and percutaneous or surgical interventions are more additive and complementary than conflicting. The respective advantages and disadvantages of the various treatment strategies are known. Unstable angina is a medical situation associated with a build-up of multiple pathophysiological processes culminating in myocardial ischemia. Interventions are often required as an adjunct to medical treatment to relieve recurrent ischemia and severe obstruction. Conversely, aggressive medical treatment is required as an adjunct to vessel closure associated with the presence of a thrombus. The procedures, at times, may be life-saving. Whether percutaneous or surgical procedures should be performed is a matter of coronary anatomy, benefit and risk of the respective procedures, and often, patient choice guided by physician experience. Percutaneous intervention first targets correction of the culprit lesion, and bypass surgery targets more complete revascularization. Angioplasty is usually preferred in one-vessel disease. Comparison of the respective merits of bypass surgery versus angioplasty in patients with multivessel disease is an indication for bypass surgery, and proximal left anterior descending coronary artery stenosis is also often best treated by internal mammary artery graft surgery. In the Bypass Angioplasty Revascularization Investigation (BARI) trial, treated diabetic patients with multivessel disease had a significantly better five-year survival with bypass surgery than with balloon angioplasty when at least one internal mammary graft implant was performed [7].

The technical advances and increased safety of percutaneous interventions with adjunctive GP IIb/IIIa inhibition, stent implantation, and a search for optimal angiographic results have significantly reduced the previously reported high failure rates of early interventions. A new era in bypass surgery has also opened with minimally invasive surgery. This progress has led more to timely use of interventions, greater expertise, development of widespread facilities, and networks for patient referral to tertiary centers. The relative advantage of medical therapy versus intervention therapy is best evaluated at present in the context of risk and benefit for individual patients and optimal use of medical resources. These resources differ between countries and between regions in the same country. One approach generally recommended consists of initial medical therapy tailored to risk, with rapid progression to invasive management when ischemia is not adequately controlled.

TAILORED THERAPEUTIC MODALITIES AND INTENSITY TO RISK PROFILE

The majority of patients with unstable angina are well controlled with medical therapy, with no recurrent ischemia, and have a favorable risk profile [8, 9]. These patients do not need routine angiography and are adequately stratified with proactive testing, including imaging techniques when available. A negative exercise test rules out ischemia associated with severe stenosis and is associated with a low event rate during follow-up. ST-segment depression or a transient perfusion defect indicates significant stenosis. Treatment may be medical if the modifications are not severe or are manifested at a high level of exercise or invasive if more severe or occurring at low level of exercise.

In summary, patients with angina in the early phase of MI, those with electrocardiographic ST-segment depression, those with elevated cardiac biomarkers, or those with persistence of instability on medical treatment are at high risk. They should have early coronary angiography with the goal of identifying a critical coronary stenosis suitable for correction by an intervention. Recurrent ischemia indicates lack of control of the disease state, presence of a critical stenosis, or more extensive disease. Patients with non ST-segment elevation ACS whose clinical symptoms stabilize with intensive medical therapy should be treated aggressively with a GP IIb/IIIa agent with fractionated or unfractionated heparin followed by a 'deferred catheterization and revascularization'. Low-risk ACS patients (those without elevated cardiac markers, no ST-segment depression and stabilized symptoms) should be non-invasively risk stratified, using exercise or pharmacologic vasodilator stress, preferably with sestamibi myocardial perfusion imaging. Thus, continued emphasis on non-invasive risk stratification guided by the presence or absence of ischemia in patients whose condition has stabilized seems prudent in order to identify those individuals whose subsequent therapy can be tailored to their level of risk.

REFERENCES

1. Braunwald E, Jones RH, Mark DB et al. Diagnosing and managing unstable angina, *Circulation* 1994; **90**:613–622.
2. Aguirre FV, Younis LL, Chairman BR et al. Early and one-year clinical outcomes of patients evolving non-Q wave versus myocardial infarction after thrombolysis: results from the TIMI II study, *Circulation* 1995; **91**:2541–2548.
3. Hultgren HN, Pfeifer JF, Angel WW et al. Unstable angina: comparison of medical and surgical patients, *Am J Cardiol* 1977; **39**:734–740.
4. Luchi RJ, Scott SM, Deupree RH. Principal investigators and their associates of Veterans Administration Cooperative Study No. 28. Comparison of medical and surgical treatment for unstable angina pectoris, *N Engl J Med* 1987; **316**:977–984.
5. TIMI IIIB Investigators. Effects of tissue plasminogen activator and a comparison of early invasive and conservative strategies in unstable angina and non-Q wave myocardial infarction: results of the TIMI IIIB trial, *Circulation* 1994; **89**:1545–1556.
6. The Veterans Affairs Non-Q Wave Infarction Strategies in Hospital (VANQWISH) study. Results presented at the European Heart Association Meeting. Stockholm, Sweden, August 25, 1997.
7. The BARI Investigators. Influence of diabetes on five-year mortality and morbidity in a randomized trial comparing CABG and PTCA in patients with multivessel disease: the Bypass Angioplasty Revascularization Investigation (BARI), *Circulation* 1997; **96**:1761–1769.
8. Grines CL, Lytle BW, McCauley KM et al. Diagnosing and managing unstable angina, *Circulation* 1994; **90**:613–622.
9. Cairns J, Theroux P, Armstrong P et al. Unstable angina: report from a Canadian expert roundtable, *Can J Cardiol* 1996; **12**:1279–1292.
10. Szatmary LJ, Marco J, Fajadet J et al. The combined use of diastolic counterpulsion and coronary dilation in unstable angina due to multivessel disease under unstable hemodynamic conditions, *Int J Cardiol* 1988; **19**:59–66.

Section III: Comparative trials of CABG versus PCI

11

Bypass Angioplasty Revascularization Investigation (BARI)

Martial G Bourassa

CONTENTS • Introduction • Methods • Results • Discussion

INTRODUCTION

Previous clinical trials comparing coronary bypass surgery with medical therapy have identified high-risk patient subgroups with multivessel coronary disease which may derive long-term benefit from coronary artery bypass grafting (CABG). Among these subgroups are those with left main coronary disease, triple-vessel disease with impaired ventricular function, proximal left anterior descending artery stenosis, and other major risk factors [1–5].

Several prospective randomized trials have compared percutaneous transluminal coronary angioplasty (PTCA) to coronary bypass surgery in patients with multivessel disease during the last decade. Although these trials have greatly contributed to our current knowledge of the incidence of cardiac events, angina status, and need for repeat procedures after either coronary angioplasty or bypass surgery, most of them reported only short-term results and, with the exception of the Bypass Angioplasty Revascularization Investigation (BARI), none of them was large enough to reliably assess the influence of coronary interventions on total mortality [6, 7]. BARI was designed to test the hypothesis that long-term clinical outcome of

patients with multivessel disease and severe angina or ischemia (relatively high-risk patients) suitable for treatment with either PTCA or CABG is not compromised when PTCA is chosen as the initial treatment strategy [8–11]. Although cumulative total mortality, the primary end-point of BARI, was similar for both procedures after an average of 5.4 years of follow-up, subgroup analysis revealed that total mortality was significantly higher in patients with treated diabetes mellitus assigned to coronary angioplasty [12]. The purpose of this report is to describe and discuss the primary and secondary outcome measures of the BARI trial, overall and within patient subgroups.

METHODS

Study design

The aim of the Bypass Angioplasty Revascularization Investigation (BARI) was to compare PTCA with CABG in patients with multivessel coronary disease and severe angina or ischemia who required coronary revascularization and who were suitable for both interventions. The hypothesis tested in BARI was that an initial strategy of PTCA in these eligible patients compared with CABG did not compromise clinical outcome during a five-year follow-up period [8–10].

Mortality was the primary outcome measure of the trial. However, several other major secondary end-points were also deemed to be of critical importance, especially if there was no difference in mortality between the two treatment strategies. The large sample size provided sufficient power to examine treatment differences not only in mortality, but also in rates of myocardial infarction (MI), repeat revascularization, and recurrent severe angina or ischemia. Distribution by treatment assignment of exercise capacity, ventricular function, and need for medication were also compared at selected time intervals during follow-up. The economic and quality of life impacts of coronary angioplasty and bypass surgery were compared during follow-up in an ancillary Study of Economics and Quality Of Life (SEQOL) conducted at seven participating BARI sites [11]. In addition to SEQOL, data on the number of cardiac hospitalizations, employment status, and limitations of activities were collected for all BARI patients.

BARI also provided comparative data for predetermined patient subgroups. Four baseline clinical and angiographic characteristics: severity of angina or ischemia, number of vessels diseased, lesion complexity according to the American College of Cardiology/American Heart Association (ACC/AHA) classification, and left ventricular function, were prespecified for subgroup analysis. In 1992, because of concerns raised by a previous study about the outcomes of coronary angioplasty in diabetics, the Data Safety Monitoring Board requested that diabetic patients be also monitored [12].

New interventional devices such as stents were not used during the initial coronary angioplasty. The protocol stipulated that the initial coronary angioplasty and bypass surgery had to be performed within two weeks after randomization.

Inclusion and exclusion criteria

To be eligible for BARI, patients had to meet several clinical and angiographic criteria documenting their need and suitability for coronary revascularization. Clinical eligibility required the presence of severe angina or ischemia defined as follows: unstable angina or non-Q wave MI stabilized for four hours to six weeks; stable class III or IV angina pectoris; stable class I or II angina with severe ischemia on non-invasive testing, Q wave MI stabilized for 24 hours to 30 days, or resting ejection fraction (EF) < 0.50; and no angina during the six weeks prior to entry, but severe ischemia on non-invasive testing and either prior Q wave MI or history of prior angina. Severe ischemia on non-invasive testing was defined as follows: exercise-limiting angina or exercise-induced severe ST-segment response with a final exercise stage less than Bruce stage 3; multiple reversible defects or one single reversible and one fixed defect with increased lung uptake on exercise or dipyridamole radionuclide myocardial scintigraphy; decline in left ventricular EF of at least 0.05 (from resting EF > 0.50) on exercise radionuclide ventriculography [8–10].

Angiographic eligibility required the presence of multivessel coronary disease judged by an angioplasty operator to be suitable for PTCA and by a cardiovascular surgeon to be suitable for CABG. Because the BARI investigators recognized the limitations of trying to prospectively describe all the features that define suitability for PTCA and CABG, the final evaluation for eligibility involved the subjective judgement of both the surgeon and angioplasty operator. Although complete revascularization was not a requirement, the protocol called for anticipation of successful relief of the major areas of ischemia.

Some patient subgroups were excluded from screening such as: age < 17 and > 80 years, single-vessel disease, prior PTCA or CABG, or primary congenital, valvular, or myocardial disease. Exclusions from randomization included insufficient angina or myocardial ischemia, left main coronary stenosis > 50%, unstable angina or MI requiring emergency revascularization, geographic inaccessibility for follow-up, clinical contraindication to PTCA or CABG, competing clinical studies, and other miscellaneous reasons.

Definitions

Chronic stable angina was graded according to the Canadian Cardiovascular Society (CCS) classification. Unstable angina was defined as pain accelerating in frequency, severity, or duration; occurring at rest; lasting at least 20 minutes; or continuing within 14 days post-infarction. Q wave MI was diagnosed as a two-step worsening of the Q wave Minnesota code or a new left bundle branch block on the electrocardiogram (ECG), associated with a two-fold increase in total creatine phosphokinase and a positive MB fraction. Non-Q wave MI was diagnosed when cardiac enzymes were elevated with chest pain for > 20 minutes or with the appearance of new ECG changes. Cardiac enzymes were not used to define an MI within 96 hours after coronary revascularization. Cause of death was classified as cardiac, non-cardiac but related to atherosclerotic disease, or non-cardiac medical causes. Cardiac death was defined as death < 1 hour after onset of cardiac symptoms, within 30 days after documented or probable MI, or due to intractable congestive heart failure (CHF), cardiogenic shock, or other documented cardiac causes.

Left ventricular and coronary angiographic findings were analyzed by a central radiographic laboratory using a quantitative angiographic coding system. Multivessel disease was defined by caliper measurement as diameter reduction of ⩾ 50% of two or more arteries of ⩾ 1.5 mm diameter supplying at least two of the three major coronary artery perfusion territories (anterior, lateral, posterior/inferior). Lesion complexity was categorized as type A, B or C according to the previous guidelines of the ACC/AHA Task Force [13]. The amount of

myocardium jeopardized by coronary artery stenoses or global percent jeopardy score was calculated as the ratio of left ventricular territory subtended by terminal coronary segments compromised by lesions with diameter stenosis ⩾ 50% to the sum of all left ventricular territory supplied by major terminal coronary branches [14].

A successful dilatation was defined as a reduction in luminal diameter narrowing ⩾ 20% with final lumen diameter narrowing < 50% and TIMI grade 3 flow.

Data collection

Baseline data included a demographic, clinical and angiographic profile, angina status for the preceding six-week period, a 12-lead ECG, medication use, behavioral risk factors, functional status and quality of life measures. During hospitalization, ECG information was obtained pre- and post-procedure and in the setting of a suspected MI. Follow-up visits were conducted at the clinics at weeks 4–14 after study entry and at one, three and five years, with telephone contacts at six months, and two and four years. During office visits, blood pressure, weight, blood samples for lipid analysis, and resting and exercise ECGs were obtained. Angina status, current medication use, and quality of life data were collected at all follow-up points. Details for intervening hospitalizations, angiographic procedures, coronary revascularizations, suspected MIs, and death were recorded.

All rest and exercise ECGs were interpreted at a central ECG and MI classification core laboratory and all coronary angiograms were read by a central radiographic laboratory. A Data Coordinating Center was responsible for study administration, data management and statistical analysis. An independent Mortality and Morbidity Classification Committee classified major end-point events and an independent Data Safety Monitoring Board regularly reviewed interim study results.

RESULTS

Patient population

Between August 1988 and August 1991, 1829 patients from 18 participating clinical sites entered the BARI randomized trial: 915 were assigned to PTCA and 914 to CABG (Table 11.1). From patients screened but not randomized, two registry populations were defined for follow-up: 2013 patients eligible for randomization by clinical and angiographic criteria, but not randomized; and 422 patients (a 6.3% random sample) eligible for randomization by clinical criteria, but excluded on the basis of angiographic characteristics unsuitable for either coronary angioplasty or bypass surgery.

Only the randomized population of 1829 patients is the subject of the present report.

Baseline characteristics

The baseline clinical and angiographic characteristics of the randomized patients clearly show that they represent a population at relatively high risk for future cardiac events (Table 11.1). The primary clinical indications for revascularization were non-Q wave MI, unstable angina or stable class III or IV angina in 85% of the patients (Fig. 11.1). Of the 12% of patients randomized with class I or II angina, a severe ischemic response on non-invasive testing was present in the majority of patients (182 of 223

Table 11.1 Baseline demographic, clinical and angiographic characteristics of the BARI population		
	CABG (n = 914)	PTCA (n = 915)
Age (mean years)	61.1	61.8
Females	26%	27%
Race		
White	89%	91%
Black	7%	5%
Other	3%	4%
History of		
Myocardial infarction	55%	54%
Diabetes	25%	24%
Hypertension	49%	49%
Congestive heart failure	9%	9%
Three-vessel disease	41%	41%
Myocardium at jeopardy	61.3%	61.5%
Ejection fraction (mean)	57.6%	57.2%
Ejection fraction < 50	21%	23%
Proximal LAD stenosis ≥ 50%	37%	36%

CABG, coronary artery bypass grafting; PTCA, percutaneous transluminal coronary angioplasty; LAD, left anterior descending artery.

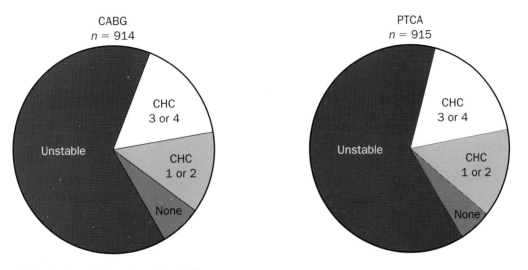

Figure 11.1 Angina at time of randomization.

patients). Of the 3% without angina at the time of randomization but with a severe ischemic response on exercise testing, 40 of 45 had a prior MI. Mean age was 61.5 years, and 39% were > 65 years of age. A history of MI or hypertension was present in one half, of diabetes mellitus in one fourth and of CHF in one tenth of the patients. Angiographically, 41% had three-vessel disease, 77% had a significant proximal or mid left anterior descending artery stenosis (preseptal in 37%), 40% had one or more type C lesions, 22% had a depressed EF and, on the average, 62% of the myocardium was jeopardized by a coronary stenosis > 50%.

The randomized PTCA and CABG treatment arms were well matched for baseline demographic, clinical and angiographic criteria (Table 11.1).

Procedural and in-hospital outcome

Among the 904 patients who underwent coronary angioplasty as assigned, dilatation was attempted for an average of 2.4 lesions. Multilesion angioplasty was attempted in 78% of the patients, and multivessel angioplasty in 70%. At least one lesion was successfully dilated in 88% of the patients, and all were successfully dilated in 57%. Immediate angiographic success was achieved in 78% of attempts, with the mean degree of stenosis reduced from 67% to 31%. Therefore an average of 1.9 of 3.5 clinically important lesions were successfully dilated (54%). The median hospital stay after PTCA was three days [12].

Among the 892 patients who received bypass surgery as assigned, an average of 3.1 coronary arteries were bypassed with a mean of 2.8 grafts. All intended vessels were grafted in 91% of patients. At least one internal thoracic artery (ITA) graft was used in 82% of patients. The median hospital stay after surgery was seven days [12].

The rate of in-hospital mortality was similar in the two treatment groups: 1.1% for coronary angioplasty and 1.3% for bypass surgery (Table 11.2). Patients assigned to angioplasty were less likely to sustain a Q wave MI than those assigned to surgery: 2.1% versus 4.6% ($p = 0.004$). However, patients assigned to angioplasty were more likely to require early reintervention: 12.8% had additional procedures during hospitalization, and 6.3% required

Table 11.2 In-hospital procedure outcomes

	CABG	PTCA
Death	1.3%	1.2%
Q wave MI	4.6%	2.1%
Stroke	0.8%	0.2%
Emergency CABG	0.1%	6.3%
Emergency PTCA	0.0%	2.2%

CABG, coronary artery bypass grafting; PTCA, percutaneous transluminal coronary angioplasty; MI, myocardial infarction.

emergency bypass surgery. Abrupt closure occurred in the laboratory in 86 angioplasty patients. In 35, all stenotic lesions were reopened; of the 51 with vessels not reopened, 30 (59%) required bypass surgery [12]. In-hospital event rates did not differ among patients with and without diabetes mellitus.

Five- and seven-year outcomes

Survival and survival free of MI
At an average follow-up of 5.4 years, cumulative survival rates were not significantly different in the two treatment groups: 86.3% for coronary angioplasty and 89.3% for bypass surgery ($p = 0.174$) (Fig. 11.2a). Rates of survival free of Q wave MI also did not differ significantly between treatment groups: 78.7% for

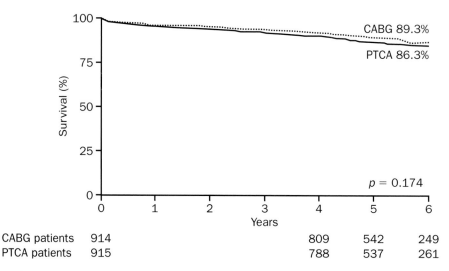

(a)

CABG patients	914			809	542	249
PTCA patients	915			788	537	261

Figure 11.2 (a) BARI primary end-point: five-year survival.

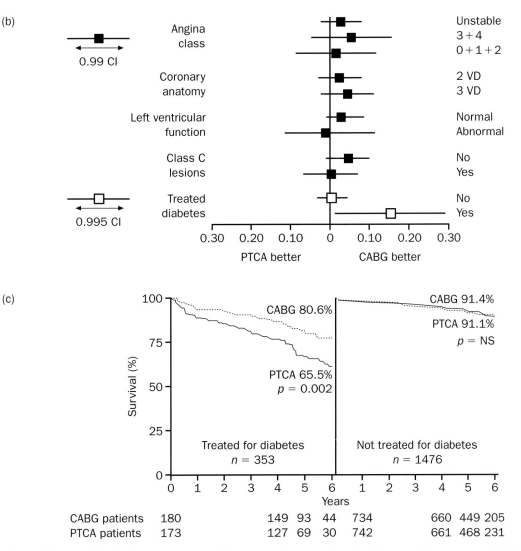

Figure 11.2 *contd.* (b) Five-year survival difference in five monitored subgroups. (c) Influence of treated diabetes on five-year survival in BARI randomized patients.

angioplasty and 80.4% for bypass surgery ($p = 0.84$) [12]. Although patients receiving coronary angioplasty had a lower incidence of Q wave MI during the initial hospitalization, cumulative rates of Q wave MI were not different between treatment groups at 5 years: 10.9% for angioplasty patients versus 11.7% for bypass surgery patients ($p = 0.45$).

The only significant mortality difference occurred in the subgroup of patients with treated diabetes mellitus (Fig. 11.2b). Five-year survival was 65.5% among patients with treated diabetes who were assigned to coronary angioplasty, as compared with 80.6% among diabetics assigned to bypass surgery (Fig. 11.2c). The difference between groups was 15.1 percentage points, with a 99.5% confidence interval (CI) of 1.4–28.9% ($p = 0.003$). For the 1476 other patients (81% of the BARI population), five-year survival was essentially identical in the two treatment groups: 91.1% versus 91.4% respectively ($p = 0.73$) [12, 15, 16].

At an average of 7.2 years of follow-up, a steady divergence persisted between the survival curves of the 915 patients randomized to coronary angioplasty and that of the 914 patients randomized to bypass surgery ($p = 0.043$) [17]. Overall, seven-year survival rates were 80.9% for PTCA and 84.4% for CABG. Again, the observed difference was due to a statistically significant treatment difference in the subgroup of the 353 patients with treated diabetes mellitus ($p = 0.0011$). Estimates of seven-year survival were 55.7% for diabetic patients assigned to PTCA and 76.4% for those assigned to CABG. Among the 1476 patients without treated diabetes at baseline, cumulative seven-year survival was virtually identical: 86.8% for the angioplasty group, and 86.4% for the bypass surgery group ($p = 0.7155$).

In diabetic patients, an advantage of bypass surgery was observed overall and among all subgroups [15–17]. For diabetic patients who underwent bypass surgery, those who received at least one ITA graft had a better seven-year survival (83.2%) compared with those who received only saphenous vein grafts (SVG) (54.5%). The survival rate in this latter group was almost identical to that of diabetic patients who received coronary angioplasty (55.5%). Among the non-diabetic patients, the three corresponding groups had nearly identical survival rates: 86.5% versus 85.2% versus 86.8%.

In addition, as compared with prior coronary angioplasty, prior bypass surgery had a highly favorable influence on five-year survival after MI in patients with diabetes mellitus, and a smaller beneficial effect among diabetics who did not suffer an MI [18]. The risk of death during five-year follow-up after spontaneous Q wave MI was greatly reduced in diabetic patients (relative risk [RR], 0.09; 95% CI, 0.03–0.29). Among diabetic patients with prior bypass surgery who did not suffer a Q wave MI, the corresponding relative risk of death was

0.65 (95% CI, 0.45–0.94). Among the patients without diabetes, no protective effect of bypass surgery was evident.

Seven-year rates of freedom from death and Q wave MI were not different between the two treatment groups: 73.5% versus 75.3% for PTCA and CABG, respectively ($p = 0.46$). Among diabetic patients, there was a statistically significant advantage of bypass surgery over coronary angioplasty in freedom from death and Q wave MI: 65.2% versus 50.0% ($p = 0.049$), whereas among non-diabetic patients, the rates were similar: 78.9% for PTCA and 77.8% for CABG ($p = 0.57$) [17].

MI events and cardiac mortality

The cumulative cardiac mortality rate at five years was 8.0% in the angioplasty group versus 4.9% in the bypass surgery group (RR, 1.55; $p = 0.022$) [19]. However, the cumulative rate for the composite end-point of cardiac mortality or MI was 20.2% in the angioplasty group and 17.5% in the bypass surgery group, and this difference between the two treatment groups was not statistically significant (RR, 1.15; $p = 0.23$). Myocardial infarction events occurring during the index hospitalization and after the initial procedure were greater after bypass surgery than after coronary angioplasty (41 versus 19 Q wave MI events; $p = 0.004$). Conversely, MI events occurring after the index hospitalization discharge were greater in the angioplasty group than in the surgical group (122 versus 75 MI events; $p < 0.001$). The RR for cardiac mortality after MI was 5.9 ($p < 0.001$) for patients who sustained a first MI during follow-up, and it increased to 13.2 ($p < 0.001$) for those who sustained a second MI. The impact of MI on cardiac mortality was comparable between the two treatment groups. The RR was similar by patient subgroups with the exception of diabetic patients. The RR of angioplasty versus surgery was 3.12 for cardiac mortality ($p < 0.001$) in the 353 diabetic patients, whereas cardiac mortality was virtually identical for both treatment groups in the non-diabetic population (RR = 1.04; $p = 0.91$).

Cardiac mortality rates were 20.6% and 5.8% for PTCA and CABG, respectively, among diabetic patients, compared with 4.8% and 4.7%, respectively, for other BARI patients. Among patients receiving CABG, cardiac mortality of diabetic patients was 2.9% when at least one ITA graft was used, and 18.2% when only SVG were used. The latter rate was similar to that of patients receiving PTCA (20.6%). Post-randomization MI rates of diabetic and non-diabetic patients were comparable for all three groups (19.3% after ITA grafts, 15.2% after SVG only, and 19.4% after PTCA in diabetic patients versus 12.4% after ITA grafts, 12.3% after SVG only, and 14.2% after PTCA in non-diabetic patients). However, ITA use was associated with much lower post-MI cardiac mortality rates in both diabetic and non-diabetic patients.

Reintervention

Eight percent of the patients assigned to bypass surgery underwent additional revascularization procedures in the first five years: 1% underwent CABG and 7% PTCA. In the coronary angioplasty group, 54% underwent at least one subsequent procedure: 31% underwent a subsequent CABG, and 34% underwent a second PTCA (11% underwent both) (Fig. 11.3). Unlike patients assigned to bypass surgery, most patients assigned to coronary angioplasty who underwent a second revascularization did it in the first year of follow-up.

Seven-year rates of repeat revascularization were 59.7% for PTCA and 13.1% for CABG ($p < 0.001$) [17]. Among the surgical patients, repeat revascularization rates were not different for those who received at least one ITA conduit as compared with those who received only SVG: 13.2% versus 10.9%. Repeat revascularization rates were higher in the angioplasty group during the first year of follow-up, but cumulative rates increased at a similar pace over subsequent years.

Bypass surgery was used as the repeat procedure in 35.5% of PTCA patients and in 1.7% of CABG patients, whereas coronary angioplasty was performed in 37.3% of PTCA patients and in 12.1% of CABG patients. Both

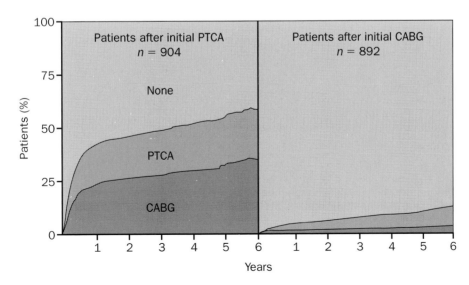

Figure 11.3 Time to secondary procedure in BARI randomized patients.

procedures were performed in 12% of PTCA patients [12].

Among patients assigned to coronary angioplasty, repeat revascularization rates were higher for diabetic patients than for nondiabetic patients: 69.95% versus 57.8% ($p = 0.0078$), with higher rates of subsequent bypass surgery: 48.0% versus 33.3% ($p = 0.014$). Among bypass surgery patients, repeat revascularization rates were similar for patients with or without treated diabetes mellitus: 11.1% versus 13.5% ($p = 0.45$) [12].

Clinical and functional outcomes

Relief of angina
Patients assigned to coronary angioplasty and bypass surgery had similar angina status at baseline: 63% had unstable angina, 30% had stable angina, and 7% had no angina or angina associated only with an MI. Substantial relief of angina occurred by early follow-up in both treatment groups and was maintained through-

out five years (Fig. 11.4). Angina reported during follow-up was primarily stable and predominantly class I or II. At each follow-up interval, a larger proportion of the surgical group was angina-free compared with the angioplasty group. At 4–14 weeks, 73% of PTCA patients reported no angina as compared with 95% of CABG patients. This difference gradually decreased throughout follow-up, and at five years, 78% of PTCA patients were angina-free compared with 86% of CABG patients ($p = 0.011$). Among these asymptomatic patients, 48% of those receiving angioplasty had no additional procedures during follow-up, 15% had only one additional PTCA, and the remaining 37% underwent two or more additional procedures, with approximately the same total number of PTCAs and CABGs. Of the corresponding surgical cases, 94% did not require additional revascularization procedures and the remaining 6% underwent mostly percutaneous coronary interventions [20].

Angina status was no longer significantly different between treatment groups among

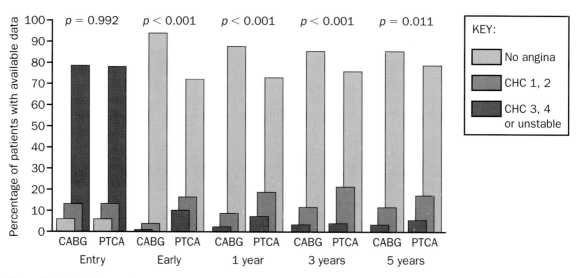

Figure 11.4 Angina in BARI randomized patients.

survivors at seven-year follow-up: 15.1% PTCA versus 11.4% CABG ($p = 0.075$). The angina reported was mainly stable class I or II angina [17].

Improvement in exercise parameters
With the exception of the 4–14 week visit, when less surgical cases were able to reach Bruce stage 3, there was no significant treatment difference in work capacity during the five-year follow-up [20]. Angioplasty patients experienced more frequent abnormal exercise-induced ST-segment changes than surgical patients; however, the difference narrowed from 11% at 4–14 weeks (PTCA = 31% versus CABG = 20%, $p < 0.001$) to a non-significant 3% (PTCA = 31% versus CABG = 28%) at five years. Exercise-induced angina was also more frequent in coronary angioplasty than in bypass surgery patients at 4–14 weeks (16% versus 5%, $p < 0.001$) and at three years (12% versus 6%, $p < 0.001$), but not at five years (10% versus 7%).

Use of anti-ischemic medication
Use of anti-ischemic medication was similar at baseline between the treatment groups. During follow-up, the angioplasty group was more likely to be treated with anti-ischemic medication [20]. At the 4–14 weeks follow-up, 89% of angioplasty patients were prescribed at least one anti-ischemic medication compared with 44% in the surgical group ($p < 0.001$). This difference narrowed to 76% versus 57% by the fifth year, but remained statistically significant ($p < 0.001$).

Work status and limitations of activities
Forty-one percent of coronary angioplasty patients and 47% of bypass surgery patients were employed at baseline. At the 4–14 week follow-up, return-to-work rates were 55% for angioplasty patients and 36% for surgical patients ($p < 0.001$). At one year follow-up, return-to-work rates had increased to 72% for bypass surgery patients versus 69% for coronary angioplasty patients, and were no longer significantly different [20, 21]. Patients in the angioplasty group, however, were more likely

to report limitations in household work, sex life, and interests, and to rate their own health as fair or poor ($p < 0.05$ for all comparisons).

Modifications in other risk factors
At baseline, approximately 25% of both groups were smokers. At the 4–14 week follow-up, smoking was reduced to 12% of angioplasty patients and 8% of surgical patients ($p < 0.001$). Smoking rates were no longer different by one year, and at five years, 14% of patients in both treatment groups reported smoking. The percentage of patients who reported regular exercise increased from 16% at baseline to 42% at five years for both treatment groups. Overall, blood lipids and blood pressure levels showed mild and usually non-significant variations throughout the five years of follow-up [20].

Medical care costs and quality of life
A total of 934 patients participated in the SEQOL at 7 of the 18 participating BARI clinical sites. Of these, 465 were assigned to PTCA, and 469 to CABG. The mean follow-up period was 5.5 years. The baseline characteristics and event rates during follow-up in these patients were comparable to those of the whole BARI population [21].

- Quality of life: the functional status of the patients, as assessed by the Duke Activity Status Index (DASI), improved by 5.7 units ($p < 0.001$) after one year. The functional status of bypass surgery patients improved significantly more than that of coronary angioplasty patients during follow-up. Improvement at one year was 7.0 versus 4.4 units ($p < 0.02$), and at three years 5.6 versus 3.2 units ($p = 0.04$). However, the difference was no longer significant at four (4.3 units versus 2.6 units, $p = 0.17$), and at five years (3.6 units versus 2.0 units, $p = 0.27$) (Fig. 11.5). Emotional health, as measured by the RAND Mental Health Inventory, also improved significantly after coronary revascularization, with no difference between the treatment groups throughout follow-up [21].

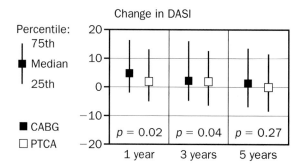

Figure 11.5 Study of Economics and Quality of Life (SEQOL): improvement in physical function.

- Medical costs: the initial cost of coronary revascularization was significantly lower in the angioplasty than in the bypass surgery group, with mean hospital costs and physicians' fees of $21,023 as compared with $32,347 ($p < 0.0001$) (Fig. 11.6a). The difference of $11,324 in the initial cost (a 35% difference) narrowed progressively over the next three years, but the cost of angioplasty remained significantly lower than that of bypass surgery throughout follow-up. The total cost after five years of follow-up was $2,175 less (5% lower) in the angioplasty than in the bypass surgery group ($54,898 versus $57,073, $p = 0.047$) (Fig. 11.6b). Cost-effectiveness ratio for bypass surgery became progressively more favorable over the course of follow-up: $478,609 per year of life added at one year; $97,032 at two years; $37,876 at three years; $29,740 at four years; and $26,117 at five years. Among the diabetic patients, bypass surgery led to lower costs and longer life expectancy than did angioplasty; among the remaining patients, surgery had higher costs than angioplasty, with a similar life expectancy [21]. The number of diseased vessels was the only baseline clinical factor that had a significant interaction with treatment assignment with respect to four-year cumu-

lative costs ($p < 0.001$). The lowest cost was in patients in the angioplasty group who had two-vessel disease; in the remaining patients, costs were 17–22% higher [21].

DISCUSSION

Major findings of the BARI trial

The initial BARI results, published in 1996, showed that overall five-year survival, the primary end-point of the trial, and survival free of MI were not significantly different between the coronary angioplasty and bypass surgery randomized treatment arms, confirming the original BARI hypothesis that an initial strategy of coronary angioplasty, compared to an initial strategy of bypass surgery, did not compromise five-year clinical outcome [12]. This was consistent with the then published results of several smaller trials which showed no significant difference, at 1–3 year follow-up, in major cardiac events such as mortality or MI between the two treatment groups [6, 7]. Moreover, the BARI data did not show any significant treatment difference within subgroups of randomized patients, with the exception of treated diabetic patients. At five years in BARI, there was a trend for better survival with coronary bypass surgery, and this became a significant advantage in favor of bypass surgery at seven years [12, 17]. However, these differences were accounted for solely by an excess mortality among treated diabetics assigned to an initial PTCA strategy (65% and 56% survival rates at five and seven years versus 81% and 76% for patients initially treated with CABG). Conversely, survival rates in non-diabetics were almost identical for both treatment arms at five and seven years (91% for both arms at five years, and 86% for CABG versus 87% for PTCA at seven years). Since the publication of the initial BARI results, several groups have compared long-term mortality rates after CABG and PTCA in databases from observational studies [22–24] and from randomized trials [25,

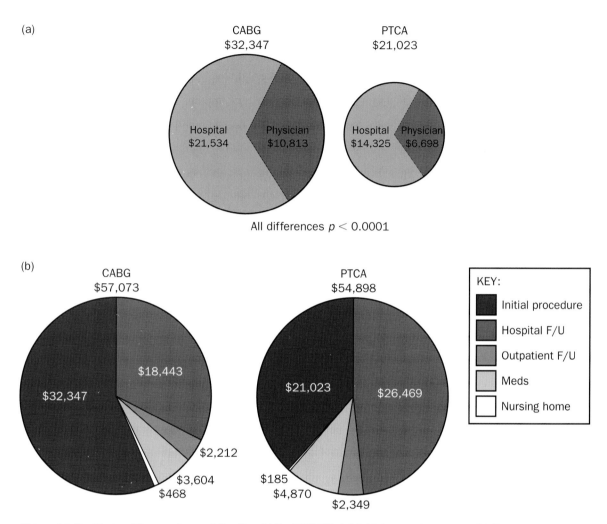

(a)

CABG
$32,347

PTCA
$21,023

Hospital
$21,534

Physician
$10,813

Hospital
$14,325

Physician
$6,698

All differences $p < 0.0001$

(b)

CABG
$57,073

PTCA
$54,898

KEY:

■ Initial procedure

■ Hospital F/U

■ Outpatient F/U

□ Meds

□ Nursing home

$18,443

$32,347

$2,212

$3,604

$468

$21,023

$26,469

$185

$4,870

$2,349

Figure 11.6 Study of Economics and Quality of Life (SEQOL). (a) Initial procedure costs. (b) Five-year costs by category.

26]. The results of these comparisons have been inconsistent; some studies have supported and others have challenged the BARI diabetes findings. Retrospective subgroup analysis, selection biases and small numbers of diabetics available for analysis probably account to a large extent for the discrepancies between these studies.

Although the mechanisms for the better survival rates of diabetic patients following bypass surgery have not been clearly established, the survival benefit in BARI was entirely due to a significant decrease in cardiac mortality and it was limited to patients who received an ITA graft usually to the left anterior descending artery [15–17]. In addition, a recent analysis of the BARI data suggests that, in patients who suffer an MI after coronary revascularization, bypass surgery has a greater protective effect against subsequent cardiac events than does coronary angioplasty [18]. Although CABG did not alter the incidence of spontaneous Q wave MI in either diabetic or non-diabetic patients, it greatly reduced the high mortality rate after the event in diabetic patients, an effect not seen in non-diabetics.

As in the other prospective randomized trials comparing the two techniques of revascularization, BARI also showed a much higher rate of repeat revascularization when coronary angioplasty, the less invasive procedure, was chosen as the initial treatment strategy. Compared to bypass surgery, coronary angioplasty was associated with a 6.8-fold increase in the need for repeat revascularization at five years, and a 4.6-fold increase at seven years [12, 17]. As expected, repeat revascularization rates were higher in the angioplasty group during the first year of follow-up, but cumulative rates increased at a similar pace over subsequent years. Among patients assigned to coronary angioplasty, repeat revascularization rates were higher for diabetic patients than for non-diabetic patients, with higher rates of subsequent bypass surgery; among bypass surgery patients, repeat revascularization rates were similar for patients with or without treated diabetes mellitus.

As seen in Fig. 11.4, although both procedures relieved angina pectoris in a large number of BARI patients, at each follow-up interval, a larger proportion of the surgical group was angina-free compared to the angioplasty group. However, this difference gradually decreased throughout follow-up and, at the seven-year follow-up, angina status was no longer significantly different between treatment groups [17, 20].

In the SEQOL ancillary study, CABG improved the functional status of patients undergoing revascularization to a greater extent than PTCA for the initial three years; subsequently, the improvement was similar in both groups [21]. The other quality of life measures were equally improved in both treatment groups. As expected, PTCA patients returned to work five weeks sooner than CABG patients; but long-term work status was similar between the two treatment groups [21]. The cost data in this substudy were particularly interesting. The

initial costs of PTCA were only 65% of CABG; however, they rose progressively to 95% of CABG by five years [21].

Strengths of the BARI trial

BARI is unique among the prospective randomized trials of PTCA versus CABG for several reasons. First, it is the only trial of patients with multivessel coronary disease in which the sample size was large enough to allow five-year mortality to be chosen as the primary end-point of the study. Secondly, BARI provided important information on post-revascularization rates of MI, which was an important secondary end-point of the study. It used rigorous methodology and a central ECG and MI classification laboratory to obtain accurate data on symptomatic Q wave and non-Q wave MI, as well as silent Q wave MIs. Thirdly, the large ancillary SEQOL provided exceptional long-term data on quality of life and costs of procedures. Other important features of BARI are the registries and the angiographic substudy.

Most importantly, however, in the context of this book, BARI is unique by the fact that it targeted patients at relatively high risk for subsequent cardiac events. As shown in Fig. 11.1, the entry criteria were aimed at selecting patients with severe symptoms (class III or IV angina, unstable angina and non-Q wave MI). The minority (15% overall) of patients with mild or no symptoms had evidence of profound ischemia on non-invasive testing and prior Q wave MI. Additional evidence of high-risk coronary disease is provided, as shown in Table 11.1, by the presence of older age, prior MI, history of hypertension, diabetes and CHF, and severity of disease at angiography. Finally, BARI patients with or without treated diabetes mellitus differed substantially at study entry [15–17]. Diabetics were more often women and blacks, and they had a higher proportion of patients with a history of CHF, hypertension, chronic renal failure, and peripheral vascular disease. In addition, they had higher triglyceride levels and body mass indexes. The extent of coronary disease was also greater, as shown by the presence of three-vessel disease and more distal lesions, and left ventricular EF was lower in diabetics than in non-diabetics.

Limitations of the BARI trial

Coronary revascularization in BARI was performed with the 1990–1991 technology, and only balloon dilatation was allowed as the initial angioplasty procedure. Both coronary angioplasty and bypass surgery have undergone significant refinements during the last decade. Although at least one ITA graft anastomosis was achieved in 82% of the BARI patients, the use of both ITAs and of additional arterial grafts is more frequent now than 10 years ago. In addition, more and more bypass surgery patients are now managed with minimally invasive surgical procedures. Among patients undergoing percutaneous coronary interventions, coronary stenting has been shown to reduce restenosis, and stent implantation is now commonly used. Newer antiplatelet drugs such as glycoprotein IIb/IIIa platelet receptor inhibitors may also reduce complications in high-risk patients undergoing percutaneous coronary intervention. Although several prospective randomized trials comparing stents to coronary bypass surgery in patients with multivessel disease are currently ongoing, long-term results allowing definite conclusions are not yet available.

The seven-year results of the BARI trial were published recently [17]. However, in order to further elucidate the relative benefits of PTCA and CABG, since graft failure and disease progression may substantially influence long-term outcome, all patients are currently being followed for a minimum of at least 10 years.

Finally, although the BARI data strongly suggest that bypass surgery should be the preferred revascularization procedure in diabetic patients who meet its eligibility criteria and although these data are supported by those of

other trials, this diabetic subgroup analysis must be viewed mainly as a major hypothesis-generating conclusion which requires further confirmation. Moreover, recent advances in percutaneous coronary intervention, bypass surgery, and medical therapy, as mentioned above, call for further properly controlled randomized trials to determine the best treatment strategy for patients with diabetes mellitus. The BARI 2 trial in diabetics (BARI 2D) supported by the National Heart, Lung, and Blood Institute (NHLBI) is one such trial which was initiated recently. This randomized multicenter clinical trial uses a 2×2 factorial design to examine the effects of revascularization plus aggressive medical therapy versus aggressive medical therapy alone, as well as insulin-providing versus insulin-sensitizing strategies for tight glycemic control. A total of 2600 diabetic patients with coronary artery disease, stable angina, or documented ischemia, and suitability for revascularization by at least one method will be enrolled. The results of this trial are expected in the year 2008.

REFERENCES

1. Takaro T, Hultgren HN, Lipton MJ, Detre KM, for Participants in the Study Group. The VA Cooperative Randomized Study of Surgery for Coronary Arterial Occlusive Disease, II: subgroup with significant left main lesions, *Circulation* 1976; **54** (suppl III):III107–III117.
2. The Veterans Administration Coronary Artery Bypass Surgery Cooperative Study Group. Eleven-year survival in the Veterans Administration randomized trial of coronary bypass surgery for stable angina, *N Engl J Med* 1984; **311**:1333–1339.
3. Passamani E, Davis KB, Gillespie MJ, Killip T, and the CASS Principal Investigators and their associates. A randomized trial of coronary artery bypass surgery. Survival of patients with a low ejection fraction, *N Engl J Med* 1985; **312**: 1665–1671.
4. Alderman EL, Bourassa MG, Cohen LS et al for the CASS Investigators. Ten-year follow-up of survival and myocardial infarction in the

randomized coronary artery surgery study, *Circulation* 1990; **82**:1629–1646.

5. Varnauskas E and the European Coronary Surgery Study Group. Twelve-year follow-up of survival in the randomized European Coronary Surgery Study, *N Engl J Med* 1988; **319**:332–337.

6. Sim I, Gupta M, McDonald K, Bourassa MG, Hlatky MA. A meta-analysis of randomized trials comparing coronary artery bypass grafting with percutaneous transluminal coronary angioplasty in multivessel coronary artery disease, *Am J Cardiol* 1995; **76**:1025–1029.

7. Pocock SJ, Henderson RA, Rickards AF et al. Meta-analysis of randomized trials comparing coronary angioplasty with bypass surgery, *Lancet* 1995; **346**:1184–1189.

8. Protocol for the Bypass Angioplasty Revascularization Investigation, *Circulation* 1991; **84** (suppl V):V1–V27.

9. Bourassa MG, Roubin GS, Detre KM et al and the BARI Study Group. Bypass angioplasty revascularization investigation: patient screening, selection, and recruitment, *Am J Cardiol* 1995; **75**:3C–8C.

10. Rogers WJ, Alderman EL, Chaitman BR et al and the BARI Study Group. Bypass Angioplasty Revascularization Investigation (BARI): baseline clinical and angiographic data, *Am J Cardiol* 1995; **75**:9C–17C.

11. Hlatky MA, Charles ED, Nobrega F et al and the BARI Study Group. Initial functional and economic status of patients with multivessel coronary artery disease randomized in the Bypass Angioplasty Revascularization Investigation (BARI), *Am J Cardiol* 1995; **75**:34C–41C.

12. The Bypass Angioplasty Revascularization Investigation (BARI) Investigators. Comparison of coronary bypass surgery with angioplasty in patients with multivessel disease, *N Engl J Med* 1996; **335**:217–225.

13. Ryan TJ, Faxon DP, Gunnar RM et al. Guidelines for percutaneous transluminal coronary angioplasty. A report of the American College of Cardiology/American Heart Association Task Force on Assessment of Diagnostic and Therapeutic Cardiovascular Procedures (Subcommittee on Percutaneous Transluminal Coronary Angioplasty), *J Am Coll Cardiol* 1988; **12**:529–545.

14. Alderman EL, Stadius M. The angiographic definitions of the Bypass Angioplasty Revascu-

larization Investigation, *Coron Artery Dis* 1992; **3**:1189–1207.

15. The BARI Investigators. Influence of diabetes on five-year mortality and morbidity in a randomized trial comparing CABG and PTCA in patients with multivessel disease. The Bypass Angioplasty Revascularization Investigation (BARI), *Circulation* 1997; **96**:1761–1769.

16. Detre KM, Guo P, Holubkov R et al. Coronary revascularization in diabetic patients. A comparison of the randomized and observational components of the Bypass Angioplasty Revascularization Investigation (BARI), *Circulation* 1999; **99**:633–640.

17. The BARI Investigators. Seven-year outcome in the Bypass Angioplasty Revascularization Investigation (BARI) by treatment and diabetic status, *J Am Coll Cardiol* 2000; **35**:1122–1129.

18. Detre KM, Lombardero MS, Brooks MM et al for the Bypass Angioplasty Revascularization Investigation Investigators. The effect of previous coronary-artery bypass surgery on the prognosis of patients with diabetes who have acute myocardial infarction, *N Engl J Med* 2000; **342**:989–997.

19. Chaitman BR, Rosen AD, Williams DO et al on behalf of the BARI Investigators. Myocardial infarction and cardiac mortality in the Bypass Angioplasty Revascularization Investigation (BARI) randomized trial, *Circulation* 1997; **96**:2162–2170.

20. Alderman EL, Andrews K, Bourassa MG et al on behalf of the Bypass Angioplasty Revascularization Investigation (BARI) Investigators. Five-year clinical and functional outcome comparing bypass surgery and angioplasty in patients with multivessel coronary disease. A multicenter randomized trial, *JAMA* 1997; **277**:715–721.

21. Hlatky MA, Rogers WJ, Johnstone I et al for the Bypass Angioplasty Revascularization Investigation (BARI) Investigators. Medical care costs and quality of life after randomization to coronary angioplasty or coronary bypass surgery, *N Engl J Med* 1997; **336**:92–99.

22. Barsness GW, Peterson ED, Ohman EM et al. Relationship between diabetes mellitus and long-term survival after coronary bypass and angioplasty, *Circulation* 1997; **96**:2551–2556.

23. Weintraub WS, Stein B, Kosinski A et al. Outcome of coronary bypass surgery versus coronary angioplasty in diabetic patients with

multivessel coronary artery disease, *J Am Coll Cardiol* 1998; **31**:10–19.

24. Niles NW, McGrath PD, Malenka D et al for the Northern New England Cardiovascular Disease Study Group. Survival of patients with diabetes and multivessel coronary artery disease after surgical or percutaneous coronary revascularization: results of a large regional prospective study, *J Am Coll Cardiol* 2001; **37**:1008–1015.

25. Henderson RA, Pocock SJ, Sharp SJ et al. Long-term results of RITA-1 trial: clinical and cost comparisons of coronary angioplasty and coronary-artery bypass grafting. Randomized Intervention Treatment of Angina, *Lancet* 1998; **352**:1419–1425.

26. King SB, Kosinski AS, Guyton RA, Lembo NJ, Weintraub WS for the Emory Angioplasty Versus Surgery Trial (EAST) Investigators. Eight-year mortality in the Emory Angioplasty Versus Surgery Trial (EAST), *J Am Coll Cardiol* 2000; **35**:1116–1121.

12

The RITA trials

Robert A Henderson

CONTENTS • Introduction • RITA-1 • RITA-2 • Summary

INTRODUCTION

Percutaneous transluminal coronary angio-plasty (PTCA) was introduced into routine clinical practice during the late 1970s, and since then the role of the procedure in patients with coronary artery disease has been the subject of intense debate. Early experience established PTCA as an effective treatment for selected patients with single vessel disease, and over time the indications for the technique expanded to include patients with more complex coronary anatomy. Encouraged by these favourable results some cardiologists promoted PTCA as an alternative to coronary artery bypass surgery (CABG), but other clinicians expressed concerns about the paucity of long-term follow-up data and called for formal assessment of the benefits of PTCA [1, 2]. The interventional cardiology community responded by initiating randomized clinical trials of PTCA versus alternative medical and surgical treatment strategies [3].

In the UK the first Randomized Intervention Treatment of Angina (RITA) trial was designed to compare initial treatment strategies of PTCA and CABG in patients in whom equivalent revascularization could be achieved by either treatment method [4]. The second RITA trial is comparing the long-term effects of an initial strategy of PTCA with an initial conservative (medical) strategy in patients for whom early revascularization is not considered essential.

RITA-1

In 1985 Edgar Sowton and colleagues at Guy's Hospital conducted a pilot study of PTCA versus CABG in patients with coronary artery disease considered suitable for either method of revascularization. The pilot study demonstrated the feasibility of randomizing patients to such different interventions and led to the development of the RITA-1 trial protocol. A steering committee of interested clinicians was formed and the first patient was randomized in RITA-1 during March 1988.

Trial protocol

The trial design including patient entry criteria, intervention procedures and outcome measures has been described in detail [4]. Patients with arteriographically proven coronary artery disease were considered for randomization if myocardial revascularization was considered necessary on clinical grounds. Eligible patients were not required to have angina if revascularization was considered appropriate for reasons other than symptom relief. Patients with left main stem disease, previous myocardial revascularization, haemodynamically significant valve disease, or systemic disease likely to limit long-term prognosis were all excluded from the study.

A register of all patients undergoing coronary arteriography under the care of participating cardiologists was maintained during the recruitment period to identify suitable patients [5]. A participating cardiologist and cardiac surgeon reviewed the coronary arteriograms of potentially eligible patients and were required to agree that equivalent revascularization could be achieved by either treatment method. As part of this process the surgeon identified up to three major epicardial vessels (estimated to supply 20% or more of the left ventricular myocardium) that would be grafted, and the cardiologist had to agree to attempt dilatation of all important stenoses in the same vessels. The intention to achieve equivalent revascularization could include occluded vessels provided the cardiologist was prepared to attempt to reopen the vessel by angioplasty and the surgeon intended to graft the distal vessel, but the trial did not mandate treatment of all diseased vessels. Coronary stenoses were considered significant if there was a reduction in luminal diameter of at least 70% in one angiographic view or 50% reduction in two views.

Eligible patients who consented to participate in the trial were randomly assigned to initial treatment by coronary angioplasty or coronary artery bypass surgery, with prospective stratification by number of treatment vessels. The trial was designed as a pragmatic comparison of contemporary surgical and interventional techniques and no attempt was made to standardize operative methods. Multivessel angioplasty could be staged over several procedures, but it was intended that all assigned revascularization procedures be completed within three months of randomization.

During follow-up patients were reviewed one, six and twelve months after the assigned intervention procedure, and two, three, four and five years after randomization. The primary trial end-point was the combined incidence of death and definite non-fatal myocardial infarction. Definite myocardial infarction was defined as (i) the appearance of new pathological Q waves within seven days of an intervention procedure (procedure related myocardial infarction), or (ii) a convincing clinical history at least seven days after any intervention procedure, associated with the appearance of new pathological Q waves or elevation of the serum level of two cardiac enzymes (or creatine kinase MB fraction alone) to twice the upper limit of normal. Silent myocardial infarction was defined as the appearance of new pathological Q waves on a follow-up electrocardiogram, without an accompanying clinical event.

Results

During the first 34 months of the recruitment period the coronary arteriogram register recorded 27,975 patients with arteriographically proven coronary artery disease. The management plan for these patients included CABG (43%), PTCA (16%) and randomization in the RITA trial (3%) [5]. The trial was designed with a recruitment target of 1000 patients and from March 1988 to November 1991, 1011 patients were randomized.

The baseline clinical characteristics of the 510 patients assigned to PTCA and the 501 patients assigned to CABG were comparable. The median age was 57 years, 19% were women, 43% had previous myocardial infarction, and 6.1% had diabetes mellitus. Single-vessel disease was present in 45% of patients, while 12% had three-vessel disease [6].

The assigned CABG and PTCA procedures were carried out in 490 (98%) and 493 (97%) patients respectively. The assigned revascularization procedure was not carried out in 28 patients (CABG 11, PTCA 17), but five patients received PTCA instead of the intended CABG and seven patients received CABG instead of the intended PTCA. On the 'intention to treat' principle, these patients were included in the original randomized groups for all analyses [6].

Among patients who underwent CABG all vessels selected for treatment at randomization were grafted in 97%. For 160 CABG patients (33%) the number of grafts was greater than the number of vessels selected for treatment, reflecting the need to graft all diseased vessels at a single operation. An internal mammary artery graft was used in 74%.

Among patients assigned to PTCA, dilatation was attempted in fewer vessels than were selected for treatment at randomization in 62 patients (13%). All patients assigned to PTCA were treated by conventional balloon angioplasty, apart from one patient in whom a chronically occluded artery was treated by a low-speed rotational device. In total, angioplasty was attempted in 779 vessels in 493 patients, with angiographic success (final diameter stenosis $< 50\%$) in 672 vessels (87%). At least one vessel was successfully dilated in 90% of the 493 PTCA-treated patients, but emergency CABG was required in 4.5% and repeat PTCA before discharge in 1%. Of the 226 PTCA patients with multi-vessel dilatation 15 (7%) required more than one hospital admission to complete the procedure [6].

During a median 6.5 years follow-up there were 45 non-cardiac deaths (24 CABG, 21 PTCA) and 39 cardiac deaths (21 CABG, 18 PTCA), including seven deaths (5 CABG, 2 PTCA) related to the assigned revascularization procedures. All cause mortality was 9.0% in the CABG group and 7.6% in the PTCA group ($p = 0.51$). Non-fatal myocardial infarction occurred in 55 PTCA patients (10.8%) and 37 CABG patients (7.4%) ($p = 0.08$), of which 18 and 12, respectively, occurred during hospital admission for the assigned revascularization procedure.

Overall there was no difference between the two treatment groups in the primary end-point, and at seven years the cumulative risk of death or myocardial infarction was 17.1% in the PTCA group and 16.0% in the CABG group. This risk was substantially higher during the first year after randomization than during subsequent years in both treatment groups, mainly due to the assigned revascularization procedures. The effect of the randomized interventions on the risk of death or myocardial infarction was similar for subgroups with single and multi-vessel disease [7].

In the subgroup of 62 patients with diabetes mellitus there were 10 deaths, of which two (6.9%) occurred in the PTCA group and eight (24.2%) in the CABG group (interaction test $p = 0.09$). Death or non-fatal myocardial infarction occurred in five diabetic patients in the PTCA group and 12 in the CABG group (17.2% versus 36.4%, interaction test $p = 0.055$) [7].

During follow-up there have been 304 repeat coronary arteriograms in the PTCA group and 113 in the CABG group. In total 134 (26%) PTCA patients have had subsequent CABG, and 138 (27%) have had an additional non-assigned PTCA. Of the 501 patients assigned CABG 14 (3%) have had a second operation and 47 (9%) required PTCA. Stents were used during 14 of 210 subsequent non-assigned PTCA procedures. During the first year of follow-up 28% of the PTCA group required at least one additional non-assigned intervention, but by years 3–5 the re-intervention rate in the PTCA group had decreased to 3% per year (of which 1.4% were CABG operations). In the CABG group the re-intervention rate averaged 2% per year with no clear trend over time (Fig. 12.1).

Among patients assigned to PTCA, those with multi-vessel disease had a higher rate of subsequent CABG than those with single-vessel disease (31% versus 21%, $p = 0.01$), but the rate of repeat PTCA was 27% in both groups. Among patients assigned to CABG the re-intervention rates were similar amongst those with single and multi-vessel disease.

Angina was graded using the Canadian Cardiovascular Society Classification [8]. At randomization 59% of patients had grade III or IV angina, and following the assigned revascularization procedures there was a striking

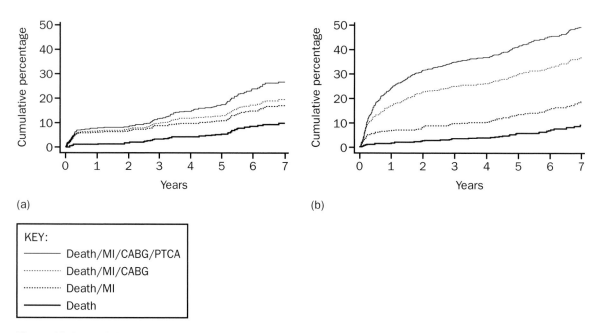

KEY:
———— Death/MI/CABG/PTCA
·········· Death/MI/CABG
············ Death/MI
———— Death

Figure 12.1 (a) RITA-1 patients assigned to CABG: cumulative risk of PTCA, CABG, myocardial infarction (MI) or death; (b) RITA-1 patients assigned to PTCA: cumulative risk of PTCA, CABG, myocardial infarction (MI) or death.

improvement in angina in both treatment groups. Nevertheless, throughout follow-up there was a persistent excess of angina in the PTCA group compared with the CABG group. For instance, six months after randomization 11.0% of CABG patients had angina compared with 31.6% of PTCA patients (relative risk 0.35, 95% CI 0.26–0.47, $p < 0.001$). Thereafter the prevalence of angina increased in both treatment groups, and between one and five years the prevalence of limiting (grade II or higher) angina increased from 20.6% to 25.6% in the PTCA group, and from 10.8% to 16.6% in the CABG group. These treatment differences in prevalence of angina occurred among patients with single-vessel (9% after CABG, 29% after PTCA at six months) and multi-vessel disease (12% after CABG, 34% after PTCA at six months). In both treatment groups the prevalence of angina during follow-up was greater in

patients with severe (grade III or IV) angina at baseline. Overall the prevalence of grade II or worse angina at five years was 25.5% for patients with grade III or IV angina at baseline but 14.9% for patients with grade II or less at baseline.

At randomization, 97% of patients in both groups were taking at least one anti-anginal drug (beta-blocker, calcium antagonist or long acting nitrate) and 38% were taking three anti-anginal drugs. During follow-up patients assigned to PTCA had considerably greater use of anti-anginal drugs than patients assigned to CABG. For instance, six months after their procedure 75% of PTCA patients were taking at least one anti-anginal drug and 11% were on triple drug therapy. By contrast six months after CABG 28% were taking one or more anti-anginal drugs with just two such patients on triple drug therapy. This treatment difference attenuated over time but at five years was still statistically significant with 63% of PTCA patients and 45% of CABG patients taking at least one anti-anginal drug [7].

Breathlessness was assessed on a six-point scale ranging from not breathless to breathless at rest. At randomization 35% of patients complained of severe breathlessness, but this fell to around 11% after revascularization with no evidence of a treatment difference over five years.

Physical activity was scored on a five-point scale ranging from sedentary (confined indoors) to vigorously active (regular exercise or heavy physical work). At baseline 26% of patients were physically active (vigorous or moderately active) but there was a considerable increase in the extent of reported physical activity over time in both treatment groups. One month after CABG there were fewer physically active patients than one month after PTCA (38% versus 52%) but there was no evidence of a treatment difference thereafter. At one year 65% of patients were physically active but this decreased to 55% at five years.

Symptom limited exercise treadmill tests were performed using the modified Bruce protocol [9], unless contraindicated by unstable angina or co-morbidity. At randomization the mean exercise times in the CABG and PTCA groups were 10.3 mins (SEM 0.25 mins) and 10.9 mins (SEM 0.24 mins) respectively. One month after revascularization the mean increase in exercise time was 2.3 mins in the PTCA group and 1.6 mins in the CABG group ($p = 0.0002$). At all subsequent follow-up visits up to five years mean exercise time was increased by approximately 3 minutes with no statistically significant difference between the two treatment groups [7].

Health-related quality of life was assessed with the Nottingham Health Profile (NHP), a standardized self-administered questionnaire [10]. Compared with the baseline assessment, at six months and two years there was a marked improvement in all six dimensions of the NHP (energy, pain, emotional reactions, sleep, social isolation and physical mobility) in both treatment groups. Nevertheless there was a close link between angina and impaired health related quality of life, and patients in the PTCA group had slightly greater impairment of quality of life, reflecting their significantly higher chances of having angina during follow-up [11].

Employment status was analyzed for men aged less than 60 years at randomization. Patients beyond normal retirement age and women (whose employment intentions may be difficult to ascertain) were excluded from analysis. At randomization 47% of such men were not working due to coronary disease. Two months after the assigned intervention 39% of PTCA patients and 9% of CABG patients were back at work, but by five months 52% and 50%, respectively, had returned to work. Thereafter there was a trend towards greater coronary-related unemployment rate in the PTCA group that falls short of statistical significance.

The health service costs of the two revascularization strategies were estimated by combining resource use data with unit cost data provided by two of the participating centres. The cost analyses included data on the initial assigned revascularization procedures, all subsequent coronary arteriograms and additional revascularization procedures, all inpatient care, and consumption of anti-anginal medication. The initial average cost of treating a patient randomized to PTCA was 52% of the cost of a patient assigned to CABG, but this increased to 80% after two years and 95% after five years, mainly because of the greater need for additional interventions in the PTCA group [7, 12].

Discussion

The first RITA trial compared the long-term results of PTCA and CABG in patients with angina considered suitable for either method of revascularization. The trial included patients with single- and multi-vessel disease and overall the enrolled patients were at moderate cardiovascular risk with a death rate around 1%

per year in both treatment groups. Several other randomized trials of PTCA versus CABG only recruited patients with multi-vessel disease at higher cardiovascular risk. For example in the Emory Angioplasty Surgery Trial (EAST) mortality at eight years was 21.7% in the PTCA group and 17.3% in the CABG group ($p = 0.40$) [13]. In the Bypass Angioplasty Revascularization Investigation (BARI) seven-year mortality was 15.6% in the CABG group and 19.1% in the PTCA group, a difference which just reaches statistical significance ($p = 0.043$) [14]. In total, nine trials of PTCA versus CABG recruited 5200 patients and currently available data indicate that a major difference in mortality is unlikely, but a small prognostic advantage of CABG cannot be excluded [15, 16].

The number of diabetic patients in RITA-1 was small and only 16% died during follow-up, but over 6.5 years there was a trend towards lower mortality in the PTCA group (6.9% versus 24.2%). By contrast other trials have reported higher mortality rates among diabetic patients treated by PTCA [13, 17]. In BARI seven-year mortality in diabetic patients was 23.6% in the CABG group but 44.3% in the PTCA group and this difference was attributed to lower cardiac mortality among diabetic patients who received an internal mammary artery graft during the coronary bypass operation [14, 18]. These subgroup analyses must be interpreted cautiously, because they were not pre-specified and are not consistent with data from other sources [19, 20]. Nevertheless in the recently published ARTS trial comparing multi-vessel percutaneous coronary stenting with bypass surgery, diabetic patients treated by multi-vessel stenting had a worse one-year outcome than patients assigned to surgery or non-diabetic patients treated by stenting [21, 22]. Overall the accumulating data suggest that patients with diabetes and multi-vessel coronary disease have less favourable outcomes when treated by PTCA, but the magnitude of this effect is uncertain and may have been over-estimated in BARI. At present the optimal treatment strategy for patients with diabetes who require myocardial revascularization remains uncertain and further evaluation of contemporary percutaneous techniques in diabetic patients is required.

Although the objective in RITA-1 was to achieve equivalent revascularization, an initial strategy of CABG provided more complete revascularization. This reflects an intrinsic difference between the two revascularization procedures, and in the trial surgeons grafted most target vessels at the initial operation, but many cardiologists apparently accepted partial revascularization rather than subject patients to the increased risk of multi-vessel angioplasty. This difference in the extent of myocardial revascularization, combined with the effects of restenosis, account for the substantially higher rates of repeat coronary arteriography and re-intervention in the PTCA group during the first year of follow-up, and similar results have been reported elsewhere [13, 23]. Thereafter the low intervention rate probably reflects a slow rate of disease progression in both groups and the gradual appearance of disease in saphenous vein bypass grafts in the CABG group.

In RITA-1 both revascularization procedures improved angina but at every follow-up assessment there was small excess of mild angina in the PTCA group. Overall around 30% of PTCA patients remained symptomatic and a substantial proportion required long-term anti-anginal medication. By contrast, one month after surgical revascularization only 2% of patients complained of angina, and although angina gradually recurred amongst surgically-treated patients a significant treatment difference persisted for six years. The BARI trial also reported an excess of mild angina among patients assigned to PTCA but in both trials there was little difference in the prevalence of severe (grade III–IV) angina between the two treatment groups [24]. The higher prevalence of angina in the PTCA group is probably at least partly due to incomplete revascularization at the initial procedure, and in BARI the extent of revascularization (assessed by a myocardial jeopardy score) was predictive of angina at one year [25].

These data suggest that CABG is a more effective treatment for angina in the medium term, but in RITA-1 surgical revascularization did not improve other measures of functional capacity. As expected one month after revascularization surgically-treated patients had shorter exercise times, more breathlessness, lower levels of physical activity and a lower rate of return to work. Thereafter there was no treatment difference in these assessments of functional capacity and the small differences in health related quality of life score could be largely explained by the differences in angina.

RITA-1 randomized a selected group of patients in whom equivalent revascularization was considered possible by either treatment method. Nevertheless we estimate that the results of RITA-1 (which included patients with single-vessel disease) may be applicable to 21% of patients undergoing percutaneous or surgical revascularization [5]. The BARI Investigators estimate that their results are relevant to about 12% of patients undergoing revascularization for multi-vessel disease [26]. The results of the revascularization trials are therefore not applicable to all patients with coronary artery disease but are relevant to a substantial subgroup judged clinically and angiographically suitable for either intervention.

RITA-1 and other trials of revascularization procedures provide clinicians with valuable information on which decisions about patient management can be based. Overall there is no evidence of a difference in mortality, risk of myocardial infarction or economic cost between the two treatment strategies, and patients deemed suitable for either method of revascularization can therefore be offered a choice. On the one hand, an initial strategy of PTCA usually involves a short admission to hospital, followed by a rapid return to normal activity. Although PTCA relieves symptoms, in the medium term patients are more likely to complain of angina, require anti-anginal medication, and undergo repeat coronary arteriography and additional myocardial revascularization. On the other hand, the more invasive CABG operation usually involves a longer initial hospitalization and subsequent convalescence. Thereafter surgically-treated patients enjoy slightly better relief from angina and require fewer anti-anginal drugs, at least over 5–7 years. When choosing a revascularization procedure physicians and their patients must also consider the impact of new technologies on the relative risks and benefits of percutaneous and surgical treatment strategies. RITA-1 recruited patients before the widespread use of stents and glycoprotein IIb/IIIa receptor antagonists and these adjuncts have had a major impact on the acute and long-term results of balloon angioplasty [21, 27].

RITA-2

Randomized clinical trials are required to determine whether patients in whom myocardial revascularization is not considered essential should be treated by a policy of early angioplasty, or whether revascularization can be safely deferred. The second Randomized Intervention Treatment of Angina (RITA-2) trial was designed to compare the long-term effects of initial treatment strategies of coronary angioplasty and conservative (medical) care in patients deemed suitable for either treatment method.

Trial protocol

Patients with arteriographically proven coronary artery disease were considered for RITA-2 if the supervising cardiologist was uncertain about the optimal treatment method, and thought that continued medical therapy and coronary angioplasty were clinically acceptable alternatives. Patients were not required to have current symptoms but patients with severe symptoms were potentially eligible if they were prepared to accept an initial strategy of conservative treatment. Patients with multi-vessel disease, impaired left ventricular or recent unstable angina were eligible for randomization. Patients in whom early myocardial revascularization was considered necessary for symptoms or for prognosis, and patients with previous myocardial revascularization, left main stem disease, haemodynamically significant valve or life threatening non-cardiac disease were also excluded [28].

Before randomization the coronary arteriograms of eligible patients were reviewed by an interventional cardiologist who identified at least one significant coronary stenosis in a major epicardial vessel, which was suitable for interventional treatment. A significant coronary lesion was defined as a 50% or greater diameter stenosis in at least two radiographic projections, or 70% diameter stenosis in one projection. Major coronary vessels were defined as the left anterior descending artery and large diagonal branches, or the circumflex artery and large obtuse marginal branches, or a balanced or dominant right coronary artery.

Patients who satisfied the eligibility criteria and provided informed consent were assigned to initial treatment strategies of coronary angioplasty or continued medical care. Interventional methods were not standardized during an assigned angioplasty procedure and stents and other coronary interventional techniques could be used if the initial angioplasty result was unsatisfactory. There was no requirement for all coronary stenoses to be dilated, but multi-vessel dilatation could be staged over more than one procedure. Following assigned intervention clinicians were encouraged to discontinue anti-anginal medication unless the patient complained of angina. During follow-up coronary arteriography and additional intervention procedures were carried out when clinically indicated.

Patients assigned to an initial treatment strategy of non-interventional (medical) therapy were prescribed anti-anginal medication for symptom relief. During follow-up coronary arteriography was only repeated for compelling clinical reasons, and myocardial revascularization procedures were reserved for patients whose symptoms were not adequately controlled by optimal medical therapy, which usually included a beta-adrenoceptor blocking agent, with a calcium antagonist and/or long-acting nitrate preparation in maximally tolerated doses.

Patients were assessed at baseline, and three months, six months and yearly intervals after randomization. The primary trial end-point was predefined as the combined incidence of death (from all causes) and definite non-fatal myocardial infarction. Definite myocardial infarction was diagnosed if new pathological Q waves ($> 30\,ms$ in duration) appeared on an electrocardiogram: (i) within seven days of any myocardial revascularization procedure or (ii) during subsequent follow-up. Definite myocardial infarction was also diagnosed if a convincing clinical history was associated with electrocardiographic changes compatible with non-Q wave infarction and the serum activities of at least two cardiac enzymes were above twice the upper limit of normal. All data were analyzed according to the original treatment assignment (intention-to-treat) [28].

Results

During the recruitment period around 70,000 patients underwent coronary arteriography at the participating centres, of whom 2750 were considered eligible for randomization. From July 1992 to May 1996 a total of 1018 patients (37%) were recruited, and patient refusal was the reason why half of the remaining eligible patients were not randomized.

The baseline characteristics of the 504 patients assigned to coronary angioplasty and the 514 patients assigned to continued medical treatment were comparable. The mean age was 57 years and 18% were women. Angina grade III or worse was present in 21% of patients, 10% had recent unstable angina, 47% had previous myocardial infarction and 9% were treated diabetics. Single-vessel disease was present in 60% of patients, two-vessel disease in 33% and three-vessel disease in 7%. The majority of patients had normal or mildly impaired left ventricular function and 28% of patients had a significant stenosis in the proximal left anterior descending artery.

The assigned angioplasty procedure was not carried out in 33 (7%) patients because of symptom improvement, disease progression or regression, and patient refusal. Overall 642 stenoses were dilated in 471 patients with an angiographic success rate of 93%. The trial recruited patients before the widespread use of stents, which were used during 44 (9%) assigned interventional procedures. Emergency coronary artery bypass surgery was required in seven patients (1.5%), and nine patients underwent CABG instead of the intended randomized PTCA.

During a median 2.7 years follow-up there were 11 deaths in the PTCA group and seven in the medical group ($p = 0.32$). The cause of death was cardiac in five PTCA patients (including one randomized-procedure-related death) and three medical patients. There was an excess of definite non-fatal myocardial infarct in the PTCA group (21 versus 10) which is largely explained by seven non-fatal infarcts related to the randomized procedure. Overall death or definite myocardial infarction occurred in 32 PTCA patients (6.3%) and 17 medical patients (3.3%), an absolute treatment difference of 3.0% (relative risk 1.92, 95% CI 1.08–3.41, $p = 0.02$).

Additional coronary arteriograms have been required in 133 PTCA patients and 92 medical group patients. Since randomization CABG has been carried out in 40 patients assigned to

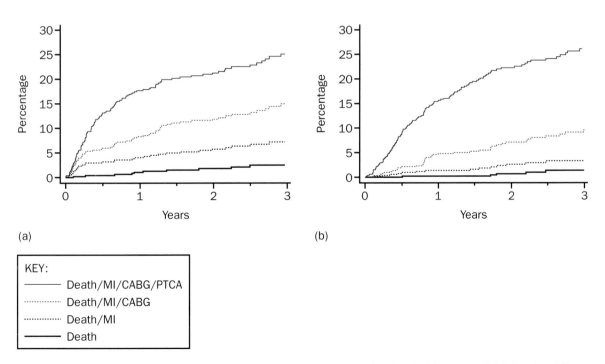

(a)

(b)

KEY:
——— Death/MI/CABG/PTCA
·········· Death/MI/CABG
············ Death/MI
——— Death

Figure 12.2 (a) RITA-2 patients assigned to PTCA: cumulative risk of PTCA, CABG, myocardial infarction (MI) or death; (b) RITA-2 patients assigned to medical treatment: cumulative risk of PTCA, CABG, myocardial infarction (MI) or death. Reproduced with permission from *Lancet* 1997; **350**:461–468.

PTCA (7.9%) and 30 patients assigned to medical treatment (5.8%). A non-randomized PTCA was required in 62 PTCA patients and 101 medical patients. After two years the cumulative risk of death, myocardial infarction, or CABG was 12.3% and 7.1% in the PTCA and medical groups, respectively (Fig. 12.2). The accumulating risks of death, myocardial infarction, or any non-assigned revascularization procedure are also shown in Fig. 12.2.

Of the 117 medical group patients who have undergone revascularization, 75% had grade III or IV angina and 83% were taking two or more anti-anginal drugs at the time of the change in treatment strategy. As expected the use of coronary stents during non-assigned PTCA increased from 9% in 1993–1994 to 47% in 1996.

Angina was assessed using the Canadian Cardiovascular Society classification [7]. Following randomization angina improved in both groups, with substantially greater improvement among PTCA patients. At baseline 80% of patients in both groups complained of angina but at three months this had decreased to 36% in the PTCA group and 62% in the medical group. Thereafter about one third of patients in the PTCA group continued to have angina, but anginal symptoms in the medical group gradually improved. By three years the prevalence of any angina was 31% and 45% in the PTCA and medical groups, respectively. The difference in the prevalence of limiting angina was less marked, and at three months there was a 16.5% excess of grade II+ angina in the medical group ($p < 0.001$), but this attenuated to 7.6% after two years ($p = 0.02$). This trend can be partly explained by the fact that patients with worsening symptoms underwent cardiac interventions in both treatment groups. Treatment by PTCA also improved symptoms of breathlessness (42% at three months vs 57% in the medical group, $p < 0.001$), but these differences became less marked over time.

At baseline the majority of patients were taking one (41%) or two (37%) anti-anginal drugs but 7% were on no anti-anginal medication.

During follow-up patients in the medical group required more anti-anginal drugs, and at two years 87% of the medical group but 69% of the PTCA group were taking at least one anti-anginal drug. There was no difference between the two treatment groups in the use of aspirin or lipid-lowering drugs.

Symptom limited exercise treadmill tests were carried out using the Bruce protocol and at baseline the mean exercise time was 7 min 41 s in both groups (SD 2 min 47 s). Following randomization exercise times increased, but at three months the improvement in the PTCA group exceeded that in the medical group by a mean of 35 s (95% CI 20–451 s). This attenuated over time and at three years there was no difference in exercise time between the two treatment groups.

Subgroup analyses demonstrated that the beneficial effects of PTCA on angina and exercise time were mainly confined to patients with severe angina and poor exercise tolerance at baseline. For instance among patients with grade III or IV angina at baseline 58% of medical patients and 36% of PTCA patients had limiting (grade II+) angina at six months. By contrast among patients with grade 0 or I angina at baseline 17% of medical patients and 14% of PTCA patients had limiting angina at six months.

Health related quality of life was assessed with the Short-Form 36 (SF-36) self-administered questionnaire [29]. After randomization both the PTCA and medical treatment groups showed substantial improvements in most aspects of quality of life. The PTCA group had significantly greater improvements in physical functioning, vitality and general health at both three months and one year compared with the medical group, but there was no treatment difference in any of the eight SF-36 scores at three years. These treatment differences could be explained by the greater improvements in angina, breathlessness and exercise treadmill time in the PTCA group [30].

At baseline 32% of males aged less than 65 were unemployed due to coronary disease.

Following randomization coronary related unemployment decreased to around 25% in both groups with no significant treatment difference over three years.

The mean three-year costs of the two treatment strategies in RITA-2 have been estimated [31]. The cost of an initial strategy of PTCA exceeded the cost of an initial strategy of medical management by 74% over 3 years.

Discussion

The RITA-2 trial is a pragmatic comparison of initial treatment policies of PTCA and medical care in patients with coronary artery disease who were considered suitable for either treatment method. The randomized patients are therefore not representative of all patients undergoing percutaneous coronary intervention, but the trial results are likely to be relevant to a substantial subgroup for whom either medical therapy or angioplasty appear appropriate and for whom optimal treatment is uncertain. Other trials of PTCA and medical care have also reported results, but these trials are small and have limited statistical power to compare the two strategies for risk of death and myocardial infarction [32–34].

Most RITA-2 patients had mild symptoms, one or two-vessel coronary artery disease and preserved left ventricular function, and would be predicted to be at low cardiovascular risk [35]. Nevertheless the policy of early PTCA was associated with an excess hazard mainly due to procedure-related myocardial infarction. By contrast the risk of myocardial infarction in the medical group was low, even though all patients had a significant stenosis in a major epicardial artery. These data are consistent with evidence that myocardial infarction is often not due to pre-existing flow-limiting stenoses [36] and as yet RITA-2 provides no evidence that successful PTCA reduces the risk of myocardial infarction. The long-term implications of procedure-related myocardial infarction in RITA-2 are uncertain but in other studies even

small elevations of cardiac enzyme levels after percutaneous intervention appear to be of prognostic significance [37]. These data suggest that PTCA should not be carried out for 'prognostic' reasons in asymptomatic patients and the early use of PTCA in some low-risk patients may be inappropriate.

RITA-2 demonstrated that PTCA improves angina, breathlessness, exercise tolerance and health related quality of life scores in the medium term. These treatment differences attenuate over 2–3 years, partly because patients with severe symptoms in the medical group eventually underwent revascularization. Symptomatic improvement in the medical group may also be partly due to modification of anti-anginal treatment, disease regression and development of coronary collaterals, as well as regression to the mean.

Subgroup analyses clearly demonstrated that the benefits of PTCA are mainly confined to patients with limiting angina or impaired exercise tolerance at baseline, and these analyses have important implications for clinical practice. Patients without limiting angina did not benefit substantially from PTCA, and in these patients revascularization might reasonably be deferred unless more severe symptoms supervene. Furthermore exercise times did not improve significantly in patients with good baseline exercise times, and since such patients are generally at low cardiovascular risk they are unlikely to gain a major prognostic benefit from coronary angioplasty. Patients with more severe angina and with limited exercise tolerance at baseline may gain appreciable benefit from PTCA, but this must be balanced against the small procedure related hazard and the additional economic cost.

SUMMARY

The RITA-1 and RITA-2 trials have provided valuable insights into the role of coronary balloon angioplasty in patients with coronary artery disease. The trials provide no evidence that 'plain old' balloon angioplasty reduces cardiovascular risk, and in RITA-2 there was a procedure-related excess risk of myocardial infarction. Nevertheless in both trials an initial policy of percutaneous intervention provided effective relief of angina over several years, albeit at the clinical and economic cost of additional revascularization procedures.

Since the results of the RITA trials were published the practice of interventional cardiology has developed rapidly. The use of coronary stents and glycoprotein IIb/IIIa receptor antagonists is now widespread and these adjuncts have been shown to improve the short and long-term results of percutaneous interventions [21, 27]. Although the problem of restenosis has not been fully resolved the results of intracoronary brachytherapy and drug-coated stents appear promising [38, 39]. There have also been major advances in the medical treatment of patients with coronary artery disease, including the use of new antiplatelet agents and HMGCoA reductase inhibitors for managing hypercholesterolaemia [40]. In addition the importance of the glycaemic control in patients with diabetes is increasingly recognized [41, 42]. The extent to which these advances in medical practice will influence the results of percutaneous coronary interventions in the 21st century can only be determined by additional randomized clinical trials of contemporary percutaneous coronary intervention versus alternative medical and surgical treatment strategies.

REFERENCES

1. Mock MB, Reeder GS, Schaff HV et al. Percutaneous transluminal coronary angioplasty versus coronary artery bypass. Isn't it time for a randomized trial? *New Engl J Med* 1985; **312**:916–919.
2. Ryan TJ. Multilesion angioplasty: progress and a plea for proof, *J Am Coll Cardiol* 1989; **13**:289–290.
3. Editorial. BARI, CABRI, EAST, GABI and RITA: coronary angioplasty on trial, *Lancet* 1990; **335**:1315–1316.
4. Henderson RA for the Randomized Intervention Treatment of Angina Trial. The Randomized Intervention Treatment of Angina (RITA) trial protocol: a long-term study of coronary angioplasty and coronary artery bypass surgery in patients with angina, *Br Heart J* 1989; **62**: 411–414.
5. Henderson RA, Raskino CL, Hampton JR. Variations in the use of coronary arteriography in the UK: the RITA trial coronary arteriogram register, *Q J Med* 1995; **88**(3):167–173.
6. RITA Trial Participants. Coronary angioplasty versus coronary artery bypass surgery: the Randomized Intervention Treatment of Angina (RITA) trial, *Lancet* 1993; **341**:573–580.
7. Henderson RA, Pocock SJ, Sharp SJ et al. Long-term results of RITA-1 trial: clinical and cost comparisons of coronary angioplasty and coronary-artery bypass grafting. Randomized Intervention Treatment of Angina, *Lancet* 1998; **352**(9138):1419–1425.
8. Campeau L. Grading of angina pectoris, *Circulation* 1976; **54**:522–523.
9. Sheffield LT. *Exercise testing and training of apparently healthy individuals. A handbook for physicians*, (American Heart Association: 1972) 35–38.
10. Backett EM, McEwen J, Hunt SM. Report to the Social Science Research Council. *Health and Quality of Life* (London: Social Science Research Council, 1981).
11. Pocock SJ, Henderson RA, Seed P, Treasure T, Hampton JR. Quality of life, employment status and anginal symptoms after coronary angioplasty or bypass surgery: three-year follow-up in the Randomized Intervention Treatment of Angina (RITA) trial, *Circulation* 1996; **94**:135–142.
12. Sculpher MJ, Seed P, Henderson RA et al. Health service costs of coronary angioplasty and coronary artery bypass surgery: the Randomized Intervention Treatment of Angina (RITA) trial, *Lancet* 1994; **344**:927–930.
13. King SB III, Kosinski AS, Guyton RA, Lembo NJ, Weintraub WS. Eight-year mortality in the Emory Angioplasty versus Surgery Trial (EAST), *J Am Coll Cardiol* 2000; **35**(5):1116–1121.
14. The BARI Investigators. Seven-year outcome in the Bypass Angioplasty Revascularization Investigation (BARI) by treatment and diabetic status, *J Am Coll Cardiol* 2000; **35**(5):1122–1129.
15. Pocock SJ, Henderson RA, Rickards AF et al. Meta-analysis of randomized trials comparing

coronary angioplasty with bypass surgery, *Lancet* 1995; **346**(8984):1184–1189.

16. Henderson RA. Coronary angioplasty and coronary artery bypass surgery. In: Pitt B, Julian D, Pocock S, eds, *Clinical Trials in Cardiology* (London: WB Saunders Company Ltd, 1997) 203–220.

17. Bertrand ME. Long-term follow-up of European revascularization trials. Presented at the 68th Scientific Sessions. Plenary Session XII, American Heart Association, Anaheim, California, 1995.

18. The BARI Investigators. Influence of diabetes on five-year mortality and morbidity in a randomized trial comparing CABG and PTCA in patients with multivessel disease: the Bypass Angioplasty Revascularization Investigation (BARI), *Circulation* 1997; **96**(6):1761–1769.

19. Feit F, Brooks MM, Sopko G et al. Long-term clinical outcome in the Bypass Angioplasty Revascularization Investigation Registry: comparison with the randomized trial. BARI Investigators, *Circulation* 2000; **101**(24):2795–2802.

20. Weintraub WS, Stein B, Kosinski A et al. Outcome of coronary bypass surgery versus coronary angioplasty in diabetic patients with multi-vessel coronary artery disease, *J Am Coll Cardiol* 1998; **31**(1):10–19.

21. Serruys PW, Unger F, Sousa JE et al. Comparison of coronary-artery bypass surgery and stenting for the treatment of multi-vessel disease, *N Engl J Med* 2001; **344**(15):1117–1124.

22. Abizaid A, Costa MA, Centemero M et al. Clinical and economic impact of diabetes mellitus on percutaneous and surgical treatment of multi-vessel coronary disease patients: insights from the arterial revascularization therapy study (ARTS) trial, *Circulation* 2001; **104**(5):533–538.

23. The Bypass Angioplasty Revascularization Investigation (BARI) Investigators. Comparison of coronary bypass surgery with angioplasty in patients with multi-vessel disease, *New Engl J Med* 1996; **335**:217–225.

24. The Bypass Angioplasty Revascularization Investigation (BARI) Investigators. Five-year clinical and functional outcome comparing bypass surgery and angioplasty in patients with multi-vessel coronary disease. A multicenter randomized trial. Writing Group for the Bypass Angioplasty Revascularization Investigation (BARI) Investigators, *JAMA* 1997; **277**:715–721.

25. Whitlow PL, Dimas AP, Bashore TM et al. Relationship of extent of revascularization with angina at one year in the Bypass Angioplasty Revascularization Investigation (BARI), *J Am Coll Cardiol* 1999; **34**(6):1750–1759.

26. Detre KM, Rosen AD, Bost JE et al. Contemporary practice of coronary revascularization in US hospitals and hospitals participating in the Bypass Angioplasty Revascularization Investigation (BARI), *J Am Coll Cardiol* 1996; **28**:609–615.

27. Kong DF, Califf RM, Miller DP et al. Clinical outcomes of therapeutic agents that block the platelet glycoprotein IIb/IIIa integrin in ischemic heart disease, *Circulation* 1998; **98**(25):2829–2835.

28. RITA-2 Trial Participants. Coronary angioplasty versus medical therapy for angina: the second Randomized Intervention Treatment of Angina (RITA-2) trial, *Lancet* 1997; **350**:461–468.

29. Ware JE, Sherbourne CD. The SF-36 short-form health status health survey: 1. conceptual framework and item selection, *Medical Care* 1992; **30**:473–483.

30. Pocock SJ, Henderson RA, Clayton T, Lyman GH, Chamberlain DA. Quality of life after coronary angioplasty or continued medical treatment for angina: three-year follow-up in the RITA-2 trial. Randomized Intervention Treatment of Angina. *J Am Coll Cardiol* 2000; **35**(4):907–914.

31. Sculpher MJ, Smith DH, Clayton RA et al. Coronary angioplasty versus medical therapy for angina. Health service costs based on the second Randomized Intervention Treatment of Angina (RITA-2) trial, *Eur Heart J* 2002; in press.

32. Folland ED, Hartigan PM, Parisi AF. Percutaneous transluminal coronary angioplasty versus medical therapy for stable angina pectoris: outcomes for patients with double-vessel versus single-vessel coronary artery disease in a Veterans Affairs Cooperative randomized trial. Veterans Affairs ACME Investigators, *J Am Coll Cardiol* 1997; **29**:1505–1511.

33. Parisi AF, Folland ED, Hartigan P. A comparison of angioplasty with medical therapy in the treatment of single-vessel coronary artery disease, *New Engl J Med* 1992; **326**:10–16.

34. Sievers B, Hamm CW, Herzner A, Kuck KH. Medical therapy versus PTCA: a prospective, randomized trial in patients with asymptomatic coronary single vessel disease (abstract), *Circulation* 1993; **88**:1–296.

35. Ringqvist I, Fisher LD, Mock M et al. Prognostic value of angiographic indices of coronary artery disease from the coronary artery surgery study, *J Clin Invest* 1983; **71**:1854–1866.

36. Giroud D, Li JM, Urban P, Meier B, Rutishauser W. Relation of the site of acute myocardial infarction to the most severe coronary arterial stenosis at prior angiography, *Am J Cardiol* 1992; **39**:729–732.

37. Califf RM, Abdelmeguid AE, Kuntz RE et al. Myonecrosis after revascularization procedures, *J Am Coll Cardiol* 1998; **31**(2):241–252.

38. Sousa JE, Costa MA, Abizaid A et al. Lack of neointimal proliferation after implantation of sirolimus-coated stents in human coronary arteries: a quantitative coronary angiography and three-dimensional intravascular ultrasound study, *Circulation* 2001; **103**(2):192–195.

39. Teirstein PS, Massullo V, Jani S et al. A subgroup analysis of the Scripps Coronary Radiation to Inhibit Proliferation Poststenting Trial. *Int J Radiation Oncology, Biology, Physics* 1998; **42**(5):1097–1104.

40. Scandinavian simvastatin survival study group. Randomized trial of cholesterol lowering in 4444 patients with coronary heart disease: the Scandinavian simvastatin survival study (4S), *Lancet* 1994; **344**:1383–1389.

41. United Kingdom Prospective Diabetes Study (UKPDS) Group. Intensive blood-glucose control with sulphonylureas or insulin compared with conventional treatment and risk of complications in patients with type 2 diabetes (UKPDS 33), *Lancet* 1998; **352**(9131):837–853.

42. Diabetes Control and Complications Trial Research Group. The effect of intensive treatment of diabetes on the development and progression of long-term complications in insulin-dependent diabetes mellitus, *New Engl J Med* 1993; **329**(14):977–986.

13

Emory angioplasty versus surgery trial

Spencer B King III

CONTENTS • Introduction • Methods • Screening procedures • Results • Discussion • Conclusion

INTRODUCTION

When Andreas Gruentzig first developed coronary angioplasty in 1977, the goal was to apply this technology to relatively discrete lesions primarily in single vessels. Shortly after the development of the procedure, more complex lesions were attempted and in the early 1980s, it became evident that angioplasty would be challenging coronary bypass surgery [1]. In following the initial cohort of patients treated in Zurich for ten years, it became evident that single vessel disease patients had a superior outcome to those with multi-vessel disease [2]. A number of cardiologists began to perform angioplasty, not only in multiple vessels, but in multiple lesions within those vessels [3–6]. The NHLBI Registry of angioplasty, first organized in the late 1970s, was redone in 1985–1986 [7]. The number of patients having multi-vessel angioplasty increased in the latter registry to almost 50% of the patients treated. Our group and others were interested in comparing angioplasty to bypass surgery, however with the initial equipment available, angioplasty had not reached adequate maturity to be tested against such an established procedure. Following the development of steerable guidewires in 1982, it became possible to reach most stenoses that required therapy and with the advent of higher pressure balloons, it became possible to dilate those lesions. Gruentzig advocated for a randomized trial as early as 1983. Although that trial was not funded following revisions, we did begin the EAST trial in 1987. This became the first NHLBI-sponsored comparison of angioplasty versus bypass surgery. The goal of this trial would be to randomize patients with multi-vessel disease to a strategy of balloon angioplasty dilating the lesions felt to be responsible for ischemia and to bypass surgery performing the accepted techniques available at that time.

METHODS

The Emory Angioplasty Surgery Trial was a single-center, randomized trial of patients who had been referred for revascularization because of symptoms and/or extensive ischemia felt to require revascularization. The primary endpoint of the trial was to be a composite of clinically relevant adverse events. Those were death, Q wave myocardial infarction, or the presence of a significantly extensive ischemic defect on thallium stress testing at the defined end-point of the trial. These end-points were selected because power to detect the difference in mortality would have required far more patients than could be generated, and it was judged that death or unequivocal myocardial infarction would be highly clinically relevant, and the presence of extensive ischemic defects identified on thallium scanning would signal failure to achieve or to maintain adequate revascularization. The thallium defect was also judged to be an important future prognostic marker and therefore would be clinically relevant. More sensitive markers of myocardial infarction were rejected as an end-point because of the expectation that these would be much more common in the surgical cohort and there was not data to support the relevance of the post-surgical CK changes. The defined follow-up end-point was three years and with additional support from the NHLBI, a five year extension of the study was obtained to provide long-term follow-up for survival and other features.

In addition to periodic clinical follow-ups, follow-up angiograms and stress thallium scans were scheduled for all patients at one and three years. In addition to those tests and electrocardiograms, extensive collection of risk factor data was obtained at baseline, one and three years. Unassigned serum and plasma samples were also frozen for future analysis. The structure and baseline features of this trial have been previously reported [8].

SCREENING PROCEDURES

All patients being referred for catheterization or presenting with angiograms already obtained for consideration of revascularization to the Emory University Hospitals were screened for eligibility in the trial. There were 5118 patients with multi-vessel disease without a prior history of angioplasty or bypass surgery. If these patients were being considered for revascularization, a search was made for any defined exclusions which would eliminate them from consideration. The most common exclusions preventing patients from consideration in the trial were chronic total occlusions more than eight weeks old, left main disease > 30%, two or more total occlusions, and an ejection fraction

< 25%. In addition, if patients were judged to have insufficient ischemia to warrant consideration for surgery or insufficient symptoms to warrant revascularization, these patients were not considered further. Additional exclusions were myocardial infarction within the preceding five days and non-cardiac illness threatening survival over the ensuing three years. All eligible patients were reviewed by a cardiologist investigator and a surgeon investigator. If either investigator felt that their procedure could not be performed with a reasonable degree of safety, then the patient was excluded. Eight hundred and forty-two (16.5%) of the screened population were found to be eligible. The patient's attending physician was consulted and if permission was granted to approach the patient, the patient was informed of the trial and asked if they would volunteer. Ultimately, 392 patients consented and were randomized, and 450 patients were entered into a parallel registry because either the attending physician or the patient refused to consent.

The baseline features of these patients have been previously described [8], and the pertinent ones are listed in Table 13.1. In the entire cohort of eligible patients and in the randomized trial, 40% had 3 vessel disease and 60% 2 vessel disease.

RESULTS

Analyses that have been performed on the EAST trial include the three year defined end-point analyses of the primary end-point and its components, the requirement for revascularization over the three year period, the economic and quality of life analyses, detailed angiographic assessments, and the predictors of restenosis and progression of disease, a comparison of the outcomes in the randomized trial, the eight year completed follow-up of these patients, and the correlation of some non-traditional risk factors utilizing the stored blood component samples [9–14].

The baseline features of this study, which

Table 13.1 Baseline characteristics of randomized and registry patients

Characteristic	Randomized (n = 392)	Registry (n = 450)	p value
Age (years)	61.6 ± 10.0	61.8 + 0.4	0.73
Men	289 (73.7)	355 (78.9)	0.078
White race†	367 (93.6)	426 (95.1)	0.32
College education†	75 (19.1)	114 (26.0)	0.019
Three-vessel disease	156 (39.8)	180 (40.0)	0.95
No. of narrowings ⩾ 70% in diameters	1.7 ± 1.1	2.0 ± 1.3	0.008
Proximal LAD stenosis ⩾ 70%	153 (39.0)	164 (36.4)	0.44
Totally occluded vessel	8 (2.0)	21 (4.7)	0.037
Ejection fraction (%)‡	61.4 ± 11.7	60.2 ± 11.9	0.21
Prior myocardial infarction	160 (40.8)	174 (38.7)	0.52
Congestive heart failure	13 (3.3)	16 (3.6)	0.85
CCS class III or IV angina†	302 (79.7)	305 (73.3)	0.035
Diabetes mellitus†	90 (23.0)	92 (20.5)	0.38
Systemic hypertension†	206 (52.7)	234 (52.2)	0.90
Cigarette smoking†	251 (64.5)	293 (65.1)	0.86
Total serum cholesterol (mg/dl)‡	221 ± 47	218 ± 51	0.13
Medication			
Intravenous heparin	124 (31.6)	101 (22.4)	0.003
Intravenous nitroglycerin	46 (11.7)	38 (8.4)	0.11
Beta-blockers†	135 (34.5)	173 (38.4)	0.24
Calcium antagonists	297 (75.8)	308 (68.4)	0.018
Topical nitrates	195 (49.7)	151 (33.6)	< 0.001
Aspirin	193 (49.2)	203 (45.1)	0.23

Plus-minus values are means ± SD; all other values are numbers of patients with percentages given in parentheses. To convert values for cholesterol to mmol/l, multiply by 0.02586. †Few missing values were present and percentages were calculated based on available data. ‡Total number of patients: ejection fraction, 385 of 446 for randomized and/or registry. CCS, Canadian Cardiovascular Society; LAD, left anterior descending artery.

were pertinent for an average age of 62 with 74% men, 72% involvement of the proximal LAD, overall ejection fraction of 61%, and Canadian Cardiovascular Class Angina III or IV in 80% of the patients, indicates that these patients represented a fairly broad spectrum with the majority of the patients representing neither the highest risk nor lowest risk patients for revascularization.

The initial revascularization procedures resulted in four deaths, two in the angioplasty group and two in the surgery group, for a 1% mortality overall. At the completion of the three year follow-up, the primary end-point was not significantly different between the groups (freedom from death, Q wave MI, or extensive thallium ischemic defect being 27.3% in the surgery group and 28.8% in the PTCA group, $p = 0.81$). The components of the end-point also did not differ (93.8% surgery and angioplasty 92.9%), Q wave myocardial infarction (19.6% surgery and 14.6% angioplasty), or the extensive ischemic defect (5.7% surgery and 9.6% angioplasty).

It was anticipated that the angioplasty group would require more revascularization than the surgery group over the ensuing years. This was indeed true as at three years while 13% of the surgery group had undergone repeat procedures, 41% of the angioplasty group had had repeat revascularization. Some of the revascularization in the angioplasty group was due to surgery at the time of the initial procedure. Ten per cent of the patients underwent surgery within the initial hospitalization because of either urgent need to do so or failure to achieve adequate revascularization by angioplasty leading to elective surgery.

The angiographic findings were reviewed in a subsequent publication [10]. In order to assess the degree of revascularization, a scheme of 'index segments' was developed. These were segments that supplied important segments of the left ventricular myocardium and were pre-defined (Fig. 13.1). Revascularization was more complete initially in the surgery group. At the time of the index procedure in the angioplasty group, 85% of the pre-specified index segments were attempted, whereas 98% of the surgery segments were attempted. At one year the follow-up angiogram revealed that 88% of the surgery segments remained revascularized compared to 59% of the angioplasty segments. By three years that gap had been reduced with 87% of the surgery segments now patent compared to 70% of the angioplasty segments. This improvement was due to repeat revascularization in the angioplasty group. The degree of revascularization was also reviewed as to the completeness of 'functional revascularization'. When the index segments were analyzed for their freedom from severe stenosis ($\geqslant 70\%$) and when the artery involved was larger than 2 mm, the groups did not differ in terms of three year completeness of revascularization (93% for PTCA patients and 75% for CABG patients) [10].

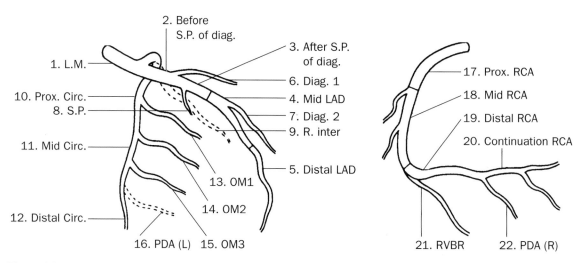

Figure 13.1 Identification of segments that, if obstructed, were considered index segments on the baseline, one-year and three-year angiograms.

At three years angina was more common in the angioplasty group. Canadian Cardiovascular Society Angina of Class II, III, or IV was present in 20% of the angioplasty group compared to 12% of the surgery group.

Comparison of randomized patients and the registry patients

In the 450 patients who were eligible but were not entered into the trial, the clinical and angiographic characteristics were almost identical to those patients who were actually randomized. The one exception was a higher education level and socioeconomic status in the patients in the non-randomized registry. Despite the strong similarity of the baseline features between the randomized trial and the registry, there was significant physician judgment toward selecting patients for surgery with more extensive disease. Of the patients in the registry with three-vessel disease, 84% had surgery and of the patients with two-vessel disease, 54% had angioplasty. There were obviously other subtle differences that influence the decision for surgery or angioplasty. At the end of three years, the overall survival was slightly better for the registry cohort (96.4%) as compared to the randomized patients (93.4%). The relief of angina was similar between the angioplasty and surgery patients in the registry. When the randomized and registry cohorts were followed out to eight years, there was no significant difference in the survival curves. We believe that the registry supports the randomized trial and confirms that there was no bias toward selecting low-risk patients for the randomized trial.

Economics and quality of life

The cost of the two strategies was of significant interest as was the continuing quality of life. Analysis of the costs was done utilizing the uniform billing 82 conversions and adding on physician charges. Although costs were higher

in the surgery group initially, that advantage was largely lost by three years due to repeat procedures in the angioplasty group [11]. At eight years there was no additional change with the costs remaining comparable between the two strategies over the entire follow-up period. The three year quality of life questionnaire indicated that surgery patients believed they had recovered more completely, however the question regarding optimism about their health favored the angioplasty group. Overall there was little difference between the groups and their quality of life measures.

Eight year follow-up

All of the patients in the randomized trial were followed for at least eight years [15]. This late follow-up did not include all the end-points that were adjudicated at the three year follow-up but rather concentrated on survival and repeat procedures. Follow-up was accomplished by annual questionnaires and follow-up phone calls when the questionnaires were not answered completely. At the end of eight years, survival in the surgery group was 82.7% and in the angioplasty group 79.3% ($p = 0.40$) (Fig. 13.2). An analysis was made of the diabetic cohort and although there were only 59 treated diabetics in the EAST trial, the directionality was similar to the BARI trial [16]. Also similar to the BARI trial, the patients without diabetes had identical eight-year survival regardless of the group to which they were initially assigned.

Repeat procedures, which were markedly different at one and three years, remained relatively parallel between three and eight years (Fig. 13.3).

Progression of disease

The performance of routine angiograms at one and three years allowed for quantitative angiographic assessment of disease progression. Patients were divided into those who had new

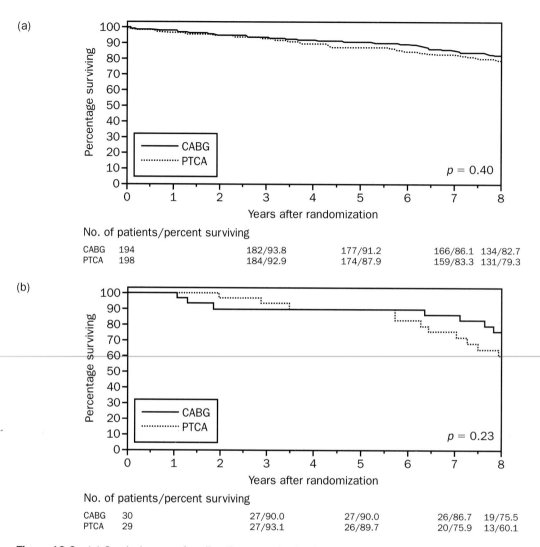

Figure 13.2 (a) Survival curves for all patients randomized to surgery or angioplasty in the EAST trial. (b) Survival curves for patients with diabetes randomized to angioplasty or surgery.

lesions developing versus those who did not. Risk factors for new lesion development included low density lipoprotein:high density lipoprotein (LDL:HDL) ratio, diabetes mellitus, hypertension, total cholesterol, baseline ST-segment depression > 0.1 mV, recurrent chest pain, and baseline systolic blood pressure. The lesions dilated by balloon angioplasty also had a high incidence of restenosis. The one year angiogram revealed that 44% of the lesions initially dilated underwent restenosis with greater than 50% stenosis at follow-up. Fifty six percent of the patients had no restenosis, 28% had between 50% and 70% stenosis, and 16% had greater than 70% stenosis within the first year. Blood products were maintained in −70° refrigerators throughout the course of this trial. Because of interest in less traditional risk factors, gradient

(c)

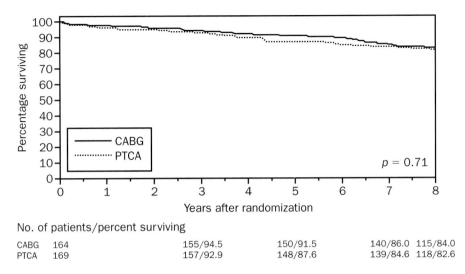

No. of patients/percent surviving

CABG	164	155/94.5	150/91.5	140/86.0	115/84.0
PTCA	169	157/92.9	148/87.6	139/84.6	118/82.6

Figure 13.2 *contd.* (c) Survival curves for patients without diabetes randomized to angioplasty or surgery.

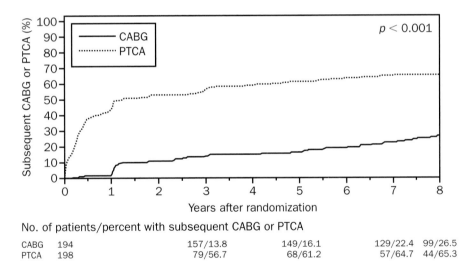

No. of patients/percent with subsequent CABG or PTCA

CABG	194	157/13.8	149/16.1	129/22.4	99/26.5
PTCA	198	79/56.7	68/61.2	57/64.7	44/65.3

Figure 13.3 Cumulative frequency of first repeat PTCA or CABG in the two randomized groups.

gel electrophoresis was undertaken to look for LDL phenotypes. It was found that there was a significant correlation between the pattern B (small dense LDL particle size) and coronary artery disease progression [14]. Additionally it was discovered that homocysteine levels correlated with eight year mortality [13].

DISCUSSION

The EAST trial was not structured to detect a difference in survival. On the other hand, the endpoints selected were highly clinically relevant and reflected the kind of events that revascularization therapy was designed to avoid. The long-term results of the EAST trial have been highly informative. Regardless of the initial therapy selected, survival overall has been similar. Revascularization, which was dramatically different between the two groups at three years largely due to restenosis, has remained unchanged beyond that time. That revascularization in the angioplasty group was due to a combination of early surgery to manage emergencies and to perform elective surgery to further revascularize patients who were felt to be inadequately revascularized by angioplasty. Newer studies utilizing stenting, such as ARTS [17] and SOS [18], have virtually eliminated the early need for reparative surgery in the angioplasty cohort and have also reduced restenosis. The reduction in repeat events has been approximately 50% in those two trials compared to EAST.

The parallel registry has been instructive in that patients in that group had slightly better survival at three years than the randomized cohort, however by eight years those curves no longer differ. The selection of surgery for the more difficult patients in that randomized trial parallels current selection as well. Lessons learned from EAST and from BARI have helped inform new trials, such as BARI 2D, which will not randomize angioplasty and surgery but will utilize information and apply judgments learned from the EAST and BARI trials in selecting the revascularization strategy that will be the most effective and most efficacious.

Numerous improvements have been added to both surgery and angioplasty since this trial was completed. On the angioplasty side, stenting technology has been the most evident change. At the time of the EAST trial, no patients received stents, whereas in the latest NHLBI Dynamic Registry experience, 80% of the patients received stents. The stent technology has made the placement of stents at least as easy and perhaps easier than performing balloon angioplasty. The stents have largely eliminated acute closure and have reduced emergency surgery rates to approximately 1%. Stenting also has reduced restenosis in many subsets. Whether the use of stents will alter the

long-term outcome of patients undergoing percutaneous intervention, however, remains to be discovered since long-term follow-up of these patients is not yet available.

The EAST trial also supports the finding of the BARI trial that diabetic patients with multivessel disease have fared better with surgery than with balloon angioplasty. Although the numbers are small, the directional change in the EAST trial is almost identical to that seen in BARI at seven and eight years [19]. Glycoprotein IIB/IIIa receptor blockers have also perhaps decreased some of the complications of angioplasty. The EPISTENT trial raises the question of whether target vessel revascularization has also been reduced in diabetic patients undergoing stent placement [20]. Certainly the use of thianopyridines has made stenting practical and also perhaps reduced some of the complications.

Most importantly, however, careful observation of the survival curves in the EAST trial would suggest an ongoing attrition of these patients due to progression of disease. To that end, major changes have occurred in secondary preventive therapy for vascular disease patients. The use of lipid lowering therapies, hypertensive control, as well as glycemic control for the diabetic patients has improved significantly since the late 1980s. It is hoped that these measures will contribute materially to the long-term survival curves that were present in the EAST trial. The surgery patients have also benefited from improved technology. The use of arterial conduits, although high in the EAST trial, has become almost universal, especially for bypassing the anterior descending coronary. Multiple arterial conduits are now frequently used and shorter hospital stays have undoubtedly improved the initial economic disadvantage that surgery patients had. In addition, the secondary prevention measures applied in surgery patients has changed over the years. The same management of lipids, hypertension, diabetes, etc., that should be helpful for the angioplasty patients, will also prove beneficial for the surgery patients of the future.

CONCLUSION

EAST was the first US trial to compare angioplasty and bypass surgery. This was a crucial step in the development of a new technology and the assessment of its proper place in the management of coronary disease patients. Many lessons were learned regarding survival, symptomatic improvement, degree of revascularization, and the economic impact of repeat procedures. Additional lessons have involved the understanding of restenosis and the impact of traditional and non-traditional risk factors on disease progression. The two American trials, EAST and its younger but bigger brother BARI, have provided the benchmark platform for multi-vessel disease intervention. Improvements in technology and the continuum of care for such patients should build on this experience for improving the outcomes of patients undergoing both revascularization strategies.

REFERENCES

1. Gruentzig A. Transluminal dilatation of coronary-artery stenosis, *Lancet* 1978; **1**:263.
2. King SB III, Schlumpf M. Ten-year completed follow-up of percutaneous transluminal coronary angioplasty: the early Zurich experience, *J Am Coll Cardiol* 1993; **22**:353–360.
3. Cowley MJ, Vetrovec GW, DiSciascio G, Lewis SA, Hirsch PD, Wolfgang TC. Coronary angioplasty of multiple vessels: short-term outcome and long-term results, *Circulation* 1985; **72**: 1314–1320.
4. Myler RK, Topol EJ, Shaw RE et al. Multiple vessel coronary angioplasty: classification, results, and patterns of restenosis in 494 consecutive patients, *Cathet Cardiovasc Diagn* 1987; **13**:1–15.
5. Vandormael MG, Deligonul U, Kern MJ et al. Multilesion coronary angioplasty: clinical and angiographic follow-up, *J Am Coll Cardiol* 1987; **10**:246–252.
6. O'Keefe JH Jr, Rutherford BD, McConahay DR et al. Multi-vessel coronary angioplasty from 1987 to 1989: procedural results and long-term outcome, *J Am Coll Cardiol* 1990; **16**:1097–1102.
7. Detre K, Holubkov R, Kelsey S et al and the co-investigators of the NHLBI PTCA Registry. Percutaneous transluminal coronary angioplasty in 1985–1986 and 1977–1981: The NHLBI Registry, *N Engl J Med* 1988; **318**:265–270.
8. King SB III, Lembo NJ, Hall EC for the East Investigators. The Emory Angioplasty vs Surgery Trial (EAST): analysis of baseline characteristics, *AM J Cardiol* 1995; **75**:42–59.
9. King SB III, Lembo NJ, Weintraub WS et al for the Emory Angioplasty Versus Surgery Trial (EAST). A randomized trial comparing coronary angioplasty with coronary bypass surgery, *N Engl J Med* 1994; **331**:1044–1050.
10. Zhao XQ, Brown G, Stewart DK et al. Effectiveness of revascularization in the Emory Angioplasty Versus Surgery Trial. A randomized comparison of coronary angioplasty with bypass surgery, *Circulation* 1996; **93**:1954–1962.
11. Weintraub WS, Mauldin PD, Becker E, Kosinski AS, King SB III. A comparison of the costs of and quality of life after coronary angioplasty or coronary surgery for multivessel coronary artery disease. Results from the Emory Angioplasty Versus Surgery Trial (EAST), *Circulation* 1995; **92**:2831–2840.
12. King SB III, Barnhart HX, Kosinski AS et al and the EAST Investigators. Angioplasty or surgery for multivessel coronary artery disease: comparison of eligible registry and randomized patients in the EAST trial and influence of treatment selection on outcomes, *Am J Cardiol* 1997; **79**: 1453–1459.
13. Zhao XQ, Kosinski AS, Malinow R et al. Association of total plasma homocyst(e)ine levels and eight-year mortality following PTCA or CABG in EAST, *Circulation* 2000; **102**:II-699 (abstract).
14. Zhao XQ, Kosinski AS, Malinow MR et al. Association of LDL heterogeneity and native coronary disease progression at three years following PTCA or CABG in EAST, *Circulation* 2000; **102**:II-698 (abstract).
15. King SB III, Kosinski AS, Guyton RA, Lembo NJ, Weintraub WS for the Emory Angioplasty Versus Surgery Trial (EAST) Investigators. Eight year mortality in the Emory angioplasty vs surgery trial, *J Am Coll Cardiol* 2000; **35**: 1116–1121.
16. The BARI Investigators. Influence of diabetes on five-year mortality and morbidity in a randomized trial comparing PTCA and CABG in

patients with multi-vessel disease. The Bypass Angioplasty Revascularization Investigation (BARI), *Circulation* 1997; **96**:1761–1769.

17. Serruys PW, Unger F, Sousa JE et al for the Arterial Revascularization Therapies Study Group. Comparison of coronary-artery bypass surgery and stenting for the treatment of multi-vessel disease, *N Engl J Med* 2001; **344**:1117–1124.

18. Stables RH. The Stent or Surgery Trial (SOS): a randomized controlled trial to compare coronary artery bypass grafting (CABG) with percutaneous transluminal coronary arteriography supported by stent implantation. Presented at the American College of Cardiology Annual Scientific Session, March 2001, Orlando, FL, USA.

19. BARI Investigators. Seven year outcome in the Bypass Angioplasty Revascularization Investigation (BARI) by treatment and diabetic status, *J Am Coll Cardiol* 2000; **35**:1122–1129.

20. The EPISTENT Investigators. Randomized placebo-controlled and balloon-angioplasty-controlled trial to assess safety of coronary stenting with use of platelet glycoprotein IIB/IIIa blockade, *Lancet* 1998; **352**:87–92.

14

Percutaneous coronary intervention and coronary bypass surgery in high-risk patients: a look from the South

Alfredo E Rodriguez

CONTENTS • Non-Q myocardial infarction and acute coronary syndromes • Coronary artery bypass surgery and stenting in multiple vessel disease: the evidence from Argentine randomized studies • Percutaneous interventions versus surgery in the stent era: expanded indications to unprotected left main stenosis • Summary • Acknowledgments

Coronary artery bypass graft (CABG) surgery and percutaneous coronary intervention (PCI) are both effective treatments for patients with symptomatic coronary artery disease. Randomized studies and registries have objectively demonstrated the role of both techniques in treating patients with symptomatic coronary artery disease.

Several randomized comparisons of surgical and medical treatment, from the 1970–1980 period, demonstrated a long-term survival advantage with CABG, in subsets of patients with stable angina and severe coronary artery disease [1–6]. However, in patients with unstable angina, there was a higher initial surgical mortality and morbidity, and no late survival benefit with CABG (excluding patients with left main coronary stenosis) [4].

Since 1990, seven randomized comparisons of CABG and PCI have been reported [7–13]. After the recruitment of more than 4000 patients, the major finding of those studies was that there was no significant difference in terms of long-term survival, or freedom from myocardial infarction, between PCI and CABG, in patients with multiple vessel disease and non-treated diabetes. However, there were significant differences in favour of CABG, in terms of requirements for repeat revascularization procedures, as well as in the incidence of angina (Figs 14.1 and 14.2). Two of those studies, BARI and CABRI, also showed a significantly better long-term survival with surgery in patients with treated diabetes [11, 14, 15].

It is important to note that all of these trials were performed prior to the widespread use of stents or debulking procedures, and prior to the introduction of platelet glycoprotein IIb/IIIa receptor blocking drugs [16–25]. Furthermore, the majority of patients included in these studies were relatively low-risk. Only a minority of patients in these early trials had either rest angina, post myocardial infarction angina, or poor left ventricular function. Accordingly, a

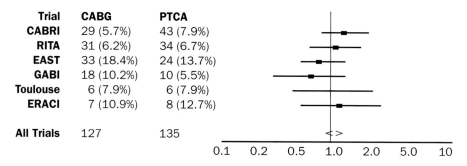

Figure 14.1 Cardiac death and myocardial infarction for PTCA group compared with CABG group in first year since randomization. Modified from S Pocock et al. *Lancet* 1995; **3435**:1184–1189.

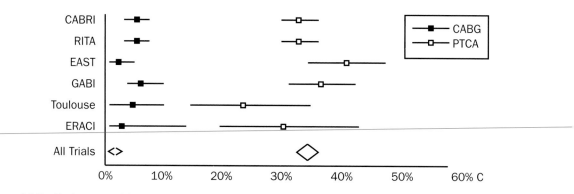

Figure 14.2 Patients requiring additional interventions (PTCA and/or CABG) during first year of follow-up in both treatment groups. Modified from S Pocock et al. *Lancet* 1995; **3435**:1184–1189.

comparison of PCI with CABG, which would include the use of stents and glycoprotein IIb/IIIa receptor blockers, among high-risk patients, was warranted. Furthermore, epidemiological studies supported the feasibility of such a trial.

NON-Q MYOCARDIAL INFARCTION AND ACUTE CORONARY SYNDROMES

Two recent studies were designed to assess the role of early intervention versus conservative therapies in patients with non-Q myocardial infarction or acute coronary syndromes: VAN-QWISH and FRISC II [26, 27]. The VANQWISH trial [26] was performed in 16 Veterans Affairs

(VA) Hospitals in the United States. Patients with non-Q myocardial infarction, and stable post-infarct symptoms were randomly allocated between routine early catheterization and revascularization, and conservative therapy with revascularization reserved for recurrent symptoms. Patients treated aggressively after a non-Q infarction, had greater 30-day mortality than those treated in the conservative arm, and those results were maintained at the one-year follow-up. However, the VANQWISH results have been questioned because of a relatively high surgical in-hospital mortality in the invasive arm. At 30 days, the CABG patients in the invasive cohort had an 11.7% mortality rate compared with only 3% among CABG patients in the conservative strategy arm (PCI therapy in the early invasive arm had no hospital or 30-day mortality).

In contrast, in the FRISC II study [27], an early invasive strategy was associated with better results compared with a more conservative strategy. However, in FRISC II, 30-day mortality with surgery in the invasive arm was only 2.1%. Similarly to VANQWISH, 30-day mortality with PCI was almost negligible in FRISC II: 0.009%).

It is not clear that the early surgical mortality in VANQWISH is inappropriately high, given that all of the VANQWISH patients had post-infarction unstable angina. Several registries have also reported higher short-term CABG associated mortality among patients operated shortly after a myocardial infarction. The ACC/AHA Guideline for coronary bypass surgery stressed that patients with unstable angina, who required surgery during the same hospitalization, had a surgical mortality in the range of 4–7% [28]. In the New York State database during the 1996–1998 period, 58,000 patients underwent CABG, and the operative mortality for the 27,589 patients with unstable angina was 3.3%, which was 2.5-fold greater than the operative mortality for the patients operated without unstable angina [29].

CORONARY ARTERY BYPASS SURGERY AND STENTING IN MULTIPLE VESSEL DISEASE: THE EVIDENCE FROM ARGENTINE RANDOMIZED STUDIES

ERACI I

During 1988–1990, 127 patients with multiple vessel disease were randomized in a single center in Buenos Aires between PTCA (without stents or glycoprotein IIb/IIa receptor blockers) and CABG. The study had a large proportion of patients with unstable angina (more than 80%). The major findings of this pre-stent era study published in 1993 were similar one-year survival and freedom from myocardial infarction between both strategies of revascularization. Nevertheless, the in-hospital mortality of patients treated with PTCA, in both the randomized and randomizable populations, was three times lower than the CABG mortality. This raised the possibility that the study was underpowered, and the absence of a statistically significant early survival difference between CABG and PTCA might represent a type II error [8] (Table 14.1). As in previous trials, significantly higher requirements for repeat revascularization procedures and higher

Table 14.1 Major in-hospital complications in randomized and randomizable but not randomized patients

	Randomized (127 pts)		Randomizable (175 pts)	
	CABG	PTCA	CABG	PTCA
Death (%)	4.6	1.5	5.2	2
AMI (%)	6.2	6.3	3.9	5
Emergency CABG (%)	—	1.5	—	2
Emergency PTCA (%)	1.5	—	—	—
Stroke (%)	3.1	1.5	2.6	0

Modified from A Rodriguez et al. *JACC* 1993; **33**:1060–1067.

rates of angina were observed in the patients treated with PCI. Repeat revascularization procedures were required in 33% of the PCI patients in the first year with 18% of PCI assigned patients crossing over to surgery. These rates were comparable to other pre-stent era trials. Cost analysis, including hospital charges, fees and honorarium for both procedures showed higher costs with surgery during hospitalization, and in the entire three years of follow-up [9].

ERACI II

The routine use of stents during coronary interventions dramatically reduced the incidence of acute PCI complications, such as acute or threatened vessel closure and emergency bypass surgery. Stent use has also been accompanied by significantly reduced rates of angiographic restenosis and target vessel failure during follow-up [16, 19, 20, 21, 30]. As stated previously, the impact of stents on acute and long-term outcomes, coupled with a need to evaluate higher risk populations, made a more contemporary trial of PCI versus CABG necessary. In October 1996, seven clinical sites in Argentina began patient recruitment for the Argentine Randomized Study between coronary stents versus surgery in patients with multiple vessel disease (ERACI II). During two years of screening, 2759 consecutive patients were identified with angiographic and clinical indication for revascularization by either stents or surgery. Of those patients, 1076 patients met the entrance criteria for randomization, and 450 patients (16.5%) consented and were included in the randomized trial.

The primary end-point of the study was major adverse cardiac events (MACE), defined as death, Q wave myocardial infarction and/or the requirement for repeat revascularization procedures (PCI or CABG) at 30 days, one, three, and five years of follow-up. During the first month, non-fatal stroke was also included in MACE. Angina class, angiographic and physiologic completeness of revascularization, and a cost effectiveness were secondary analyses of the study.

Entry criteria for the study
Patients were eligible for inclusion if they had severely limiting stable angina, unstable angina including post myocardial infarction angina, or were asymptomatic with a large area of myocardium at risk. Patients were required to have angiographic evidence of severe coronary obstruction ($\geqslant$ 70% by visual estimation) in at least one major epicardial vessel and more than 50% in other vessels, suitable for stenting. To be included in the trial, the patient's angiographic lesions had to be considered approachable by both PCI and CABG. In contrast to ERACI I, ERACI II included patients with post myocardial infarction angina, concomitant peripheral vascular disease, and even unprotected left main stenosis (at the discretion of individual operators).

Clinical profile of the patients included in the ERACI II
Baseline clinical characteristics from the patient population included in this study demonstrate the uniquely high-risk nature of this cohort of patients. As shown in Table 14.2, 91% had unstable angina class II–III or C Braunwald classification, including 10% with post acute myocardial infarction angina; 38% were older than 65 years; and 23% had concomitant severe peripheral vascular disease [31]. All of these findings have been associated with high surgical rates of adverse outcome. The ACC/AHA Task Force for Coronary Bypass Surgery recognized the high in-hospital mortality with surgery in patients with refractory unstable angina, and among patients with post acute myocardial infarction angina and ST changes consistent with subendocardial ischemia [28]. Another recent study of 5517 CABG patients [32] demonstrated higher in-hospital mortality for patients: treated within seven days of myocardial infarction (13%); with concomitant peripheral vascular disease (8%); with age $\geqslant$ 65

Table 14.2 ERACI II. Basal demographics and angiographic characteristics

	PTCA (225 pts)	CABG (225 pts)	p
Male	77.3%	81.4%	0.7
Age	62.4	61.3	0.8
Hypertension	71%	70.5%	0.9
Smokers	54.3%	49.5%	0.6
Diabetic	17.3%	17.3%	0.9
High cholesterol	62.5%	60.2%	0.8
Previous infarction	28.5%	27.7%	0.9
Obesity	28.8%	23.5%	0.4
Unstable II—III—C	92.1%	90.7%	0.7
Peripheral disease	19.1%	26.6%	0.16
Double vessels	40%	38%	
Three vessels	54.7%	58%	
Left main	5.3%	4%	

Modified from A Rodriguez et al. *JACC* 2001; **37**:51.

years (4%); or with class IV angina (5%). Older age (≥ 70 years) is a specific 'high risk' factor for coronary bypass surgery from the Veterans Affairs Surgical Registry. Concomitant vascular disease was also associated with high hospital surgical risk as reported by the BARI group (27% of MACE) [33].

For purposes of comparison, consider another recent randomized multi-national comparison between stents and surgery, the Arterial Revascularization Therapy Study (ARTS) [34]. The ARTS trial randomized patients with considerably lower risk than ERACI II, as shown in Table 14.3. Specifically, the proportions of patients with unstable angina, unstable angina Braunwald class C, peripheral vascular disease, and treated hypertension were all significantly higher in ERACI II than the larger ARTS trial. This kind of demographic difference is important to consider when comparing trial results.

Revascularization techniques
The strategies of revascularization were different with PCI and CABG. With surgery, anatomical complete revascularization was the goal of the procedure and was obtained in more than 88% of cases. With percutaneous interventions, including the liberal use of stents, anatomically complete revascularization was obtained in only 51% of the patients treated, significantly fewer than with CABG ($p = 0.02$) [7, 31]. However, complete revascularization was obtained in 89% of PCI patients where it was attempted with stents as compared with 90% where it was attempted with CABG. Accordingly, physiologic completeness of revascularization, as determined by stress thallium at 30 days, was similar with the two techniques.

In the CABG group, the left internal mammary artery was used in almost 90% of the cases, and there were 2.6 distal anastomoses per patient. With PCI, 1.4 stents per patient were

Table 14.3 Baselines characteristics in ARTS and ERACI II			
	ARTS	**ERACI II**	*p*
Unstable angina	37%	91.7%	0.0002
Unstable angina C	0%	10%	0.0002
Diabetes	17.3%	17.3%	NS
Peripheral vascular disease	5.6%	26.6%	0.0002
Previous AMI	44%	28.5%	0.0002
Cholesterolemia	58%	62%	NS
Smokers	28%	54%	0.0002
Hypertension	43%	70.5%	0.0002
Left main	0%	4.6%	0.0002
LAD	90%	91.3%	NS

LAD, left anterior descending.

used, and conventional balloon angioplasty was used in the remaining vessels; a total of 91.5% of planned vessels were successfully treated. Chronic total occlusions were usually not treated in the PCI arm. Given the high-risk clinical profile of the ERACI II patients, there was liberal use of glycoprotein IIb/IIIa receptor inhibitors [24]; 28% of patients randomized to stents received a bolus and infusion of Reopro. No patients in the CABG group received glycoprotein IIb/IIIa receptor blocking agents.

Thirty-day and long-term outcome in patients randomized in ERACI II
The 30-day results and also the six-month outcome from the patients randomized to ERACI II, demonstrated a significant survival advantage for patients randomized to PCI [29]. This is the first randomized trial reporting a significant survival advantage with PCI versus CABG in any subset. Similarly, the incidence of Q wave myocardial infarction was significantly reduced in patients treated with PTCA plus stenting. These results derived from a reduction in the incidence of death and myocardial infarction during hospitalization in the PCI arm. After

hospital discharge, the incidence of cardiac death or myocardial infarction was similar in both revascularization groups.

Are the ERACI II results the expression of a flawed initial surgical procedure?
If we consider the types of patients randomized in ERACI II, perhaps we can answer this important question. Patients with stable angina had similar acute and long-term outcomes in the PCI and CABG groups; in fact, there were no perioperative (30-day) mortalities among stable angina patients treated with CABG. In contrast, patients with unstable class II had 1.4% death with PCI versus 5.6% with CABG (*p* = ns); only patients with unstable III-C had major differences in short-term mortality between both techniques (0% vs 7.9% with PCI and CABG respectively (*p* = 0.06). Even though ERACI II was not powered to assess differences according to angina class at the time of randomization, there was a trend toward a higher mortality with surgery seen in patients who were unstable (Table 14.4). Although there are no current trials designed to assess differences in mortality according to angina class, in

Table 14.4 ERACI II. Thirty days mortality with PTCR and CABG

	Stable angina	Unstable angina class II	Unstable angina class III + C
PTCR	0% (0/17)	1.4% (2/138)	0% (0/70)*
CABG	0% (0/21)	5.6% (8/141)	7.9% (5/63)*

*$p = 0.06$. Modified from A Rodriguez et al. *JACC* 2001; **37**:51.

patients treated with PTCA or CABG, several registries have reported higher in-hospital mortality in patients having refractory unstable angina or post acute myocardial infarction angina. In this regard, 28% of ERACI II patients had angina at rest with changes in ST-segment, in the 48 hours prior to revascularization; 10% had post myocardial infarction angina. Furthermore, almost 27% of patients randomized to surgery also had peripheral vascular disease, an additional risk factor for adverse outcomes with CABG [33]. In the New York State registries for CABG, patients with unstable angina had a three-times higher procedural risk than patients without unstable angina [35]. Taken together, these demographic data suggest that the surgical mortality was not unrea-

sonably high for this type of population. Accordingly, we conclude that the survival advantage for PCI was not a result of inappropriately high perioperative mortality.

Late clinical follow-up

A mean clinical follow-up of three years was completed in all patients in the ERACI II study. The Kaplan–Meier survival curves, at 900 days demonstrate better survival with PCI compared with CABG (log rank, $p = 0.017$). Most of this difference occurred in the first 30 days, after which the curves are nearly parallel. Kaplan–Meier freedom from myocardial infarction was also better in PCI vs CABG (log rank, $p = 0.017$) (Fig. 14.4). In contrast, freedom from requirement for repeat revascularization procedures

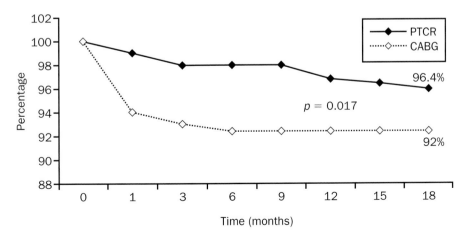

Figure 14.3 ERACI II. Follow-up survival. Log rank test. Modified from A Rodriguez et al. *JACC* 2001; **37**:51.

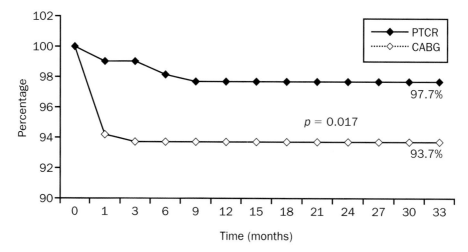

Figure 14.4 ERACI II. Freedom from myocardial infarction. Log rank test. Modified from A Rodriguez et al. *JACC* 2001; **37**:51.

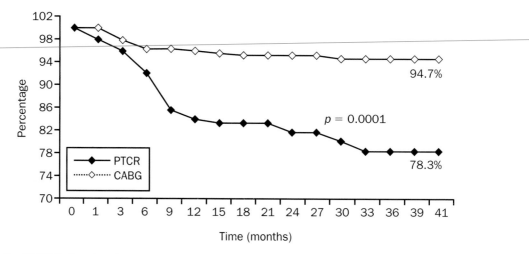

Figure 14.5 ERACI II. Freedom from repeat PTCR/CABG. Modified from A Rodriguez et al. *JACC* 2001; **37**:51.

was significantly better with CABG (log rank test, $p = 0.001$) (Fig. 14.5). Eleven patients (4.8%) assigned to PCI crossed over to CABG during the entire follow-up period. Patients assigned to CABG were also more often free of angina than patients assigned to PCI (92% versus 84.5% respectively, $p = 0.01$). However, this difference was less evident at the end of the second year, and became similar at the end of the follow up period.

Multiple vessel stenting versus surgery in three different subsets of patients: proximal left anterior descending artery disease, three-vessel disease, and treated diabetes

Previous randomized studies, excluding diabetic patients, have not shown differences in survival between PCI or CABG in any subsets of patients with multiple vessel disease [6, 10]. Nevertheless, several registries in the US have reported a survival advantage with surgery when the proximal segment of the left anterior descending artery (LAD) was involved. For example, a Duke University registry study reported better survival with surgery in those patients with two- or three-vessel disease, which included proximal stenosis of the LAD [37].

In ERACI II, from 450 patients included in the randomized population, we identified 230 patients, with severe stenosis in the osteal or proximal segment of LAD, 83 of them had two-vessel disease, whereas 147 patients had three-vessel disease [38]. Baseline clinical characteristics of these patients were similar to those of the entire ERACI group (89% had unstable angina; 40% were older than 65 years; and 21% had peripheral vascular disease) (Table 14.5). Of these 230 patients, 113 were randomized to PCI and 117 to CABG. The revascularization strategy included liberal use (93%) of the internal mammary artery in the CABG arm and stent use (97%) in the PCI arm. The in-hospital and 30-day outcomes of this cohort of patients were not different between

CABG and stent therapy. At a mean clinical follow-up of 25±6months, survival, freedom from myocardial infarction and freedom from death and myocardial infarction were similar with both strategies of revascularization (Table 14.6). The presence of more frequent angina and requirement for repeat revascularization procedures favored CABG over PTCA in this subset [38] (Fig. 14.6).

Similar findings were present in ERACI II subset with three-vessel disease [40]. Among the 254 patients with three-vessel disease included in ERACI II, survival at one year was 95% in both groups and again there were no differences in hospital mortality between PCI and CABG (1.6% and 3.8% respectively) (Table 14.7). These results are in agreement with recent findings from the BARI trial. The seven-year follow-up outcome showed no difference in survival between patients treated with old PTCA techniques (only 51% of planned vessel successfully treated) compared with CABG, excluding treated diabetic patients [14]. It is intriguing that in BARI randomized patients,

Table 14.5 ERACI II. Left anterior descending ostial or proximal. Basal demographic and clinical characteristics

	PTCR (113 pts)	CABG (117 pts)	p
Male	76.6%	77.1%	NS
Age > 65 years	48.6%	36.2%	NS
Unstable II—III—C	91%	91.5%	NS
Hypertension	69.3%	70.5%	NS
Diabetics	15.2%	13.6%	NS
High cholesterol	64%	58%	NS
Previous infarction	18%	20.5%	NS
Obesity	15.3%	19%	NS
Peripheral disease	20.1%	25.4%	NS
Two vessels	31%	29%	NS
Three or more vessels	69%	71%	NS

Table 14.6 ERACI II. Multi-vessel stenting versus surgery in patients with multiple vessel disease and ostial or proximal, left anterior descending stenosis

	PTCR (n = 113)	CABG (n = 117)	p
30-day outcome			
Death	0%	2.5%	
AMI (Q)	1%	5.1%	
MACE	2.7%	7.6%	NS
Follow-up (25 ± 6.4 months)			
Death	1%	4.3%	
AMI	2.6%	5.1%	
TVR	25.2%	3.4%	0.0002
MACE	28%	13%	

AMI, acute myocardial infarction; TVR, target vessel revascularization; MACE, major adverse cardiac events.

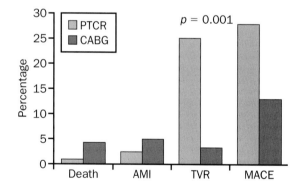

Figure 14.6 ERACI II. LAD ostial or proximal. MACE at follow-up (25 ± 6.4 months). AMI, acute myocardial infarction; TVR, target vessel revascularization; MACE, major adverse cardiac events.

there was a trend to better survival among patients with poor left ventricular function, LAD stenosis, congestive heart failure, treated with PTCA, despite the fact that these patients were treated without stents or glycoprotein IIb/IIIa receptor antagonists (Fig. 14.7).

Among the treated diabetic patients included in the ERACI II (76 patients), there were no differences in survival or freedom from myocardial infarction in favor of either revascularization procedure. Furthermore using the database of both randomized studies (ERACI I and ERACI II) (90 patients) survival and nonfatal myocardial infarction at three years of follow-up were similar in the PCI and CABG groups [41].

Hospital and follow-up costs of revascularization procedures in ERACI II: comparison with previous studies

In Argentina, there was an average cost in US dollars of $4500 for uncomplicated balloon angioplasty and $11,000 for uncomplicated coronary bypass surgery (average analysis between National or Private Social Security System with each hospital participating in the ERACI II) during the recruitment patients period (1996–1998). These costs included hospital charges, fees and honorarium. The cost of

Table 14.7 ERACI II. Multi-vessel stenting versus surgery in patients with three or more vessel disease

	PTCR (n = 124)	CABG (n = 130)	p
30-day outcome			
Death	1.6%	3.8%	NS
AMI (Q)	0.8%	5.3%	NS
One-year follow-up			
Survival	95.2%	94.6%	NS
Freedom AMI	97.6%	94%	NS
Freedom MACE	74.4%	87%	0.059
TVR	21%	1.5%	0.002

AMI, acute myocardial infarction; TVR, target vessel revascularization; MACE, major adverse cardiac events.

	CABG	PTCA	Difference
Severity of angina			
Unstable angina or non Q wave MI	86.1%	86.0%	
Stable angina (CCS class 3 or 4)	87.6%	88.5%	
Severe ischemia	86.4%	88.2%	
Left ventricular function			
Normal	88.9%	88.7%	
Abnormal	75.9%	82.5%	
Type of vessel disease			
Double	86.1%	88.0%	
Triple	86.7%	85.0%	
Type C lesion			
Absent	88.8%	86.8%	
Present	82.9%	86.7%	
Proximal LAD disease			
Absent	86.4%	85.1%	
Present	86.3%	89.7%	
History of diabetes			
None or not treated	86.4%	86.8%	
Treated	76.4%	55.7%	

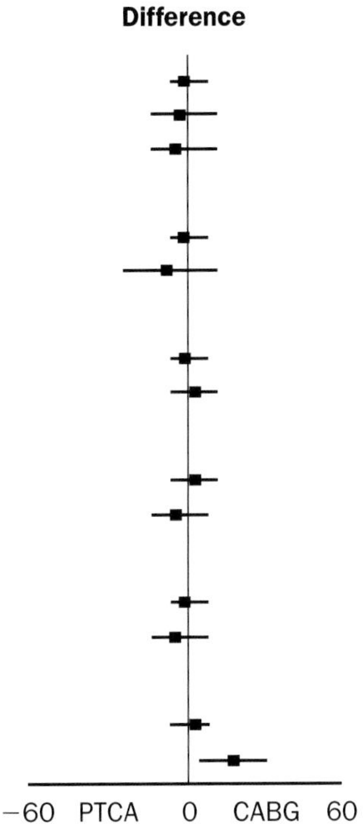

−60   PTCA   0   CABG   60

Figure 14.7   The BARI Investigators. Seven-year outcome in Bypass Angioplasty Revascularization Investigation (BARI) by treatment and diabetic status. Modified from *JACC* 2000; **35**:1122–1129.

the stents was $3000. These costs included two days of hospitalization for PCI patients and nine days of hospitalization for CABG patients. Each additional day in the coronary care unit added a cost of $1080. The bolus and infusion of Reopro added a total cost of $2974. Taking into account the procedural costs, and related procedural resources, and costs of complications, the 30-day final costs for both techniques were similar. During the next one-year of follow-up, requirements for repeat procedures added additional cost. By one-year follow-up, costs for both procedures showed a trend to be higher with PCI. This is in contrast to ERACI I, where despite significantly higher requirements of repeat procedures compared with ERACI II (33% vs 18% and with higher number of patients crossing over to surgery, 18% in ERACI I vs 4.8% in ERACI II), the cost at three years for conventional PCI was still lower than surgery.

These current analyses of revascularization techniques demonstrate a significant increase in costs for percutaneous interventional procedures in Argentina, especially when stents and/or glycoprotein IIb/IIIa receptor antagonists were used. This should be taking into account in the final analysis of cost effectiveness of both procedures [31].

PERCUTANEOUS INTERVENTIONS VERSUS SURGERY IN THE STENT ERA: EXPANDED INDICATIONS TO UNPROTECTED LEFT MAIN STENOSIS

The first successful saphenous vein coronary bypass graft was performed in 1964 by Garret and DeBakey and was done in a patient with severe left main stenosis [42]. After that, several randomized studies and registries showed a significant improvement in survival for patients with severe left main stenosis who were treated with bypass surgery [5, 6].

Conventional coronary angioplasty, introduced by Gruentzig in 1977 [43], was also performed in patients with severe unprotected left main stenosis. However, the incidence of acute or sub-acute closure, and/or the potential risk of high recurrence rate, dictated that this angiographic finding be a relative contraindication for conventional balloon angioplasty. Since the introduction of stents, unprotected left main stenosis intervention has become more frequent, mostly in patients who are poor surgical candidates, or during an acute myocardial infarction. The ULTIMA registry using both old and current PCI techniques showed an improvement in results when new devices were used to treat unprotected left main disease [44].

Barragan [45] and Marco [46] reported acceptable long-term outcomes with stents in treating patients with unprotected left main stenosis. In their series, acute success in elective indications was almost 100%; and survival was higher than 90% at one-year of follow-up. Park reported a larger series, with almost 100% acute success and long-term outcome, which was even better than the previously reported French experiences. Park used debulking techniques in addition to stenting [47]. The recurrence rate in his series was about 15%. However late sudden death, presumably related to restenosis and/or late reocclusion has been reported, and remains the major concern of this technique.

In our experience, beginning in 1995, 124 patients with unprotected left main stenosis have been treated with stents [48, 49]. A single stent procedure to left anterior descending artery was the preferred approach in the majority of patients (Fig. 14.8). Debulking techniques were used in less than 5% of cases. The use of a sequential stent to the circumflex artery (T stent technique) was used in only 7.5% of patients. Acute and 30-day mortality has, thus far, only been observed among patients treated during acute myocardial infarction or among patients who were poor surgical candidates.

We identified a cohort of 93 patients defined as potentially good surgical candidates using clinical and angiographic parameters (patients with ejection fraction less than 35%, concomitant illness, and/or acute myocardial infarction were excluded). In these good surgical candidate

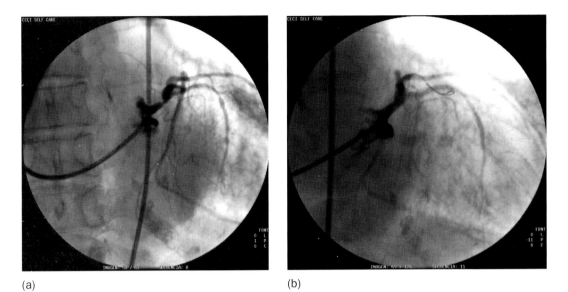

(a)   (b)

Figure 14.8   Severe stenosis in left main and ostial LAD, treated with single stent in main and LAD. (a) left main lesion before stent, (b) left main lesion after stent.

patients, we have had no periprocedural major complication (death or acute myocardial infarction). At long-term clinical follow-up (14.6 ± 11.3 months), freedom from death was 94.2%, freedom from cardiac death was 93.2% and freedom from death and non-fatal myocardial infarction was 90% (Fig. 14.9). Target lesion revascularization was required during follow-up in 21.2%, and appears to be associated with initial stent technique: 15% versus 75% without and with an additional T stent to the circumflex artery. Although Park reported better long-term outcome associated with aggressive debulking prior to stenting in patients with bifurcation left main stenosis [47], we use debulking techniques infrequently. These 14.6 months follow-up

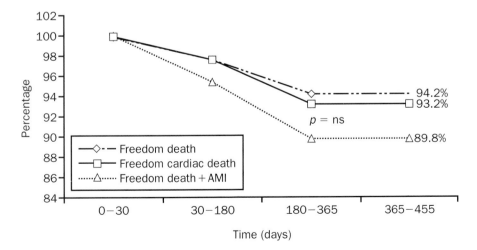

Figure 14.9   Unprotected left main angioplasty in stent era. Long-term outcome (14.6 months). Good surgical candidates patients (89 pts).

survival with stents in good surgical candidates patients are highly competitive with the results with conventional bypass surgery, and support the need for a randomized comparison of PCI versus CABG in this cohort of patients.

SUMMARY

In ERACI II, patients with acute coronary syndromes randomized between a PCI versus CABG strategy, had a lower risk of major procedural complications when they were treated with current interventional percutaneous techniques compared with conventional coronary bypass surgery. The use of stents and glycoprotein IIb/IIIa receptor blocking drugs are likely important differences from previous CABG versus PCI randomized trials. The presence of high-risk unstable angina, defined as recurrent angina or post myocardial infarction angina, identified a cohort of patients at high-risk of adverse outcomes with conventional coronary bypass surgery. Even in those patients with more complex anatomy, previously associated with better results with surgery (such as osteal or proximal LAD stenosis, three-vessel disease, or unprotected left main stenosis) current PCI techniques achieved similar one-year survival and freedom from myocardial infarction as CABG. Similarly, we found no difference in survival or freedom from infarction between CABG and PCI among our treated diabetic subset. Taken together, these data support the use of PCI as an alternative to CABG among some patients with unstable angina who were previously only considered for CABG. The comparisons of risk/benefit and cost/benefit must be made on an individual patient basis.

ACKNOWLEDGMENTS

The author wishes to thank Dr Oberdan Andrin, Dr Cesar Vigo, Dr Douglass Morrison, and Ms Marta Biagioni for their help in preparing this manuscript.

REFERENCES

1. European coronary surgery study group. Coronary bypass surgery in stable angina pectoris, *Lancet* 1979; **1**:889–893.
2. European Coronary Artery Surgery Study Group. Coronary bypass surgery in stable angina pectoris. Survival at two years, *Lancet* 1979; **1**:889–893.
3. Hultgren HN, Shettigar UR, Miller DC. Medical versus surgical treatment of unstable angina. *Am J Cardiol* 1982; **50**:663–670.
4. Unstable angina pectoris study group. Unstable angina pectoris: National Cooperative Study Group to compare medical and surgical therapy – II. In-hospital experience and initial follow-up results in patients with one-, two- and three-vessel disease. *Am J Cardiol* 1978; **42**:839–848.
5. Detre K, Peduzzi P, Murphy ML et al. Effect of bypass surgery on survival of patients in low- and high-risk subgroups delineated by use of simple clinical variables, *Circulation* 1981; **63**:1329–1338.
6. Takaro T, Hultgren HN, Lipton MJ, Detre KN. The VA cooperative randomized study of surgery for coronary arterial occlusive disease II. Subgroup with significant left main lesions, *Circulation* 1976; **54** (suppl III):III-10717.
7. Pocock S, Henderson R, Rickards A et al. Meta-analysis of randomized trials comparing coronary angioplasty with bypass surgery, *Lancet* 1995; **3435**: 1184–1189.
8. Rodríguez A, Boullon F, Pérez Baliño N et al. Argentine randomized trial of percutaneous transluminal coronary angioplasty versus coronary artery bypass surgery in multi-vessel disease (ERACI): in-hospital results and one-year follow-up, *J Am Coll Cardiol* 1993; **33**:1060–1067.
9. Rodriguez A, Mele E, Peyrene E et al. Three-year follow-up the Argentine randomized trial of percutaneous transluminal coronary angioplasty versus coronary artery bypass surgery in multi-vessel disease (ERACI), *J Am Coll Cardiol* 1996; **27**:1178–1184.
10. The Bypass Angioplasty Revascularization Investigation (BARI) Investigators. Comparison of coronary bypass surgery with angioplasty in patients with multi-vessel disease, *N Engl J Med* 1996; **335**:217–225.
11. CABRI trial participants. Coronary Angioplasty vs Bypass Revascularization Investigation

(CABRI) results during the first year, *Lancet* 1995; **346**:1179–1183.

12. RITA trial participants. Coronary angioplasty versus coronary artery bypass surgery: the Randomized Intervention Treatment of Angina (RITA) trial, *Lancet* 1993; **341**:573–580.

13. King SB III, Lembo NJ, Weintraub WS et al. A randomized trial comparing coronary angioplasty with coronary bypass surgery. Emory Angioplasty versus Surgery Trial (EAST), *N Engl J Med* 1994; **331**:1044–1050.

14. The BARI Investigators. Seven-year outcome in the Bypass Angioplasty Revascularization Investigation (BARI) by treatment and diabetic status, *J Am Coll Cardiol* 2000; **35**:1122–1129.

15. King SB, Kosinski AS, Blyton RA et al. Eight-year mortality in the Emory Angioplasty versus Surgery Trial (EAST), *J Am Coll Cardiol* 2000; **35**:1116–1121.

16. Roubin GS, Cannon AD, Agrawal SK et al. Intracoronary stenting for acute and threatened closure complicating PTCA, *Circulation* 1992; **85**:916–927.

17. George BS, Voorhees WD, Roubin GS et al. Multi-center investigation of coronary stenting to treat acute or threatened closure after PTCA; clinical and angiographic outcomes, *J Am Coll Cardiol* 1993; **22**:135–143.

18. Sutton JM, Ellis SG, Roubin GS et al. Major clinical events after coronary stenting; the multi-center registry of acute and elective Gianturco-Roubin stent placement. The Gianturco-Roubin Intracoronary Stent Investigator Group, *Circulation* 1994; **89**:1126–1137.

19. Serruys PS, de Jaegere P, Kiemeneij F et al for the Benestent Study Group. A comparison of balloon expandable stent implantation with balloon angioplasty in patients with coronary artery disease, *N Engl J Med* 1994; **331**:489–495.

20. Fischman DL, Leon MB, Baim DS et al. A randomized comparison of coronary-stent placement and balloon angioplasty in the treatment for coronary disease, *N Engl J Med* 1994; **331**:496–501.

21. Rodriguez AE, Santaera O, Larribau M et al. Coronary stenting decreases restenosis in lesions with early loss in luminal diameter 24 hours after successful PTCA, *Circulation* 1995; **91**:1397–1402.

22. Moussa L, Di Mario C, Moses J et al. Coronary stenting following rotational atherectomy in calcified and complex lesions: angiographic and clinical follow-up results, *Circulation* 1997; **96**:128–136.

23. Baim DS, Cutlip DE, Sharma SK et al. Final results of the Balloon vs Optimal Atherectomy Trial (BOAT): six months angiography and one-year clinical follow-up, *Circulation* 1998; **97**:322–331.

24. The EPISTENT investigators. Randomized placebo-controlled and balloon-angioplasty controlled trial to assess safety of coronary stenting with use of platelet glycoprotein IIb/IIIa blockade, *Lancet* 1998; **352**:87–92.

25. The Platelet Receptor Inhibition for Ischemic Syndrome Management in Patients Limited by Unstable Signs and Symptoms (PRISM-PLUS) Trial Investigators. Inhibition of the platelet glycoprotein IIb/IIIa receptor with tirofiban in unstable angina and non-Q wave myocardial infarction, *N Engl J Med* 1998; **338**:1488–1497.

26. Boden WE, O'Rouke RA, Crawford MH et al for the Veterans Affairs Non-Q Wave Infarction Strategies in Hospital (VANQWISH) Trial Investigators. Outcome in patients with acute non-Q wave myocardial infarction randomly assigned to an invasive as compared with a conservative strategy, *N Engl J Med* 1998; **338**:1785–1792.

27. FRISC II investigators. Invasive compared with non-invasive treatment in unstable coronary-artery disease, *Lancet* 1999; **354**:708–715.

28. Eagle K, Guyton R. ACC/AHA Guidelines for Coronary Artery Bypass Graft Surgery; A Report of the American College of Cardiology/American Heart Association Task Force on Practice Guidelines, *J Am Coll Cardiol* 1999; **34**:1262–1347.

29. Ryan TJ. Present-day PTCR versus CABG: a randomized comparison with a different focus and a new result, *J Am Coll Cardiol* 2001; **37**:59–61.

30. Rodriguez A, Ayala F, Bernardi V et al. Optimal coronary balloon angioplasty with provisional stenting versus primary stent (OCBAS): immediate and long-term follow-up results, *J Am Coll Cardiol* 1998; **32**:1351–1357.

31. Rodriguez A, Bernardi V, Navia J et al. Argentine randomized study: coronary angioplasty with stenting versus coronary bypass surgery in patients with multiple-vessel disease (ERACI II): 30-day and one-year follow-up results, *J Am Coll Cardiol* 2001; **37**:51.

32 Magovern JA, Sakert T, Magovern GJ et al. A model that predicts morbidity and mortality after coronary artery bypass graft surgery, *J Am Coll Cardiol* 1996; **28**:1147–1153.

33. Burek K, Sutto-Tyrrell K, Brooks M et al. Prognostic importance of lower extremity arterial disease in patients undergoing coronary revascularization in the bypass angioplasty revascularization investigation (BARI), *J Am Coll Cardiol* 1999; **34**:716–721.

34. Serruys PW, Unger F, Sousa EJ et al. Comparison of coronary artery bypass surgery and stenting for the treatment of multivessel disease (ARTS), *N Engl J Med* 2001; **344**:1117–1124.

35. Hannan El, Raez MJ, McCallister BD et al. A comparison of three-year survival after coronary artery bypass graft surgery and percutaneous transluminal coronary angioplasty, *J Am Coll Cardiol* 1999; **33**:63–72.

36. Kereiakes D, Lincoff M, Miller DP et al. Abciximab therapy and unplanned coronary stent deployment, *Circulation* 1998; **97**:857–864.

37. Jones RH, Kesler K, Phillips HR III et al. Long-term survival benefits of coronary artery bypass grafting and percutaneous transluminal angioplasty in patients with coronary artery disease, *J Thorac Cardiovasc Surg* 1996; **111**:1013–1025.

38. Rodriguez A, Saavedra S, Fernández C et al. Percutaneous transluminal coronary revascularization versus coronary bypass surgery in patients with multiple vessel disease and proximal left anterior descending artery stenosis: results from the ERACI II study, *J Am Coll Cardiol* 2000; **79–7**:9A (abstract).

39. Loop FD, Lytle BW, Cosgrove DM et al. Influence of the internal mammary-artery graft on 10-year survival and other cardiac events, *N Engl J Med* 1986; **314**:1–6.

40. Rodriguez A, Rodriguez Alemparte M, Bernardi V et al. Patients with three or more vessel disease treated with percutaneous interventions achieved similar safety long term outcome to those treated with conventional CABG: one-year follow-up results from ERACI II study, *JACC* 2001.

41. Fernández Pereira C, Bernardi V, Martinez J et al. Diabetic patients with multi-vessel disease treated with percutaneous coronary revascularization had similar outcome to those treated with surgery: one-year follow-up results from two Argentine randomized studies (ERACI I–ERACI II), *J Am Coll Cardiol* 2000; **1019–85**:3A (abstract).

42. Garret HE, Dennis EW, DeBakey ME. Aortocoronary bypass with saphenous vein graft: Seven-year follow-up, *JAMA* 1973; **223**:792–794.

43. Gruentzig AR, King SB, Schlumpf M et al. Long-term follow-up after percutaneous transluminal coronary angioplasty: the early Zurich experience, *N Engl J Med* 1987; **316**:1127–1132.

44. Ellis S. ULTIMA multi-center registry in unprotected left main stenosis. TCT Meeting October 1999 (personal communication).

45. Silvestri M, Barragan P, Sainsous J, Bayet G et al. Unprotected left main coronary artery stenting: immediate and medium-term outcomes of 140 elective procedures, *JACC* 2000; **35**:1543.

46. Marco J, Fajadet J, Brunel P et al. Stenting of unprotected left main stenosis, *JACC* 1996; **27** (suppl):227A (abstract).

47. Park S-J, Park S-W, Lec SW, Hong M-K et al. Long-term outcome for unprotected left main stenting, *Am J Cardiol* 1998; **82** (suppl 7A):TCT 30 (abstract).

48. Mauvecin C, Bernardi V, Fernández C J et al. Unprotected left main angioplasty in stent era, *Am J Cardiol* 1998; **82** (suppl 7A):TCT 30 (abstract).

49. Bernardi V, Fernández P, Saavedra S et al. Angioplastia coronaria en lesiones no protegidas de tronco de arteria coronaria izquierda: resultados intrahospitalarios y al seguimiento en la era del stent, *Rev Argent Cardiol* 1998; **66** (6):627–634.

15

The MASS trials

Luiz A Machado César and Whady A Hueb

CONTENTS • Introduction • MASS-1 • MASS-2

INTRODUCTION

Coronary artery disease (CAD) has a broad variety of clinical presentations and evolves differently in patients. Those presenting with chronic coronary disease may have stable angina or may have no symptoms at all even though they test positive for ischemia or they have stenosis documented by angiography. Patients may experience sudden death or may have stable angina that lasts for years. Based on the results of non-randomized and necropsy studies [1–5], we assume an unfavorable prognosis in patients with proximal left anterior descending (LAD) artery stenosis. Therefore, more aggressive therapy has been recommended, because this artery supplies blood to an important myocardial area [6, 7]. The danger of LAD stenosis causes a dilemma for cardiologists who have to choose the best treatment for each individual patient. Since the development of coronary artery bypass graft surgery (CABG) in the late 1960s, many patients have been operated on because it was supposed that they would survive longer and have fewer symptoms. They would also have the advantage of needing less medication and would thus have a better quality of life. This kind of thinking was

reasonable considering what was known about the disease at that time, including single-vessel disease compromising the left anterior descending artery [8]. However, the publication of the results of the Coronary Artery Surgery Study (CASS) [9] raised doubts about that line of thinking and shed new light on the physio-pathology and natural history of CAD. In CASS, medical treatment was compared with CABG. Patients undergoing bypass surgery were more frequently free of symptoms at the five-year follow-up, but, except for certain sub-groups, they had no better survival. We must remember that at the time of the study, only beta-blockers and nitrates were prescribed as a rule although aspirin and anti-coagulants also played a role. Patients with poor left ventricular function received the greatest benefits. Subsequent analysis of CASS [10] revealed that those patients with stenosis of the proximal left anterior descending coronary artery and disease in one other vessel, or those with three-vessel disease also had better mortality rates with surgical treatment, but patients with single-vessel or double-vessel disease without a compromised left anterior descending artery did not. It is important to point out that patients with vessels > 50% stenosed were considered for inclusion in CASS. Similar results were also observed especially in patients with multi-vessel disease.

Angioplasty was developed as an alternative to surgery in the 1980s [6, 11–18] and brought with it a new disease, restenosis [19]. Although this complication can be managed by performing a new angioplasty procedure, restenosis is considered a new event when it occurs during the course of the disease and may possibly cause myocardial infarction and death. Since restenosis began occurring, surgeons and interventional cardiologists have been competing aggressively to demonstrate who has found the best treatment. The controversy is almost never ending because new surgical approaches and new catheters and stents are introduced almost monthly, which are claimed to improve the results of both treatments. Along with these innovations, new drugs are being developed based on physiopathological concepts. It is now possible to disrupt the progression of and even promote the regression of atherosclerotic lesions, which means it is possible to dramatically change the natural history of CAD. The results of the Scandinavian Simvastatin Survival Study (4S) [20] published in 1994 documented amazing reductions in coronary mortality (42%), all-cause mortality (35%), and the need for revascularization procedures in patients with chronic stable coronary disease during a follow-up of 4.4 years. Concomitantly, the Collaborative Trialists' Collaboration [21], a systematic meta-analysis of aspirin, reported a 20% reduction in mortality for coronary patients. It is now very difficult to analyze all data together because new drugs are being developed, and the results of new trials are published regularly making it increasingly difficult to solve the puzzle of which treatment is the best for an individual patient. However, the major concern is for patients with chronic stable angina and normal left ventricular function. Among causes, single-vessel disease continues to motivate discussion although multi-vessel disease is not out of the picture. Furthermore, long-term studies comparing outcomes of treat-

ment with medicine, percutaneous transluminal coronary angioplasty (PTCA), and CABG were not available before our first study. The purpose of our study, the Medicine, Angioplasty, or Surgery Study (MASS) and subsequent MASS-2, is to compare the outcomes of these three therapeutic strategies.

MASS-1

We evaluated in a randomized prospective manner, medical treatment, angioplasty, and bypass surgery in patients with a single proximal left anterior descending (LAD) artery lesion and compared the occurrence of: (1) angina and angiographically documented coronary atherosclerosis progression at the end of the study; (2) myocardial infarction and congestive heart failure occurring at any time during follow-up, and (3) survival in each group after a five-year follow-up. The study model, patient selection criteria, and randomization procedure have been previously published [22].

MASS-1 began enroling patients in 1988 and completed enrolment in 1991. At that time, no agreement existed about hypercholesterolemia treatment, so patients were given only nutritional advice. At the end of the study, in 1998, only certain patients were receiving medication to treat their dyslipidemia. In addition to nutritional advice, patients were encouraged to stop smoking, to start exercising, and to lower their weight. Aspirin, propranolol, and nitrates were prescribed to all patients in the three groups. Calcium antagonists were added when necessary or as a substitute when propranolol was contraindicated. The treatment in the angioplasty group did not include stenting.

To ensure the feasibility of the study, all angiograms were first analyzed by the interventional cardiologist team to determine which patients met the inclusion criteria. Patients with stable angina whose angiograms identified a single stenotic lesion in the proximal third of the LAD, before the diagonal branch, were selected. Eligible patients could not have had prior coronary bypass surgery or PTCA. The artery had to be at least 80% occluded on visual evaluation, and the lesion length had to measure $\leqslant 12$ mm to be adequate to receive the 3.0 mm or larger catheter balloon.

The specific angiographic criteria for exclusion from the study were: (1) lesions > 12.0 mm in length; (2) a $\leqslant 2.5$ mm involvement in the artery ostium or artery diameter, or (3) an occluded, tortuous, or calcified artery. Patients with $\geqslant 50\%$ occlusion of the left main coronary artery were also excluded.

It is important to mention that angioplasty was performed by the same interventional cardiologist and surgery by the same surgeon. This gives strong support to the results obtained in both interventional strategies. On the other hand, this is an important limitation, because results cannot be universalized. As in many other trials nearly a third of patients were excluded, and the leading cause (52.8%) was the refusal to participate.

The study population was 214 patients, almost evenly distributed among the three treatment strategies. Characteristics of the patients are shown in Table 15.1. All patients were followed-up for five years, and examinations were performed every three months. The surgical procedure in all patients was a left internal mammary artery anastomosis with the descending anterior artery upon extracorporeal circulation in accordance with the conventional technique and with a $2.0–2.4$ L/min/m^2 perfusion and mild systemic hypothermia of

Table 15.1 Baseline characteristics of the study patients according to treatment group			
	Medical (*n* = 72)	PTCA (*n* = 72)	Surgery (*n* = 70)
Clinical			
Age (years)	58 ± 7	54 ± 9	58 ± 11
Male Sex (*n*)	59	58	58
Hypertension (%)	38	34	30
Diabetes (%)	20	15	18
Current smoker (%)	36	36	37
Employed (%)	89	88	90
Laboratory			
Total cholesterol (mg/dL)	240 ± 40	213 ± 49	230 ± 45
LDL-cholesterol (mg/dL)	162 ± 36	141 ± 42	155 ± 36
HDL-cholesterol (mg/dL)	41 ± 9	38 ± 9	37 ± 8
Triglycerides (mg/dL)	199 ± 111	192 ± 126	200 ± 110
Positive TI 201 stress scintigraphic results (%)	86	82	84
Angiographic findings			
Mean stenosis (%)	89	86	88
Ejection fraction (%)	75.0 ± 6.3	74.7 ± 6.4	74.9 ± 6.5

Unless otherwise indicated, data presented are mean value ± SD. HDL, high-density lipoprotein; LDL, low-density lipoprotein; PTCA, percutaneous transluminal coronary angioplasty; TI, thallium.

34–35°C. The initial success of angioplasty was defined as the reduction to less than 50% of the residual stenosis, with clinical improvement, and without myocardial infarction during hospitalization. Currently, this definition for 'success' is used for procedures at our institution. Repeat angiograms were to be performed in the angioplasty group at six months, two years, and five years after the procedure, or whenever necessary in case of an ischemic event. A final angiogram was performed in all living patients at the five-year follow-up. The study design allowed for patients to cross-over from one treatment to another, based on the occurrence of symptoms anytime during the study. Patients with unstable angina in the follow-up who were randomized to the medical therapy group would be changed to the angioplasty or surgery group, if necessary. Those patients with unstable angina or acute myocardial infarction who were randomized to the angioplasty group received surgical intervention or medical therapy. Patients who underwent surgery were considered for medical treatment after the occurrence of acute myocardial infarction or unstable angina; they were referred for angioplasty in the presence of stenosis at the site of anastomosis or upon the appearance of a new lesion requiring a catheterization procedure.

All living patients complied with the follow-up. The primary end-point was the combination of cardiac death, myocardial infarction, and refractory angina requiring revascularization. We also analyzed the angina status and the progression of coronary atherosclerosis at the end of the study.

Statistical analysis

The primary end-point was defined as one of the following events: cardiac-related death, acute myocardial infarction, and refractory angina requiring revascularization. The event-free survival time was defined as the interval between randomization and the occurrence of a primary end-point or the last follow-up.

Cardiac-related death time was considered as the interval between randomization and death or last follow-up. The likelihood of occurrence of events in each group was estimated by the Kaplan–Meier method and compared using the log-rank test.

Continuous variables were compared among the three groups using one-factor analysis-of-variance, followed by multiple comparisons. Fisher's exact test and the chi-square test were used to compare the three groups concerning qualitative variables. All analyses were made according to the intention-to-treat principle. P values less than 0.05 were considered significant. Statistical analyses were performed using the Statistical Analysis System (SAS).

Event-free survival

The rates of event-free survival were significantly different among the three groups ($p = 0.001$ by the log-rank test). Patients assigned to PTCA had more events (defined as additional revascularization, myocardial infarction, or death) than patients treated with medical therapy and surgery. In the PTCA group, 29 patients had events. Seventeen events occurred in the group treated with medical therapy. Only six patients in the surgery group had events. The cumulative event-free survival rates at one year were 98.6% for patients who underwent surgery, 63.9% for patients who underwent PTCA, and 88.9% for patients receiving medical therapy (Fig. 15.1). No significant difference occurred in the cumulative cardiac-related death curves for the three treatment groups (Fig. 15.2). Four deaths occurred in the PTCA group; two in the surgery group, and two in the medically-treated group ($p = 0.622$ by the log-rank test). The cumulative survival rates at five years were 94.3% in the PTCA group, 97.1% in the surgery group, and 97.1% in the medical treatment group.

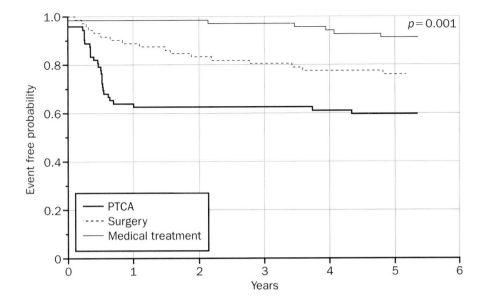

Group	No of patients	No of events	Years	Event-free probability	Standard error	Patients at risk
Surgery	70	6	1	0.986	0.014	69
			3	0.971	0.020	68
			5	0.914	0.033	56
PTCA	72	29	1	0.639	0.057	46
			3	0.625	0.057	45
			5	0.597	0.058	34
Medical treatment	72	17	1	0.889	0.037	64
			3	0.804	0.047	57
			5	0.761	0.051	44

Figure 15.1 Survival free from additional revascularization, myocardial infarction, or death. Patients assigned to PTCA are indicated by solid thick lines, patients assigned to surgery by solid thin lines, and patients assigned to medical therapy by dashed lines.

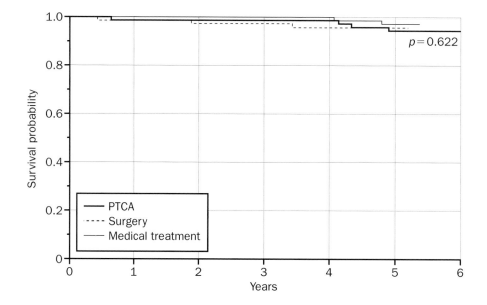

Group	No of patients	No of events	Years	Event-free probability	Standard error	Patients at risk
Surgery	70	2	1	1.000	–	70
			3	1.000	–	70
			5	0.971	0.020	59
PTCA	72	4	1	0.986	0.014	71
			3	0.986	0.014	70
			5	0.943	0.057	57
Medical treatment	72	2	1	0.986	0.014	71
			3	0.971	0.019	68
			5	0.971	0.024	55

Figure 15.2 Probability of absence of cardiac-related death. Patients assigned to PTCA are indicated by solid thick lines, patients referred to surgery by solid thin lines, and patients referred to medical therapy by dashed lines.

Medical therapy group

Three of the 72 patients had uncomplicated acute myocardial infarctions; eight were referred for surgery, and four for angioplasty because they showed signs of unstable angina. Two cardiac and four non-cardiac deaths were recorded. The cardiac deaths were related to acute myocardial infarction, and the non-cardiac deaths were related to cancer (three patients) and stroke (one patient).

CABG group

In the 70 patients referred for surgery, one patient had a perioperative acute myocardial infarction. No in-hospital deaths occurred in this group; however, one patient died on his way to the hospital as a result of unstable angina after 43 months of follow-up, and one patient developed cardiogenic shock and died during evolution of an acute myocardial infarction. Non-fatal myocardial infarction was observed in three patients and stroke in one patient. None of these patients required angioplasty during the follow-up period. No neoplasia were diagnosed in this group until the end of the study.

PTCA group

The success rate was 96%. Emergency surgery was required in one patient because of an acute myocardial infarction during the procedure, and it was not possible to dilate the stenotic artery in three patients. During the follow-up period, 27 (39.1%) of the 69 patients in this group underwent repeat catheterization due to unstable angina, and 20 (29.9%) required one or two additional angioplasty procedures for treatment of restenosis. Elective cardiac surgery was necessary in eight patients due to the development of unstable angina, and none of these required further surgery during the first six months of follow-up. Four patients died

during follow-up; one died of sudden death at home, and the other three died during acute myocardial infarctions. A stroke and immuno-deficiency syndrome were the causes of non-cardiac deaths in two patients. Non-fatal myocardial infarctions occurred in four patients during the follow-up period.

Anginal symptoms

Patients treated with CABG were the most likely to be free of anginal symptoms at the conclusion of the study, but a marked increase was observed in anginal symptoms among patients randomized to medical therapy. Only 17 (25.8%) patients in the medically-treated group were free of such symptoms at the end of the study, compared with 48 (72.7%) in the surgery group and 44 (64.7%) in the angioplasty group. A statistically significant benefit was found for angioplasty as compared with medical therapy ($p < 0.001$). None of the study patients in any of the groups presented with refractory angina (functional class III or IV) at final follow-up. When coronary flow is ameliorated by an intervention, it is expected that angina and quality of life will improve. Treadmill testing performed on 161 patients (80%) at the end of the study period revealed that 46% of those in the medical therapy, 66% of those assigned to angioplasty, and 72% of the patients randomized to surgery were free from ischemia in the final ergometric test ($p = 0.008$). Interestingly, nearly 50% of patients treated medically have no ischemia. It is well known that other methods, like myocardial perfusion scintigraphy and stress echocardiography with dobutamine are more sensitive for detecting ischemia than ergometric testing. However, in patients with single-vessel disease and with no previous myocardial infarction, ergometric testing has moderate-to-high sensitivity and specificity [23] and can be used as a good test for ischemia surveillance.

Progression of atherosclerosis

At the end of the study, 191 patients underwent coronary angiography; 96 (50.3%) patients had evidence of stenosis (> 50% occlusion in vessels that had been normal at the beginning of the study). We observed progression of atherosclerosis in 27 of the 63 patients assigned to the surgery group who had completed follow-up, 30 of the 63 patients in the angioplasty group, and 38 of the 65 patients who received medical treatment ($p = 0.193$). No relationship existed between the baseline and follow-up levels of total serum cholesterol or its fractions in patients who developed coronary atherosclerosis, nor did a difference exist in cholesterol levels between patients with and without atherosclerosis. Baseline and final cholesterol levels were 239 ± 49 and 236 ± 52 mg/dL, respectively, for patients who developed new stenoses; and 224 ± 15 and 228 ± 476 mg/dL, respectively, for those who did not develop new stenoses ($p = 0.077$). It is clear that cholesterolemia control was not effective with dietary advice alone.

At the end of the study, 49 (75.4%) patients assigned to medical treatment had vessel diameter stenosis between 70% and 99%, and 10 (15.4%) patients had an occluded LAD artery. Thirty-six (58.1%) angioplasty-referred patients had < 70% vessel diameter stenosis, and 11 (17.7%) had stenosis between 70% and 99%. Twelve (19.4%) patients had total occlusion of the LAD artery. Two (3.2%) patients assigned to surgery had lesions with < 70% occlusion, 17 (27.4%) patients had stenosis between 70% and 99%, and 41 (66.1%) had LAD occlusion. The left internal mammary artery was free from significant atherosclerosis in all patients, except for one who had occlusion at the end of the study.

Ventricular function

At admission, left ventricular ejection fraction (LVEF) was $75 \pm 6\%$ and at the end of the study it was $71 \pm 7\%$ for patients assigned to medical treatment; $75 \pm 6\%$ and $68 \pm 10\%$ for patients assigned to angioplasty, and $75 \pm 6\%$ and $72 \pm 6\%$ for patients assigned to surgical treatment ($p = 0.136$ among the groups). This is a very important result because, despite severe lesions, patients treated medically and without statin therapy did not have deterioration in left ventricular function and, as we know, ventricular function is the most important predictor of mortality in cardiac disease as well as in coronary heart disease. When indicating a revascularization procedure, we also have in mind preserving ventricular function. This study does not support using these procedures for preserving ventricular function as the main strategy, but only to relieve symptoms and reduce ischemia, at least for a five-year period.

Employment status

No difference was observed among the groups in terms of the ability to return to regular employment after randomization. Fifty-six (84.8%) patients randomized to medical treatment, 46 (69.7%) referred to angioplasty, and 56 (82.3%) patients in the surgical group were employed at the end of the study ($p = 0.072$). The majority of patients did not do heavy work, but at least 50% did perform moderate exercise in their jobs.

General considerations

Percutaneous transluminal coronary angioplasty was introduced in the late 1970s. It was a less invasive alternative for revascularization of the ischemic myocardium [16]. By the early 1990s, more than 300,000 procedures had been carried out in the US, mostly in patients with single-vessel coronary disease. Recent comparative studies observed the effects of treatment with implantation of expandable-balloon stents and balloon-catheter angioplasty in patients with single-vessel coronary disease. Although outcomes were initially the same for both strategies, improvement in material and stent shape have produced better results. Today, at least 70% of patients referred for catheter intervention are treated with stenting instead of angioplasty alone. This is true in the US as well as in Europe and Brazil. All patients referred for angioplasty in our study were treated with the balloon-catheter alone. Therefore, it is not clear whether interventional techniques used during that period, i.e. the catheter alone, have provided any major benefits thus far.

Moreover, few studies have compared coronary angioplasty and surgical bypass in different subgroups of coronary disease [13–15, 17, 18]. In addition, it is not clear whether myocardial bypass even results in a better short-term or long-term prognosis than medical treatment alone. The need for comparisons among the different therapeutic strategies is clear.

The results of the MASS-1 trial are in accordance with the data recently published from the 'Angioplasty Compared to Medical (ACME) Trial' [16], which indicated that patients with single-vessel coronary disease, including the LAD, and who were treated with angioplasty, had better symptomatic relief than patients treated pharmacologically. However, all three therapeutic strategies in our study led to the elimination of limiting angina, and the additional symptomatic benefit in the surgical bypass or catheter groups may not be clinically significant. Surgical treatment, when compared with other treatments, was significantly superior in terms of the estimated probability of the absence of events. This superiority probably resulted from the low perioperative complication rate, the absence of conditions that could lead to re-operation, and the improvement in symptoms.

Our results were similar to those of other studies in patients with single LAD stenosis who received surgical treatment [11]. The results of a randomized comparative study of coronary angioplasty versus surgical bypass for treatment of patients with proximal LAD stenosis were recently published by Goy et al [15]. In this study, which included a homogenous group of 134 patients with stable angina, the authors observed that 86% of the patients who received surgical bypass and 43% of those treated with angioplasty were free from adverse events after an average follow-up period of 2.5 years. In comparison, our results demonstrate a significantly higher estimated probability of absence of events among patients referred for surgery (97%) in relation to patients treated with angioplasty (64%) ($p = 0.001$). However, we found no significant differences between the occurrences of death or myocardial infarction between the surgery and angioplasty groups.

The observed relatively benign evolution in patients with non-revascularized critical LAD stenosis observed in the present study may be partially attributed to the preserved ventricular function and also to the remission of anginal symptoms. Studies by Klein et al [2] in clinically-treated patients with LAD stenosis revealed an estimated survival of 97% in an average follow-up period of 17 months. In fact, it was the impaired ventricular function that determined the poor outcome. Another study by Califf et al [1] in patients with preserved ventricular function and single LAD stenosis revealed an estimated survival of 98% at five-year follow-up when the stenosis was after the first septal branch, and 90% when it was before this branch. Although the prognosis is less optimistic in patients with LAD involvement, when compared with the involvement of other arteries, however, a consensus exists that patients with single-vessel disease and preserved ventricular function have a fairly favorable long-term prognosis.

Progression of atherosclerosis

At the end of out study, the final angiographic examination revealed that 96 (50%) patients who were free of apparent obstructive disease at baseline had developed stenosis of > 50% occlusion. However, LAD stenosis in the patients randomized to the medical treatment group remained stable, without progression, in 75% of the patients.

Few prospective and randomized studies exist that are aimed at determining atherosclerotic disease progression, irrespective of the treatment provided [24]. So the recognition of the development of stenosis in apparently normal vessels and plaque 'stabilization' in previously lesioned vessels in the same patient offers new perspectives for consideration and fuels the debate about coronary atherosclerosis progression and its physiopathologic role. Ultimately we can consider that coronary artery bypass surgery using the left internal mammary artery in patients with angina, proximal LAD stenosis, and normal ventricular function produces a significant benefit in terms of the estimated probability of the absence of events. This was largely due to reintervention in the angioplasty group, either surgically or via balloon catheter, during the five years of outpatient follow-up. However, the rate of coronary atherosclerosis progression was not insignificant in vessels that did not undergo intervention and apparently were free from obstructive processes at the beginning of the study. Moreover, the three groups demonstrated similar results in relation to the occurrence of myocardial infarction and death during follow-up. Therefore, the atherosclerotic involvement of coronary arteries other than the left anterior descending coronary artery transforms the status of these patients from single-vessel to multivessel disease, which could significantly influence progression, the clinical course, and treatment strategies adopted. Therefore, future cost-effectiveness analyses with longer clinical follow-up are necessary for the thorough establishment of patients' prognoses. Finally, a meta-analysis [25] of all randomized studies may supply important information about the main outcomes of the current therapeutic modalities for this disease. These considerations lead us to the second study, the MASS-2 trial.

MASS-2

We used the MASS-1 design for MASS-2, except for the following criteria: (1) patients with previous myocardial infarction were not excluded as they had been in MASS-1 and (2) any interventional cardiologist from the angioplasty team and any surgeon from the surgery team could perform the procedure. This was different from MASS-1 where only one particular interventional cardiologist or surgeon did the procedures. By allowing various physicians to perform the procedures, the results can be applied to other centers, without the bias of the procedures being performed by the same person. After all entry criteria were satisfied, the interventional cardiology team did the last procedure, watching the angiograms and deciding whether the obstructed main arteries were prone to angioplasty and whether angioplasty would approximate the results of surgery in terms of revascularizing the extent of myocardium at risk. Angioplasty was performed with a stent in at least one artery in 143 (70%) patients. Patients were chosen randomly.

The selection of patients started in June 1995 and ended in March 2000. A total of 611 patients were randomized, 203 for medical, 205 for PTCA/stent, and 203 for surgery treatments. Characteristics of all three groups are in Table 15.2. We can see that normal left ventricular function as the main inclusion criteria was achieved. Mean ejection fraction is within normal limits and near 0.68 in all groups. Nearly 37% of the patients were aged 65 years or more with a mean age of 60 ± 9, the majority being men (423 patients, 69.2%). In MASS-1, the mean age was 57. Certainly ages 65 and greater indicate an elderly population, many of whom had retired because of their disease. A striking difference existed between these patients and those of MASS-1 regarding employment status and history of hypertension. Only 179 (29.3%) had a job and 232 (59.2%) had hypertension, but in MASS-1 88% were employed and 35% had hypertension. Laboratory values show lower total cholesterol (near 218 mg/dL) and low

Table 15.2 Characteristics of all patients according to treatment in MASS-2 trial

Characteristic	Medical (*n* = 203)	Surgery (*n* = 203)	Angioplasty (*n* = 205)
Gender			
Male *n* (%)	140 (69)	146 (72)	138 (67)
Female *n* (%)	63 (31)	57 (28)	67 (33)
Age (years)			
Mean ± SD	60 ± 9	60 ± 9	60 ± 9
% of pts ⩾ 65	36	34	38
Employed (%)	29	24	27
History			
Previous MI, *n* (%)	79 (39)	84 (41)	105 (51)
Current smoker, *n* (%)	67 (33)	65 (32)	55 (27)
Hypertension, *n* (%)	111 (55)	127 (63)	124 (60)
Diabetes, *n* (%)	73 (36)	59 (29)	54 (26)
Angina class II or II, *n* (%)	158 (78)	172 (85)	156 (76)
Positive ETT, *n* (%)	80 (39)	98 (48)	89 (43)
Laboratory values (mg/dL)			
Total cholesterol	222 ± 39	220 ± 41	214 ± 42
LDL-cholesterol	148 ± 34	147 ± 36	143 ± 36
HDL-cholesterol	37 ± 0	38 ± 10	37 ± 10
Angiographic findings			
Mean ejection fraction (%)	68 ± 7	67 ± 8	67 ± 9
Double-vessel disease	84	85	85
Triple-vessel disease	119	120	118
LAD disease (%)	32	34	44

density lipoprotein (LDL)-cholesterol levels (146 mg/dL) compared with those in MASS-1. This may reflect antilipemic treatment, at least in the 268 (43.8%) patients with a previous myocardial infarction. The majority of patients, 357 (58.4%), had triple-vessel disease, and 223 (36.5%) had LAD obstruction. Except for normal left ventricular function, this is a high-risk population, considering coronary arteries with obstructions alone. Taking into account the presence of risk factors, diabetes in 186 (30.4%) and hypertension in 232 (59.2%), this would suppose a high event rate even during the one-year period for patients in the medical therapy group. Follow-up over one year shows no significant difference in the rates of death in the three groups, 1.5% in the medical group, 4.5% in the surgery group, and 3.5% in the angioplasty group (Fig. 15.3). The cumulative probability curve of being free of non-fatal myocardial infarction is presented in Fig. 15.4. These results show a

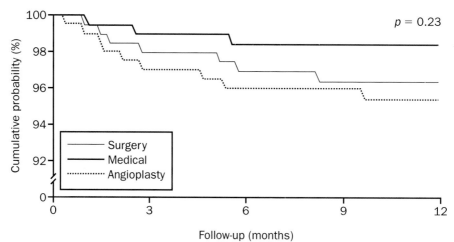

Figure 15.3   First year survival curve in MASS-2

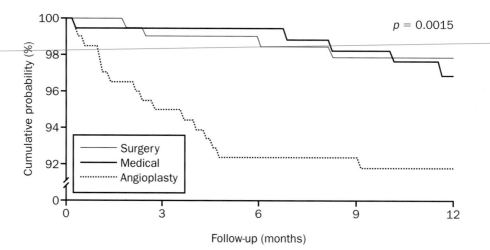

Figure 15.4   First year free of non-fatal AMI follow-up in MASS-2.

higher event rate in the angioplasty group ($p < 0.0015$).

We will need to wait until the five-year follow-up is completed to know more about the MASS-2 trial. If the results are similar to those of MASS-1, we will really need to change our approach to coronary heart disease patients in terms of invasive treatments.

REFERENCES

1. Califf RM, Tomabechi Y, Lee KL et al. Outcome in one-vessel coronary artery disease, *Circulation* 1983; **67**:283–290.
2. Klein LW, Weintraub WS, Agarwal JB et al. Prognostic significance of severe narrowing of the proximal portion of the left anterior descending coronary artery, *Am J Cardiol* 1986; **58**:42–46.

3. European Coronary Surgery Study Group. Long-term results prospective randomized study of coronary artery bypass surgery in stable angina pectoris, *Lancet* 1982; **2**:1173–1180.

4. Shuster EH, Griffith LS, Bulkley BH. Preponderance of acute proximal left anterior descending coronary artery lesions in fatal myocardial infarction: a clinico-pathologic study, *Am J Cardiol* 1981; **47**:1189–1196.

5. Rahimtoola SH. Left main equivalence is still an unproved hypothesis but proximal left anterior descending coronary artery disease is a 'high-risk' lesion, *Am J Cardiol* 1984; **53**:1719–1721.

6. Ellis SG. Percutaneous coronary intervention in the 1990s. Results in patients with single or multi-vessel disease, *Herz* 1992; **17**:18–26.

7. Gruentzig A. A transluminal dilatation of coronary artery stenosis, *Lancet* 1978; **1**:263.

8. Tyras DH, Kaiser GC, Barner HB et al. The rationale for operative therapy of symptomatic single-vessel coronary artery disease, *J Thorac Cardiovasc Surg* 1980; **80**:73–78.

9. CASS Principal Investigators and their associates. Myocardial infarction and mortality in the coronary artery surgery study (CASS) randomized trial, *N Engl J Med* 1984; **310**:750–758.

10. Chaitman BR, Davis KB, Kaiser GC et al. The hole of coronary bypass surgery for 'left main equivalent' coronary disease: the coronary artery surgery study registry, *Circulation* 1986; **74** (suppl III):17–25.

11. Kramer JR, Proudfit WL, Loop FD et al. Late follow-up of 781 patients undergoing percutaneous transluminal coronary angioplasty or coronary artery bypass grafting for an isolated obstruction in the left anterior descending coronary artery, *Am Heart J* 1989; **118**:1144–1153.

12. Ellis SG, Fisher L, Dushman-Ellis S et al. Comparison of coronary angioplasty with medical treatment for single- and double-vessel coronary disease with left anterior descending coronary involvement: long-term outcome based on an Emory-CASS registry study, *Am Heart J* 1989; **118**:208–219.

13. Rodriguez A, Boullon F, Perez-Balino N et al. Argentine randomized trial of percutaneous transluminal coronary angioplasty versus coronary artery bypass surgery in multivessel disease (ERACI): in-hospital results and one-year follow-ups. ERACI groups, *J Am Coll Cardiol* 1993; **22**:1060–1067.

14. RITA Trial Participants. Coronary angioplasty versus coronary bypass surgery: the Randomized Intervention Treatment of Angina (RITA) trial, *Lancet* 1993; **341**:573–580.

15. Goy JJ, Eeckout E, Burnand B et al. Coronary angioplasty versus left internal mammary artery grafting for isolated proximal left anterior descending artery stenosis, *Lancet* 1994; **343**:1449–1453.

16. Parisi AF, Folland ED, Hartigan P. A comparison of angioplasty with medical therapy in the treatment of single-vessel coronary artery disease, *N Engl J Med* 1992; **326**:10–16.

17. Hamm CW, Reimers J, Ischinger T et al. A randomized study of coronary angioplasty compared with bypass surgery in patients with symptomatic multi-vessel coronary disease. German Angioplasty Bypass Surgery Investigation, *N Engl J Med* 1994; **331**:1037–1043.

18. King SB III, Lembo JN, Weintraub SW et al. A randomized trial comparing coronary angioplasty with coronary bypass surgery. Emory Angioplasty versus Surgery Trial, *N Engl J Med* 1994; **331**:1044–1050.

19. Lange RA, Willard JE, Hillis LD. Southwestern Internal Medicine Conference: restenosis: the Achilles heel of coronary angioplasty, *Am J Med SCI* 1993; **306** (4):265–275.

20. Scandinavian Simvastatin Survival Study (4S). *Lancet* 1994; **344**:1383–1389.

21. Antiplatelet Trialists' Collaboration. Collaborative overview of randomised trials of antiplatelet therapy—I: prevention of death, myocardial infarction, and stroke by prolonged antiplatelet therapy in various category of patients, *BMJ* 1994; **308**:81–106.

22. Hueb WA, Belloti G, Oliveira SA et al. The Medicine, Angioplasty or Surgery Study (MASS): a prospective, randomized trial of medical therapy, balloon angioplasty or bypass surgery for single proximal left anterior descending artery stenosis, *J Am Coll Cardiol* 1995; **26**:1600–1605.

23. Gianrossi R, Detrano R, Mulvihill D et al. Exercise-induced ST depression in the diagnosis of coronary artery disease: a meta-analysis, *Circulation* 1989; **80**:87.

24. Alderman EL, Corley SD, Fisher LD et al and the CASS participating investigators and staff. Five year angiographic follow-up of factors associated with progression of coronary artery disease

in the coronary artery surgery study (CASS), *J Am Coll Cardiol* 1993; **22**:1141–1154.

25. Pocock SJ, Henderson RA, Rickards AF et al. Meta-analysis of randomized trials comparing coronary angioplasty with bypass surgery, *Lancet* 1995; **346**:1184–1189.

16

The AWESOME trial

Douglass A Morrison, Jerome Sacks, William G Henderson and Gulshan Sethi

CONTENTS • Introduction • Study methods • Results • Discussion • What did AWESOME teach us that we did not already know?

INTRODUCTION

The Angina With Extremely Serious Operative Mortality Evaluation (AWESOME) randomized trial, and prospective registry began enrollment in February 1995 and completed enrollment on March 31, 2000. Over the five-year period, 16 Veterans Affairs Medical Centers participated, with 11 sites enrolling throughout the entire period, and five enrolling for periods of 2–3 years [1, 2]. The trial was designed to compare long-term survival with a percutaneous coronary intervention (PCI) strategy that could include stents, with a strategy of coronary artery bypass graft surgery (CABG). The registries of (a) patients directed to one or the other option rather than permitting random allocation (physician directed) and of (b) eligible patients who were offered random allocation but declined (patient choice), were intended to provide further insight into relative advantages and disadvantages of the two revascularization options for patients with medically refractory myocardial ischemia and one or more of five risk factors for adverse outcome with CABG (age > 70; left ventricular ejection fraction [LVEF] < 0.35; prior CABG; myocardial infarction [MI] within seven days; or intra-aortic balloon pump [IABP] required) [3].

Are PCI and CABG appropriate revascularization options for the relief of medically refractory, high-risk unstable angina?

Coronary artery bypass graft (CABG) surgery and percutaneous coronary intervention (PCI) are associated with relief of symptoms and enhanced survival in selected patients with coronary artery disease (CAD) [4–17]. Direct comparison of PCI and CABG in randomized trials suggests that long-term survival is comparable, albeit with more frequent repeat revascularization, among patients randomized to PCI [17–27]. In some cases, better symptom relief has been observed among patients randomly assigned to CABG [17–27].

Current guidelines recommend CABG as the preferred revascularization option for high-risk patients, where risk is determined largely based on extent of anatomic coronary disease and left ventricular function [4, 17]. In practice, high risk is determined not only by extent of anatomic coronary disease and left ventricular function but also by other factors such as urgency of revascularization, co-morbidity, hemodynamic instability and prior CABG. Previous randomized comparisons of CABG and PCI frequently excluded patients with unfavorable coronary anatomy and significant co-morbidity [17–27] and all revascularization trials prior to the AWESOME trial excluded patients with prior CABG, severe left ventricular function (LVEF < 0.25 and in most trials < 0.35), very recent or ongoing myocardial infarction (< 24 hours and in most trials < seven days), and patients requiring emergency revascularization [4–29]. Some of these high-risk patients were at prohibitive risk for CABG. PCI remained the only revascularization option, and a therapy strategy for these high-risk patients had to be formulated in the absence of randomized trial experience. Confronted with this situation, we began, in 1988, offering 'salvage angioplasty' without surgical standby to selected patients with medically refractory ischemia who had been refused CABG [30] and found that PCI provided substantial relief for those patients who were at prohibitive risk for CABG. As experience with 'salvage angioplasty' increased, the question was raised 'whether some patients at increased but not prohibitive risk of adverse outcomes with CABG be better served with PCI, even though CABG remained an option. This 'salvage angioplasty' experience resulted in a proposed randomized clinical trial to compare CABG and PCI for the revascularization of patients with medically refractory ischemia and high but not prohibitively high, risk of adverse outcome with CABG [1]. From the Veterans Affairs Continuous Improvement in Cardiac Surgery Program database, we identified five variables associated with increased 30-day postoperative mortality: prior heart surgery; age > 70 years; left ventricular ejection fraction < 0.35; intra-aortic balloon pump prior to surgery; myocardial infarction < seven days prior to CABG [31, 32]. These factors, which were often exclusions in the earlier trials, were inclusion factors for the proposed trial [33]. The Cooperative Studies Evaluation Committee (CSEC) approved the proposed study, enrollment began in February 1995 and ended on March 31, 2000.

The study results, which parallel earlier studies, indicate CABG and PCI are both reasonable options for these patients [1, 2]. The rest of this chapter will present, in detail, the primary study findings and by comparing patient selection, methods, and results with other trials, place the results of AWESOME in context.

STUDY METHODS

Patient screening and accrual

Patient screening took place in a five-step process. The first three steps consisted of identifying clinically eligible patients who had medically refractory myocardial ischemia and one or more of the high risk factors.

Myocardial ischemia was defined by the presence of at least one of the following:

- Rest angina with reversible electrocardiographic changes.
- Rest angina in a patient with prior myocardial infarction or angiographically confirmed coronary artery disease.
- Recurrent rest angina.
- Rest angina with seven days of an acute myocardial infarction.
- Angina which had been stabilized medically, with a subsequent positive provocative test for ischemia.

Medically refractory was defined as ischemia, which persisted despite a regimen that included aspirin and/or intravenous heparin and at least one of the following:

- Heart rate < 60 beats/min and systolic blood pressure < 120 mmHg on no anti-anginal drug.
- Enough anti-anginal drug so that resting heart rate < 70 beats/min and/or systolic blood pressure < 150 mmHg.
- Intra-aortic balloon pump required to stabilize.
- Significant clinical contraindication to both beta-blocking and calcium-blocking agents.

These criteria were selected so as to be flexible enough for potential application to patients > 80 years of age and with LVEF < 0.35.

High-risk patients had at least one of five high-risk factors chosen from the Veterans Affairs Continuous Improvement in Cardiac Surgery Program database [31, 32] that predicted high 30-day surgical mortality:

- Prior heart surgery.
- Age > 70.
- Left ventricular ejection fraction < 0.35.
- Intra-aortic balloon pump required.
- Myocardial infarction within the previous seven days (could include ongoing infarction).

Patients who met the three clinical eligibility criteria (myocardial ischemia; medically refractory; high risk of adverse outcomes) underwent coronary angiography which was reviewed by both a surgeon and an interventional cardiologist. The protocol called for the surgeon and interventional cardiologist to achieve consensus regarding suitability for random assignment. In practice, referring physicians and non-invasive cardiologists often also became involved in this decision. Specific exclusions from the randomized trial included any of the following: no graftable or dilatable vessels; co-morbidity likely to limit the patient's life to a greater extent than the coronary disease; angioplasty within six months.

Clinically eligible patients with a coronary anatomy deemed acceptable for random assignment between the two revascularization strategies were approached for informed consent to participate in the trial.

Table 16.1 outlines patient flow through the screening process at the 16 VA hospitals. A total of 22,662 patients were screened and of these patients, 7278 did not meet criteria for myocardial ischemia, 5783 failed to meet criteria for medically refractory, and 10,030 had none of the high-risk factors. There were 2431 clinically eligible patients, who met all three criteria. After coronary angiography had been reviewed by both an interventional cardiologist and a surgeon, a total of 781 (32%) were acceptable to both operators as candidates for random allocation and 454 (58%) consented to a randomized choice of revascularization. The 327 patients who refused random allocation and the 1650 patients for whom physician consensus would not allow random assignment constitute a prospectively gathered registry experience.

Given the rapidly changing nature of both PCI and CABG, the decision was made to allow operators to use whatever techniques, technologies, or drugs were available during the course of the study [1, 2].

Randomization was under the direction of the study biostatistician at the Hines Veterans Affairs Cooperative Studies Program Coordinating Center. Patients were stratified by hospital, age (≤ 70, > 70 years), and prior heart surgery (yes, no). The co-chairmen and local principal investigators were blinded from the study results throughout the course of the study.

Table 16.1 Patient flow through 16 participating Veteran Affairs medical centers

Patient flow	Number	Percent
Screened	22662	—
Clinically eligible	2431	100
Turned down for CABG	649	27
Turned down for PCI	681	28
Turned down for both	320	13
Angiographically eligible	781	32
Eligible for randomization	781	100
Patient refused	327	42
Patient consented	454	58
Randomization assignments	454	100
CABG	232	51
PCI	222	49

CABG, coronary artery bypass graft surgery; PCI, percutaneous coronary intervention.

Outcome variables

The primary outcome of the trial was survival. Death records were filled out on each patient who died during the course of the trial by the research nurse coordinators. Patient records were matched with VA death records recorded in the Veterans Affairs Beneficiary Identification and Record Locator Subsystem (BIRLS) database to check survival information [34]. Repeat hospitalization, repeat catheterization, and repeat CABG and PCI were obtained from the clinically scheduled follow-up visits and rechecked against the Patient Treatment File (PTF), an independent database maintained by the Veterans Administration. Unstable angina, defined as either progressive, new-onset, or occurring at rest, was also recorded from both clinic records and the PTF.

Statistical methods

The primary end-point, long-term survival, was estimated by the Kaplan–Meier procedure, survival curves were plotted for visual comparisons and global differences between the CABG and PCI plots were evaluated by log-rank tests. In addition, the annual survival rate post six months and its standard error were estimated by maximum likelihood estimate (MLE). The secondary end-points, survival free from unstable angina and survival free from unstable angina or repeat revascularization were also evaluated by the Kaplan–Meier procedure. Survival curves were plotted for visual comparisons, and global differences between the CABG and PCI plots were evaluated by log-rank tests. Annual survival rates post six months were estimated by maximum likelihood (MLE). All comparisons are based on cohorts specified by the intention-to-treat principle.

RESULTS

Baseline comparability of CABG and PCI cohorts

Table 16.2 presents selected clinical and angiographic baseline variables for the randomly allocated CABG and PCI cohorts. Table 16.3 presents clinical and angiographic baseline variables for the overall randomly allocated and registry cohorts. Table 16.4 presents selected clinical and angiographic baseline variables for the cohorts assigned by physicians or by patient selection to PCI or CABG. The CABG and PCI profiles are similar for all baseline variables and there are no significant differences between the mean values for the clinical variables comparing the cohort randomized to CABG versus the cohort randomized to PCI. In contrast, physicians did use several clinical and angiographic parameters to help choose between revascularization options [3]. Overall, patients chose PCI by a 2 : 1 margin, but appeared to do so more independently of clinical parameters [3].

CABG and PCI methods

The numbers of distal anastamoses performed were relatively stable at 2.9 across the five years of the study. The use of arterial conduits increased somewhat with average use over the five years as follows: left internal mammary use at 70.3% and right internal mammary use at 3.3%, radial artery at 2.8% and gastroepiploic artery use at 0%. Overall, 92.7% of operated patients received myocardial preservation with large intra-hospital variations in cold versus warm, and anterograde versus retrograde cardioplegia.

Stent use increased from 26% of cases in 1995, to 88% of cases in 1999/2000. The use of glycoprotein IIb/IIIa receptor blocking agents as adjuncts to PCI increased from 1% in 1995, to 52% in 1999/2000. Conversely, the use of intra-aortic balloon counter-pulsation decreased from

Table 16.2 Baseline comparison of clinical variables of patients randomly assigned to CABG or to PCI (with permission from reference 2)

Baseline	CABG	PCI
Number of patients	232	222
Age	67 years	67 years
Males	99%	99%
White	88%	82%
Black	5%	6%
Married	66%	63%
Medical therapy		
ASA	88%	88%
Heparin	64%	61%
Beta-blocker	76%	76%
Calcium blocker	36%	27%
High-risk factors		
Age > 70	53%	50%
Prior CABG	32%	30%
Myocardial infarction < seven days	32%	35%
LVEF < 0.35	23%	18%
IABP required	2%	2%
Two or more high risk factors	35%	32%
Other risk factors		
Current smoker	24%	25%
Hypertension	69%	67%
Diabetes	34%	29%
Prior PCI	22%	17%
Prior myocardial infarction	71%	70%
Prior stroke	14%	9%
Left ventricular ejection fraction	0.44	0.47
Native coronary disease		
One-vessel CAD	17%	20%
Two-vessel CAD	33%	40%
Three-vessel CAD	50%	40%
Left anterior descending > 70%	88%	87%
Thrombus containing lesions	11%	21%*
Calcified lesions by angiography	27%	32%
Total lesion length > 70 mm	11%	11%
Highest ACC/AHA class:		
A	5%	4%
B	36%	38%
C	59%	59%

CABG, coronary artery bypass graft; IABP, intra-aortic balloon pump required; PCI, percutaneous coronary intervention; LVEF, left ventricular ejection fraction; CAD, coronary artery disease; PCI, percutaneous coronary intervention; ACC/AHA, American College of Cardiology/American Heart Association; *, $p < 0.01$.

Table 16.3 Baseline comparisons of randomized, total registry, physician-directed and patient-choice cohorts (with permission from reference 3)

Variable		Random	Registry	Physician directed	Patient choice
Patients	number	454	1977	1650	327
Age	mean	67	67	68	67
Age > 70	%	52	53	53	52
Prior PCI	%	23	24	24	23
Prior CABG	%	31	42*	44	36[++]
Prior MI	%	57	57	57	59
MI < 7 days	%	33	32	31	39[+]
LVEF < 0.35	%	21	18	18	16
LVEF	mean	42	44	43	46
IABP	%	2	5	5	3
Smoker	%	35	30	30	35
Diabetes	%	33	33	34	28
Hypertension	%	70	67	68	64
Prior CHF	%	61	69	71	57[++]
Prior stroke	%	13	12	12	9
Aspirin	%	94	96	96	95
Heparin	%	84	84	82	90
Beta blocker	%	79	78	78	77
Calcium blocker	%	33	37	37	33
One-vessel	%	18	22	20	30
Two-vessel	%	41	33	33	37
Three-vessel	%	41	44	47	33[++]
Native CAD	%	99	98	98	97
Graft CAD	%	26	33*	35	26[++]
Left anterior descending > 70%	%	89	83	83	83
L. main > 50%	%	7	18*	19	12[++]
ACC/AHA class C	%	75	78	80	67[++]
NYHA class 3/4	%	61	69*	71	57[++]

*, statistically significant difference between random and registry: $p < 0.01$; [+], statistically significant difference between physician directed and patient choice registry subsets: $p < 0.05$; [++], statistically significant difference between physician directed and patient choice registry subsets: $p < 0.01$.

Table 16.4 Baseline comparison of clinical and angiographic variables for physician-directed and patient-choice cohorts by intervention (with permission from reference 3)

| | | Physician directed | | Patient choice | |
		CABG	PCI	CABG	PCI
Patients	n	692	651	95	207
Age	years	69	66	68	66
Age > 70	%	63	42**	58	50
Prior PCI	%	17	32**	17	26
Prior CABG	%	22	55**	34	36
Prior MI	%	51	65**	54	61
MI < 7 days	%	28	35**	36	41
LVEF < 0.35	%	17	19	21	14
LVEF	mean	43	43	45	46
IABP	%	5	7	3	3
Smoker	%	28	32	33	36
Diabetes	%	36	31	22	32
Hypertension	%	69	66	66	64
Prior CHF	%	83	57**	47	60*
Prior stroke	%	11	11	7	9
Three-vessel	%	57	39**	35	30
Native CAD	%	98	98	97	98
SVG CAD	%	21	40**	20	26
Left anterior descending > 70%	%	92	78**	86	80
L. main > 50%	%	34	11**	15	10
TIMI no flow	%	44	54*	51	37
ACC/AHA class C	%	84	75**	57	70*
NYHA class 3/4	%	83	57**	47	60*

*, statistically significant difference between CABG and PCI: $p < 0.05$; **, statistically significant difference between CABG and PCI: $p < 0.01$.

21% of PCI cases in 1995, to 10% in 1999/2000. There was no use of cardiopulmonary support or heart-lung bypass as an adjunct for PCI throughout the course of the study. By 1998, there was no further use of directional atherectomy.

Short-term outcomes

Table 16.5 presents the CABG and PCI short-term outcomes. Of the 232 patients randomized to receive CABG, 227 (98%) were revascularized and five (2%) were not revascularized (the surgeon declined post-randomization due to high risk [$n = 2$], the patient refused surgery post-randomization [$n = 2$]; no reason [$n = 1$]).

Table 16.5 Short-term outcomes of patients randomly assigned to CABG or PCI (with permission from reference 2)

Index revascularization	Number		Percent	
	CABG	PCI	CABG	PCI
Randomized	232	222	100	100
Revascularized	227	221	98	99.5
Received only CABG	215	1	93	0.5
Received only PCI	10	213	4	96
Received CABG and PCI	2	7	1	3
Complications				
Renal	3	4	1	2
Stroke	3	2	1	1
In-hospital death	8	2	4	1

In-hospital mortality of the CABG cohort was 4% ($n = 8$) and the 30-day mortality was 5%. Of the 222 patients randomized to PCI, 221 (99.5%) were revascularized and one patient (0.5%) died before a scheduled PCI. In-hospital mortality in the PCI cohort was 1% ($n = 2$) and 30-day mortality was 3%.

Within 30 days of revascularization, none of the patients randomized to CABG underwent repeat CABG but four patients (2%) underwent PCI. Within 30 days of revascularization, five (2%) of the patients randomized to PCI underwent repeat PCI and nine (4%) underwent CABG.

Long-term outcomes

Table 16.6 presents Kaplan–Meier estimates of 36-month survival, survival free of unstable angina, and survival free of unstable angina or repeat revascularizations for the cohorts which were randomly allocated, physician-directed and chosen by the patients. The CABG–PCI differences and standard errors are also shown.

CABG and PCI survival rates at one, six and 36 months are similar as are the annual survival rates post six months. Figure 16.1 shows the

five-year Kaplan–Meier survival curves for the CABG and PCI cohorts in the randomized trial. The two plots are similar and the global log-rank test is not statistically significant ($p = 0.46$). Figure 16.2 shows the five-year Kaplan–Meier plot of survival for CABG versus PCI for the patients in the physician-directed registry. Figure 16.3 shows the five-year Kaplan–Meier plot of survival for CABG and PCI patients in the patient-choice registry.

DISCUSSION

PCI and CABG are appropriate revascularization options for the relief of medically refractory, high risk, unstable angina

The Angina With Extremely Serious Operative Mortality Evaluation (AWESOME) study was designed to compare long-term survival with PCI versus CABG for patients with medically refractory myocardial ischemia and high risk of adverse outcomes with CABG. The primary result of this trial was comparable CABG and PCI three-year survival for patients randomly allocated, directed by physicians and allowed

Table 16.6 CABG and PCI 36 month survival, survival free of unstable angina (UA) and survival free of unstable angina or repeat revascularizations (with permission from reference 3)

Outcome	CABG (%)	PCI (%)	CABG–PCI difference (%)	Standard error (%)
Survival				
Randomized	79	80	1	5.6
Physician directed	76	76	0	2.8
Patient choice	80	89	−9	5.9
Survival free of unstable angina				
Randomized	65	59	−6	8.4
Physician directed	66	51	15*	5.0
Patient choice	63	64	−1	11
Survival free of unstable angina or repeat revascularization				
Randomized	61	48	13	10
Physician directed	63	46	17	12
Patient choice	60	57	3	5

*, statistically significant difference: $p < 0.01$.

patient choice. The additional finding that PCI survival free of unstable angina was not significantly different from the CABG survival free of unstable angina also supports the primary hypothesis. The finding of more frequent repeat revascularization with a PCI strategy is consistent with all previous CABG versus PCI comparisons and reflects the differences in restenosis and completeness of revascularization which are implicit in the two methods [4–29].

The results from this trial are compatible with the 'salvage angioplasty' experience with medically refractory unstable angina patients who were at a prohibitively high risk for CABG and extends the PCI option to patient groups at high but not prohibitively high risk of adverse outcomes with CABG [1–3, 30]. Furthermore, the survival results from this trial are consistent with other randomized clinical trials, which

also report comparable CABG and PCI survival [17–29]. The general conclusion is that CABG and PCI are both reasonable revascularization options with regard to survival but they differ in other important aspects. The final choice will obviously depend on a patient and physician decision based on the specific situation.

Comparison of AWESOME with BARI (Tables 16.7–16.10)

BARI was designed to compare CABG and PTCA long-term outcome in selected patients with multi-vessel coronary disease. A number of steps were taken in an extraordinary effort to assess as broad a sample of multi-vessel disease patients as possible. These steps included: (1) a registry of patients who refused randomization, (2) a survey of all patients with multi-vessel

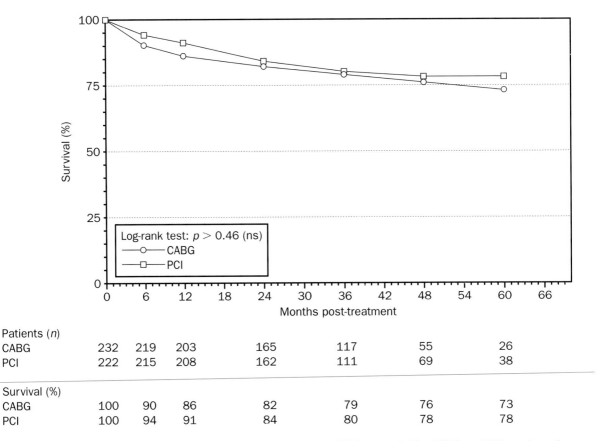

Patients (n)							
CABG	232	219	203	165	117	55	26
PCI	222	215	208	162	111	69	38

Survival (%)							
CABG	100	90	86	82	79	76	73
PCI	100	94	91	84	80	78	78

Figure 16.1 Kaplan–Meier survival plot of CABG (circles) versus PCI (squares). The CABG and PCI number of patients (n) and the percentage surviving for each time period are shown at the bottom of the plot. (With permission from reference 2.)

disease undergoing revascularization at the respective institutions (BARI universe), and (3) a survey of US non-BARI hospitals [24, 25].

AWESOME compared CABG and PCI long-term survival for patients with medically refractory ischemia and high risk of adverse outcomes with CABG. In both cases, planners wished to limit their enquiry to patients with a 'need for revascularization' (BARI terminology) or 'medically refractory ischemia' (AWESOME wording). BARI emphasized 'suitability for revascularization' which in part, emphasized the anatomic limitations of the equipment available for PTCA in 1988–1991. AWESOME, which occurred 4–7 years later (1995–2000) was addi-

tionally focused on patients for whom CABG presented a higher than usual risk of 30-day mortality.

Because multi-vessel disease was a specific inclusion, BARI began screening after the patient's coronary anatomy was known. BARI also excluded from screening, patients with prior CABG or prior PCI. By contrast, AWE-SOME screened prior to coronary angiography for patients with medically refractory myocardial ischemia and one or more risk factors for adverse outcomes with CABG.

With regard to risk factors for adverse outcome with either CABG or PCI, the AWESOME average age of 67 years was six years older than

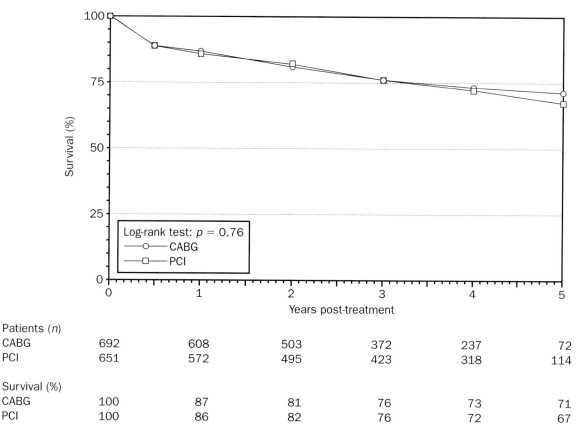

Patients (n)						
CABG	692	608	503	372	237	72
PCI	651	572	495	423	318	114
Survival (%)						
CABG	100	87	81	76	73	71
PCI	100	86	82	76	72	67

Figure 16.2 Kaplan–Meier plot of survival for CABG (circles) versus PCI (squares) for the physician-directed registry patients. The CABG and PCI number of patients (n) and the percentage surviving free of unstable angina for each time period are shown at the bottom of the plot. (With permission from reference 3.)

the average age in BARI [15–22]. The AWE-SOME mean left ventricular ejection fraction (0.45) was 0.12 lower than the mean value for BARI (0.57). Prior CABG (31% of AWESOME patients) and prior PCI (20% of AWESOME) were excluded from BARI. Both AWESOME and BARI enrolled recent myocardial infarction patients, but BARI excluded acute myocardial infarction patients if they were felt to need emergency revascularization.

With regard to processes of medical care, of the patients coming to diagnostic angiography prior to enrollment in the AWESOME randomized trial, 86% were receiving aspirin, 62% were receiving heparin, 90% were receiving nitrates, 75% were receiving beta-blockers, and 31% were receiving calcium-channel blockers. This is in contrast to aspirin use (45%), heparin use (31%), beta-blocker use (50%), and calcium-channel blocker use (76%) in BARI [18, 21, 22].

With regard to surgical processes of care, 70% of AWESOME surgical patients received left internal mammary grafts, 3.3% received right internal mammary grafts, 2.8% received radial artery grafts. In contrast, 84% of BARI patients received internal mammary grafts [18, 21].

With regard to percutaneous interventional

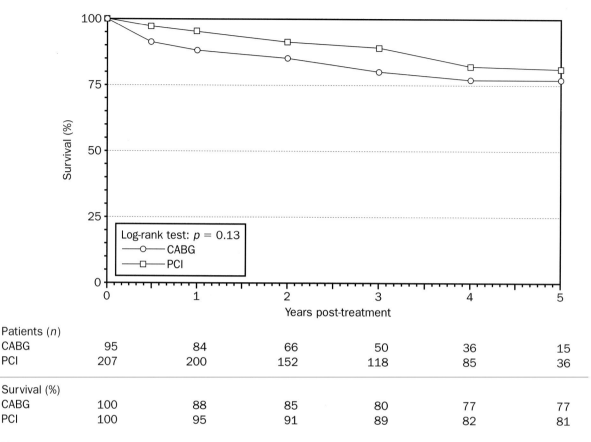

Patients (n)						
CABG	95	84	66	50	36	15
PCI	207	200	152	118	85	36

Survival (%)						
CABG	100	88	85	80	77	77
PCI	100	95	91	89	82	81

Figure 16.3 Kaplan–Meier plot of survival for CABG (circles) versus PCI (squares) for the patient-choice registry patients. The CABG and PCI number of patients (n) and the percentage surviving free of unstable angina or repeat revascularizations for each time period are shown at the bottom of the plot. (With permission from reference 3.)

processes of care, the average stent use over the five year AWESOME study was 54% with an increase from 26% in 1995 to 88% in 1999/2000. Overall, 11% of AWESOME PCI patients received glycoprotein IIb/IIIa receptor blocking agents with an increase from 1% in 1995 to 52% in 1999/2000. Neither stents nor glycoprotein IIb/IIIa receptor blocking agents were available when BARI was conducted [18, 21].

BARI did not find an overall difference in survival or freedom from infarction between the CABG and PCI groups up to five years. After five years the survival curves diverge with CABG having higher average survival but the divergence is driven entirely by a relative survival advantage for CABG among treated diabetic patients (see chapters in this text on BARI by Bourrasa and Fye, and diabetes by Sedlis and Lorin). CABG did not have any survival advantage among the non-treated diabetic patients.

Another important point emphasized in the chapter on BARI in this text, is that in order to compare myocardial infarction, as an unbiased outcome, between CABG and PTCA, the BARI trialists specified uniform ECG and enzyme sampling and had core laboratories to avoid measurement error for those parameters.

Table 16.7 Comparison of AWESOME with selected trials of CABG versus PTCA or PCI

Trial	Age (years)	LVEF (mean)	Prior MI (%)	Diabetes (%)	Hypertension (%)
AWESOME	67	0.45	71	33	70
ARTS	61	0.60	43	18	45
BARI	61	0.57	55	25	49
CABRI	60	0.63	42	12	36
EAST	62	0.61	41	23	53
ERACI I	57	0.61	50	—	—
ERACI II	62	—	28	17	71
GABI	59	0.56	47	13	41
RITA	57	—	42	—	—

Table 16.8 Comparison of AWESOME with selected trials of CABG versus PTCA or PCI

Trial	Single-vessel (%)	Two-vessel (%)	Three-vessel (%)
AWESOME	18	41	41
ARTS	2	68	30
BARI	0	59	41
CABRI	2	57	41
EAST	0	60	40
ERACI I	0	55	45
ERACI II	5	39	56
GABI	0	82	18
RITA I	45	43	12

Table 16.9 Stents, glycoprotein IIb/IIIa and medial therapy among randomized patients in RCTs comparing CABG and PCI

Trial	Aspirin (%)	Heparin (%)	Beta-blockers (%)	Calcium (%)	GP IIb/IIIa (%)	Stents (%)
AWESOME	94	84	79	33	11	54
BARI	45	31	50	76	0	0
CABRI	96	12	63	66	0	0
EAST	49	32	35	76	0	0
ERACI II	—	—	—	—	28	100
RITA	72	—	75	72	0	0

Table 16.10 Risk subsets included in CABG versus PCI RCT			
Risk subsets	**RCT**		
Prior CABG	AWESOME		
MI ongoing or < 24 hours	AWESOME	ERACI II	
MI < seven days	AWESOME	ERACI II	EAST
Emergency revascularization (including IABP)	AWESOME		
Stent use in RCT	AWESOME	ERACI II	ARTS SOS
Glycoprotein IIb/IIIa	AWESOME	ERACI II	

Comparison of AWESOME with EAST

The stated aim of EAST was 'to determine if the strategy of beginning with PTCA in patients with multi-vessel disease requiring revascularization is as safe and effective as starting with coronary bypass surgery'. Accordingly and as in BARI, screening began with patients who had had coronary angiography demonstrating multi-vessel coronary artery disease (CAD). Angiographic exclusions included a number of features felt to put the patient at higher risk of a technically unsuccessful PTCA. The clinical criteria used to assure that revascularization was warranted appear to be comparable to the AWESOME definition of medically refractory. As in BARI, a number of the EAST exclusions overlap with the risk factor *inclusions* of AWESOME; specifically, prior CABG; LVEF < 0.25; MI within five days.

Like BARI, the medical processes of care were very different between EAST and AWESOME, in part reflecting the differences made by approximately five years of clinical trials. In EAST, aspirin use was 49%, heparin use was 32%, beta-blocker use was 34%, and calcium-channel blocker use was 76% [18, 21, 22]. EAST patients treated surgically received internal mammary grafts in 86% of cases [18, 21]. Neither stents nor glycoprotein IIb/IIIa receptor blocking agents were used in EAST [18, 21].

EAST found no significant difference between patients randomized to CABG versus PCI in their three-year composite end-point of death, Q wave myocardial infarction, and a large ischemic defect on thallium scanning.

Comparison of AWESOME with CABRI, ERACI I, GABI, RITA

CABRI was a large (1054 patients) multi-national (26 European centers) randomized comparison of PTCA versus CABG in multi-vessel patients. CABRI specifically set out to include a broader range of multi-vessel disease patients by permitting incomplete revascularization and by not excluding patients based on the presence of occluded vessels. Given these criteria, it is not surprising that in terms of freedom from angina and freedom from subsequent revascularization, CABRI demonstrated an advantage for CABG. As in all the previous trials, the survival and myocardial infarction rates were not different between CABG and PTCA.

GABI was a German study, which randomized 359 patients between CABG and PCI, at about the same time as EAST. In addition, patients with prior CABG; with MI within four weeks, with total occlusions and patients who were felt to have lesions which would jeopardize > 50% of their myocardium were all excluded. At one year, patients in the two groups had comparable survival and relief of angina, but the PTCA cohort required more drugs and repeat revascularizations to achieve a comparable symptomatic outcome.

ERACI I was a trial of 127 patients conducted in Argentina and one-year outcomes were reported in 1993. Again as in all other trials, CABG and PCI survival and freedom from myocardial infarction were comparable.

RITA was a large (1011 patients randomized between CABG and PCI) trial from the UK in the 'pre-stent era' (1993 report of 2.5 years). RITA included patients with one-vessel coronary disease (45%) and only 12% of its randomly allocated cohort had three-vessel disease. Patients displayed a broad spectrum of myocardial ischemia ranging from no symptoms in 7% to rest angina in 59%. Medical treatment, in terms of proportions of patients on aspirin, beta-blockers, calcium blockers, and nitrates, and multiple drugs, were comparable to AWESOME. Again as in all other trials, RITA found no differences in CABG and PCI survival or definite infarction, but repeat revascularization was greater with PTCA.

Comparison of AWESOME with ERACI II

ERACI II is an Argentine study which randomized 450 patients between CABG and PCI, including the Gianturco-Roubin II stent and adjunctive abciximab. The objective was to compare CABG with 'current PCI' in multivessel disease patients. Patients with prior CABG, MI within 24 hours, and LVEF < 0.35 were excluded. On the other hand, this study included a very high proportion of patients with unstable angina, and patients with considerably greater anatomic complexity, including unprotected left main stenoses, than nearly any CABG versus PCI trial.

ERACI II, like AWESOME, included the use of stents and glycoprotein IIb/IIIa receptor blocking agents and focused on patients with unstable syndromes. It differed from AWESOME in extending the risk application specifically to unprotected left main and single

chronic total occlusion patients. The ERACI II trial reported a PCI survival advantage relative to CABG out to one year.

Comparison of AWESOME with ARTS

ARTS is a recently reported randomized trial of 1205 patients from The Netherlands. Modern stents were used but adjunctive glycoprotein IIb/IIIa receptor blocking agents were not used. Patients with multi-vessel disease were randomized between CABG and PCI. It did not extend the comparison into the risk groups targeted by AWESOME. Mean age was 61 years and mean LVEF was 0.61. Exclusions included prior CABG, LVEF < 0.30, MI within one week, and major co-morbidity. ARTS demonstrated comparable CABG and PCI one-year survival and freedom from myocardial infarction. ARTS reported a narrowing of the repeat revascularization differential between CABG and PCI and it demonstrated cost savings with PCI.

WHAT DID AWESOME TEACH US THAT WE DID NOT ALREADY KNOW?

First, AWESOME supports the application of either PCI or CABG for high-risk categories of patients that had not previously been subject to random allocation namely: (1) post CABG; (2) within 24 hours of acute myocardial infarction; (3) with LVEF < 0.35 and (4) patients requiring emergency revascularization. This conclusion is consistent with all other RCT comparing CABG and PCI survival, and extends the result to important high-risk groups.

These data are important because throughout the US and the world, surgeons and interventionists are taking on higher-risk patients, and reporting reduced rates of short-term mortality.

Second, the attempt to define medically refractory has further refined the clinical definition of syndromes which merit revascularization. It has also likely resulted in better medication strategies for the high-risk patients. More aggressive medical therapy contributed to the low in-hospital mortality rates (1% with PCI; 4% with CABG) for the oldest cohort, with the lowest LVEF, and highest rates of diabetes, hypertension, and prior MI randomly allocated between CABG and PCI. Interestingly, this approach of aggressive medical therapy with revascularization is being specifically considered in the ongoing COURAGE trial (see Chapter 9).

Finally, as has been the case with both CASS and BARI, it is likely that the AWESOME registry will also contribute to the knowledge base of revascularization for high-risk patients. The 1977 prospectively gathered cohort includes patients who could not be randomly allocated either because of physician-direction or patient-choice. Factors which patients and physicians used to choose between CABG and PCI in high-risk patients with refractory ischemia may be identified from further study of this registry experience.

REFERENCES

1. Morrison DA, Sethi G, Sacks J et al. A multi-center, randomized trial of percutaneous coronary intervention versus bypass surgery in high-risk unstable angina patients, *Controlled Clinical Trials* 1999; **20**:601–619.

2. Morrison DA, Sethi G, Sacks J et al for the investigators of the Angina With Extremely Serious Operative Mortality Evaluation (AWESOME). Percutaneous coronary intervention versus coronary artery bypass graft surgery for patients with medically refractory myocardial ischemia and risk factors for adverse outcome with bypass, *J Am Coll Cardiol* 2001; **38**:143–149.

3. Morrison DA, Sethi G, Sacks J et al for the AWESOME Investigators. Percutaneous coronary interventions versus coronary bypass graft surgery for patients with medically refractory myocardial ischemia and risk factors for adverse outcomes with bypass. The VA AWESOME multicenter registry: comparison with the randomized clinical trial, *J Am Coll Cardiol* 2002; **39**:266–273.

4. Kirklin JW, Akins CW, Blackstone EH et al. ACC/AHA Task Force Report. Guidelines and indications for coronary artery bypass graft surgery, *J Am Coll Cardiol* 1991; **17**:543–589.

5. Luchi RJ, Scott SM, Deupree RH and the Principal Investigators and their Associates of Veterans Administration Cooperative Study No 28. Comparison of medical and surgical treatment for unstable angina pectoris, *N Engl J Med* 1987; **316**:977–984.

6. Scott SM, Luchi RJ, Deupree RH and the Veterans Administration Unstable Angina Cooperative Study Group. Veterans Administration Cooperative Study for treatment of patients with unstable angina, *Circulation* 1988; **78**: (Suppl I):I113–I121.

7. Parisi AF, Khuri S, Deupree RH et al. Medical compared with surgical management of unstable angina five year mortality and morbidity in the Veterans Administration Study, *Circulation* 1989; **80**: 1176–1189.

8. Russell RO, Moraski RE, Kouchoukos N et al. Unstable angina pectoris: National Cooperative Study Group to compare medical and surgical therapy I. Report of protocol and patient population, *Am J Cardiol* 1976; **37**:896–902.

9. Russell RO, Moraski RE, Kouchoukos N et al. Unstable angina pectoris: National Cooperative Study Group to compare surgical and medical therapy II. In-hospital experience and initial follow-up results in patients with one-, two-, and three-vessel disease, *Am J Cardiol* 1978; **42**: 839–848.

10. Russell RO, Moraski RE, Kouchoukos N et al. Unstable angina pectoris: National Cooperative Study Group to compare surgical and medical therapy III. Results in patients with ST-segment elevation during pain, *Am J Cardiol* 1980; **45**: 819–824.

11. The Veterans Administration Coronary Artery Bypass Surgery Cooperative Study Group. Eleven year survival in the Veterans Administrations randomized trial of coronary bypass surgery for stable angina, *N Engl J Med* 1984; **319**:332–337.

12. Varnauskas E and the European Coronary Study Group. Twelve year follow-up of survival in the randomized European Coronary Surgery study, *N Engl J Med* 1988; **319**:332–337.

13. Coronary Artery Surgery Study (CASS) principal investigators and associates. CASS: a randomized trial of coronary bypass surgery, *Circulation* 1983; **68**:939–950.

14. Parisi AF, Folland ED, Hartigan P on behalf of the Veterans Affairs ACME Investigators. A comparison of angioplasty with medical therapy in the treatment of single-vessel coronary artery disease, *N Engl J Med* 1992; **326**:10–16.

15. RITA-2 trial participants. Coronary angioplasty versus medical therapy for angina: the second Randomized Intervention Treatment of Angina (RITA-2) trial, *Lancet* 1997; **350**:461–468.

16. Ryan TJ, Klocke FJ, Reynolds WA and the ACP/ACC/AHA task force on clinical privileges in cardiology. Clinical competence in percutaneous transluminal coronary angioplasty, *JACC* 1990; **15**:1469–1474.

17. Ryan TJ, Bauman WB, Kennedy JW et al. Guidelines for percutaneous transluminal coronary angioplasty: a report of the American College of Cardiology/American Heart Association task force on assessment of diagnostic and therapeutic cardiovascular procedures (committee on percutaneous transluminal coronary angioplasty), *JACC* 1993; **22**(7):2033–2054.

18. Lembo NJ, King SB III. Randomized trials of percutaneous transluminal coronary angioplasty, coronary artery bypass grafting surgery, or medical therapy in patients with coronary artery disease, *Cor Art Dis* 1990; **1**:449–454.

19. RITA trial participants. Coronary angioplasty versus coronary artery bypass surgery: the Randomized Intervention Treatment of Angina (RITA) trial, *Lancet* 1993; **341**:573–580.

20. CABRI trial participants. First year results of CABRI (Coronary Angioplasty vs Bypass Revascularization Investigation), *Lancet* 1995; **346**:1179–1184.

21. King SB, Lembo NJ, Kosinski AS et al. A randomized trial comparing coronary angioplasty with coronary bypass surgery, *N Engl J Med* 1994; **331**:1044–1050.

22. Hamm CW, Riemers J, Ischinger T et al. A randomized study of coronary angioplasty compared with bypass surgery in patients with symptomatic multi-vessel coronary disease, *N Engl J Med* 1994; **331**:1037–1043.

23. Rodriguez A, Boullon F, Perez-Balino N et al. Argentine randomized trial of percutaneous transluminal coronary angioplasty versus coronary artery bypass surgery in multi-vessel disease (ERACI): in-hospital results and one year follow-up, *J Am Coll Cardiol* 1993; **22**:1060–1067.

24. BARI Investigators. Protocol for the Bypass Angioplasty Revascularization Investigation, *Circulation* 1991; **84** (Suppl V):1–27.

25. Frye RL, King SB III, Sopko G, Detre KM. A symposium: multi-vessel PTCA versus CABG. Baseline data from the Bypass Angioplasty Revascularization Investigation (BARI) and the Emory Angioplasty Surgery Trial (EAST), *Am J Cardiol* 1995; **75**:1C–59C.

26. Pocock SJ, Henderson RA, Rickards AF et al. Meta-analysis of randomized trials comparing coronary angioplasty with bypass surgery, *Lancet* 1995; **346**:1184–1189.

27. Sim I, Gupta M, McDonald K, Bourassa M, Hlatky MA. A meta-analysis of randomized trials comparing coronary artery bypass grafting with percutaneous transluminal coronary angioplasty in multi-vessel coronary artery disease, *Am J Cardiol* 1995; **76**:1025–1029.

28. Rodriguez A, Bernardi V, Navia J et al for the ERACI II Investigators. Argentine randomized study: coronary angioplasty with stenting versus coronary bypass surgery in patients with multiple-vessel disease (ERACI II), 30-day and one-year follow-up results, *J Am Coll Cardiol* 2001; **37**: 51–58.

29. Serruys PW, Unger F, Sousa JE et al for the Arterial Revascularization Therapies Study Group. Comparison of coronary artery bypass surgery and stenting for the treatment of multi-vessel disease, *N Engl J Med* 2001; **344**:1117–1124.

30. Morrison DA, Barbiere CC, Johnson R et al. Salvage angioplasty for unstable angina? *Cath and CV Diag* 1992; **27**:169–178.

31. Grover FL, Hammermeister KE, Burchfeil C and the cardiac surgeons of the Department of Veterans Affairs. Initial report of the Veterans Administration preoperative risk assessment study for cardiac surgery, *Ann Thorac Surg* 1990; **50**:12–28.

32. Grover FL, Johnson RR, Marshall G, Hammermeister KE and the Department of Veterans Affairs Cardiac Surgeons. Factors predictive of operative mortality among coronary artery bypass subsets, *Ann Thorac Surg* 1993; **56**:1296–1307.

33. Morrison DA, Sacks J, Barbiere CC, Sethi G. Editorial: PTCA comes to the bifurcations in the road. What the VA has to offer, *J Am Coll Cardiol* 1997; **29**:1512–1514.

34. Ohman R. Interactive database management (IDM). *Computer Methods in Biomedicine* 1995; **47**:221–227.

17

Randomized comparison of coronary artery bypass surgery and stenting for the treatment of multi-vessel disease

Patrick W Serruys and Felix Unger

INTRODUCTION

While the latest worldwide survey of coronary revascularization showed 583,000 coronary artery bypass surgeries performed in 1995 [1], European statistics estimate the annual need for balloon angioplasties to be 739 per million inhabitants [2]. Approximately 60% of these patients have multi-vessel disease and may be treated either by bypass surgery or balloon angioplasty [3]. Despite the publication of a number of trials [4–10], the question of the most appropriate treatment is still subject to debate. These trials suggest that the results are similar in terms of survival and myocardial infarctions but that patients who undergo bypass surgery need fewer re-interventions. However, when interpreting the results from these past trials, it is important to realize that improvements in both percutaneous and surgical techniques have occurred which call into question the current validity of these earlier conclusions. This may be especially true for angioplasty since several studies have shown that coronary stenting leads to better results than balloon angioplasty [11–15], particularly with respect to the need for repeat revascularization. Therefore, while surgery may still be seen as the most appropriate technique for multi-vessel disease when compared to conventional balloon angioplasty, that may not be true when stent placement — the current standard practice [16, 17] — is added to the angioplasty procedure.

A second reason to reconsider the comparison between surgery and percutaneous techniques is the rising cost of health care. While stenting may still be expected to be less effective than surgery in terms of the need for repeat revascularization, stenting may lead to cost savings [18–21]. In an era in which new treatments are increasingly assessed in terms of the balance between additional costs and additional effects [22–27], one might question whether the additional effects of bypass surgery are still worth the additional cost compared to stenting. Therefore Arterial Revascularization Therapies Study (ARTS) was designed to compare not only clinical outcomes but also the cost and cost-effectiveness of bypass surgery versus stenting. As such, ARTS combines end-points which are of great relevance to health care administrators as well as physicians treating individuals with coronary artery disease not responding to medical therapy.

METHODS

Study design

Arterial Revascularization Therapies Study (ARTS) is a randomized trial based on a consensus of the surgeon and the interventional cardiologist as to equivalent 'treatability' of the patient by either technique, with analysis of clinical effectiveness, costs, cost-effectiveness and quality of life at short (30 days), medium (one year), and long-term (three and five years). Detailed description of the protocol has been reported elsewhere [28].

Selection of patients

Patients with angina or ischemia but no prior bypass surgery or angioplasty were selected after agreement between surgeons and cardiologists, randomized after written informed consent via a central telephone service and treated by either surgery or stented angioplasty. These patients had stable (Canadian Cardiovascular Society I, II, III or IV) [29] or unstable (Braunwald class IB, IC, IIB, IIC, IIIB, IIIC) [30] angina pectoris or silent ischemia and were eligible for coronary revascularization if they had at least two de novo lesions (located in different vessels and in different territories) potentially amenable to stent implantation, but without left main stem stenosis.

One totally occluded major epicardial vessel or side branch could be included and targeted as long as one other major vessel had a significant stenosis amenable to stented angioplasty, provided that the age of the occlusion was believed to be less than one month old (based on the clinical history). Conventional balloon angioplasty without stent implantation was permitted as complementary treatment of vessels smaller than 2.75 mm provided that at least two of the other targeted lesions were amenable to stenting and were intended to be stented. The number of stents to be implanted per patient was not restricted but needed to exceed

one. The indication for stenting in lesions at a bifurcation, with a fresh thrombus, calcification, very long obstruction (> 20 mm), complex anatomy or stenting of side branches was left to the operator's own discretion. Left ventricular ejection fraction needed to be at least 30% and overt congestive heart failure was excluded. Patients with a history of prior cerebrovascular accident, transmural myocardial infarction within the previous week, severe hepatic or renal disease, diseased saphenous veins or patients who needed concomitant major surgery (e.g. valve surgery or resection of aortic or left ventricular aneurysm, carotid endarterectomy, abdominal aortic aneurysm surgery, etc.), were also excluded. Finally, patients with intolerance or contraindication to acetyl salicylic acid or ticlopidine, and those with neutropenia or thrombocytopenia were also excluded.

General management consideration and operator certification

Surgery and cardiac interventions were performed together at 67 sites. The institution involved in the ARTS trial, had to perform at least 400 coronary cases per year, in which the mammary artery was used in 80% of the cases [31]. As standard procedure the internal mammary artery had to be used for revascularization of the left anterior descending coronary artery and/or the diagonal branches during extra corporeal circulation. The use of other arterial conduit material was discouraged. The remaining vessels could be bypassed by use of the greater saphenous vein in whatever configuration the surgeon deemed appropriate. Anesthetic techniques as well as the type of cardioplegic solution were not standardized.

A minimum of 500 angioplasty cases per center and a minimum of 100 procedures per year per operator were required to qualify as an ARTS participant.

Concomitant risk factor modification was an important aspect of treatment for all ARTS patients. All smokers were counseled in and assisted with smoking cessation. Patients with hypertension were required to have their blood pressure lowered to less than 140/90 mmHg. Diabetic patients had to be treated with diet, exercise, oral agents and insulin, as clinically indicated. According to the most recent European guidelines [32], pharmacological treatment was instituted for patients with total cholesterol above 5.5 mmol/l.

Endpoints

The objective of the present study was to compare coronary stent implantation employing the Cordis Palmaz-Schatz™ Crown and/or the Crossflex™ stent to bypass surgery, in patients with multi-vessel disease.

The primary end-point was defined as the absence of any of the following major adverse cardiac and cerebrovascular events within 12 months after randomization: death; cerebrovascular event; documented non-fatal myocardial infarction; revascularization by percutaneous intervention or bypass surgery. In the primary comparison of the two treatment strategies, all deaths (cardiac and non-cardiac) were reported. Cerebrovascular events were classified into three major categories: stroke, transient ischemic attacks and reversible ischemic neurologic deficits [28].

After randomization, all myocardial infarctions were counted as events, whether they occurred spontaneously or in association with angioplasty or coronary bypass graft surgery procedures. The Minnesota code for pathological Q waves was used [33]. The serum levels of creatine kinase and creatine kinase MB were sampled at six, 12 and 18 hours post-intervention and their ratios were calculated. Within the first seven days post-intervention, a definite diagnosis of myocardial infarction was made if new Q waves were documented together with one sampled ratio of creatine kinase MB/total cardiac enzyme greater than 0.1 or one plasma level of creatine kinase MB being five times the upper limit of normal. After seven days, either Q wave or enzymatic elevation were sufficient as criteria for myocardial infarction. This specific definition of myocardial infarction was agreed upon to cope with the difficulty in determining a myocardial infarction following surgery [34, 35]. Myocardial infarctions were confirmed only after the relevant ECGs were analyzed by the electrocardiographic core laboratory and adjudicated by a clinical event committee. Every subsequent revascularization procedure was recorded, including the reasons why that procedure was performed.

Secondary objectives of the study were to compare both strategies at one year with respect to: anginal status, medication use, costs, cost-effectiveness, quality of life; the combined end-point death, myocardial infarction and stroke; and the itemized outcomes death, myocardial infarction, stroke or revascularization procedure. Events were counted from the time of the randomization, whereas the clinical status was assessed at predetermined times of one month, six months and 12 months after the procedure.

Costs, effectiveness and cost-effectiveness

Costs were limited to the direct medical costs per patient, assessed from a societal perspective. Costs per patient were calculated as the product of each patient's use of resources and the corresponding unit costs. Data on the use of resources comprised a selection of so called 'big-ticket' items: hospital days, postoperative intensive care, coronary care, non-intensive/non-coronary care, diagnostic and therapeutic procedures (e.g. outpatient visits; angiography, intra-aortic balloon pumping; rehabilitation, etc.). Additionally, data were collected concerning medication and the items (balloons, wires, catheters, stents) that were used during the revascularizations as well as data about the duration of the various procedures. All data were collected on the case report form, but patients were also given a 'passport' so that the corresponding information could be recorded if they were treated at other hospitals. Unit costs were estimated (before analysis of the data) on the basis of detailed information from the Dijkzigt hospital, Rotterdam, The Netherlands, as reported earlier [15, 20]. The costs per procedure, excluding the costs of those items that were specifically recorded, were estimated as the product of (1) the duration of the procedure in minutes and (2) an estimate of the costs per procedure-minute.

For purposes of calculating cost-effectiveness, effectiveness was expressed in terms of the primary end-point, event-free survival. Additionally, differences in effectiveness were assessed by means of the EuroQol questionnaire [36]. Within this questionnaire, patients grade their health status on a thermometer using values between 0 (worst possible health state) and 100 (best possible health state) (the EuroQol Thermometer). Additionally, patients score themselves on five dimensions (mobility, self-care, usual activity, pain/discomfort and anxiety/depression) each with three modalities, grading from 'no problems' to 'severe problems'. The patients' scores on the five dimensions were summarized by the A-1 tariff as estimated by Dolan et al [36] (the EuroQol summary). The balance between costs and effects was expressed in terms of the incremental cost-effectiveness ratio by calculating the additional costs per additional event-free survivor after one year.

Statistical analysis

At the outset of the study, the size of the required sample (2×600 patients) was determined based on the hypothesis that the difference in major adverse cardiac and cerebrovascular events (event-free) at one year would not be less than seven percentage points in favor of bypass surgery. Assuming a two-sided type I error level (α) of 0.05, a power of 92% is achieved with the current sample size. Expectations about costs and cost-effectiveness

have been reported previously [28].

Continuous variables were expressed as means ± SD and were compared using the unpaired Student's t-test. The Fisher's exact test was used for categorical variables. The Wilcoxon scores were used for categorical variables with an ordinal scale. Discrete variables were expressed as counts and percentages and were compared in terms of relative risks (for surgery as compared to stenting) with 95% confidence intervals calculated by the formula of Greenland and Robins [37]. All statistical tests were two-tailed.

Event-free survival was estimated according to the Kaplan–Meier method and the differences were assessed using the log-rank test. A multivariate logistic regression model was built using baseline clinical and angiographic characteristics as well as procedure-related variables to identify independent risk factors for the primary endpoint (one-year event-free) of the ARTS trial. The method of revascularization (stent or surgery) was also entered into the model as a variable.

Incremental cost-effectiveness ratios were expressed with 95% confidence intervals using Fiellers approximation [38]. Incremental cost-effectiveness ratios were also expressed using confidence ellipses.

RESULTS

Patient characteristics and study flowchart

Between April 1997 and June 1998, 1205 patients were randomly assigned to stent implantation (600 patients) or bypass surgery (605 patients) at 67 participating centers. Table 17.1 presents the baseline demographic and angiographic characteristics. As indicated in Table 17.2, five patients did not undergo coronary revascularization and remained on pharmacological treatment. The average time elapsed between randomization and treatment was 27 ± 39 days (range 0–362 days) for the surgical patients and 11 ± 16 days (range 0–173 days)

Table 17.1 Baseline characteristics of the 1205 patients included in the intention-to-treat-analysis

	Stented angioplasty (n = 600)	Coronary arterybypass grafting (n = 605)
Male gender	77%	76%
Age, years (range)	61 ± 10 (30–83)	61 ± 9 (32–82)
Body mass index	27.2 ± 3.7	27.4 ± 3.7
Previous conditions		
Q-wave myocardial infarction	26%	24%
Non Q-wave myocardial infarction	18%	18%
Angioplasty*	2%	2%
Diabetes mellitus	19%	16%
Insulin dependent	4%	3%
Transcient ischemic attack[†]	1%	1%
Hypertension	45%	45%
Hypercholesterolemia	58%	58%
Carotid surgery[†]	1%	1%
Family history	39%	42%
Peripheral vascular disease	6%	5%
Chronic obstructive pulmonary disease	5%	5%
Smoking history		
Never smoked	28%	28%
Previous smoker	44%	47%
Current smoker	28%	26%
Stable angina	57%	60%
CCS classification[‡]		
1	5%	5%
2	26%	28%
3	23%	24%
4	4%	3%
Unstable angina	37%	35%
Braunwald classification[§]		
IB	6%	6%
IIB	13%	13%
IIIB	8%	7%
IC	3%	1%
IIC	6%	6%
IIIC	1%	2%
Silent ischemia	6%	5%
Ejection fraction (%)	61 ± 12%	60 ± 13%
Segments DS > 50%	2.8 ± 1.1	2.8 ± 1.1
Number of vessels diseased		
One	1.5%	0.3%
Two	68.1%	66.6%
Three	30.4%	33.1%
Vessel territory[¶]		
Right coronary artery	71.2%	72.4%
Left anterior descending artery	89.9%	90.5%
Left circumflex artery	71.2%	72.4%
Left main stem artery[†]	0.2%	0.2%
Lesion type[¶]		
A	7%	7%
B1	30%	31%
B2	55%	55%
C	8%	8%
Bifurcation or sidebranch involved[¶]	34%	31%
Total occlusion[¶]	3%	5%

*Protocol amendment: PTCA procedure of the target vessel in past history or PTCA procedure of the non-target vessel in the past year. [†]Protocol violation. [‡]CCS: according to the classification system of the Canadian Cardiovascular Society [29]. [§]According to reference [30]. [¶]Assessed by an independent angiographic core laboratory.

Table 17.2 Study flowchart

	Stented angioplasty (n = 600)	Coronary artery bypass grafting (n = 605)
Patients randomized	600	605
Medical treatment only	1	4
Death on waiting list	0	3
Cross-over from stent to CABG*	6	–
Cross-over from CABG to stent†	–	19
Treated according to randomization	593 (98.8%)	579 (95.9%)
Average time on waiting list	11 ± 16 days (0–173)	27 ± 39 days (0–362)

* Three patients withdrew consent, two patients had significant left main disease, and in one patient inappropriate patient selection occurred. † Eight patients withdrew consent, in eight patients the inclusion criteria were not met, in one patient there was a miscommunication between the investigator and the study co-ordinator about the randomization, one patient developed a Q wave myocardial infarction on the waiting list and one patient developed unstable angina on the waiting list and was treated by stented angioplasty.

for the percutaneous group. Three patients assigned to surgery died on the waiting list. Six patients allocated to the stent arm crossed over to the surgical treatment whereas 19 surgical candidates were treated with stent implantation. During the initial hospital stay, 14 patients initially assigned to stenting underwent surgical revascularization, three urgently and 11 electively, following complicated or unsatisfactory percutaneous treatment. Similarly two surgical patients underwent angioplasty during their hospital stay. Ninety-nine percent of the patients in the stent group and 96% in the surgical group were treated according to their assigned treatment.

Assessment of revascularization and post-procedural enzyme release

In the stent group 2.8 ± 1.1 stenotic lesions (diameter stenosis greater than 50%) were detected on the diagnostic angiogram and 2.7 ± 1.1 lesions were actually stented (89%) or treated with balloon angioplasty alone (11%). In the surgical group 2.8 ± 1.1 lesions were present and 2.7 ± 1.1 anastomoses were performed using 2.5 ± 0.7 conduits. At least one arterial conduit was used in 93% of the patients; the left anterior descending artery was revascularized with an arterial conduit in 95%. In the stent group the average length of stents implanted per patient was 47.5 mm ± 21.8 mm with 27% of single stents being longer than 15 mm. The duration of the surgical procedure was 248 ± 76 minutes whereas the percutaneous procedure lasted for 93 ± 51 minutes. In the first 24 hours following the intervention, an abnormal level of creatine kinase MB iso-enzyme was measured in 61% of the surgical patients and in 31% of the stented patients. A plasma level of creatine kinase iso-enzyme more than five times the upper limit of normal was measured in 12.6% of the surgical patients and in 6.2% of the stented patients (Fig. 17.1).

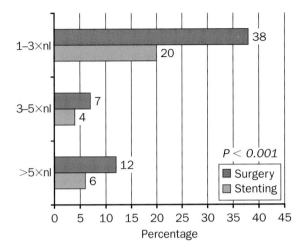

Figure 17.1 Frequency of elevation of creatine kinase MB after bypass surgery and stenting, according to the pre-stratified categories of creatine kinase MB levels: 1–3 times normal (1–3×nl), 3–5 times normal (3–5×nl) and more than 5 times normal (>5×nl).

Clinical outcome at 12 months

Events per patient and ranking of clinical events at 12 months follow-up are shown in Table 17.3. The primary clinical end-point (major adverse cardiac and cerebrovascular events) was reached by 158 (26.3%) of the 600 patients assigned to stented angioplasty compared with 74 (12.2%) of the 605 patients assigned to bypass surgery (relative risk 0.39 [95% confidence interval 0.29, 0.53]). Freedom from death, stroke and myocardial infarction was similar in both groups (91.2% versus 90.5%, relative risk 0.92 [95% confidence interval 0.62, 1.35]). In fact, the difference in clinical outcomes between the study groups at 12 months is entirely due to the need for more repeat revascularizations in the stented patients.

In patients free of death, stroke and myocardial infarction the need for additional revascularization after percutaneous treatment was 13 percentage points higher than after surgery. This difference in clinical outcome is shown in

the Kaplan–Meier estimates of event-free survival for both treated groups as well as for the freedom from death, stroke and myocardial infarction (Fig. 17.2). The improved one-year outcome in the surgical group is also partially reflected in the difference in anginal status and anti-anginal medication use between the two groups (Table 17.4). At the 12-month follow-up, 89% of the surgical patients were asymptomatic as compared to 79% of the stented patients. Independent risk factors for late clinical outcome in the total ARTS population and in each treatment group are displayed in Table 17.5.

Quality of life

Table 17.4 presents an indication of the differences in quality of life. Although more patients were free of angina after surgery throughout the 12-month period, the EuroQol instrument, encompassing more than just chest pain, shows a significantly better quality of life in favor of stenting after one month, no difference after six months and a one point difference in favor of surgery after 12 months.

Costs and cost-effectiveness

Table 17.6 presents the difference in costs. The initial costs were significantly higher in the patients assigned to bypass surgery versus stented angioplasty (EUR 10,653 versus EUR 6441). The difference in the costs of the initial procedure was mainly related to the cost of the procedural time and the cost associated with the length of hospitalization. However, part of the initial difference in costs (EUR 4212) was lost due to more repeat revascularizations at follow-up in the stent group. At one year the net difference in favor of the percutaneous treatment was EUR 2973. It is estimated that the additional cost per additional event-free survivor at one year would have been EUR 21,329, if a policy of elective bypass surgery had been applied to every patient enrolled in this trial.

Table 17.3 Frequency of primary clinical endpoints at one year (365 days) in descending order of severity and total number of events

	Ranking*		Patients with events†		p value
	SA (n=600)	CABG (n=605)	SA (n=600)	CABG (n=605)	
Death	15 (2.5%)	17 (2.8%)	15 (2.5%)	17 (2.8%)	0.858
Cerebrovascular accident	9 (1.5%)	12 (2.0%)	10 (1.7%)	13 (2.1%)	0.675
Myocardial infarction	32 (5.3%)	24 (4.0%)	37 (6.2%)	29 (4.8%)	0.313
Q wave MI	28 (4.7%)	22 (3.6%)	32 (5.3%)	26 (4.3%)	0.422
Non-Q wave MI	4 (0.7%)	2 (0.3%)	5 (0.8%)	3 (0.5%)	0.505
Any repeat revascularization	101 (16.9%)	21 (3.5%)	126 (21%)	23 (3.8%)	
CABG	28 (4.7%)	3 (0.5%)	40 (6.7%)	4 (0.7%)	<0.001
PTCA	73 (12.2%)	18 (3.0%)	94 (15.7%)	20 (3.3%)	<0.001
Event free†	443 (73.8%)	531 (87.8%)	–	–	
Any event§			157 (26.2%)	74 (12.2%)	<0.001

Events on waiting list. In the stented-angioplasty arm one patient developed a myocardial infarction on the waiting list whereas in the CABG arm three patients died on the waiting list, one patient developed a cerebrovascular accident and four patients suffered from myocardial infarction.

SA, stented angioplasty; CABG, coronary artery bypass grafting; PTCA, percutaneous transluminal coronary angioplasty. *Ranking, frequency of primary clinical endpoints in descending order of severity. †Patients with events, if a patient required repeat angioplasty and later coronary-artery bypass grafting, the total count at 365 days would reflect both events, not just the first that occurred). ‡Wilcoxon rank sum test (p value = 0.0001) §Relative risk: 2.14 (95% confidence interval: 1.66–2.75).

Figure 17.3 indicates both costs and effects in a two-dimensional plane together with the estimated uncertainties.

DISCUSSION

The ARTS trial shows no significant difference in terms of death, stroke and myocardial infarction between the two groups, a 13% difference in favor of surgery in repeat revascularization, and lower costs (EUR 2973) at 12 months in favor of percutaneous intervention.

When compared to previous trials using balloon angioplasty in a similar population [4–10], it is seen that the need for urgent surgical revas-

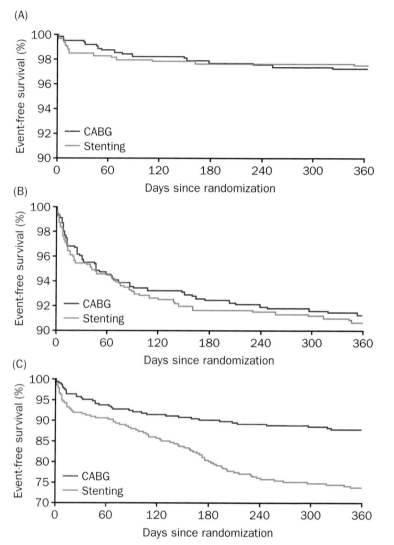

Figure 17.2 One-year event-free survival curves of patients enrolled in the ARTS trial. (A) Actuarial survival rate for patients assigned to stenting versus bypass surgery ($p = 0.75$). (B) Kaplan–Meier event-free survival curves for death, myocardial infarction or cerebrovascular events of patients assigned to stenting versus bypass surgery ($p = 0.71$). (C) Kaplan–Meier event-free survival curves for death, cerebrovascular events, myocardial infarction or any repeat revascularization of patients assigned to stenting versus bypass surgery ($p = 0.0001$).

cularization following failed or complicated balloon angioplasty is reduced from an incidence of 4.6% [10] to 0.5% and that the gap in clinical outcome between the surgical and percutaneous approach has been reduced by approximately 50%. The improvement in clinical outcome when stenting is added to the balloon angioplasty is illustrated in Figure 17.4, which compares the clinical outcome at one year in the ARTS and CABRI trials [39]. The considerable improvement in the percutaneous approach shown is likely explained by increased safety and partial prevention of restenosis provided by the stent. In addition, the degree of revascularization achieved in the group treated with multi-vessel stenting is now comparable to the surgical cohort. In this trial 2.7 out of 2.8 stenotic lesions detected on the diagnostic angiogram were successfully treated, whereas in the CABRI trial [7] 2.1 out of 3.4 and in the BARI trial [5] 1.9 out of 3.5 stenotic lesions were successfully treated.

Table 17.4 Anginal status, medication status and health status of surviving patients

| | Baseline | | | 1 month | | | 6 months | | | 12 months | |
	SA	CABG	p value	SA	CABG	p value	SA	CABG	p value	SA	CABG	p value
Angina-free	0%	0%		87.2%	95.5%	<0.001	75.5%	92.7%	<0.001	78.9%	89.5%	<0.001
Angina medication-free	7.5%	4.6%		16.4%	29.4%	<0.001	18.6%	39.0%	<0.001	21.1%	41.5%	<0.001
Angina and medication-free	0%	0%		14.9%	28.6%	<0.001	14.6%	36.3%	<0.001	19.1%	38.4%	<0.001
EuroQol thermometer	58±19	59±18		75±16	71±16	<0.001	78±15	78±15	0.62	78±15	79±15	0.17
EuroQol summary	69±20	68±20		84±16	78±17	<0.001	86±16	86±15	0.47	86±16	87±16	0.35

SA, stented angioplasty; CABG, coronary artery bypass grafting

Table 17.5 Independent correlates with one-year major cardiac and cerebrovascular events

Independent risk-factors	Total population (n=1205)		Stent (n=600)		CABG (n=605)	
	p	Odds ratio	p	Odds ratio	p	Odds ratio
Assignment to bypass surgery	0.0001	0.31				
Elevated creatine kinase MB	0.0001	1.36			0.0001	1.73
Treatment according to randomization	0.0002	0.19				
Diabetes mellitus	0.001	1.85	0.002	2.1		
Use of digitalis	0.038	2.8				
Treatment of distal RCA*	0.049	2.62				
Maximal balloon pressure in the LAD†			0.002	0.95		
Number of stents implanted in mid RCA*			0.004	1.43		
Stenosis in distal RCA*			0.02	4.53		
Number of unsuccessful treated segments			0.03	1.27		
Increasing age					0.0023	1.06
Use of heparin					0.003	2.66
Abnormal hematocrit					0.013	2.56
Intra-aortic balloon pump					0.035	9.44
Anastomosis in distal RCA*					0.04	0.4

*Right coronary artery; †left anterior descending; ‡successful treatment: less than 50% diameter stenosis after balloon angioplasty or less than 20% diameter stenosis after stented angioplasty by visual assessment.

For patients who were eligible for this trial the practitioner faces the dilemma of the most appropriate treatment in terms of patient benefit and cost-effectiveness. On the one hand angioplasty with stenting is less invasive, is associated with a quicker recovery and a better quality of life at one month. On the other hand, bypass surgery is associated with less angina, fewer anti-anginal medications, and fewer re-interventions at one year. However, the choice is also affected by budgetary constraints. When the choice is made in favor of bypass surgery, this will cost approximately EUR 3000 more than with angioplasty. In return there will be 0.14 additional event-free survivors per treated patient, reflecting the 14% difference in event-free survival observed in this trial. Stated

otherwise one needs to treat seven patients with surgery to get one (7 × 0.14) additional event-free patient and this will cost approximately EUR 21,000 (7 × EUR 3000), an incremental cost-effectiveness ratio of EUR 21,000 per additional event-free survivor. Whether this is acceptable may be subject to debate. However, it should be noted that these figures are substantially higher than those for the use of abciximab in PTCA patients [40] or for primary balloon angioplasty after myocardial infarction [41, 42].

Another factor to consider in the ultimate balance between surgery and percutaneous revascularization is that the time elapsed between randomization and treatment was approximately three times longer for the surgical cohort; eight major adverse cardiac events

Table 17.6 One-year results: average resource use per patient, effectiveness, costs & cost-effectiveness

	Average resource use (units)			Costs (Euro)		
	CABG (n = 600)	STENT (n = 605)	Unit costs	CABG (n = 600)	Stent (n = 605)	p*
Procedure						
Cathlab occupation time (minutes)	2.56	97.79	16	42	1.581	< 0.001
OR occupation time (minutes)	234.41	1.94	27	6.330	54	< 0.001
				6.372	1.635	< 0.001
Endarterectomy	0.01	0.00	1.044	10	0	0.015
Guiding catheter	0.05	2.06	82	4	168	< 0.001
Guide wire	0.05	1.98	95	5	188	< 0.001
Balloon	0.06	2.53	368	21	931	< 0.001
Mounted stent	0.03	1.47	817	26	1.203	< 0.001
Non-mounted stent	0.04	1.46	454	19	662	< 0.001
Rotablator	0.00	0.01	908	0	8	0.082
Other atherectomy	0.00	0.01	1.044	0	10	0.315
Laser-catheter	0.00	0.00	1.395	2	2	0.995
Doppler	0.00	0.00	483	0	1	0.315
Intravascular ultrasound catheter	0.00	0.02	545	0	13	< 0.001
Cardiopulmonary support	0.00	0.00	908	0	2	0.315
Intra-aortic balloon pump catheter	0.01	0.05	635	5	34	< 0.001
Abciximab	0.00	0.03	1.021	0	27	< 0.001
Contrast medium (ml)	11	390	0	5	177	< 0.001
Procedure related events	0.06 (n=38)	0.02 (n=13)	2.366	155	45	0.010
Procedure costs				6622	5106	<0.001
CCU days	0.45	0.66	856	386	564	<0.001
ICU days	1.89	0.13	941	1.781	118	<0.001
Non-CCU/ICU days	6.11	2.14	305	1.864	653	<0.001
Total procedure costs				10,653	6441	<0.001
One-year follow-up						
(Re)-PTCA†	0.03 (n=21)	0.19 (n=114)	3.053	107	579	<0.001
CABG†	0.01 (n=4)	0.07 (n=40)	6.622	44	441	<0.001
Transfusion	0.02 (n=13)	0.02 (n=9)	53	1	1	0.280
Vascular surgery	0.00 (n=1)	0.01 (n=4)	3.861	6	19	0.313
Thrombolysis	0.00 (n=2)	0.03 (n=18)	1.134	4	32	0.002
Angiography	0.08 (n=46)	0.21 (n=123)	1.934	147	396	<0.001
Computer tomography-scan	0.02 (n=11)	0.02 (n=10)	142	3	2	0.841
Other procedure-related events	0.07 (n=40)	0.02 (n=9)	2.265	174	10	<0.001
CCU days	0.33	0.61	856	285	525	<0.001
ICU days	0.33	0.15	941	314	144	0.067
Non-CCU/ICU days	2.50	3.30	305	762	1005	<0.001
Rehabilitation days	3.42	1.00	145	496	145	<0.001
Total follow up costs				2343	3299	<0.001
Medication				642	925	<0.001
Total 1 year direct medical costs				13,638	10,665	<0.001

*Mann–Whitney rank sum test; †number of events (target and non-target vessel, where applicable).

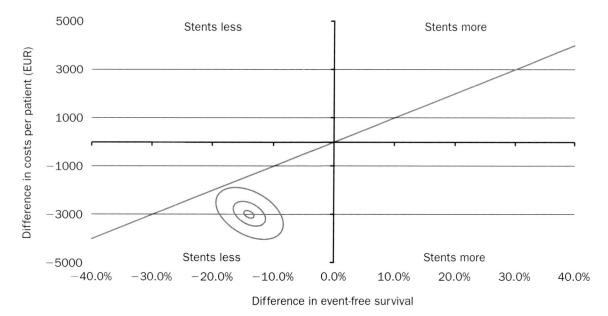

Figure 17.3 Average and Incremental cost-effectiveness. Outer ellipse, smallest area containing, with 95% probability, average costs and effects; middle ellipse, that area with 50% probability; inner ellipse, that area with 5% probability; center of ellipses, point estimate of both average costs and effects.

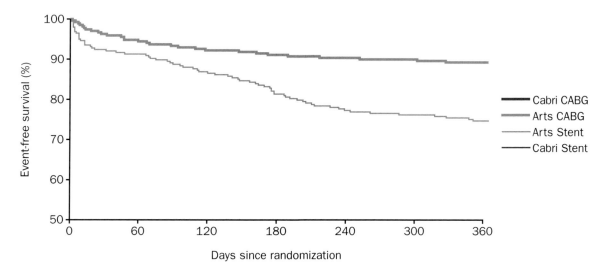

Figure 17.4 One-year event-free survival curves of patients enrolled in the ARTS and CABRI trials. Kaplan–Meier event-free survival curves for death, myocardial infarction or any repeat revascularization in the surgical cohort 91% versus 89% and in the percutaneous treatment group 59% versus 75% of the CABRI and ARTS patients, respectively.

occurred in the surgical group versus one in the stent group during that time. There are reports that the 'waiting list for cardiac surgery engender (sic) high risks for the patients' [43–45].

The ARTS trial was designed in April 1996, initiated in April 1997, and patient recruitment was completed in June 1998. Since practice evolves continuously, it is relevant to critically analyze the differences between the techniques as performed during this study and what is now considered to be state of the art [46]. Beside total arterial revascularization there are new developments in coronary revascularization such as: off-pump surgery and a minimally invasive approach [47–52]. Although these techniques may affect our future practice they do not represent the current practice except at some centers of excellence [31, 53, 54]. At the same time, there are new developments in percutaneous interventions: direct stenting without balloon pre-dilatation, and intra-coronary radiation therapy [55–57]. It is worth noting that 40% of the 30-day events in the stent group were due to stent thrombosis, which occurred in 1.1% of the stented lesions, but in 2.8% of the patients. These events might have been prevented by the use of a glycoprotein receptor blocker [58] and/or heparin coated stents [15]. Again these therapies, although promising, cannot yet be considered as standard practice. While these therapies may be more effective, they are also likely to be more costly and hence affect the balance between costs and effects.

It has been pointed out that most randomized trials recruit eligible patients who represent only a small fraction of the population amenable to surgical revascularization [59]. However in this trial, a prospective universe analysis has shown that, in any given week, between 0–33% of patients with multi-vessel disease at the participating institution were actually enrolled in the ARTS trial. This wide range is attributable both to the restrictive eligibility criteria for the study as well as local logistical considerations. In essence these trials [4–9] should be viewed as scientific experience testing concepts, expanding our knowledge of the field of revascularization and unraveling the need for improvement.

In this regard, logistic regression analyses of each arm of the trial showed that an elevated creatine kinase MB subfraction was the main determinant of clinical outcome in the surgical cohort, whereas diabetes mellitus was the key predictor of a bad clinical outcome in the percutaneous cohort. On the one hand this observation will further fuel the debate on the prognostic and the pathophysiologic significance of cardiac enzyme release during surgical revascularization; on the other hand it corroborates the findings of the BARI trial with respect to the adverse clinical impact of diabetes in patients treated with percutaneous intervention. These observations indicate future directions for research to yield even better outcomes.

In summary, this trial has tipped the scales of cost-effectiveness in favor of the percutaneous approach by substantially reducing the gap in outcomes following surgical versus percutaneous interventions. The essence of the debate remains whether an endoluminal treatment is a more physiological and permanent means of revascularization than a bypass conduit that supplies the myocardium with blood but does not restore the natural pathway of the coronary circulation.

ACKNOWLEDGEMENTS

We thank B Firth and P Marshall for their careful review of the manuscript and for their constructive comments. This study was conducted under the auspices of the European Academy of Sciences and Arts, patronage: Mr Jacques Santer, former President, European Commission in Brussels. Sponsored by Cordis, a Johnson & Johnson Company. Safety and data monitoring was conducted by Stuart Pocock (UK), Tom Ryan (USA), and Ken Taylor (UK). The board of governors comprised Marvin Woodall (International Vice President, Johnson & Johnson, USA), Brian Firth (Vice President,

Worldwide Medical Affairs and Health Economics, Cordis, a Johnson & Johnson Company, USA), Felix Unger (European Heart Institute, Professor of Cardiac Surgery, Austria), Patrick Serruys (Chairman Executive Steering Committee, Professor of Interventional Cardiology, The Netherlands), and Paul Hugenholtz (Past President European Society of Cardiology, The Netherlands). The Executive Steering Committee comprised a subgroup of investigators and representatives from both the sponsor and the coordinating center.

• Surgery: Felix Unger (Chairman, Austria), Lex van Herwerden (The Netherlands), Friedrich Mohr (Germany), Jochen Cremer (Germany), and Gusta Petterson (Denmark).

• Interventional cardiology: Patrick Serruys (Chairman, The Netherlands), Rudiger Simon (Germany), William Wijns (Belgium), Hans Bonnier (The Netherlands), Antonio Colombo (Italy), Marie-Claude Morice (France), O Madonna (Cordis, a Johnson & Johnson company) and GA van Es (Cardialysis). The Critical Event Committee was composed of JJ Bredee (The Netherlands), O Hess (Switzerland), WJ Morshuis (The Netherlands), W Wijns (Chairman, Belgium). The Angiographic Committee was composed of M van den Brand (Chairman, The Netherlands), B Rensing (The Netherlands) and C van de Wiel (The Netherlands).

All ECGs collected for the study are assessed by an independent core laboratory, located at Cardialysis, Rotterdam, The Netherlands. The data coordinating center is also located at Cardialysis, Rotterdam, The Netherlands (H Hennessey, A-M Hoogenboom, M Kuypers, M-A Morel, V de Valk). The trial is being monitored by Parexel (I Kuit). Data analysis was carried out by W Lindenboom and B Koens. BA van Hout (The Netherlands) carried out the health economic analysis.

The following institutions and investigators participated in the study. The number of patients enrolled at each center is given in parentheses: Instituto Dante Pazzanese de Cardiologia, Sao Paulo, Brazil: JE Sousa, A Jatene (66); Catharina Ziekenhuis, Eindhoven, The Netherlands: JJRM Bonnier, JPAM Schönberger (61); The Queen Elizabeth Hospital, Birmingham, UK: N Buller, R Bonser (54); CHU Sart Tilman, Liège, Belgium: V Legrand, R Limet (47); AZR Dijkzigt, Thoraxcentrum, Rotterdam, The Netherlands: PW Serruys, L van Herwerden (47); St Paul's Hospital, Vancouver, Canada: R Carere, S Lichtenstein (46); Herzzentrum Leipzig, Leipzig, Germany: G Schuler, FW Mohr (43); Medisch Centrum 'De Klokkenberg', Breda, The Netherlands: PCH Roose, ThR van Geldorp (39); Hospital Clinico San Carlos, Madrid, Spain: C Macaya, JL Castañon (32); Landeskrankenanstalten Salzburg, Salzburg, Austria: G Heyer, F Unger (30); Hospital Universitario de Valladolid, Valladolid, Spain: F Fernandez-Avilès, J Herreros Gonzáles (28); Ziekenhuis De Weezenlanden, Zwolle, The Netherlands: H Suryapranata, M Haalebos (27); Onze-Lieve Vrouw Ziekenhuis, Aalst, Belgium: W Wijns, F Wellens (26); London Chest Hospital, London, UK: MT Rothman, R Balcon, J Wright (26); Unicor Hospital, Sao Paulo, Brazil: E Ribeiro, E Buffolo (26); Rambam Medical Center, Haifa, Israel: R Beyar, S Milo (25); Christian Albrechts Universität, Kiel, Germany: R Simon, D Regensburger (25); St James's Hospital, Dublin, Ireland: P Crean, E McGovern (22); Academisch Ziekenhuis Middelheim, Antwerp, Belgium: P van den Heuvel, C van Cauwelaert (21); Vancouver Hospital and Health Science Centre, Vancouver, Canada: I Penn, GFO Tyers (20); Harefield Hospital, Uxbridge, UK: C Ilsley, M Yacoub (19); Skejby Sygehus, Arhus, Denmark: T Toftegaard Nielsen, P Kildeberg Paulsen (18); Onze Lieve Vrouwe Gasthuis, Amsterdam, The Netherlands: F Kiemeney, L Eysmann (17); Algemeen Ziekenhuis St Jan, Genk, Belgium: M Vrolix, G Fransen (17); Hôpital de la Citadelle, Liège, Belgium: P Materne, G de Koster (17); Hospital Santa Cruz, Linda-A-Velha, Portugal: R Seabra-Gomes, J Queiróz E Melo (17);

Montreal Heart Institute, Montreal, Canada: L Bilodeau, M Carrier (17); Fundación Favaloro, Buenos Aires, Argentina: HF Londero, V Caramutti (16); Universitair Ziekenhuis Gent, Gent, Belgium: Y Taeymans, G van Nooten (16); Herzzentrum Bodensee, Kreuzlingen, Switzerland: M Pieper, D Maass (16); Northern General Hospital, Sheffield, UK: D Cumberland, F Ciulli, G Cooper (16); Wessex Cardiology Centre, Southampton, UK: K Dawkins, S Livesey (16); Academisch Ziekenhuis Maastricht, Maastricht, The Netherlands: FWHM Bär, K Prenger (15); Royal North Shore Hospital of Sydney, Sydney, Australia: GIC Nelson, D Marshman (15); Hospital Clínic i Provincial, Barcelona, Spain: A Betriu, JL Pomar (14); Academisch Ziekenhuis Groningen, Groningen, The Netherlands: AJ van Boven, PW Boonstra (14); Onassis Cardiac Surgery Center, Athens, Greece: V Voudris, G Stavridis (13); Rigshospitalet, Copenhagen, Denmark: K Saunamäki, K Sander-Jensen (13); Centro Hospitalar de Gaia, Vila Nova de Gaia, Portugal: V Gama Ribeiro, MDMS Guerreiro (13); Universitätsklinikum Charité, Berlin, Germany: W Rutsch, W Konertz (11); Prince Charles Hospital, Brisbane, Australia: JHN Bett, P Tesar (11); Hôpital Henri Mondor, Créteil, France: JL Dubois-Rande, D Loisance (11); Ospedale di Circolo, Varese, Italy: G Binaghi, G Tarelli (11); Allgemeines Krankenhaus der Stadt Wien, Vienna, Austria: P Probst, E Wolner, G Laufer (11); I Medizinische Klinik RWTH Aachen, Aachen, Germany: P Hanrath, B Messmer (10); Instituto Malattie Cardiovascolare, Policlinico S Orsola-Malpighi, Bologna, Italy: G Piovaccari, C Marrozzini, G Marinelli (10); Hadassah University Hospital, Jerusalem, Israel: C Lotan, G Merion (10); Tel Aviv Medical Center, Tel Aviv, Israel: S Braun, R Mor (10); Institut Cardiovasculaire Paris-Sud, Institut Hospitalier Jacques Cartier, Massy, France: MC Morice, P Donzeau-Gouge (9); Hôpital Universitaire de Mont Godinne, Yvoir, Belgium: E Schroeder, JC Schoevaerdts (9); Shaare Zedek Medical Center, Jerusalem, Israel: D Tzivoni, D Bitran (8); Ospedale Maggiore, Trieste, Italy: A Salvi, L Dreas, B Branchini (8); Städtische Kliniken Dortmund, Dortmund, Germany: B Lösse, MJ Polonius (7); Centre Universitaire Vaudois, Lausanne, Switzerland: JJ Goy, LK von Segesser (7); Academisch Ziekenhuis St Radboud, Nijmegen, The Netherlands: H Gehlmann, S Singh (7); Centro Cuore Columbus, Milan, Italy: A Colombo, C Santoli (6); Instituto Scientifico H San Raffaele, Milan, Italy: I Sheiban, O Alfieri (6); University Hospital, Zürich, Switzerland: T Lüscher, M Turina (6); UCL Saint-Luc, Brussels, Belgium: C Hanet, R Dion (5); Universitätsklinikum Rudolf Virchow, Franz-Volhard Klinik, Berlin Buch, Germany: DC Gulba, B Schübel (4); Clinique Générale St Jean, Brussels, Belgium: M Vandormael, P Bettendorf (4); Green Lane Hospital, Auckland, New Zealand: J Ormiston, P Ruygrok, A Kerr (3); Instituto cardiovascular de Buenos Aires, Buenos Aires, Argentina: J Belardi, D Navia (3); Zentrum für Innere Medizin, Universitätsklinikum Essen, Essen, Germany: R Erbel, M Haude, J Chr. Reidemeister (3); Academisch Medisch Centrum, Amsterdam, The Netherlands: K Koch, BAJ de Mol (2); Klinikum Grosshadern, Munich, Germany: S Nikol, B Reichart (2); Deutsches Herzzentrum München, Munich, Germany: A Schömig, Meisner, K Holper (1).

REFERENCES

1. Unger F. Worldwide survey on coronary interventions 1995. Report of the European Heart Academy of Sciences and ARTS, *Cor Europaeum* 1999; **7**:128–146.
2. Unger F. Cardiac interventions in Europe 1997: coronary revascularization procedures and open heart surgery, *Cor Europeaum* 1999; **7**:177–186.
3. Rigter H, Meijler AP, McDonnell J, Scholma JK, Bernstein SJ. Indications for coronary revascularisation: a Dutch perspective, *Heart* 1997; **77**:211–218.
4. Rodriguez A, Mele E, Peyregne E et al. Three-year follow-up of the Argentine Randomized Trial of Percutaneous Transluminal Coronary Angioplasty Versus Coronary Artery Bypass

Surgery in Multivessel Disease (ERACI), *J Am Coll Cardiol* 1996; **27**:1178–1184.

5. Comparison of coronary bypass surgery with angioplasty in patients with multivessel disease. The Bypass Angioplasty Revascularization Investigation (BARI) Investigators, *N Engl J Med* 1996; **335**:217–225.

6. Coronary angioplasty versus coronary artery bypass surgery: the Randomized Intervention Treatment of Angina (RITA) trial. *Lancet* 1993; **341**:573–580.

7. First-year results of CABRI (Coronary Angioplasty versus Bypass Revascularisation Investigation). CABRI Trial Participants, *Lancet* 1995; **346**:1179–1184.

8. Hamm CW, Reimers J, Ischinger T et al. A randomized study of coronary angioplasty compared with bypass surgery in patients with symptomatic multivessel coronary disease. German Angioplasty Bypass Surgery Investigation (GABI), *N Engl J Med* 1994; **331**:1037–1043.

9. King SB III, Lembo NJ, Weintraub WS et al. A randomized trial comparing coronary angioplasty with coronary bypass surgery. Emory Angioplasty versus Surgery Trial (EAST), *N Engl J Med* 1994; **331**:1044–1050.

10. Pocock SJ, Henderson RA, Rickards AF et al. Meta-analysis of randomized trials comparing coronary angioplasty with bypass surgery. *Lancet* 1995; **346**:1184–1189.

11. Serruys PW, de Jaegere P, Kiemeneij F et al. A comparison of balloon-expandable-stent implantation with balloon angioplasty in patients with coronary artery disease. Benestent Study Group, *N Engl J Med* 1994; **331**:489–495.

12. Fischman DL, Leon MB, Baim DS et al. A randomized comparison of coronary-stent placement and balloon angioplasty in the treatment of coronary artery disease. Stent Restenosis Study Investigators, *N Engl J Med* 1994; **331**:496–501.

13. Versaci F, Gaspardone A, Tomai F et al. A comparison of coronary-artery stenting with angioplasty for isolated stenosis of the proximal left anterior descending coronary artery, *N Engl J Med* 1997; **336**:817–822.

14. Macaya C, Serruys PW, Ruygrok P et al. Continued benefit of coronary stenting versus balloon angioplasty: one-year clinical follow-up of Benestent trial. Benestent Study Group, *J Am Coll Cardiol* 1996; **27**:255–261.

15. Serruys PW, van Hout B, Bonnier H et al.

Randomized comparison of implantation of heparin-coated stents with balloon angioplasty in selected patients with coronary artery disease (Benestent II), *Lancet* 1998; **352**:673–681.

16. Eeckhout E, Wijns W, Meier B, Goy JJ. Indications for intracoronary stent placement: the European view. Working Group on Coronary Circulation of the European Society of Cardiology, *Eur Heart J* 1999; **20**:1014–1019.

17. Malenka DJ, O'Connor GT. The Northern New England Cardiovascular Disease Study Group: A regional collaborative effort for continuous quality improvement in cardiovascular disease, *J Comm J Qual Improv* 1998; **24**:594–600.

18. Califf RM. Restenosis: the cost to society, *Am Heart J* 1995; **130**:680–684.

19. Cohen DJ, Breall JA, Ho KK et al. Evaluating the potential cost-effectiveness of stenting as a treatment for symptomatic single-vessel coronary disease. Use of a decision-analytic model. *Circulation* 1994; **89**:1859–1874.

20. Van Hout BA, van der Woude T, de Jaegere PP et al. Cost-effectiveness of stent implantation versus PTCA: the BENESTENT experience, *Semin Interv Cardiol* 1996; **1**:263–268.

21. Peterson ED, Cowper PA, DeLong ER et al. Acute and long-term cost implications of coronary stenting. *J Am Coll Cardiol* 1999; **33**:1610–1618.

22. Hlatky MA, Rogers WJ, Johnstone I et al. Medical care costs and quality of life after randomization to coronary angioplasty or coronary bypass surgery. Bypass Angioplasty Revascularization Investigation (BARI) investigators, *N Engl J Med* 1997; **336**:92–99.

23. Vaitkus PT, Witmer WT, Brandenburg RG, Wells SK, Zehnacker JB. Economic impact of angioplasty salvage techniques, with an emphasis on coronary stents: a method incorporating costs, revenues, clinical effectiveness and payer mix, *J Am Coll Cardiol* 1997; **30**:894–900.

24. Sculpher MJ, Seed P, Henderson RA et al. Health service costs of coronary angioplasty and coronary artery bypass surgery: the Randomised Intervention Treatment of Angina (RITA) trial, *Lancet* 1994; **344**:927–930.

25. Freeman VG, Rathore SS, Weinfurt KP, Schulman KA, Sulmasy DP. Lying for patients: physician deception of third-party payers, *Arch Intern Med* 1999; **159**:2263–2270.

26. Weintraub WS, Craver JM, Jones EL et al.

Improving cost and outcome of coronary surgery, *Circulation* 1998; **98:**II23–II28.

27. van Hout BA, Goes ES, Grijseels EW, van Ufford MA. Economic evaluation in the field of cardiology: theory and practice, *Prog Cardiovasc Dis* 1999; **42:**167–173.

28. Serruys PW, Van Hout BA, Van den Brand MJB et al. The ARTS (Arterial Revascularization Therapies Study): background, goals and methods, *Int J Cardiovasc Interventions* 1999; **2:**41–50.

29. Campeau L. Grading of angina pectoris, *Circulation* 1976; **54:**522–523.

30. Braunwald E. Unstable angina. A classification, *Circulation* 1989; **80:**410–414.

31. Eagle KA, Guyton RA, Davidoff R et al. ACC/AHA Guidelines for Coronary Artery Bypass Graft Surgery: A Report of the American College of Cardiology/American Heart Association Task Force on Practice Guidelines (Committee to Revise the 1991 Guidelines for Coronary Artery Bypass Graft Surgery). American College of Cardiology/American Heart Association, *J Am Coll Cardiol* 1999; **34:**1262–1347.

32. Wood D. European and American recommendations for coronary heart disease prevention, *Eur Heart J* 1998; **19 Suppl A:**A12–A19.

33. Edlavitch SA, Crow R, Burke GL, Baxter J. Secular trends in Q wave and non-Q wave acute myocardial infarction. The Minnesota Heart Survey, *Circulation* 1991; **83:**492–503.

34. Hodakowski GT, Craver JM, Jones EL, King SB, 3rd, Guyton RA. Clinical significance of perioperative Q-wave myocardial infarction: the Emory Angioplasty versus Surgery Trial, *J Thorac Cardiovasc Surg* 1996; **112:**1447–1454.

35. Califf RM, Abdelmeguid AE, Kuntz RE et al. Myonecrosis after revascularization procedures, *J Am Coll Cardiol* 1998; **31:**241–251.

36. Dolan P. Modeling valuations for EuroQol health states, *Med Care* 1997; **35:**1095–1108.

37. Greenland S, Robins JM. Estimation of a common effect parameter from sparse follow-up data, *Biometrics* 1985; **41:**55–68.

38. Cox DR. Fieller's theorem and a generalization, *Biometrika* 1967; **54:**567–572.

39. Van der Brand MJBM, Breeman A, Rensing B et al. Comparison of the extent of revascularization and event free survival in the angioplasty arms of two randomized trials of coronary angioplasty versus surgery for multivessel coronary artery disease, *Eur Heart J* 1999; **20:**153 (abstract).

40. Topol EJ, Mark DB, Lincoff AM et al. Outcomes at one year and economic implications of platelet glycoprotein IIb/IIIa blockade in patients undergoing coronary stenting: results from a multicentre randomized trial. EPISTENT Investigators. Evaluation of platelet IIb/IIIa inhibitor for stenting, *Lancet* 1999; **354:**2019–2024.

41. Lieu TA, Gurley RJ, Lundstrom RJ et al. Projected cost-effectiveness of primary angioplasty for acute myocardial infarction, *J Am Coll Cardiol* 1997; **30:**1741–1750.

42. Parmley WW. Cost-effectiveness of reperfusion strategies, *Am Heart J* 1999; **138:**142–152.

43. Bernstein SJ, Rigter H, Brorsson B et al. Waiting for coronary revascularization: a comparison between New York State, The Netherlands and Sweden, *Health Policy* 1997; **42:**15–27.

44. Teo KK, Spoor M, Pressey T et al. Impact of managed waiting for coronary artery bypass graft surgery on patients' perceived quality of life, *Circulation* 1998; **98:**II29–II34.

45. Jackson NW, Doogue MP, Elliott JM. Priority points and cardiac events while waiting for coronary bypass surgery, *Heart* 1999; **81:**367–373.

46. Unger F, Frommer P, Hetzer R et al. Standards and concepts in cardiac interventions. Coronary artery disease: revascularization, *Cor Europaeum* 1997; **6:**32–39.

47. Moshkovitz Y, Lusky A, Mohr F. Coronary artery bypass without cardiopulmonary bypass: analysis of short-term and mid-term outcome in 220 patients, *J Thorac Cardiovasc Surg* 1995; **110:**979–987.

48. Borst C, Jansen EW, Tulleken CA et al. Coronary artery bypass grafting without cardiopulmonary bypass and without interruption of native coronary flow using a novel anastomosis site restraining device ('Octopus'), *J Am Coll Cardiol* 1996; **27:**1356–1364.

49. Calafiore AM, Di Giammarco G, Teodori G et al. Mid-term results after minimally invasive coronary surgery (LAST operation), *J Thorac Cardiovasc Surg* 1998; **115:**763–771.

50. Benetti F, Mariani MA, Sani G et al. Video-assisted minimally invasive coronary operations without cardiopulmonary bypass: a multicenter study, *J Thorac Cardiovasc Surg* 1996; **112:**1478–1484.

51. Gu YJ, Mariani MA, van Oeveren W, Grandjean

JG, Boonstra PW. Reduction of the inflammatory response in patients undergoing minimally invasive coronary artery bypass grafting, *Ann Thorac Surg* 1998; **65:**420–424.

52. Bergsma TM, Grandjean JG, Voors AA et al. Low recurrence of angina pectoris after coronary artery bypass graft surgery with bilateral internal thoracic and right gastroepiploic arteries, *Circulation* 1998; **97:**2402–2405.

53. Borst C, Grundeman PF. Minimally invasive coronary artery bypass grafting: an experimental perspective, *Circulation* 1999; **99:**1400–1403.

54. Loop FD. Coronary artery surgery: the end of the beginning, *Eur J Cardiothorac Surg* 1998; **14:**554–571.

55. Pentousis D, Guerin Y, Funck F et al. Direct stent implantation without predilatation using the MultiLink stent, *Am J Cardiol* 1998; **82:**1437–1440.

56. Condado JA, Waksman R, Gurdiel O et al. Long-term angiographic and clinical outcome after percutaneous transluminal coronary angioplasty and intracoronary radiation therapy in humans, *Circulation* 1997; **96:**727–732.

57. Teirstein PS, Massullo V, Jani S et al. Catheter-based radiotherapy to inhibit restenosis after coronary stenting, *N Engl J Med* 1997; **336:**1697–1703.

58. The EPISTENT Investigators. Randomized placebo-controlled and balloon-angioplasty-controlled trial to assess safety of coronary stenting with use of platelet glycoprotein-IIb/IIIa blockade. Evaluation of Platelet IIb/IIIa Inhibitor for Stenting, *Lancet* 1998; **352:**87–92.

59. Detre KM, Rosen AD, Bost JE et al. Contemporary practice of coronary revascularization in US hospitals and hospitals participating in the bypass angioplasty revascularization investigation (BARI), *J Am Coll Cardiol* 1996; **28:**609–615.

Section IV: Differential risks/differential benefits: patient subsets

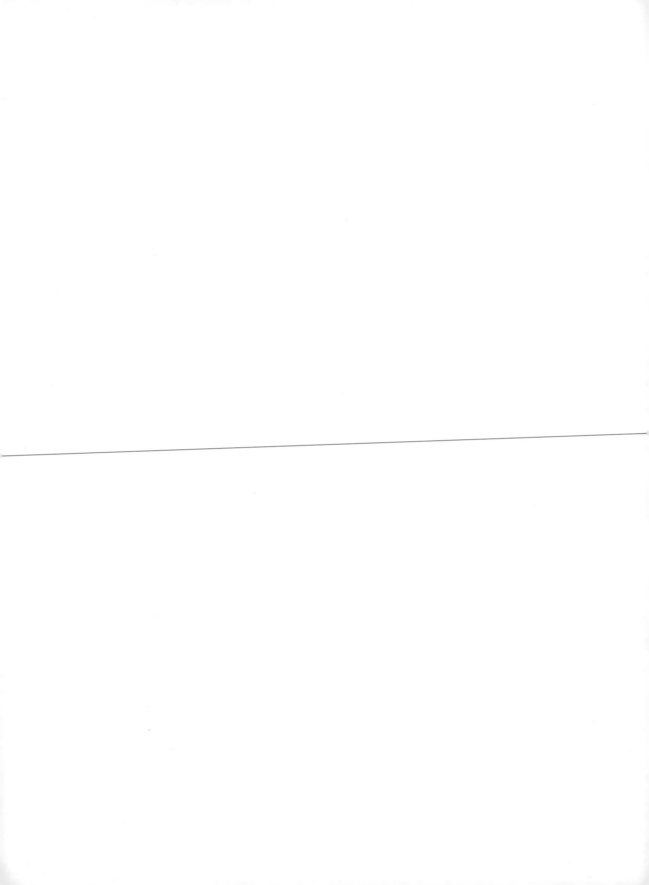

18

Re-operative revascularization

Bruce W Lytle

CONTENTS • **The evolution of coronary re-operations: patient population and surgical strategies** • **Evaluation for coronary re-operation** • **Technical aspects of re-operations** • **Off-pump surgery** • **Risk of re-operations** • **Late outcomes after re-operation** • **Multiple coronary re-operations** • **Conclusion**

Patients with previous bypass surgery who develop recurrent ischemia are different to patients who undergo primary operations. For reoperative candidates, areas of myocardium are often dependent upon saphenous vein grafts, and jeopardized by vein graft pathologies that are distinct from native vessel coronary atherosclerosis (vein graft atherosclerosis and intimal fibroplasia). Also, although in situ arterial to coronary bypass grafts rarely develop pathologic changes, they are commonly a critical source of myocardial perfusion and may be at risk during repeat surgery. There are other characteristics that are not unique but are more common when patients have had prior bypass surgery. Diffuse cardiac and non-cardiac atherosclerosis are extremely common in patients many years after undergoing initial surgery for extensive coronary artery disease. Availability of bypass conduits is rarely a problem for patients undergoing primary surgery but commonly is an issue during reoperation. Abnormal left ventricular function is also more common in most reoperative series. All these characteristics tend to increase risk and, in addition to increasing the risk of coronary bypass reoperations, they also make pharmacologic or percutaneous treatment less likely to

be successful, and decision-making more difficult.

A major difficulty in recommending therapy for patients with previous bypass surgery is the relative lack of data concerning the natural history of well-defined angiographic and clinical subsets of these patients. None of the randomized studies of bypass surgery versus medical management included reoperative candidates, and there are not randomized studies of surgery versus PTCA currently available that deal with any significant numbers of patients with previous surgery.

To investigate the impact of vein graft pathology on outcomes we conducted two non-randomized, retrospective studies of patients who had undergone bypass surgery followed by repeat coronary angiography (usually performed for symptoms). In the first study we compared outcomes for patients who were found to have at least one stenotic vein graft with patients who had no vein graft stenosis [1]. For patients studied less than five years after operation, having a stenotic vein graft did not predict a worse survival. However, when patients were found to have late vein graft stenoses (more than five years after operation) the presence of those stenoses predicted an increased late mortality rate for patients who did not undergo repeat surgery.

It is likely that at least part of the difference in the survival of patients with early vs late vein graft stenoses is based on a difference in the types of pathology found at those postoperative intervals [2–4]. Vein graft stenoses within five years of operation are usually caused by intimal fibroplasia, a concentric diffuse lesion that is initially cellular but with time becomes more fibrous. Intimal fibroplasia appears to occur to some extent in most vein grafts but in a few it creates specific stenotic lesions. Late vein graft stenoses are usually caused by vein graft atherosclerosis. Vein graft atherosclerosis is distinct from native vessel atherosclerosis. Native vessel atherosclerosis is based on the media, usually encapsulated by the intima, eccentric, proximal and segmental. Vein graft atherosclerosis is diffuse, circumferential, superficial, and unencapsulated. Vein graft atherosclerosis appears to be a much more active lesion than either intimal fibroplasia or native vessel atherosclerosis. Embolization of atherosclerotic debris from vein grafts more than five years after operation has been clinically documented at the time of interventions or repeat operation and may occur spontaneously. Vein graft atherosclerosis accounts for some of the risks encountered by patients with previous bypass surgery regardless of treatment choice.

Our first study of patients with vein graft disease established that late vein graft stenoses predicted an increased risk of death without surgery. Our second study was designed to see whether or not re-operation decreased that mortality rate [5]. We found that patients with early vein graft stenoses did not have an improvement in their already favorable survival with re-operation although those patients who underwent repeat surgery did experience more symptom relief. Patients with late vein graft stenoses, however, did have an improved survival rate if they underwent re-operation and that improvement was particularly dramatic if they had stenosis in a vein graft to the

left anterior descending (LAD) coronary artery. Thus, situations where there is an atherosclerotic vein graft subtending the LAD coronary artery or a heavily dominant circumflex or right coronary artery, or patients with multiple stenotic atherosclerotic vein grafts constitute anatomic indications for re-operation.

These retrospective angiographic and followup studies did not assess functional testing, but Lauer et al have investigated that issue with an analysis of 873 symptom-free patients who underwent exercise thallium-201, SPECT testing [6]. Stress abnormalities were predictors of subsequent adverse cardiac events. Impaired exercise capacity (≤ 6 METS) was strongly predictive of subsequent death or non-fatal myocardial infarction.

The arrival of percutaneous procedures offered another possibility for the anatomic treatment of vein graft lesions. However, the percutaneous treatment of vein graft lesions has been less effective than the treatment of native vessel atherosclerotic disease. Early studies showed that balloon angioplasty was not a very successful treatment of vein graft lesions and that success was also relative to the age of those lesions [7]. Angioplasty of early vein graft lesions was relatively safe and resulted in a lower restenosis rate than angioplasty of old vein grafts, although even with early lesions more than 50% of the patients exhibited restenosis. The treatment of late atherosclerotic lesions in vein grafts with balloon angioplasty alone was very unsuccessful, encountering an increased risk of peri-procedural myocardial infarction and death with restenosis rates that approached 80%. A variety of other percutaneous devices including atherectomy catheters, extraction devices, and laser, also produced outcomes that were unfavorable.

The use of intracoronary stents has appeared to provide superior results to other percutaneous treatments [8]. However, there still is a substantial risk of in-stent restenosis. A greater problem, however, is the progression of atherosclerosis in non-stented areas of the vein graft. If a recurrence of a stenosis at any location in the graft is considered the combined incidence of restenosis and clinical events is quite high. Furthermore, vein graft restenosis continues to recur well beyond the first post-procedure year.

What are the indications for re-operation versus percutaneous treatment of patients with previous surgery? Logic would seem to dictate that patients with atherosclerotic vein grafts, significantly stenotic ($\geq 50\%$) that subtend large areas of myocardium or who have multiple jeopardized vein grafts, should undergo re-operation. Percutaneous treatments have not been reliable enough over time to justify their use for this subpopulation. Patients with early stenoses in vein grafts who are not highly symptomatic probably can be treated with medical therapy or with percutaneous techniques if they become significantly symptomatic. Patients who develop recurrent ischemic syndromes based on progression of native vessel coronary artery disease are often effectively treated with percutaneous techniques and patients with old vein grafts that subtend relatively small areas of myocardium but from which they are symptomatic often can be effectively palliated with percutaneous techniques. Unstable syndromes based on vein graft disease also may be effectively treated with percutaneous techniques since long-term outcomes are less important in that setting and the short-term risks of emergency operation are increased for patients undergoing a re-operation.

THE EVOLUTION OF CORONARY RE-OPERATIONS: PATIENT POPULATION AND SURGICAL STRATEGIES

In the early years of bypass surgery, the 1970s, patients often underwent primary operations for limited coronary artery disease, internal thoracic artery grafts were not common and risk factor modification was often haphazard. The need for re-operation during those early years was usually caused by progression of native vessel disease in ungrafted vessels, early vein graft failure, or technical errors [9]. Re-operative candidates usually had reasonably favorable risk profiles because the same was true of patients undergoing primary coronary bypass operations.

By the early 1980s the randomized studies of bypass surgery and medical management had shown that patients with more extensive disease had the most to gain from bypass surgery, particularly in regard to survival, and techniques had progressed to the point where the risk of surgery for patients with severe coronary artery disease had decreased. Thus, few patients were undergoing primary operations for single vessel disease and the likelihood of patients needing re-operation solely for the treatment of progression of a native vessel atherosclerosis was diminishing. However, the spectre of vein graft atherosclerosis as a cause of graft failure was raising its ugly head. Therefore, as time progressed, the interval between primary and repeat surgery was lengthening and most re-operations were caused by a combination of progressive native vessel disease and graft atherosclerosis. Furthermore, patient age and co-morbidity was increasing. The risks of coronary re-operations have always exceeded those for primary surgery but despite a higher patient risk profile increased surgical experience with re-operations tended to keep overall risks relatively constant [9, 10]. Myocardial protection, always the most important issue during re-operation, became much more consistent by the development of blood cardioplegia and retrograde cardioplegia delivery systems. It began to become recognized that retrograde cardioplegia was particularly useful in avoiding embolization from atherosclerotic vein grafts and in protecting areas of the myocardium supplied by patent internal thoracic artery (ITA) grafts.

In recent years the population of re-operative patients has continued to demonstrate increasing high-risk characteristics, particularly that of advancing age. Also, more patients are undergoing repeat surgery after having had multiple previous operations [11]. Surgical techniques have expanded to deal with the technical challenges, in particular the use of multiple arterial grafts (radial artery, gastroepiploic artery, right internal thoracic artery) sometimes used as composite grafts, alternative incisions, and off-pump bypass surgery have been useful during re-operations. During the decade of the 1990s substantial progress was also made in percutaneous interventions, a trend that has removed, at least temporarily, some patients from the immediate re-operation population. Those patients still needing surgery have continued to exhibit increasing numbers of high-risk characteristics.

EVALUATION FOR CORONARY RE-OPERATION

The first step in a successful coronary re-operation is a complete and accurate coronary angiogram. That is not quite as simple as it sounds. Graftable coronary arteries may be supplied by grafts from the ascending aorta, innominate artery, or descending aorta, in situ arterial grafts, coronary to coronary collaterals, and non-coronary collaterals. Unless the proper angiographic studies are obtained, grafts may be missed and the anatomy may be misunderstood. It is important that angiography define all the coronary vessels. Old operative notes and old angiograms are often useful in helping the angiographer and surgeon to define and understand the coronary anatomy. Coronary arteries do not disappear and myocardium is not created without a blood supply. Some patients considered 'inoperable' have just not had a complete angiogram.

The next step is to be certain that jeopardized coronary arteries supply viable myocardium. There are multiple imaging techniques available to assess the state of the myocardium. At The Cleveland Clinic Foundation we tend to use positron emission tomography to document metabolic activity in the myocardium and dobutamine stress echo cardiography to assess contractile reserve. These techniques are particularly useful for patients with abnormal left ventricular function. In addition to deciding whether jeopardized myocardium is in fact viable, and whether or not improvement in left ventricular function might be possible after operation, myocardial viability studies may also help to direct revascularization strategies in situations where bypass conduits are limited.

The assessment of availability of bypass conduits prior to a re-operation is essential. It is not wise to discover in the operating room that adequate grafts are not available. Angiographic studies of re-operative candidates should include angiograms of the internal mammary arteries. Doppler flow studies of the ITAs may be useful but angiographic definition is more certain. In situations where a graft to the right coronary artery is important, a gastroepiploic angiogram may also be helpful. Radial arteries may be used for grafts as long as ulnar artery flow is sufficient to supply the hand. This can be assessed by an Allen's test or formal perfusion indices. A satisfactory Allen's test does not always mean that the radial artery will be a good graft as the distal radial artery may be damaged from previous arterial monitoring catheters. In addition we perform venous Doppler studies of greater and lesser saphenous vein systems for all re-operative candidates.

Assessment of peripheral vascular atherosclerosis is important for multiple reasons. First, peripheral atherosclerosis is common in re-operative candidates. Second, carotid stenosis, particularly if bilateral, is associated with an increased risk of stroke. The management strategies for carotid stenosis are multiple and a detailed discussion of this issue is beyond the scope of this chapter, but recognition is important. Third, alternative cannulation sites must be defined in case the presence of ascending aortic atherosclerosis makes aortic cannulation risky.

TECHNICAL ASPECTS OF RE-OPERATIONS

Adverse outcomes during coronary re-operations are most commonly related to perioperative myocardial infarction, stroke, or injury to cardiovascular structures. Thus, the surgeon must avoid these negative events while trying to enhance the long-term outcomes by achieving as complete a revascularization as possible with the use of effective grafts, hopefully the internal thoracic arteries. At times compromise must be reached between avoiding the negative and accentuating the positive.

Although limited or alternative incisions can be useful in selected re-operations, most patients are best approached through a median sternotomy because of the need for grafting multiple cardiac territories and access to all bypass conduits.

We perform the repeat median sternotomy with an oscillating saw after dividing the sternal wires anteriorly but not removing the posterior wires until the bone has been divided. The posterior aspect of the wires help protect underlying structures from damage. If a lateral chest x-ray indicates adherence of the sternum to underlying structures, a CT scan may help to define the anatomy with more precision. When severe difficulties with a repeat sternotomy are expected, arterial and venous access is obtained. In situations where the right ventricle or the aorta appear to be adherent to the sternum, a small right thoracotomy may allow separation of these structures from the sternum. It is often wise to have radial artery and venous bypass conduits prepared before performing the median sternotomy, particularly in high-risk situations.

Once the median sternotomy is performed the underlying structures are dissected away and the ITA grafts are dissected from the chest wall. The right aorta and ventricle are then dissected out in preparation for cannulation.

Aortic atherosclerosis is common in re-operative candidates. We perform trans-esophageal echocardiography during the operation and if this provides evidence of aortic atherosclerosis or if aortic palpation is suspicious we also employ epi-aortic echocardiography [12]. Atherosclerosis or calcification of the ascending aorta, a problem that may be com-

bined with a lack of space on the ascending aorta due to the presence of old vein grafts, is an indication for alternative cannulation. In that setting we usually employ the innominate or axillary artery in order to avoid retrograde perfusion through an atherosclerotic descending aorta. Venous cannulation is usually accomplished with a small two-stage venous cannula placed in the right atrium along with the retrograde cardioplegia cannula. An antegrade cardioplegia needle is placed in the aorta.

Cardiopulmonary bypass is established, the aorta is cross clamped, antegrade and retrograde blood cardioplegia are given, and the left side of the heart is then dissected out. Dissection of the left ventricle with the heart relaxed allows accuracy in dissection and decreases the manipulation of stenotic or patent grafts. Patent left internal mammary artery grafts are dissected out and occluded with non-traumatic clamps. If retrograde cardioplegia is being delivered well that route is employed throughout the rest of the case.

OFF-PUMP SURGERY

Off-pump or 'beating heart' surgery can be useful during re-operations. Specific indications for re-operative off-pump bypass grafting are situations that make the use of cardiopulmonary bypass extremely risky. The most common of these situations are severe aortic atherosclerosis, heparin-induced coagulation abnormalities, recent stroke and known cerebral vascular disease. When performing off-pump surgery as a re-operation the use of partial occlusion aortic clamps for the construction of proximal anastomoses may be difficult or dangerous. Alternatives to partial aortic clamping during off-bypass surgery include using new or old ITA grafts as inflow anastomotic sites or the use of non-clamping 'connectors', devices that are newly commercially available. The other disadvantage of off-pump surgery as a strategy for patients with multiple patent but atherosclerotic vein grafts is the danger of atherosclerotic embolization during dissection of the beating heart.

Off-pump surgery is often effective in situations where single-vessel or single-area revascularization is all that is needed. For example, an atherosclerotic vein graft to the LAD system can be treated with a left internal thoracic artery (LITA) to LAD graft placed distal on the anterior descending to the old vein graft through a minimally invasive direct coronary artery bypass (MIDCAB) type small incision approach. Also, vessels in the circumflex territory can be grafted with off-pump operations performed through a left thoracotomy.

RISK OF RE-OPERATIONS

As a group, re-operations have been carried out at an increased risk relative to primary procedures. From the decade of 1980–1990 The Society of Thoracic Surgeons database documented mortality rates of 2.2% for 58,364 elective primary operations and 5.3% for 4954 elective re-operations. Updated statistics (1997–2000) from this voluntary database indicate risks of 1.91% for 340,458 elective primary procedures and 5.2% for 35,768 elective re-operations.

Of all the specific factors that increase the risk of a re-operation, the clearest is emergency status. For example, the 1997–2000 data from The Society of Thoracic Surgeons (STS) notes a risk of 9.14% for patients in the 'urgent/emergent/salvage' categories. Definitions of 'emergency' vary and in the STS registry 19% of re-operations were placed in the 'urgent/emergent/salvage' category. Absolute levels of risk during emergency operation will depend upon the definition of 'emergency' but all authors who have addressed this issue have documented a substantial increment in risk for emergency re-operations.

Other factors noted to be associated with increased risk of re-operation include congestive heart failure, advanced stage, female gender, and the presence of multiple atherosclerotic vein grafts [10, 13].

A factor that consistently impacts upon the risks and effectiveness of re-operation is diffuse coronary artery disease or 'bad vessels'. 'Bad vessels' is a variable that is difficult to quantify and, therefore, difficult to analyze. 'Bad vessels' represent a spectrum and the limits of graftability vary among institutions and surgeons. This variable is the most common reason surgeons feel patients are not candidates for re-operation and it is associated with in-hospital risk both because it makes revascularization imperfect and also because it tends to correlate with the presence of severe atherosclerosis in other vessels. The concept of 'complete revascularization' is rarely applicable to re-operative candidates. An incomplete or incompletely effective revascularization is a cause of perioperative myocardial ischemia or myocardial infarction.

The presence of patent arterial grafts has not been associated with an increased risk of re-operation. Reviewing patients with patent left ITA grafts we found a risk of in-hospital mortality of 3% and a risk of ITA damage of 3.3% [10]. Patients with previous bilateral ITA grafts have been at a slightly increased risk (four in-hospital deaths of 36 patients) in a small series [14]. The use of arterial grafts at a re-operation does not increase the risk of surgery in experienced hands. Patients receiving single or bilateral ITA grafts at re-operation were at a slightly lower risk in our series. Because many re-operative candidates have very diffuse coronary disease, arterial grafts often offer significant long-term advantages over vein grafts.

The one situation where the use of aterial grafts is awkward during a re-operation is if patients have vein grafts that are atherosclerotic but not severely stenotic [15]. In this situation if a patent vein graft is removed and replaced with an arterial graft there is a definite risk of hypoperfusion based on the difference in size and flow of arterial and venous grafts. On the other hand, if a vein graft is left in place and the arterial graft is grafted to the same vessel there is a danger of competitive flow leading to an

ITA 'string sign' if the vein graft lesion is not severe. If the vein graft lesion is severe ($\geq 50\%$) and the ITA is grafted to the same vessel, the likelihood is that the vein graft will become occluded and the ITA graft will stay functioning. Thus, when atherosclerotic vein grafts are not severely stenotic we usually replace them with vein grafts. When atherosclerotic vein grafts are severely stenotic we place arterial grafts distal to the vein grafts and leave the vein grafts in place.

Coronary re-operations are a type of operation where experience apparently lowers risk, and reports from centers performing a substantial volume of re-operations note lower risks than those general surveys of countrywide outcomes contained in the STS database. For example, review of The Cleveland Clinic Foundation data shows a hospital risk for an isolated coronary re-operation following a primary isolated coronary operation has been approximately 3.5% from the 1970s through to 1993. In more recent years the mortality rate has been 2.3% during 1999 (seven of 306) and 1.2% (three of 257) during 2000.

LATE OUTCOMES AFTER RE-OPERATION

In general the survival rates and symptom status of patients after re-operation are not quite as favorable as those after primary surgery. Due to diffuse coronary artery disease the degree of anatomic correction at re-operation tends to be not quite as 'perfect' as it is during primary procedures. The symptom status of patients after any treatment for coronary artery disease is a function of time and follow-up of patients after a first coronary re-operation has shown that five years later 40–50% of patients have some degree of symptoms [16]. However, in a relatively small number of cases are those patients severely symptomatic. Likewise, survival rates are not quite as favorable since five years after repeat surgery approximately 90% of patients are sill alive and 10 years after operation that figure

has dropped to 69% [9, 16]. However, it is important to remember that many of these patients undergo their re-operation more than 10 years after a previous procedure. Specific factors predicting a decreased later survival are left ventricular dysfunction, age, and risk factors for the development of further atherosclerosis including the presence of peripheral vascular disease, hypertension, and cigarette smoking. Also, the lack of internal thoracic artery grafts predicts a decrease in late survival.

MULTIPLE CORONARY RE-OPERATIONS

Patients with multiple previous procedures have all the risk factors of patients with a single previous operation, only more so. Lack of bypass conduits is a particularly consistent problem after multiple previous procedures and it is often necessary to employ radial arteries, the gastroepiploic artery, and/or lesser saphenous vein grafts. We have found that for our overall experience in third coronary re-operations that in-hospital mortality was 7% (33 of 469 patients through 1995). In more recent years (1993–1995) the mortality rate dropped to 4.3% and it was very low for patients less than 70 years of age (approximately 1%). However, for the elderly (> 70 years) risks were still greater than 10%. Long-term survival was also age-dependent. Approximately 80% of patients < 70 years of age were alive five years after a third operation compared with a 50% survival rate for patients over 70 years. Obviously, the prospect of recommending a third operation for someone over 70 should be carefully considered and should be undertaken only if the patient is highly and consistently symptomatic or in a life-threatening situation.

CONCLUSION

In coronary surgery, in-hospital risk is very much related to re-operation. Even in countrywide surveys, the short-term risks of primary procedures are low except in the setting of acute myocardial infarction or overwhelming co-morbid conditions. Much technical progress has been made toward increasing the safety of re-operation, but, with time, higher risk patients have been recruited into the re-operative population. The more extensive use of arterial grafts at primary operations, increased pharmacologic control of atherosclerosis, and more effective percutaneous procedures, may decrease the need for re-operation or at least delay re-operation for many patients. However, in the near future coronary re-operations will continue to give coronary surgeons their most difficult challenges.

REFERENCES

1. Lytle BW, Loop FD, Taylor PC et al. Vein graft disease: the clinical impact of stenoses in saphenous vein bypass grafts to coronary arteries, *J Thoracic Cardiovasc Surg* 1992; **103**:831–840.
2. Bourassa MG, Campeau L, Lesperance J. Changes in grafts and in coronary arteries after coronary bypass surgery, *Cardiovasc Clin* 1991; **21**:83–100.
3. Lytle BW, Cosgrove DM. Coronary artery bypass surgery. In: Wells SA, ed, *Current Problems in Surgery* (Philadelphia: WB Saunders, 1992) 733–807.
4. Neitzel GF, Barboriak JJ, Pintar K et al. Atherosclerosis in aortocoronary bypass grafts. Morphologic study and risk factor analysis six to 12 years after surgery, *Arteriosclerosis* 1986; **6**:594–600.
5. Lytle BW, Loop FD, Taylor PC et al. The effect of coronary re-operation on the survival of patients with stenoses in saphenous vein bypass grafts to coronary arteries, *J Thorac Cardiovasc Surg* 1993; **105**:605–614.
6. Lauer MS, Lytle B, Pashkow F, Snader CE, Marwick TH. Prediction of death and myocardial infarction by screening exercise-thallium testing after coronary-artery-bypass grafting, *Lancet* 1998; **351**:615–622.
7. Platko WP, Hollman J, Whitlow PL, Franco I. Percutaneous vs transluminal angioplasty of saphenous vein graft stenosis: long-term follow-up, *JACC* 1989; **14**:1645–1650.
8. Savage MP, Douglas JS, Fischman DL et al. Stent placement compared with balloon angioplasty for obstructed coronary bypass grafts, *N Engl J Med* 1997; **337**:740–747.
9. Loop FD, Lytle BW, Cosgrove DM et al. Re-operation for coronary atherosclerosis: changing practice in 2509 consecutive patients, *Ann Surg* 1990; **212**:378–386.
10. Lytle BW, McElroy D, McCarthy PM et al. The influence of arterial coronary bypass grafts on the mortality in coronary reoperations, *J Thorac Cardiovasc Surg* 1994; **107**:675–683.
11. Lytle BW, Navia JL, Taylor PC et al. Third coronary artery bypass operations: risks and costs, *Ann Thorac Surg* 1997; **64**:1287–1295.
12. Savage RM, Lytle BW, Aronson S et al. Intraoperative echocardiography is indicated in high-risk coronary artery bypass grafting, *Ann Thorac Surg* 1997; **64**:368–374.
13. Perrault L, Carrier M, Cartier R et al. Morbidity and mortality of re-operation for coronary artery bypass grafting: significance of atherosclerotic vein grafts, *Can J Cardiol* 1991; **7**:427–430.
14. Joyce FS, McCarthy PM, Taylor PC, Cosgrove DM, Lytle BW. Cardiac reoperation in patients with bilateral thoracic artery grafts, *Ann Thorac Surg* 1994; **58**:1353–1355.
15. Navia D, Cosgrove DM, Lytle BW et al. Is the internal mammary artery the conduit of choice to replace a stenotic vein graft? *Ann Thorac Surg* 1994; **107**:675–683.
16. Lytle BW, Loop FD, Cosgrove DM et al. Fifteen hundred coronary reoperations; results and determinants of early and late survival, *J Thorac Cardiovasc Surg* 1987; **93**:847–859.

19

Elective stenting of left main coronary artery disease

Seung-Jung Park

CONTENTS • Left main anatomy • Intervention for unprotected left main coronary artery stenosis • Device selection and technical considerations • IVUS guidance • Debulking before stenting • Angiographic restenosis • Long-term clinical outcomes • Future perspectives • Current recommendation • Intervention for protected left main coronary artery stenosis • Emergency intervention for unprotected LMCA stenosis

Coronary artery bypass graft surgery (CABG) remains the therapy of choice for left main coronary artery (LMCA) disease because of its proven benefit [1–6]. Since the first report of balloon angioplasty, percutaneous intervention has been investigated for treatment of LMCA stenosis [7–19]. Unfortunately, the initial experiences of patients undergoing unprotected LMCA interventions were discouraging because of procedural difficulty and an unacceptably high mortality. However, stenting has revolutionized the coronary intervention field, and it is widely performed in clinical practice [20–22]. Despite the initial skepticism of unprotected LMCA intervention [7–19], advances in techniques and equipment make it possible to expand the use of angioplasty to unprotected LMCA stenosis. Recently, it has been shown that stenting may be a promising alternative to bypass surgery in some patients with unprotected LMCA stenosis [23, 24]. Clearly, unprotected LMCA intervention is an attractive area for continued investigation, requiring further studies before this approach eventually translates into a practical, safe and effective therapy for patients with these lesions. In this chapter, we review and update the current literature concerning the intervention of unprotected LMCA stenosis.

LEFT MAIN ANATOMY

The LMCA is the origin of the left coronary artery, which contains three portions: the ostium, the trunk and the distal portion. Its normal diameter is 4.5 ± 0.5 mm in men, and 3.9 ± 0.4 in women. The LMCA ostium characteristically lacks adventitia and has considerable smooth muscle and elastic tissue, with aortic smooth muscle arranged perpendicular to and surrounding the ostium. There are many causes of LMCA stenosis, but most of these are related to atherosclerosis (Table 19.1). LMCA disease usually occurs with disease of the other coronary arteries, and LMCA atheroma is rarely isolated. Patients with LMCA stenosis has been traditionally classified by two subgroups: protected (a previous patent CABG to one or more major branches of the left coronary artery or good right-to-left collateral vessels) and unprotected LMCA diseases (without such bypasses or collateral vessels). The distinction between protected and unprotected LMCA stenosis plays an important role in determining treatment strategies for these patients.

INTERVENTION FOR UNPROTECTED LEFT MAIN CORONARY ARTERY STENOSIS

Balloon angioplasty—the past

LMCA stenosis may be considered as an attractive target for balloon angioplasty because of its larger caliber, short lesion length and lack of tortuosity. However, the results of balloon angioplasty were not favorable with high procedural complications, and early mortality [7–10]. For this reason, the American College of Cardiology/American Heart Association task force regarded balloon angioplasty of unprotected LMCA stenosis as an absolute contraindication [25]. Histologically, the LMCA has the most elastic tissue of the coronary vessel,

accounting for the poor response of the LMCA to simple balloon angioplasty. However, coronary stents have shown to reduce the immediate need for CABG for abrupt vessel closure and the likelihood of restenosis after balloon angioplasty [22]. At present, new devices are widely used to overcome the limitations of balloon angioplasty, and may also be useful to treat unprotected LMCA stenosis in particular groups of patients.

New devices, current status

The recent progress in techniques and equipment has driven the unprotected LMCA stenosis to the forefront of interventional cardiology, making it an inviting target for percutaneous intervention. Now, stenting of unprotected LMCA stenosis is considered as a therapeutic option in selected patients, and recent data in elective intervention are summarized in Table 19.2 and Table 19.3 [19, 23, 24, 26–32].

The ULTIMA experience

A multicenter registry from 25 centers ($n = 107$) was developed to study the initial and long-term outcome of patients who might be considered for percutaneous intervention of unprotected LMCA stenosis [18]. Technical success was achieved in 96.4%, but in-hospital death occurred in 20.6%, and non-fatal Q wave myocardial infarction in 10.1%. Furthermore, post-hospital discharge outcome was also unfavorable. However, the ULTIMA registry data had some limitations because it was composed of a very heterogeneous group: poor and good left ventricular function, different extent of the disease, different kind of intervention used. Despite this limitation, this study revealed that left ventricular function is the most important predictor of in-hospital mortality (Table 19.4) and long-term event free survival (Table 19.5).

Table 19.1 Etiology of left main coronary artery disease

Atherosclerosis

Non-atherosclerosis

    Idiopathic

    Radiation

    Takayasu's arteritis

    Syphilitic aortitis

    Rheumatoid arthritis

    Aortic valve disease

    Kawasaki disease

    Injury after left main coronary intervention or cardiac surgery

Table 19.2 In-hospital outcome of unprotected LMCA intervention

Series	n	Technical success (%)	Death (%)	Non-fatal MI (%)	Non-fatal CABG (%)
Stertzer et al [27]	12	83	0	0	16
O'Keefe et al [8]	33	NA	9	0	NA
Ellis et al [18]	91	99	12	4	1
Park et al [23]	42	100	0	0	0
Laruelle et al [28]	10	100	0	10	0
Cortina et al [29]	57	100	7	0	0
Silvestri et al [30]	51	100	4	0	0
Kosuga et al [31]	94	97	4	1.4	0
Tamura et al [32]	38	100	3	0	0

NA, not available.

Table 19.3 Long-term outcome of unprotected LMCA intervention

Series	n	Mean FU (months)	Late death (%)	Event-free survival (%)	Restenosis (%)
Stertzer et al [28]	12	40	8	50	NA
O'Keefe et al [8]	26	20	65	30	NA
Ellis et al [18]*	91	12	17	68	17
Park et al [23]**	42	10	2	78	22
Laruelle et al [28]	10	10	10	80	NA
Cortina et al [29]	57	6	9	NA	NA
Silvestri et al [30]	51	16	2	NA	NA
Kosuga et al [31]	94	34	16	NA	47
Tamura et al [32]	38	NA	10	0	0

*Restenosis data are derived from a subgroup of patients. **Angiographic restenosis data from 34 patients. Late deaths mean death after hospital discharge. Events include death, MI and revascularization from index intervention.

Asan medical center experience

The initial report from the ULTIMA registry still demonstrated relatively high subacute cardiac mortality in this heterogenous group of patients. Many of these patients were high risk or ineligible for bypass surgery, and a low left ventricular ejection fraction was inversely related to the event rate [18]. Therefore, in the current study, only patients who had a left ventricular function ≥ 40% were included.

By January 2001, unprotected LMCA stenting had been performed in 156 consecutive patients with normal left ventricular function at our institution, and typical examples are shown in Fig. 19.1. The procedural success rate was 99.1% and 17 patients (13%) received multi-vessel angioplasty during the intervention.

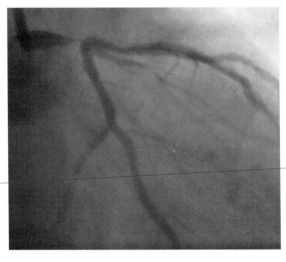

(a)

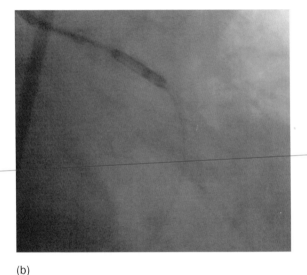

(b)

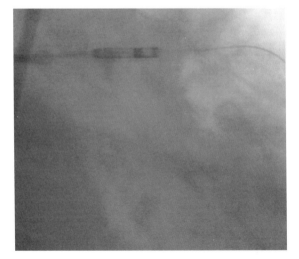

(c)

(d)

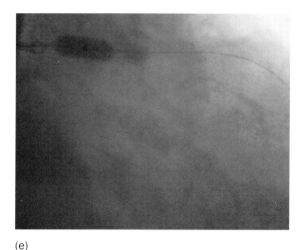

(e)

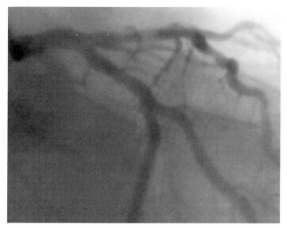

(g)

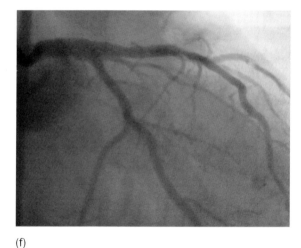

(f)

Figure 19.1   (a) Unprotected left main coronary artery bifurcation lesion. (b) Directional atherectomy at main bifurcation to LAD ostium. (c) Directional atherectomy at LCX ostium. (d) NIR (3.0 mm × 25 mm) stenting to pLAD. (e) NIR (4.0 mm × 9 mm) stenting at left main. (f) Final result showing no residual narrowing. (g) Six months follow-up angiogram showing no restenosis.

Table 19.4 Correlates of in-hospital death*

	Adjusted OR	95% CI	Multivariate *p*
Left ventricular ejection fraction	0.89	0.083–0.96	0.003
Primary treatment with stent	0.06	0.005–0.67	0.023

*Excludes patients presenting with acute myocardial infarction.

Table 19.5 Independent correlates of event-free survival*

	Est	SD	95% CI	t	p
Left ventricular ejection fraction	0.09	0.02	0.05–0.12	4.41	< 0.001
Progressive/rest angina	−1.90	0.73	−3.32−−0.48	−2.62	0.009
Treatment with DCA	1.31	0.67	0.002–2.62	1.96	0.05

DCA, debulking coronary atherectomy; *Excludes patients presenting with acute myocardial infarction.

Various types of stents were used. Tubular stents were preferred for the lesions of the left main ostium and shaft. For treatment of the LMCA bifurcation lesions, we used a combination of coil and tubular stents in a few cases. However, debulking before stenting may be more useful for these bifurcation lesions. If we can get a stent-like result after a debulking procedure on the proximal part of major arteries, we may be able to avoid multiple stenting in some cases. There were no procedure-related deaths. However, one patient developed a coronary perforation after directional coronary atherectomy, which was successfully treated with grafted stent. During the hospital stay, angiographically documented stent thrombosis occurred in one patient at day three after intervention, being complicated by a Q wave acute myocardial infarction. He was a 67-year-old man with diffuse involvement of LMCA and left anterior descending coronary artery. He underwent elective CABG 30 days after stenting, and has been well until the time of writing. In the remaining patients, the in-hospital clinical outcome was uneventful.

Angiographic follow-up data were obtained for 100 of the 104 eligible patients (follow-up rate, 96%). Restenosis was angiographically documented in 19 patients (19%).

DEVICE SELECTION AND TECHNICAL CONSIDERATIONS

Optimal lesions for intervention

The anatomic location of the stenosis should be considered before the procedure. Isolated LMCA stenosis limited to the ostium or shaft is an optimal candidate for stenting because technically it is easy. If the lesions involve the LMCA bifurcation area, CABG may be desirable because of the concern for major side branch occlusion. However, in some cases, percutaneous intervention may be considered in experienced centers if technically feasible.

Coronary stents

The high concentration of elastic fibers in the aorto-ostial and proximal segments of the LMCA has been proposed as the possible mechanism of elastic recoil and high restenosis rate of conventional balloon angioplasty at these sites. Stents have been demonstrated to reduce acute recoil and restenosis after coronary angioplasty, and it may also be true in patients with unprotected LMCA stenosis. The slotted-tube stents, instead of coil stents, are preferable for treatment of LMCA ostial disease because of their strong radial force (Fig. 19.2). Conversely, coiled stents may be considered for distal bifurcation lesion. Stent size is selected based on the reference artery size and lesion length. We usu-

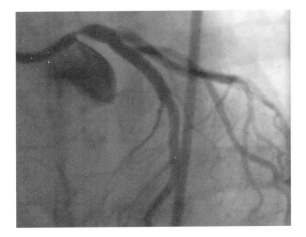

(a)

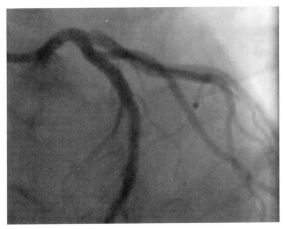

(c)

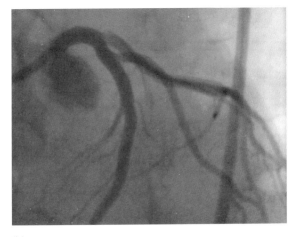

(b)

Figure 19.2 (a) Left coronary angiogram showed critical narrowing at the ostium of left main coronary artery. (b) The stent was deployed when 1–2 mm of the proximal part of the strut was hanging out into the aorta. Left coronary angiogram showed that there was no residual stenosis at left main coronary ostium after 4.0 × 9 mm new intravascular rigid (NIR) stenting. (c) Six-month angiogram showed widely patent NIR stent at left main.

ally deploy the stent so that it slightly protrudes into the aorta (1–2 mm) for treatment of LMCA ostial lesions. The predilation before stenting is usually performed with undersized, conventional angioplasty balloons. The stent is then deployed by inflating the stent delivery balloon at normal or high pressure. After the deployment of the stent, the stented segment is further dilated with high-pressure balloon inflation to achieve angiographic optimization. The balloon inflation is brief (< 30 seconds) and multiple (> 3) to avoid prolonged global ischemia and ischemia-related complications. Percutaneous

intervention of unprotected LMCA bifurcation lesion remains technically difficult.

New techniques and devices have been developed for the treatment of coronary artery bifurcation lesions with acceptable clinical outcomes [13]. These techniques can also be used for unprotected LMCA bifurcation lesions, and we usually use two strategies for this condition: strategy I (stenting alone) and strategy II (debulking atherectomy plus stenting). Strategy I is selected if the atheromatous plaque is mild or uniformly distributed. A tube stent is implanted from the LMCA to the proximal portion of the left anterior descending coronary artery if the left circumflex artery is dimunitive or its ostium is not significantly narrowed (Fig. 19.1). In contrast, Y-shaped stenting is performed if the left circumflex artery is dominant and its ostium severely narrowed: a coil stent is implanted from the LMCA to the angulated artery (left circumflex artery or left anterior descending coronary artery), and another slotted-tube stent placed into the straight artery (left anterior descending coronary artery or left circumflex artery) through the struts of coil stent. Strategy II is selected if a large eccentric plaque is present at the LMCA bifurcation site. The stenting strategy is the same as described above.

Percutaneous intervention of unprotected LMCA bifurcation lesions is technically difficult, and remains a challenging area. In our study, stenting with ($n = 34$) or without debulking atherectomy ($n = 8$) was performed in 42 patients with an unprotected LMCA bifurcation lesion and normal left ventricular function. Procedural success rate was 100%. In-hospital events did not occur in any patients. Angiographic restenosis rate was 12.5% (4/32), and target lesion revascularization was required in three patients. Stenting with or without debulking atherectomy for an unprotected LMCA bifurcation lesion may be performed with a high procedure success rate and a favorable clinical outcome in selected patients with normal left ventricular function.

IVUS GUIDANCE

Although intravascular ultrasound (IVUS) provides lots of quantitative and qualitative information on coronary artery lesions compared with stenting without use of IVUS, no study had clearly demonstrated the benefit of its performance for the long-term clinical outcome. Recently, Fitzgerald et al, reporting on the CRUISE data, suggested that IVUS-guided stent implantation may result in more effective stent expansion and less frequent target vessel

revascularization [33]. Although post-stent minimum lumen diameter (MLD) was significantly larger in IVUS-guided group (4.2 mm vs 4.0 mm, $p = 0.003$), angiographic restenosis rate and target lesion revascularization rate were not different between IVUS-guided and angiography-guided procedure in this study (Table 19.6). This finding may be explained partly by the fact that the reference vessel size in the current series was large (4.0 mm) and the post-stent MLD was also large (4.0 mm), even in the angiography-guided group. A post-stent MLD of 4.0 mm should be large enough to maintain the final MLD without angiographic restenosis at follow-up.

It is often difficult to evaluate the actual size of the LMCA on angiography [34]. Intravascular ultrasound before stenting, therefore, provides useful information about the selection of adequate size of balloons and stents, and accurate amounts and the extent of calcification [35]. In IVUS-guided stenting of ostial LMCA lesions, negative remodeling was documented in 91% in the present study. In these particular cases of ostial lesions with negative remodeling and consequently small amounts of plaque volumes, the treatment strategies should be changed from debulking with stenting to stenting only. A previous IVUS study showed that the pre-intervention IVUS procedure contributed to change in treatment modalities in 40% of non-LMCA lesions [35]. Moreover, additional high-pressure balloon dilation was done in 19.5% of 77 lesions with IVUS-guided stenting, despite angiographic optimization. This resulted in the enlargement of post-intervention stent cross-sectional area (CSA).

In any case, IVUS evaluation after stenting has a critical role in achieving the optimal stent expansion and apposition. Even though the incidence of stent thrombosis was quite low in unprotected LMCA stenting, it may potentially lead to a fatal outcome. Therefore, post-stent IVUS evaluation should be considered despite angiographic optimization.

Table 19.6 Baseline angiographic characteristics and procedural results (%)

	IVUS-guided	Angiography-guided	p
Number of lesions	77	50	
Lesion site			0.103
Os	40 (52)	19 (38)	
Body	13 (17)	6 (12)	
Bifurcation	24 (31)	25 (50)	
Debulking before stenting	30 (39)	10 (20)	0.019
Lesion morphology			0.816
A	11 (14)	5 (10)	
B1	26 (34)	15 (30)	
B2	27 (35)	20 (40)	
C	13 (17)	10 (20)	
Reference vessel diameter (mm)	4.0 ± 0.7	4.0 ± 0.6	0.463
Minimal lumen diameter (mm)			
Pre-intervention	1.2 ± 0.5	1.0 ± 0.5	0.020
Post-intervention	4.2 ± 0.6	4.0 ± 0.6	0.003
Follow-up	2.7 ± 1.0	2.7 ± 1.0	0.976
Pressure (atm)	15.1 ± 2.6	15.3 ± 2.8	0.327
Angiographic follow-up (%)	59/63 (94)	41/43 (95)	0.532
Angiographic restenosis rate (%)	11/59 (18.6)	8/41 (19.5)	0.556

DEBULKING BEFORE STENTING

In our study, the cases of rotational atherectomy as a debulking procedure were excluded. By removing the plaque, directional coronary atherectomy may facilitate successful stent placement. A recent study showed that, like non-stented lesions, residual plaque burden was also an important predictor of intimal hyperplasia in stented lesions [36], and the aggressive debulking with directional atherectomy before stenting might reduce the residual plaque burdens and subsequently the restenosis as well [37]. The degree of debulking using directional atherectomy was 30%, compatible to that of other reports [37–39]. In univariate analysis, debulking before stenting resulted in a significant reduction of angiographic restenosis. However, the benefit of debulking atherectomy was not found to be significant in multivariate analysis. Based on our data, the reference vessel size of LMCA varied from 2.3 mm to 5.8 mm and 57% of patients who had follow-up angiograms had large reference vessels of more than 4.0 mm. The most likely explanation is that the degree of debulking might be relatively insufficient in such large vessels because of the limited device size. In the large vessels, we could achieve a large MLD after stent deployment using only high-pressure balloon dilatation without debulking. Therefore, the effect of debulking seemed to be less in these vessels. Although there was no statistical significance, the benefit of debulking may be more crucial in

Table 19.7 Angiographic restenosis rate according to debulking and reference vessel size

Reference vessel size	Debulking and stenting	Stenting alone	p value
$\leqslant 3.5$	1/8 (6%)	8/20 (40%)	0.159
> 3.5	2/28 (7%)	8/44 (18%)	0.187

those vessels which are relatively small, less than 3.5 mm (Table 19.7). On the other hand, from a technical viewpoint, this debulking strategy may be more useful for treatment of distal LMCA bifurcation stenosis. The removal of a certain degree of plaque burden may lead to an improvement in initial outcome of stenting procedure by preventing plaque displacement for these lesions.

Regardless, it is notable that the debulking and stenting patients had a lower restenosis rate even though the reference diameter, quantitative coronary arteriography or angiography (QCA), final MLD, and IVUS final lumen were similar to the stenting-alone patients. This suggests that the plaque itself may contribute to the restenosis process and supports the promise that debulking and stenting may reduce restenosis.

ANGIOGRAPHIC RESTENOSIS

Decreasing reference vessel size could be related to increasing restenosis, because late lumen loss may be greater in stents implanted into small vessels rather than those implanted into large vessels [40]. As in previous studies, in non-LMCA lesions [41, 42] and protected LMCA stenting [43], the post-stent MLD and minimal lumen CSA by IVUS were the most powerful predictors of angiographic restenosis.

Although in univariate analysis there was a trend for lower restenosis rates in the debulking and large post-stent MLD group (Table 19.8), the reference artery size was the only independent predictor of angiographic restenosis in

multivariate analysis in this study. We found a clear difference in restenosis rate depending on the reference vessel size because our data included a variety of reference vessel sizes from 2.3 mm to 5.8 mm. The factor of reference vessel size shown in our study may subsume the significance of those factors (post-stent MLD, minimal lumen CSA) that have been identified previously in the literature.

Based on our current analysis, the angiographic restenosis rate was statistically higher in the group with less than 3.6 mm size of reference vessel. This cut-off level of 3.6 mm vessel size is an arbitrary lower threshold and although 31% of restenosis rate in those vessels might be slightly higher than that of non-LMCA stenting, it still is acceptable.

LONG-TERM CLINICAL OUTCOMES

In the present study the cumulative survival rate was $97.0 \pm 1.7\%$, and the cardiac event-free survival rate $86.9 \pm 3.3\%$ at two years (Fig. 19.3)—figures consistent with those reported in the low-risk group of patients [44].

One year mortality after CABG for a low-risk group similar to that identified in this study was 5.7% [45]. The mortality rate in our series over the two year follow-up was 3.1%, which could be acceptable. Among the four deaths, only one death was associated with extensive myocardial infarction immediately after CABG for treatment of restenosis. Angina recurrence generally developed within three months after stenting in 80% (12/15) of patients who had a clinical symptom recurrence, and thereafter

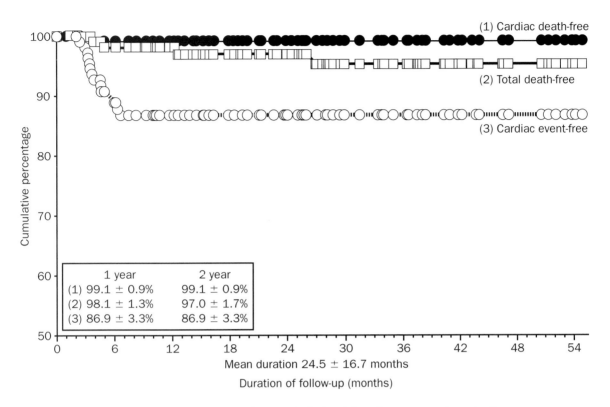

Figure 19.3 Two-year cumulative and event-free survival after left main coronary artery stenting.

most patients were free of symptoms without major adverse cardiac events.

For the patients with restenosis, CABG was recommended first. However, 47% of restenotic patients (9/19) received repeat angioplasty using rotational atherectomy. In cases of long main shaft, radiation therapy with ^{188}Re was done after rotational atherectomy. After repeat intervention, only one developed restenosis 17 months after the procedure and was subsequently operated on. The remaining eight patients who had a repeat intervention were free of symptoms over the two year follow-up.

After six months, there were no cardiac deaths or target lesion revascularizations, indicating that the long-term clinical course may be excellent after unprotected LMCA stenting in

selected patients with normal left ventricular function. This result is consistent with previously published data showing that the restenotic process after stenting is time-limited, and that little progression occurs beyond six months [46, 47].

FUTURE PERSPECTIVES

LMCA disease: is stenting an alternative to CABG?

Long-term clinical outcomes should be scrutinized before stenting is recommended as a therapeutic option for unprotected LMCA stenosis. Historical data show clear survival benefits of

CABG for LMCA disease compared to conservative therapy. Therefore, CABG has been the standard treatment for LMCA disease. However, there is still a 1.5–3% perioperative morbidity and mortality, longer hospital stay and delayed social recovery with CABG.

Our data support the feasibility of unprotected LMCA stenting in highly selected patients since there were no serious procedure-related complications and excellent long-term clinical outcomes. In the stent era, if the patients have no angiographic restenosis after six months of follow-up (80%), the patients with stenting may have long-term survival benefit compared with those patients who have had several arterial bypass grafts. However, in reality, more than half of patients who undergo CABG receive a single arterial graft and several

Table 19.8 Univariate predictors of angiographic restenosis

	Total	Restenosis	No restenosis	OR (95% CI)	p value
Angiography	**n = 100**	**n = 19**	**n = 81**		
Ref MLD (mm)	4.0 ± 0.7	3.7 ±0.6	4.1 ± 0.7	0.39 (0.17–0.87)	0.021
Pre MLD (mm)	1.1 ± 0.5	1.1 ± 0.5	1.1 ± 0.5	1.80 (0.63–5.18)	0.275
Final MLD (mm)	4.2 ± 0.6	3.9 ± 0.5	4.2 ± 0.6	0.46 (0.19–1.07)	0.072
Pressure (atm)	15.2 ± 2.7	15.1 ± 2.4	15.3 ± 2.9	0.94 (0.78–1.12)	0.480
Debulking	36	3	33	0.27 (0.07–1.01)	0.052
IVUS					
Pre-intervention	**n = 43**	**n = 9**	**n = 34**		
Distal Ref segment					
Lumen MLD	3.1 ± 0.6	2.7 ± 0.3	3.2 ± 0.6	0.11 (0.02–0.80)	0.029
Lumen CSA	9.3 ± 3.3	7.0 ± 1.4	9.9 ± 3.5	0.66 (0.45–0.97)	0.037
EEM CSA	18.2 ± 5.4	15.3 ± 3.7	18.9 ± 5.5	0.86 (0.73–1.02)	0.077
Lesion segment					
Lumen MLD	1.7 ± 0.3	1.7 ± 0.2	1.7 ± 0.3	0.92 (0.08–10.54)	0.949
Lumen CAS	2.9 ± 1.1	2.8 ± 0.7	2.9 ± 1.2	0.88 (0.43–1.81)	0.724
EEM CSA	16.5 ± 6.6	16.1 ± 6.5	16.6 ± 6.7	0.99 (0.88–1.11)	0.839
Post-intervention	**n = 59**	**n = 11**	**n = 48**		
Distal Ref segment					
Lumen MLD	3.5 ± 0.5	3.3 ± 0.5	3.5 ± 0.5	0.53 (0.15–1.85)	0.319
Lumen CSA	11.1 ± 2.8	10.0 ± 2.7	11.4 ± 2.8	0.84 (0.67–1.06)	0.138
EEM CSA	19.1 ± 5.1	17.4 ± 5.2	19.5 ± 5.0	0.92 (0.80–1.05)	0.192
Lesion segment					
Lumen MLD	3.6 ± 0.5	3.4 ± 0.3	3.6 ± 0.5	0.41 (0.11–1.59)	0.198
Lumen CSA	12.1 ± 3.0	10.8 ± 1.8	12.4 ± 3.2	0.82 (0.65–1.04)	0.103

CSA, cross-sectional area; EEM, external elastic membrane; MLD, minimal lumen diameter; Ref, reference vessel.

vein grafts. The long-term survival benefit of stenting should be compatible to that of CABG in which vein graft conduits are used.

Left main coronary artery disease is typically associated with the involvement of the other segments of the coronary arteries and the diffuse pattern in some cases. In our institution, only 35% of LMCA stenosis could be selected for elective stenting and stenting should not be generalized as a new treatment modality for most patients with unprotected LMCA stenosis. However, in highly selected patients with normal left ventricular function and who have lesions confined to the limited left main area, we believe that stenting may be a reasonable alternative to surgery.

CURRENT RECOMMENDATION

Stenting may certainly be a novel therapeutic strategy in patients with unprotected LMCA stenosis. However, it should be reserved for patients who are not candidates for CABG, who refuse CABG, or selected patients with normal left ventricular function. Stenting with or without debulking procedures appears to be a reasonable approach in these patients. Extra caution may, however, be warranted for patients with impaired left ventricular function, and an intra-aortic pump should be considered.

INTERVENTION FOR PROTECTED LEFT MAIN CORONARY ARTERY STENOSIS

Over the past 25 years, CABG has demonstrated excellent short-term and long-term clinical results for patients with LMCA disease, and the treatment of this lesion has therefore largely remained the turf of the cardiovascular surgeon. However, there is still a need for retreatment of the LMCA stenosis due to progression of native coronary artery disease or bypass graft failure [48–50]. Initial experiences with balloon angioplasty for this lesion were not good, with high procedural complications and late restenosis. Conventional balloon angioplasty may not be effective in treating this lesion because protected LMCA usually has a heavy plaque burden and calcification. In previous studies, balloon angioplasty of LMCA stenosis usually resulted in sub-optimal results, leading to restenosis and the need for repeat revascularization in 30–50% of patients, limiting the utility of this procedure [8, 10]. However, now we have stents, which reduce or eliminate elastic recoil and several studies have shown that stenting of protected LMCA stenosis can be performed safely with a high success rate and favorable clinical outcome (Table 19.9 and Table 19.10) [10, 11, 51, 52].

In a recent study [53], Kornowski et al reported that stents reduce major in-hospital complications, but may not significantly reduce repeat revascularization or major cardiac events at one year compared with non-stent LMCA procedures. In their study, diabetes mellitus (OR = 3.2, $p = 0.04$) independently predicted target lesion revascularization and the final lumen diameter (OR = 0.3, $p = 0.017$) was negatively associated with target lesion revascularization. Nevertheless, the use of stents, either alone or after initial rotational atherectomy, may certainly produce better immediate angiographic results than those in other lesion locations. Technical considerations are similar to those of unprotected LMCA intervention, and precise positioning of the stent is an important technical point to be noted as described above. In addition, pretreatment of heavily calcified LMCA lesions with rotational atherectomy may permit optimal stent expansion with a lower residual stenosis and better clinical outcome. This hypothesis of transdevice synergy appears reasonable, but remains unproven. Unfortunately, despite the widespread use of stents, no comparative data is yet available in a patient population that has had alternative treatment like repeated bypass surgery. However, we are convinced that modern stent techniques have evolved to a point that stenting may be a logical and viable option for protected LMCA stenosis.

Table 19.9 In-hospital outcome of protected LMCA intervention

Series	n	Technical success (%)	Death (%)	Non-fatal MI (%)	Non-fatal CABG (%)
Stertzer et al [27]	8	87	0	0	0
O'Keefe et al [8]	84	NA	2.4	0	NA
Eldar et al [10]	8	100	0	0	0
Crowley et al [48]	12	100	0	0	0
Lopez et al [11]	46	100	0	0	0
Chauhan et al [49]	14	100	0	0	0
Kornowski et al [41]	124	98	1	1	1

NA, not available.

Table 19.10 Long-term outcome of protected LMCA intervention

Series	n	Mean FU (months)	Late death (%)	Event-free survival (%)	Restenosis CABG (%)
Stertzer et al [27]	8	46	0	75	NA
O'Keefe et al [8]	67	20	10	78	NA
Eldar et al [10]	8	24	0	88	38
Crowley et al [48]	12	17	8	92	33
Lopez et al [11]	46	9	2	93	13
Chauhan et al [49]	14	16	14	64	43
Kornowski et al [41]	124	12	0	77	17

NA, not available; Late deaths mean death after hospital discharge. Events include death, MI and revascularization from index intervention.

EMERGENCY INTERVENTION FOR UNPROTECTED LMCA STENOSIS

Procedure-related complications

Any LMCA dissection following coronary angiography or interventional procedure is a rare but serious complication [54, 55]. Careful observation or elective CABG may be a reasonable approach for a non-flow-limiting dissection. However, emergent CABG or bail-out stenting should be performed for a flow-limiting dissection of the LMCA [15, 16]. Until now, there are few reports in the literature highlighting the optimal treatment strategies for patients with complications of LMCA instrumentation. Although elective stenting is still not recommended for unprotected LMCA stenosis, bail-out stenting appears to be very effective as a salvage procedure in these situations.

Acute myocardial infarction

Primary angioplasty has been widely performed for treatment of patients with acute myocardial infarction (AMI) because of a higher rate of recanalization and a better clinical outcome compared with thrombolysis [56, 57]. However, there is paucity of data reporting outcomes of AMI patients with acute closure of the LMCA, and therefore the role of primary angioplasty remains uncertain [51, 52, 58, 59]. Most patients initially presented with cardiogenic shock, requiring aggressive mechanical support. These patients, unlike other forms of AMI, have a high in-hospital mortality and morbidity because of left ventricular pump failure. A recent report from the ULTIMA registry suggests that primary stenting is feasible and may be the preferred initial revascularization strategy for these patients [58]. However, in-hospital cardiac death rates are still very high, occurring in > 50% of patients undergoing primary angioplasty because it cannot prevent acute left ventricular failure. Therefore, new approaches, such as early catheter-based reperfusion therapy plus left ventricular assistic device insertion, should be investigated to overcome acute left ventricular failure in this setting.

REFERENCES

1. Caracciolo EA, Davis KB, Sopko G et al. Comparison of surgical and medical group survival in patients with left main coronary artery disease: long-term CASS experience, *Circulation* 1995; **91**:2325–2334.
2. Oberman A, Harrell RR, Russel RO Jr et al. Surgical versus medical treatment in disease of the left main coronary artery, *Lancet* 1976; **2**:591–594.
3. McConahay DR, Killen DA, McCallister BD et al. Coronary artery bypass surgery for left main coronary artery disease, *Am J Cardiol* 1976; **37**:885–889.
4. Cohen MV, Gorlin R. Main left coronary artery disease. Clinical experience from 1964–1974, *Circulation* 1975; **52**:275–285.
5. Farinha JB, Kaplan MA, Harris CN et al. Surgical treatment and long-term follow-up in 267 patients, *Am J Cardiol* 1978; **42**:124–128.
6. Taylor HA, Deumite NJ, Chaitman BR et al. Asymptomatic left main coronary artery disease in the Coronary Artery Surgery Study (CASS) registry, *Circulation* 1989; **79**:1171–1179.
7. Gruentzig AR, Senning A, Siegenthaler WE. Non-operative dilatation of coronary artery stenosis, *N Engl J Med* 1979; **301**:61–67.
8. O'Keefe JH, Hartzler GO, Rutherford BD et al. Left main coronary angioplasty: early and late results of 127 acute and elective procedures, *Am J Cardiol* 1989; **64**:144–147.
9. Hartzler GO, Rutherford BD, McConohay DR, Johnson WL, Giorgi LV. High-risk percutaneous transluminal coronary angioplasty, *Am J Cardiol* 1988; **61**:33G–37G.
10. Eldar M, Schulhoff RN, Hertz I et al. Results of percutaneous transluminal coronary angioplasty of the left main coronary artery, *Am J Cardiol* 1991; **68**:255–256.
11. Lopez JJ, Ho KK, Stoler RC et al. Percutaneous treatment of protected and unprotected left main coronary stenosis with new devices; immediate angiographic results and intermediate-term follow-up, *J Am Coll Cardiol* 1997; **29**: 345–352.
12. Laham RJ, Carrozza JP, Baim DS. Treatment of unprotected left main stenoses with Palmaz-Schatz stenting, *Cathet Cardiovasc Diagn* 1996; **37**:77–80.
13. Dauerman HL, Higgins PJ, Sparano AM et al. Mechanical debulking versus balloon angioplasty for the treatment of true bifurcation lesions, *J Am Coll Cardiol* 1998; **32**:1845–1852.
14. Macaya C, Alfonso F, Iniguez A et al. Stenting for elastic recoil during coronary angioplasty of the left main coronary artery, *Am J Cardiol* 1992; **70**:105–107.
15. Sathe S, Sebastian M, Vohra J, Valentine P. Bailout stenting for left main coronary artery occlusion following diagnostic angiography, *Cathet Cardiovasc Diagn* 1994; **31**:70–72.
16. Garcia-Robles JA, Garcia E, Rico M et al. Emergency coronary stenting for acute occlusive dissection of the left main coronary artery, *Cathet Cardiovasc Diagn* 1993; **30**:227–229.
17. Tamura T, Nobuyoshi M, Nosaka H et al. Palmaz-Schatz stenting in unprotected and

protected left main coronary artery: immediate and follow-up results, *Circulation* 1996; **94**:I671.

18. Ellis SG, Tamai H, Nobuyoshi M et al. Contemporary percutaneous treatment of unprotected left main stenoses: initial results from a multicenter registry analysis 1994–1996, *Circulation* 1997; **96**: 3867–3872.

19. Karam C, Jordan C, Fajadet J et al. Six-month follow-up of unprotected left main coronary artery stenting, *Circulation* 1996; **94**:I672.

20. Colombo A, Hall P, Nakamura S et al. Intracoronary stenting without anticoagulation accomplished with intravascular ultrasound guidance, *Circulation* 1995; **91**:1676–1688.

21. Schomig A, Neumann FJ, Kastrati A et al. A randomized comparison of antiplatelet and anticoagulant therapy after the placement of coronary artery stents, *N Engl J Med* 1996; **334**:1084–1089.

22. Bittl JA. Advances in coronary angioplasty, *New Engl J Med* 1996; **335**:1290–1302.

23. Park SJ, Park SW, Hong MK et al. Stenting of unprotected left main coronary artery stenoses: immediate and late outcome, *J Am Coll Cardiol* 1998; **31**:37–42.

24. Kosuga K, Tamai H, Ueda K et al. Initial and long-term results of angioplasty in unprotected left main coronary artery, *Am J Cardiol* 1999; **83**:32–37.

25. Ryan TJ, Faxon DP, Weinber SL. Guidelines for percutaneous transluminal coronary angioplasty. A report of the American College of Cardiology/American Heart Association Task Force on the assessment of diagnostic and therapeutic cardiovascular procedures, *Circulation* 1988; **78**:486–502.

26. Kapadia SR, Ellis SG. Non-surgical management of left main coronary artery disease, *Indian Heart J* 1998; **50**:67–73.

27. Stertzer SH, Myler RK, Insel H, Wallsh E, Rossi P. Percutaneous transluminal coronary angioplasty in left main stem coronary stenosis: a five-year appraisal, *Int J Cardiol* 1985; **9**:149–159.

28. Laruelle CJ, Brueren GB, Ernst SM et al. Stenting of 'unprotected' left main coronary artery stenoses: early and late results, *Heart* 1998; **79**:148–152.

29. Cortina R, Fajadet J, Cassagneau B et al. Stenting of unprotected left main coronary artery stenosis: methodology, stent selection and clinical outcome, *J Am Coll Cardiol* 1998; **31**:180A.

30. Silvestri M, Barragan P, Roquebert PO et al. Unprotected left main coronary artery stenting: immediate and follow-up results, *Eur Heart J* 1997; **18**:27.

31. Kosuga K, Tamai H, Hsu Y-S et al. Initial and long-term results of elective angioplasty in unprotected left main coronary artery, *J Am Coll Cardiol* 1998; **31**:101A.

32. Tamura T, Kimura T, Nosaka H, Nobuyoshi M. Palmaz-Schatz stenting in unprotected left main coronary artery stenosis: immediate and follow-up results, *J Am Coll Cardiol* 1998; **31**: 273A.

33. Fitzgerald PJ, Oshima A, Hayase M et al. Final results of the Can Routine Ultrasound Influence Stent Expansion (CRUISE) study, *Circulation* 2000; **102**:523–530.

34. Hermiller JB, Buller CE, Tenaglia AN et al. Unrecognized left main coronary artery disease in patients undergoing interventional procedures, *Am J Cardiol* 1993; **71**:173–176.

35. Mintz GS, Pichard AD, Kovach JA et al. Impact of pre-intervention intravascular ultrasound imaging on transcatheter treatment strategies in coronary artery disease, *Am J Cardiol* 1994; **73**: 423–430.

36. Prati F, Di Mario C, Moussa I et al. In-stent neointimal proliferation correlates with the amount of residual plaque burden outside the stent: an intravascular ultrasound study, *Circulation* 1999; **99**:1011–1014.

37. Moussa I, Moses J, Mario CD et al. Stenting after optimal lesion debulking (SOLD) registry. Angiographic and clinical outcome, *Circulation* 1998; **98**:1604–1609.

38. Tsuchikane E, Sumitsuji S, Awata N et al. Final results of the stent versus directional coronary atherectomy randomized trial (START), *J Am Coll Cardiol* 1999; **34**:1050–1057.

39. Simonton CA, Leon MB, Baim DS et al. Optimal directional coronary atherectomy: final results of the optimal atherectomy restenosis study (OARS), *Circulation* 1998; **97**:332–339.

40. Hoffmann R, Mintz GS, Pichard AD et al. Intimal hyperplasia thickness at follow-up is independent of stent size: a serial intravascular ultrasound study, *Am J Cardiol* 1998; **82**:1168–1172.

41. Hoffmann R, Mintz GS, Mehran R et al. Intravascular ultrasound predictors of angiographic restenosis in lesions treated with Palmaz-Schatz stents, *J Am Coll Cardiol* 1998; **31**:43–49.

42. Kasaoka S, Tobis JM, Akiyama T et al. Angiographic and intravascular ultrasound predictors of in-stent restenosis, *J Am Coll Cardiol* 1998; **32**:1630–1635.

43. Hong MK, Mintz GS, Hong MK et al. Intravascular ultrasound predictors of target lesion revascularization after stenting of protected left main coronary artery stenoses, *Am J Cardiol* 1999: **83**;175–179.

44. Silvestri M, Baragan P, Sainous J et al. Unprotected left main coronary artery stenting: immediate and medium-term outcomes of 140 elective procedures, *J Am Coll Cardiol* 2000; **35**:1543–1550.

45. Ellis SG, Hill CM, Lytle BW. Spectrum of surgical risk for left main coronary stenosis: benchmark for potentially competing percutaneous therapies, *Am Heart J* 1998; **135**:335–338.

46. Kimura T, Yokoi N, Nakagawa Y et al. Three-year follow-up after implantation of metallic coronary-artery stents, *N Engl J Med* 1996; **334**:561–566.

47. Asakura M, Ueda Y, Nanto S et al. Remodeling of in-stent neointima, which became thinner and transparent over three years, *Circulation* 1998; **97**:2003–2006.

48. Loop FD, Lytle BW, Cosgrove DM et al. Atherosclerosis of the left main coronary artery: five year results of surgical management, *Am J Cardiol* 1979; **44**:195–201.

49. Campeau L, Corbara F, Crochet D, Petitclerc R. Left main coronary artery stenosis: the influence of aortocoronary bypass surgery on survival, *Circulation* 1978; **27**:1111–1115.

50. Bourassa MG, Fisher LD, Campeau L et al. Long-term fate of bypass grafts: the Coronary Artery Surgery Study (CASS) and Montreal Heart Institute experiences, *Circulation* 1985; **72** (Suppl V):V-71–V-78.

51. Crowley ST, Morrison DA. Percutaneous transluminal coronary angioplasty of the left main coronary artery in patients with rest angina, *Cathet Cardiovasc Diagn* 1994; **33**:103–107.

52. Chauhan A, Zubaid M, Ricci DR et al. Left main intervention revisited: early and late outcome of PTCA and stenting, *Cathet Cardiovasc Diagn* 1997; **41**:21–29.

53. Kornowski R, Klutstein M, Satler LF et al. Impact of stents on clinical outcomes in percutaneous left main coronary artery revascularization, *Am J Cardiol* 1998; **82**:32–37.

54. Devlin G, Lazzam L, Schwartz L. Mortality related to diagnostic cardiac catheterization: the importance of left main coronary disease and catheter induced trauma, *Int J Cardiac Imaging* 1997; **13**:379–384.

55. Kovac JD, de Bono DP. Cardiac catheter complications related to left main stem disease, *Heart* 1996; **76**:76–78.

56. Zijlstra F, Hoorntje JCA, de Boer MJ et al. Long-term benefit of primary angioplasty as compared with thrombolytic therapy for acute myocardial infarction, *N Engl J Med* 1999; **341**:1413–1419.

57. Grines CL, Cox DA, Stone GW et al for the Stent Primary Angioplasty in Myocardial Infarction Study Group. Coronary angioplasty with or without stent implantation for acute myocardial infarction, *N Engl J Med* 1999; **341**:1949–1956.

58. Marso SP, Steg G, Plokker T et al. Catheter-based reperfusion of unprotected left main stenosis during an acute myocardial infarction, *Am J Cardiol* 1999; **83**:1513–1517.

59. Spiecker M, Erbel R, Rupprecht HJ, Meyer J. Emergency angioplasty of totally occluded left main coronary artery in acute myocardial infarction and unstable angina pectoris—institutional experience and literature review, *Eur Heart J* 1994; **15**:602–607.

20

Coronary interventions in acute myocardial infarction

Vincent S DeGeare and Cindy L Grines

CONTENTS • Primary percutaneous intervention versus thrombolytic therapy • Selected patient populations • Device therapy in acute myocardial infarction • Adjunctive pharmacology • Additional benefits of primary PCI • Economic considerations • Limitations of primary percutaneous intervention • Patient selection and periprocedural care • Future insights • Conclusion

Acute myocardial infarction (MI) occurs nearly 1.5 million times and claims over 450,000 lives each year in the US [1]. In addition, many patients are severely disabled as a consequence of severe MI. Given these statistics, it is imperative that we not only continue to diminish the mortality rate associated with acute MI but also that we use whatever means are available to limit infarct size, reduce residual ischemia and preserve left ventricular function. In the early 1980s, the widespread use of thrombolytic therapy revolutionized management of MI from a mostly supportive role to one of active intervention directed at myocardial salvage. However, the use of thrombolytic therapy is limited in that many patients have important contraindications to its administration. In addition, the number of patients who fail to reperfuse the infarct-related artery or have recurrent ischemia or infarction is substantial and the incidence of severe thrombolytic-related complications is not trivial. Given these limitations of thrombolytic therapy, primary percutaneous intervention (PCI) has emerged as an acceptable alternative therapy for patients with acute

MI. Continued advances in both device therapy and adjunct pharmacotherapy have allowed for still broader application of PCI to patients with increasingly complex infarct-related coronary lesions.

PRIMARY PERCUTANEOUS INTERVENTION VERSUS THROMBOLYTIC THERAPY

The most important goal of any reperfusion therapy is to expeditiously restore meaningful antegrade flow in the infarct-related artery. Furthermore, the establishment of TIMI 3 flow has been shown to correlate inversely with mortality [2] (Fig. 20.1). Overall, mortality rates appear lower with primary PCI (Table 20.1), partly because primary percutaneous intervention can reliably restore TIMI 3 flow in greater than 90% of patients versus only 30–65% for thrombolytic therapy (on 90 min angiography) (Table 20.2). In addition, as shown in the first Primary Angioplasty in Myocardial Infarction (PAMI 1) trial, although the time from symptom onset to initiation of

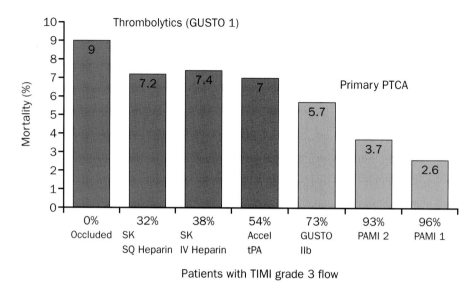

Figure 20.1 Relationship between mortality and TIMI grade 3 flow in selected thrombolytic and primary PTCA trials. Data from DeGeare et al [24].

thrombolytic therapy is less than that needed to initiate percutaneous intervention (64 min versus 101 min, $p = 0.001$), the time to symptom relief (and presumably meaningful antegrade perfusion) is less with catheter-based intervention (290 min) than with thrombolytic therapy (354 min, $p = 0.004$) [3].

The first reported cases of primary angioplasty for acute MI are from the Mid America Heart Institute (Kansas City, Missouri) in November 1980 [4]. Since these initial reports, many other institutions began to incorporate this strategy and observational data suggested that primary angioplasty was at least as effective as thrombolytic therapy and may be applicable to a wider variety of patients [5–14]. O'Keefe and colleagues reported that 96% of 1000 consecutive patients presenting with acute MI were acceptable candidates for percutaneous intervention while nearly two-thirds of the group had at least relative contraindications to thrombolytic therapy [4]. In addition, because of actual or perceived contraindications, it has been documented that over 75% of patients with acute MI are not treated with

thrombolytic therapy and that these 'lytic-ineligible' patients have a higher mortality rate (as high as 18–24% in some series) [15–17]. Primary PCI can be performed in nearly all of these patients with a success rate of greater than 90%.

There have been four major prospective, randomized trials directly comparing thrombolytic therapy and primary PCI. Gibbons et al randomized 108 patients to primary percutaneous transluminal coronary angioplasty (PTCA) or duteplase, a form of tissue plasminogen activator [18]. Both strategies provided an equal degree of myocardial salvage in this low-risk study population (only one death occurred in the trial). However, the PTCA strategy resulted in less recurrent ischemia, lower six-month follow-up costs, shorter hospital stay and lower hospital readmission rates.

Zijistra and colleagues randomly assigned 142 patients with acute MI to primary PTCA or thrombolytic therapy with streptokinase (ZWOLLE trial) [19]. Primary angioplasty resulted in higher patency rates, lower residual stenoses, higher left ventricular ejection fraction and less recurrent ischemia and recurrent MI

Table 20.1 Short-term mortality in selected trials of thrombolytic therapy and primary catheter-based intervention in (PCI) patients with acute myocardial infarction

Trial	No. of patients	Mortality (%)*
Thrombolytic trials		
GUSTO 1	41,021	
SK/SC heparin		7.2
SK/IV heparin		7.4
t-PA		6.3
t-PA/SK		7.0
GUSTO IIb	1138	
t-PA		7.0
GUSTO III [114]	15,059	
t-PA		7.5
rPA		7.2
TIMI 1 [115]	316	
t-PA		4.0
SK		5.0
TIMI 4 [116]	382	
t-PA		2.2
APSAC		8.8
t-PA/APSAC		7.2
TAMI 7 [117]	232	
A		11.0
B		6.0
C		2.0
D		7.0
E		14.0
Mayo study	103	
Duteplase		0.0
ZWOLLE	142	
SK		6.0
ISIS 2 [118]		
SK + Aspirin (ASA)	4292	8.0
ISIS 3 [119]	41,299	
t-PA		10.3
SK		10.6
APSAC		10.5
GISSI 2 [120]	12,490	
t-PA		9.0
SK		8.6
PAMI (in-hospital)	395	
t-PA		6.5
PTCA trials		
GUSTO IIb		5.7
Mayo study		0.2
ZWOLLE		0.0
PAMI 1 (in-hospital)		2.6
PAMI 2 (in-hospital)	437	3.7
Stent PAMI	900	2.7
CADILLAC (in-hospital)	2082	2.4

t-PA, tissue plasminogen activator; rPA, recombinant plasminogen activator; SK, streptokinase; APSAC, antistreplase; TIMI, thrombolysis in myocardial infarction; GUSTO, Global Utilization of Strategies to Open Occluded Coronary Arteries; TAMI, thrombolysis and angioplasty in myocardial infarction†; ISIS, International Study of Infarct Survival; GISSI, Gruppo Italiano per lo Studio della Streptochinasi nell'Infarto miocardico; PAMI, primary angioplasty in myocardial infarction. †TAMI 7 t-PA regimens: (A) 1 mg/kg over 30 min (10% bolus), then 0.25 mg/kg over 30 min. (B) 1.25 mg/kg over 90 min (20 mg bolus). (C) 0.75 mg/kg over 30 min (10% bolus), then 0.50 mg/kg over 60 min. (D) 20 mg bolus, then 30 min wait, then 80 mg over 120 min. (E) 1 mg/kg over 30 min + urokinase (1.5 million U) over 60 min.

Table 20.2 Ninety-minute TIMI flow grades in selected trials

Trial	0	0 or 1	1	2	2 or 3	3
Thrombolytic trials						
TIMI 1						
t-PA		38			62	
SK		69			31	
TIMI 4						
t-PA				24		60
APSAC				30		42
t-PA/APSAC				23		45
TEAM 2 [121]						
t-PA	20		8	12		60
SK	19		7	20		53
TAMI 5 [122]						
t-PA	17		12	18		53
UK	27		11	24		38
TAMI 7					61–83	
RAPID [123]						
t-PA				28		49
rPA 15 MU				22		41
rPA 10 + 5 MU				21		46
rPA 10 + 10 MU				22		63
RAPID II [124]						
t-PA				28		45
rPA 10 + 10 MU				23		60
PTCA trials						
GUSTO IIb						
PTCA						
Clinical site	3		2	7	3	85
Core lab	6		1	20		73
PAR [125]				2		97
PAMI 1				3		96
PAMI 2				3		93
Stent PAMI (Pilot)				5		93
Stent PAMI				8		91
CADILLAC PTCA						96
Stent						93

TEAM, Trial of Eminase in Acute Myocardial Infarction; MU, megaunits; PAR, primary angioplasty registry. Other abbreviations as in Table 20.1.

than did streptokinase. The only four deaths and the only two strokes reported in the study were in the thrombolytic group (p = NS due to small sample size). A recent follow-up study reported a sustained survival benefit in the PTCA group at a mean follow-up of five years [20].

The first Primary Angioplasty in Myocardial Infarction (PAMI 1) trial enrolled 395 patients within 12 hours of the onset of acute MI and randomized them to PTCA or front-loaded tissue plasminogen activator (t-PA) [3]. The composite end-point of in-hospital death and non-fatal MI was lower in the PTCA group (p = 0.02) as was the incidence of intracranial bleeding (0% versus 2.0%, p = 0.05). There were also significant reductions in recurrent ischemia (10.3% versus 28.0%, p = 0.001), length of hospital stay (7.6 days versus 8.4 days, p = 0.04) and total hospital charges ($26,904 versus $23,468, p = 0.04). At 6-month follow-up, the combined end-point of death plus non-fatal MI was 8.5% in the PTCA group and 16.8% in the t-PA group [21]. Patients over age 65 were especially likely to benefit from primary PTCA. Recently, it was shown that these benefits were sustained at two-year follow-up [22].

The largest prospective, randomized trial of primary PTCA versus thrombolytic therapy for acute MI is the Global Use of Strategies to Open Occluded Coronary Arteries (GUSTO) IIb Angiographic Substudy [23]. In this study, 1138 patients were randomized to primary PTCA or front-loaded t-PA (and to unfractionated heparin versus hirudin in a 2×2 factorial design). The primary end-point was a composite of death, non-fatal MI and non-fatal disabling stroke at 30 days. The end-point was reached in 13.7% of the t-PA patients and 9.6% of the PTCA group (relative risk reduction 30%, p = 0.033). Death, recurrent MI and disabling stroke all occurred more frequently in the t-PA group but the individual differences did not reach statistical significance. An important note is that many of the deaths occurred in patients randomized to PTCA who did not undergo the procedure (of these, 14.1% died and 20.7%

reached the composite end-point at 30 days). If one considers only those patients who actually underwent PTCA, the mortality rate at 30 days was only 3.2%. Of note, intracranial bleeding occurred in 1.4% of the t-PA group and 0% of the PTCA group (p = 0.004) [24].

Bleeding complications are a well known hazard of thrombolytic therapy. The most feared site of bleeding is intracranial resulting in a hemorrhagic stroke. Bleeding complications with PCI are most commonly related to the access site. However, most access site bleeding does not necessitate blood transfusion. For example, in PAMI 2 (designed to study the benefit of prophylactic intra-aortic balloon counterpulsation in high risk acute MI patients), access site bleeding was noted in 21% and 13% respectively in patients who did or did not receive a balloon pump but only 5% and 3% respectively required a blood transfusion [25].

Overall, the requirements for transfusion are slightly higher in patients undergoing PCI than for those treated with thrombolytic therapy. This likely reflects a selection bias in that many patients referred for primary PCI are considered ineligible from thrombolytic therapy due to a high bleeding risk at baseline. Despite this bias, the risk of intracranial hemorrhage is markedly reduced with primary PCI. In fact, there were no hemorrhagic strokes in the PTCA arms of the PAMI 1 or GUSTO IIb trials or in PAMI 2 (Table 20.3).

Following 'successful' thrombolysis, there often remains a high-grade lesion even if angiography reveals TIMI grade 3 flow (Fig. 20.2). The risk of early infarct-related artery reocclusion manifesting as recurrent ischemic chest pain or recurrent MI is much lower with primary PCI than with thrombolytic therapy. The incidence of recurrent ischemia was less than 10% in the PTCA arms of the PAMI, ZWOLLE and GUSTO IIb trials; much lower than that observed in thrombolytic studies (Table 20.4). Recurrent MI rates are generally < 5% with primary PTCA and between 2% and 15% with thrombolytic therapy (Table 20.5). The incorporation of intracoronary

Table 20.3 Stroke rates in selected acute MI trials (≤ 30 days)

Trial	All stroke (%)	Hemorrhagic stroke (%)
Thrombolytic trials		
GUSTO 1		
SK/SC heparin	1.2	0.5
SK/IV heparin	1.4	0.6
t-PA	1.6	0.8
t-PA/SK	1.6	1.0
GUSTO IIb		
t-PA	1.9	1.4
TIMI 4		
t-PA	1.4	0.0
APSAC	0.7	0.7
t-PA/APSAC	3.1	1.0
ISIS 2		
SK + ASA	0.6	0.1
ISIS 3		
t-PA	1.4	0.7
SK	1.0	0.2
APSAC	1.3	0.6
COBALT [126]		
Double bolus t-PA	1.9	1.2
Continuous t-PA	1.5	0.5
RAPID		
t-PA	3.9	2.6
rPA 15 MU	0.7	0.7
rPA 10 + 5 MU	0.0	0.0
rPA 10 + 10 MU	0.0	0.0
RAPID II		
t-PA	2.6	1.9
rPA 10 + 10 MU	1.8	1.2
GISSI 2		
t-PA	1.1	0.3
SK	0.9	0.3
PAMI		
t-PA	2.0	0.5
ZWOLLE		
t-PA	3.0	NA
PTCA trials		
GUSTO IIb	1.1	0.0
ZWOLLE	0.0	0.0
PAMI 1	0.0	0.0
PAMI 2	1.1	0.0
Stent PAMI	0.2	
CADILLAC	0.7	

Abbreviations as in Table 20.1.

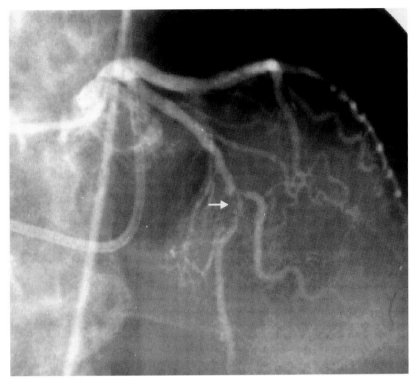

(a)

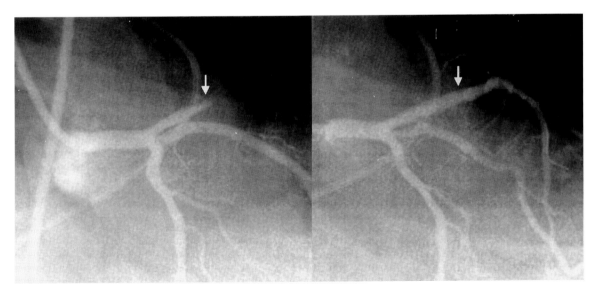

(b)

Figure 20.2 (a) Coronary angiogram revealing a high-grade residual stenosis despite TIMI grade 3 flow following 'successful' thrombolytic therapy. (b) Coronary angiogram showing < 10% residual stenosis following primary PTCA and placement of an intracoronary stent. From DeGeare et al [24].

Table 20.4 Rates of recurrent ischemia in selected trials	
Trial	**Recurrent ischemia (%)**
Thrombolytic trials	
GUSTO 1	
SK/SC heparin	20
SK/IV heparin	20
t-PA	19
t-PA/SK	19
GUSTO IIb	
t-PA	29
GUSTO III	
t-PA	29
rPA	29
TIMI 1	
t-PA	46
SK	44
TAMI 7	17–35
GISSI 2	
t-PA	11
SK	12
ZWOLLE	
SK	38
PAMI	
t-PA	24
PTCA trials	
GUSTO IIb	6
ZWOLLE	9
PAMI 1	5
PAMI 2	12
Stent PAMI (Pilot)	
PTCA	3
Stent	4
CADILLAC	3

Abbreviations as in Table 20.1.

Table 20.5 Reinfarction rates in acute MI trials ($\leq$ 30 days)	
Trial	**Reinfarction (%)**
Thrombolytic trials	
GUSTO 1	
SK/SC heparin	3
SK/IV heparin	4
t-PA	4
t-PA/SK	4
GUSTO IIb	
t-PA	7
GUSTO III	
t-PA	4
rPA	4
TIMI 1	
t-PA	12
SK	13
TIMI 4	
t-PA	7
APSAC	7
rPA/APSAC	3
TAMI 7	2–8
GISSI 2	
t-PA	2
SK	2
ISIS 2	
SK + ASA	2
ISIS 3	
t-PA	3
SK	4
APSAC	4
ZWOLLE	
SK	13
PAMI	
t-PA	7
PTCA trials	
GUSTO IIb	4
ZWOLLE	0
PAMI 1	3
PAMI 2 (incl. high risk patients)	7
Stent PAMI	< 1
PAMI No SOS	< 1
CADILLAC	< 1

Abbreviations as in Table 20.1.

stenting and adjunctive pharmacology may further reduce these complications (see below).

Late vessel reocclusion is often clinically silent but may increase ischemic burden, especially during stress. Follow-up angiography has confirmed that 3–6 month reocclusion rates are much lower following primary PCI compared to thrombolytic therapy (Fig. 20.3). This is especially true following intracoronary stenting.

Weaver and colleagues published a meta-analysis of 10 trials of primary PTCA versus thrombolytic therapy [26]. They showed a 34% relative decrease in mortality (4.4% for PTCA versus 6.5% for thrombolysis, $p = 0.02$) as well as significant reductions in death plus non-fatal MI (7.2% versus 11.9%, $p < 0.001$), non-fatal recurrent MI (2.9% versus 5.3%, $p = 0.002$), total stroke (0.7% versus 2.0%, $p = 0.007$) and hemorrhagic stroke (0.1% versus 1.1%, $p = 0.001$) (Fig. 20.4).

It must be remembered that the above data do not apply to 'rescue' PCI (performed after failure of *full-dose* thrombolytic therapy). Multiple studies have shown that PCI results in this setting are less favorable and that compli-

cations, especially bleeding, are increased (see below).

SELECTED PATIENT POPULATIONS

Elderly patients

Elderly patients are known to have a significantly increased mortality rate following acute MI. In the GUSTO 1 trial, the overall mortality rate was 7.0% but for patients > 75 years old, the mortality rate was 20.1% [27]. Elderly patients showed a similar increased incidence of stroke and intracranial hemorrhage. Therefore, a mechanical approach that achieves high rates of TIMI 3 flow with a reduction in the incidence of intracranial bleeding is particularly advantageous in elderly patients.

In the PAMI 1 trial patient age > 65 years old was an independent risk factor for the combined end-point of death and non-fatal recurrent MI if treated with t-PA instead of primary PTCA (20% versus 8.6%, $p = 0.048$) [4]. In a pooled analysis of the PAMI 1, ZWOLLE and

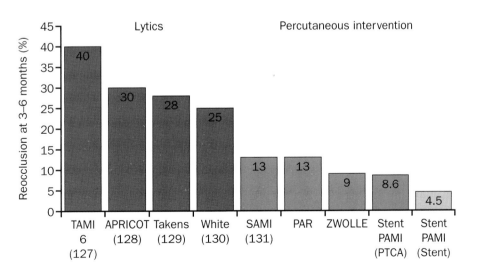

Figure 20.3 Angiographic reocclusion rates from selected thrombolytic and primary percutaneous intervention trials. Data from DeGeare et al [24].

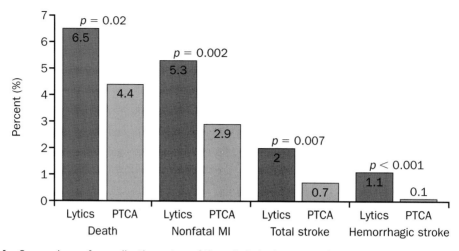

Figure 20.4 Comparison of complication rates of thrombolytic therapy and primary PTCA from a meta-analysis of 10 trials. Modified from Weaver WD et al [25].

Mayo Clinic trials, a marked reduction in mortality was noted in elderly patients treated with primary PTCA instead of thrombolytic therapy [28]. Similar reductions in death were seen in favor of primary PTCA in patients > 70 years old in the GUSTO IIb trial [11].

Six-month follow-up of 10 randomized trials of primary PTCA versus thrombolytic therapy revealed that patients > 60 years of age (and diabetics) had the greatest relative reduction in death or non-fatal reinfarction when treated with primary PTCA instead of thrombolytic therapy [29]. Another recent publication suggests that thrombolytic therapy is of limited benefit and may be detrimental in AMI patients > 75 years old [30]. This is due to increased bleeding in older patients treated with thrombolytics.

Despite these findings, elderly patients undergoing primary PCI still have a higher mortality rate than their younger counterparts [31, 32]. A recent pooled analysis of the PAMI 2, Stent PAMI and PAMI No Surgery on Site (No SOS) trials showed that patients > 75 years old had an in-hospital mortality rate five times higher than those < 75 years old (Fig. 20.5).

Cardiogenic shock

Cardiogenic shock has a very poor prognosis if coronary perfusion cannot be quickly restored. Mortality exceeds 80% without treatment. In the Multicenter Investigation of Limitation of Infarct Size (MILIS) study, 4.5% of patients presented with cardiogenic shock and 7.1% developed cardiogenic shock during their hospital course [33]. In GISSI 1 (first Gruppo Italiano per Studio della Streptochinasi nell'Infarto Miocardio), 2.5% of patients presented with shock and another 6% developed it after admission [34]. Early reports suggested a reduction in mortality with thrombolytic therapy but this was highly dependent on the ability to establish vessel patency. In the Society for Cardiac Angiography Intracoronary Streptokinase Registry, 44 patients with cardiogenic shock were identified [35]. Overall mortality was 66% but reperfusion occurred in only 19 (44%) of these patients. Of the 25 patients with occluded infarct-related arteries, mortality was 84%. In GISSI 1 and the International Study Group (ISG) trials, the mortality rate for patients with cardiogenic shock was equal to

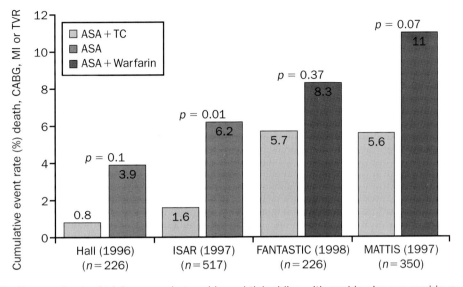

Figure 20.5 Four randomized trials comparing aspirin and ticlopidine with aspirin alone or aspirin and warfarin in patients undergoing coronary stent placement. Data from Berger PA [74].

placebo in patients treated with either t-PA or streptokinase [36, 37].

Primary PTCA has shown more promise [38, 39]. In a review of 14 series of patients with cardiogenic shock, primary PTCA resulted in reperfusion in 60–100% of cases (average 73%). Overall mortality was 44%, and in patients who had successful PTCA, death occurred in only 30%, compared to 80% without successful PCI (identical to placebo rates in other trials). O'Keefe and colleagues reported similar results in 79 unselected patients with cardiogenic shock [4].

The recently published Should We Emergently Revascularize Occluded Coronaries for Cardiogenic Shock (SHOCK) trial randomized 302 patients to emergency revascularization (PCI in 64% and/or CABG in 36%) or 'initial stabilization', which included the use of intra-aortic balloon counterpulsation and/or thrombolytic therapy [40]. Overall, all cause mortality was the same in both groups at 30 days (46.7% for early revascularization versus 56.0% for medical stabilization, $p = 0.11$) but significantly lower in the revascularization

group at six months (50.3% versus 63.1%, $p = 0.01$). Of note, patients < 75 years old benefited from early revascularization at both time end-points. Of the 161 patients who underwent PCI of the infarct-related artery (81 in the revascularization group and 20 in the medical group) the procedure was successful in 78% and those patients had a 38% mortality rate at 30 days compared to 79% in whom the procedure was unsuccessful ($p = 0.003$).

Congestive heart failure

There are no trials directly comparing thrombolytic therapy and primary PCI in patients with congestive heart failure (CHF). However, there are data to suggest that the efficacy of thrombolytic therapy is reduced in these patients [39]. This may be due to decreased cardiac output resulting in reduced levels of thrombolytic agents reaching the site of intra-coronary thrombus, especially when the drugs are given intravenously. In the GISSI 1 and ISG trials, 17–23% of patients presented in Killip Class II and 2–4% in Killip Class III [33, 34]. In GISSI 1 in-hospital mortality was reduced in class II patients but not in class III patients. At six month follow-up, there was no survival benefit over placebo in either group (mortality rates 27% versus 29% for class II and 50% versus 53% for class III). In the ISG trial, no survival benefit was seen in either group.

A recent pooled analysis of the PAMI 2, stent PAMI and PAMI No SOS databases revealed that 13.1% of enrolled patients presented in Killip Class II or Killip Class III. In-hospital and six month mortality were 7% and 16% for class II patients and 11% and 26% for class III patients, rates considerably lower than in historical controls and presentation Killip Class remained an independent predictor of mortality at both time points [41].

Patients with prior coronary artery bypass surgery

The mechanism of acute MI in patients with prior coronary artery bypass grafting (CABG) is frequently thrombotic occlusion of a saphenous vein graft (SVG) [42]. Because the thrombus is often large (> 2 cm in length), it is not surprising that thrombolytic therapy is less effective in these patients. In one small series, intravenous thrombolytic therapy only restored graft patency in 25% of cases [43]. Using primary PCI, O'Keefe et al reported successful recanalization in 86% of infarct-related SVGs. In their analysis, in-hospital mortality was the same in patients with and without prior CABG [4].

In the previously described pooled analysis of the PAMI 2, stent PAMI and PAMI No SOS trials, 4.6% of the patients had prior CABG. PCI was successful in approximately 70% of patients with infarct-related SVGs and a history of prior CABG was not associated with any increase in mortality ($p = 0.61$) [32]. The use of distal protection devices to help reduce distal embolization and no reflow may futher increase the success of SVG intervention.

'Rescue' PCI

Rescue PCI is referred to procedures performed after failure of full dose thrombolytic therapy. Multiple trials have shown that success is lower and complications are higher in this setting. The Cohort of Rescue Angioplasty in Myocardial Infarction (CORAMI) investigators attempted rescue PTCA on 72 patients who failed initial thrombolysis [44]. Procedural success was 90% and survival to hospital discharge was 96%.

The Randomized Evaluation of Salvage angioplasty with a Combined Utilization of End-points (RESCUE) trial enrolled 151 patients with a first anterior wall MI treated with thrombolytic therapy and angiographically demonstrated occlusion of the infarct-related artery within eight hours of chest pain onset. Patients were randomized to conservative therapy (aspirin, heparin and coronary vasodilators) or to this therapy plus angioplasty (± additional thrombolytic therapy). PTCA was successful in 92%. The combined end-point of death or severe heart failure at 30 days was less in the angioplasty group (6% versus 17%, $p = 0.05$) [45].

In the TIMI 4 study, 95 (24%) of patients had an occluded infarct-related vessel at 90 min angiography. Fifty-eight patients underwent rescue PTCA (90% successful). Successful rescue PTCA resulted in superior coronary flow and an adverse outcome rate of 29% compared to 83% if rescue PTCA was unsuccessful ($p = 0.01$) [46].

Ross et al studied 464 patients with failed thrombolysis enrolled in the GUSTO-1 trial compared to 1058 with successful thrombolytic therapy [47]. One hundred and ninety-eight patients underwent rescue PTCA. Patients offered PTCA were more likely to be diabetic and had lower LVEF than those managed conservatively. LVEF and 30-day mortality were similar among patients with successful rescue PTCA and those managed conservatively.

Finally, Miller et al studied the effectiveness of PTCA with or without abciximab for failed thrombolysis, in 392 patients enrolled in the GUSTO III trial. There was no difference in the composite end-point of death, stroke or reinfarction (at 30 days) although there were trends for lower 30-day mortality and increased severe bleeding in patients treated with abciximab [48]. Based on these data we generally offer catheter-based reperfusion therapy to patients with failed thrombolytic therapy, especially if any evidence of hemodynamic compromise or electrical instability is present, with the goal of symptom relief, myocardial salvage and clinical stability.

DEVICE THERAPY IN ACUTE MYOCARDIAL INFARCTION

Most of the early cases of primary PCI were performed using only balloon angioplasty. Subsequently, many interventional devices, including intracoronary stents, atherectomy devices, lasers, rheolytic thrombectomy and therapeutic ultrasound have been applied in the setting of acute MI.

Intracoronary stents

Of all of the advances in coronary angioplasty, perhaps none has had a greater impact on the success and diversification of the procedure than the widespread use of intracoronary stenting. Initially it was felt that stenting should be avoided in this setting because of the presence of intracoronary thrombus and the systemic hypercoagulable state associated with acute MI which could lead to an increased risk of acute stent thrombosis. As acute stent thrombosis was reduced with better antiplatelet therapy and reports of successful bail-out stenting during PCI for acute MI became available, randomized trials of stenting for acute MI were undertaken.

The GR II stent (Cook, Inc) in acute MI (GRAMI) trial randomized 65 patients (preliminary results) to primary PTCA with (40

patients) or without (25 patients) planned stenting. There were no technical failures, reocclusions or deaths in the stent group. The combined end-point of technical failure or death (in-hospital) was significantly lower in the stent group (0% versus 24%, $p < 0.01$) [49].

The Primary Angioplasty versus Stent Implantation in Acute MI (PASTA) trial enrolled 84 patients with infarct-related arteries greater than 2.5 mm in diameter [50]. Forty-one patients were randomized to stenting and 43 patients to PTCA alone. Patients randomized to stenting had a higher clinical success rate (93% versus 65%, $p = 0.002$) and a better three month event free rate (86.2% versus 62.4%, $p \leq 0.05$).

The Florence Randomized Elective Stenting in Acute Coronary Occlusions (FRESCO) trial randomized 150 patients with acute MI and successful PTCA to subsequent stenting versus no further intervention [51]. At six months the composite end-point of death, reinfarction or reintervention was 9% in the stent group and 28% in the PTCA group ($p = 0.003$). The incidence of angiographic restenosis or reocclusion was 17% in the stent group and 43% in the PTCA group ($p = 0.001$).

The PAMI Stent Pilot trial was a feasibility study which enrolled 312 consecutive patients with acute MI [52]. After primary PTCA, 240 patients met eligibility for stent placement and this was performed successfully in 236 (98%). At 30 days, mortality was 0.8%; reinfarction, 1.7%; recurrent ischemia, 3.8% and target vessel revascularization (TVR), 1.7%.

These and other encouraging reports led to the stent PAMI trial in which 900 patients with an infarct-related native coronary artery between 3.0 mm and 4.5 mm in diameter and lesions that could be covered with one or two 15 mm heparin-coated Palmaz-Schatz stents were randomized to PTCA only or PTCA followed by intracoronary stenting [53]. Stenting was successful in 98% of those assigned to this group. Immediately post-procedure, the stent group had a greater immediate gain in lumen size, a greater minimal luminal diameter, lower percent residual stenosis and lower incidence of angiographically evident dissection. At 6.5 months follow-up, the angiographic restenosis rate was lower in the stent group (20.3% versus 33.5%, $p < 0.001$).

Interestingly, the rate of TIMI 3 flow was slightly lower in the stent group immediately following the procedure (89.4% versus 92.7%, $p = 0.10$) but was slightly higher at follow-up angiography (90.1% versus 86.3%, $p = 0.13$). This initial flow decrement was felt to be due either to thrombus protrusion through the stent struts (resulting in distal embolization) or more likely, distal embolization caused by the rather bulky stent delivery system used in this trial.

At one month there was no significant difference in death, reinfarction or disabling stroke, but there was a slight decrease in ischemia-driven TVR in the stent group (1.3% versus 3.8%, $p = 0.02$). The composite end-point (sum of these four variables) was not different. At six months, the composite end-point was lower for the stent group (12.6% versus 20.1%, $p < 0.01$); this was entirely due to a lower incidence of ischemia-driven TVR in the stent group (7.7% versus 17.0%, $p < 0.001$).

At both six and 12 months there was a disturbing trend toward increased mortality in stented patients ($p = 0.07$ at 12 months) [54]. This finding has led to a more cautious approach by some operators in which stenting in AMI is reserved for those patients with a suboptimal angiographic result (dissection, recoil, etc.).

The largest trial of PCI in AMI to date is the Controlled Abciximab and Device Investigation to Lower late Angioplasty Complications (CADILLAC) trial [55]. In this trial, 2082 patients were randomized in a 2×2 fashion to PTCA versus stenting and abciximab versus placebo. At 30 days, the combined end-point of death, stroke, non-fatal MI or ischemia-guided TVR at 30 days was 8.6% for PTCA alone, 4.9% for PTCA plus abciximab, 5.7% for stents alone and 5.1% for stents plus abciximab ($p = 0.02$). There was no decrease in TIMI 3 flow in stented patients. At six months, the composite end-point occurred in 19.3%, 15.2%, 10.9% and 10.8% of patients respectively (once again exclusively due to a decrease in TVR with stenting). No increase in mortality was seen in stented patients (3.3% versus 3.3%). Abciximab had no effect on six month outcomes in stented patients.

These data suggest that stenting in acute myocardial infarction is feasible and safe. The worrisome trend toward increased mortality seen in stent-PAMI was not demonstrated in the larger CADILLAC trial and the need for less repeat revascularization procedures was dramatically reduced. Given the large number of procedures performed, this may result in great economic savings to the health care system.

Atherectomy devices

Rotational atherectomy
In general, rotational atherectomy (Rotablator, Scimed, Boston Scientific Corporation, Boston, MA) is not recommended in patients with acute coronary syndromes due to the presence of intracoronary thrombus at the lesion site which has been shown to result in a high incidence of distal embolization and/or the no-reflow phenomenon [56]. However, there are several scenarios where rotational atherectomy may be considered. The first is when the culprit lesion cannot be dilated using conventional techniques. Often, rotational atherectomy (even when performed using a small burr:artery ratio) can modify the lesion and facilitate PTCA with or without stenting. Another is to use rotational atherectomy to debulk proximal disease in order to allow passage of equipment through a tortuous segment of vessel to reach the target lesion. Also, if the culprit vessel is a degenerated saphenous vein graft or diminutive mammary artery graft, one may elect to intervene on a native coronary artery lesion which may be heavily calcified and benefit from rotational atherectomy. Although there are no randomized trials in this setting, the use of a glycoprotein IIb/IIIa receptor antagonist may help reduce complications in this situation.

Directional atherectomy

Directional coronary atherectomy (Devices for Vascular Intervention, Redwood City, CA) is a method of selectively removing intraluminal debris from within a coronary artery (or graft) by directing an over-the-wire cutting device toward the lesion and collecting the material in a retrievable nose-cone. There is limited data on the use of DCA as a method of primary percutaneous revascularization in the setting of acute MI. Saito and colleagues compared the results of primary DCA in 21 patients to PTCA in 43 patients with acute MI in which the culprit lesion was in the proximal portion of a non-tortuous native coronary artery (usually the LAD) and did not have fluoroscopic evidence of calcification [57]. Primary DCA was immediately successful in 18 (86%) of patients and resulted initially in a larger minimum luminal diameter than did primary PTCA (2.75 ± 0.33 mm versus 2.26 ± 0.41 mm, $p < 0.000002$). However, a high rate of restenosis and reocclusion at three month angiographic follow-up negated the beneficial effects of primary DCA. The authors concluded 'primary DCA is not a first-choice method for reperfusion therapy for acute MI'.

Extraction atherectomy

Thrombus burden is felt to be exceptionally high in cases of failed thrombolytic therapy, thrombotic saphenous vein graft occlusion and in the setting of cardiogenic shock. Transluminal extraction atherectomy (TEC, Interventional Technologies, Inc, San Diego, CA) is a method in which thrombus is aspirated from within the vessel into a extracorporeal collection chamber, thus possibly reducing the risk for distal embolization and no reflow. Kaplan et al prospectively evaluated extraction atherectomy in 100 high-risk patients (one ore more of the following: thrombolytic failure, post-infarct angina, angiographic thrombus, cardiogenic shock, thrombotic occlusion of an SVG) [58]. Procedural success occurred in 94% of patients. In-hospital events included death in 5%, CABG in 4% and blood transfusion in 18%. No patients died or required bail-out stenting or emergent CABG. Sixty-five patients underwent predischarge angiography which revealed a patent infarct-related vessel in 95%. Long-term (six-month) patency was 90% but the restenosis rate was 68% and target vessel revascularization was necessary in 38%.

The ongoing TOPIT (TEC versus PTCA in Thrombus) trial will randomize patients with acute MI to one of the above therapies. Preliminary results from 245 patients (of the 550 planned for enrollment) reveal equal efficacy (97% success in both groups) with a lower incidence of major adverse cardiac events (MACE) and fewer non-Q wave MIs in the TEC group [59]. Bail-out stenting was performed in 35% of patients in each group. The impact of combining TEC with PTCA and/or stenting and the contribution of adding a glycoprotein IIb/IIIa receptor antagonist in this setting are unknown at this time. The TEC BEfore Stenting (TECBEST) trial will assess the efficacy of performing TEC (versus PTCA) prior to stenting in patients with saphenous vein graft lesions.

Rheolytic thrombectomy

This is another method of mechanical aspiration of thrombus from within the culprit lesion. The most commonly used device is the Possis AngioJet (Possis Medical Systems, Inc) which consists of a 5F catheter that emits three high-pressure pulsatile saline jets backward from the top into an aspiration chamber [60]. The resulting vortex creates a Bernouli effect which draws the thrombus into the catheter. The largest trial of this device was the Second Vein Graft AngioJet Study (VeGAS 2 trial) [61]. In this trial 349 patients with angiographically apparent thrombus in vessels > 2.5 mm in diameter (54% in saphenous vein grafts) were randomized to thrombectomy with the AngioJet or intracoronary urokinase. The trial had originally planned to enroll 520 patients but was terminated early due to safety concerns about urokinase and poor enrollment. Preliminary results revealed a higher success rate (86.3% versus 72.7%, $p < 0.05$) and fewer complications in the AngioJet group (in-hospital event rates 13.9% versus 32.5%; bleeding complications, 5.0% versus 11.8% and vascular complications, 17.8% versus 4.4%; $p < 0.05$ for all). There was no difference in the primary composite end-point of 30-day mortality, emergency CABG, myocardial infarction or target vessel revascularization. There have been no trials directly comparing rheolytic thrombectomy and PTCA (with or without stenting) for acute myocardial infarction.

Laser angioplasty

There is very limited published experience using this debulking technique in the setting of acute MI. Estella et al reported their results using an excimer laser (Spectranetics Corporation, Colorado Springs, CO) in 12 patients (14 lesions) with thrombus-containing lesions recruited as part of a larger study [62]. They reported a clinical success rate of 58% compared to 95% in 130 patients without thrombus ($p = 0.0001$). Myocardial infarction, distal embolization and abrupt closure were all more common in the excimer laser group. At six months, the restenosis rate was 70% (compared to 51% in the patients without thrombus, $p = $ NS).

Topaz and colleagues reported the results of a multicenter registry of 2038 lesions in 1862 patients treated with a solid-state, mid-infrared holmium:YAG laser [63]. Six percent of these patients presented with acute MI. Laser plus adjunct PTCA achieved a 93% clinical success rate. However, at six months, no benefit on reducing restenosis was observed.

Ultrasound

Therapeutic ultrasound delivered at the site of a thrombus-containing lesion has been proposed as a method of selectively lysing thrombus with minimal disruption of the adjacent arterial wall.

Rosenschein et al performed ultrasound thrombolysis using the ACULYSIS system (Angiosonics, Morrisville, NC) in 15 consecutive patients with an acute anterior MI and TIMI grade 0 or 1 flow in the left anterior descending artery [64]. Ultrasound alone produced TIMI 3 flow in 87% of the patients. When coupled with adjunct PTCA, the residual diameter stenosis was $20 \pm 12\%$ and 14 patients had TIMI 3 flow and one patient had TIMI 2 flow. No adverse angiographic or clinical events occurred.

Hamm et al treated 14 patients with acute MI using pulsed intracoronary ultrasound [65]. TIMI flow grade improved at least one grade in 13/14 patients and was TIMI grade 3 following adjunctive PTCA (mean 6 ± 2 atm) in all 13 of these patients (the fourteenth patient had persistent TIMI grade 0 flow despite all measures and died from cardiogenic shock). Of the 13 successfully treated patients, two had minor distal embolization and five had non-flow-limiting dissections that did not require stenting. One patient required repeat PTCA prior to hospital discharge. At six months follow-up, 10 patients had angiography and three had stenoses > 50%. None required reintervention.

Based on these small studies, therapeutic intracoronary ultrasound appears to be safe and feasible. However, whether it has any advantage over conventional PTCA (with or without stenting) remains to be seen.

ADJUNCTIVE PHARMACOLOGY

Aspirin

All patients undergoing percutaneous coronary intervention should receive aspirin (160 mg or greater) unless there is a strong contraindication. Aspirin has been shown to decrease the risk of abrupt closure following PTCA by as much as 50% [66]. For patients who truly cannot take aspirin, and are not candidates for desensitization, clopidogrel, 75 mg daily, may be substituted.

Heparin/thrombin inhibitors

Most patients also receive unfractionated heparin (UFH) although there is evidence to suggest that the direct thrombin inhibitors (such as hirudin, leprudin and bilavirudin) are acceptable alternatives, especially in patients with a history of heparin-induced thrombocytopenia [67, 68]. Furthermore, there is research into using low molecular weight heparin (either subcutaneously or intravenously) which gives a more predictable level of anticoagulation and obviates the need to monitor activated clotting times [69].

Ticlopidine/clopidogrel

Patients who receive intracoronary stents require further antiplatelet therapy. Although initial regimens consisted of aspirin, heparin, warfarin and dextran, two large studies have now confirmed the superiority of combined antiplatelet therapy compared to anticoagulant therapy.

In 1996, Hall et al published a study of 226 patients undergoing intravascular ultrasound (IVUS)-guided stent implantation [70]. One hundred and three patients received aspirin alone and 123 received aspirin plus ticlopidine. At one month follow-up, the rate of stent thrombosis was 2.9% and 0.8% respectively.

Schomig et al published a substudy of 123 patients with AMI enrolled in the Intracoronary Stenting Antithrombotic Regimen (ISAR) study which showed a significant reduction in clinical and stent occlusion at 30 days [71]. Bleeding complications were also markedly reduced in the antiplatelet group.

The Full ANTicoagulation versus ASpirin and TIClopidine (FANTASTIC) study and the Multicenter Aspirin and Ticlopidine Trial after Intracoronary Stenting (MATTIS) trial also showed less stent thrombosis and significant reductions in bleeding and vascular complications with aspirin plus ticlopidine [72, 73]. Recently, Berger has written an excellent review of these studies [74].

More recently, another thienopyridine derivative clopidogrel has been used in place of ticlopidine. The advantages of this compound include more rapid plasma levels (and therefore platelet inhibition) following oral loading and substantially fewer side effects, most notably diarrhea, skin rash and neutropenia [75]. However, there have been reports of thrombotic thrombocytopenic purpura (TTP) with both agents [76]. Data are now emerging to show that this substitution appears safe. The Clopidogrel Aspirin Stent Interventional Cooperative Study (CLASSICS) revealed no difference in the composite end-point of death, MI or target lesion revascularization among 740 patients randomized to clopidogrel (with or without a loading dose) versus ticlopidine for 28 days (all patients received aspirin) [77].

Glycoprotein IIb/IIIa antagonists

The platelet glycoprotein IIb/IIIa receptor represents the final common pathway in the formation of thrombus. This integrin is responsible for binding to fibrinogen thereby promoting platelet aggregation. The development of drugs which can inhibit this receptor represents a major advance in antiplatelet therapy.

The first available agent in this class was abciximab, a murine antibody which irreversibly binds to the glycoprotein IIb/IIIa receptor (among others). Later, other molecules which act as competitive inhibitors of this ligand were developed (integrilin, tirofiban). Finally, orally available agents have now entered clinical trials.

Most of the studies involving these drugs have been performed in patients undergoing either elective intervention or in patients with unstable angina or non-Q wave MI, where each agent has shown some degree of efficacy in reducing acute complications [78–82]. Interestingly, the EPISTENT trial also suggested a possible restenosis benefit in diabetic patients [83]. There is little published data using these agents in the setting of primary PCI for acute ST-elevation MI.

Lefkovits et al published an analysis of a sub-group of patients in the Evaluation of c7E3 for the Prevention of Ischemic Complications (EPIC) trial [84]. Of the 2099 patients enrolled, 42 underwent primary PTCA for acute MI and 22 underwent rescue PTCA for failed thrombolysis. The composite primary end-point of death, reinfarction, repeat intervention or CABG at six months was reduced in those randomized to abciximab bolus plus 12 hour infusion when compared to placebo (47.8% versus 4.5%, $p = 0.002$). Patients receiving only a bolus of abciximab did not have a significant benefit. Of note, the greatest reduction was in the need for repeat PTCA (34.8% versus 0%, $p = 0.003$).

The Reopro and Primary PTCA Organization and Randomized Trial (RAPPORT) randomized 483 patients with acute MI to placebo versus abciximab bolus plus infusion [85]. Although the composite end-point of death, reinfarction or revascularization (urgent or elective) at six months was equivalent in both groups, abciximab significantly reduced the incidence of death, reinfarction or urgent TVR at seven, 30 and 180 days. There was no benefit on restenosis. In addition, 'bail-out stenting' was reduced by 42% (20.4% versus 11.9%, $p = 0.008$) in the treatment group.

The Abciximab Before Direct Angioplasty and Stenting in Myocardial Infarction Regarding Acute and Long-Term Follow-up (ADMIRAL) trial randomized 300 patients with acute MI undergoing PTCA with or without stenting to placebo versus abciximab bolus plus infusion [86]. Preliminary results reveal a 47% reduction in the combined end-point of death, recurrent MI or need for urgent revascularization.

The Controlled Abciximab and Device Evaluation to Lower Late Angioplasty Complications (CADILLAC) trial was a randomized trial involving 2081 patients studying PTCA versus stenting with and without abciximab in patients with acute MI [87]. Abciximab appeared to be most beneficial in patients undergoing PTCA only (with a reduction in acute closure from 1.7% to 0.6% in this group).

There was no significant impact on stented patients at 30 days and no reduction in the incidence of the composite end-point of death, stroke, non-fatal MI or ischemia driven TVR at six months.

When using abciximab, we generally reduce the heparin bolus to 70 units/kg (maximum of 7000 units) and aim to maintain the ACT between 225 and 250 seconds; a strategy which has been shown to prevent an increase in bleeding complications compared to standard dose heparin [88].

ADDITIONAL BENEFITS OF PRIMARY PCI

Up-front cardiac catheterization affords the opportunity for the acquisition of a great deal of valuable information at the time of the procedure. The status of non-infarct arteries (and any bypass grafts) can be readily assessed, and if necessary, intervened upon either immediately or in a staged procedure. Both systolic and diastolic function can be rapidly evaluated as can left-sided valvular structures and the intraventricular septum. Right-heart catheterization adds information concerning right-sided filling pressures, oximetry data and determination of cardiac output. Most hemodynamically significant congenital or acquired intracardiac shunts can be easily detected. In case of hemodynamic decompensation, an intra-aortic balloon pump can be rapidly inserted through the arterial access site.

These hemodynamic and angiographic data, when combined with clinical assessment, can be extremely useful for post-MI risk stratification. Low-risk patients (those age < 70 years old with non-anterior MI, preserved LVEF, favorable coronary anatomy and stable hemodynamics) can often avoid admission to a coronary care unit and can be discharged expeditiously [25]. Often, non-invasive testing such as exercise or pharmacologic stress testing, with or without perfusion or echocardiographic imaging, can be eliminated, thus lowering the cost of hospital admission (see below). High risk patients, especially those who will require coronary artery bypass surgery can be identified and referred before hemodynamic compromise or further ischemic complications occur.

ECONOMIC CONSIDERATIONS

Studies of the cost-effectiveness of primary percutaneous intervention for acute MI have shown this approach is no more costly than a strategy using thrombolytic therapy [89]. Gibbons et al performed a cost analysis of their study (Mayo Clinic study of PTCA versus thrombolytics) which revealed a trend toward lower hospital costs in the angioplasty group ($16,811 versus $21,400, $p = 0.09$) [18]. Six-month follow-up costs were lower in the PTCA group ($480 versus $2738, $p = 0.03$). Length of hospital stay and readmission rates were also lower in the PTCA group.

A detailed analysis of the PAMI 1 trial revealed that the charges for drugs/IV solutions, non-coronary care unit rooms, electrocardiography and radiology were higher for patients treated with t-PA leading to higher total hospital charges in this group ($26,904 versus $23,468, $p = 0.04$) [90]. When professional fees were included, the charges were similar in both groups. The ZWOLLE and GUSTO IIb trials also showed similar costs between the two treatment strategies [91].

In PAMI 2, low-risk patients (< 70 years old, no three-vessel disease, no SVG occlusion, left ventricular ejection fraction > 45%, no persistent malignant arrhythmia and an optimal PTCA result) could avoid admission to a coronary care unit and non-invasive testing and could be discharged on the third hospital day [25]. This strategy resulted in a very significant cost saving ($15,200 versus $19,400, $p = 0.001$). In addition, the diagnosis-related groups (DRG) reimbursement for patients with acute MI treated with primary PTCA is higher (relative to hospital costs) than it is for thrombolytic therapy [24].

LIMITATIONS OF PRIMARY PERCUTANEOUS INTERVENTION

Limitations of primary percutaneous intervention fall into two broad categories: medical and non-medical. There are very few medical limitations. O'Keefe et al determined that only 4% of 1000 consecutive patients with acute MI were not considered to be candidates for primary PTCA [4]. Patients with significant renal insufficiency may experience a decrement in renal function after the administration of contrast material. Diabetics and others with significant proteinuria appear to have the highest risk. However, there is strong evidence that adequate hydration (both during and after the procedure), conservation of contrast use, the use of low osmolar contrast and the administration of N-acetyl cysteine and/or fenoldopam (a selective dopamine agonist) can eliminate much of this risk [92, 93]. Occasionally, temporary or permanent renal replacement therapy is required.

The widespread use of metformin for the treatment of type 2 diabetes mellitus has led to concern about the development of lactic acidosis in patients with compromised renal function who receive intravascular contrast (especially in acute MI patients who cannot be adequately prehydrated.) However, most acute MI patients can proceed safely to emergent PCI with the immediate discontinuation of metformin and close post-procedural monitoring of renal function to ensure a return to baseline prior to restarting the drug [94].

Even with the expanded use of low osmolar contrast material, 0.2–0.4% of patients will suffer a non-life-threatening reaction requiring therapy. Anaphylactoid reactions are reported in 0.04% of patients undergoing angiography. The incidence of repeat allergic reactions in this population is 17–35% without any intervention. However, pretreatment with corticosteroids and antihistamines and changing to low osmolar contrast can lower the incidence to 0.5% [95].

Perceived non-medical limitations of primary PCI include limited availability of facilities and competent operators. In 1998, 1088 hospitals in the US performed PTCA. Ninety-one percent of these facilities had 24-hour on-call coverage for emergent procedures (SCIMED Life Systems, Inc, personal communication, February 1999).

Trials to assess the safety and efficacy of emergent transport of AMI patients to a PCI center have been performed. The Air-PAMI trial compared outcomes in lytic-eligible high-risk patients randomized either to transfer to a tertiary care center for primary PTCA or to local thrombolysis with no routine transfer [96]. Despite a delay in time to treatment due to transfer and transportation, there was a 44% decrease in the composite end-point of death, recurrent MI and disabling stroke in the PTCA group. This was not statistically significant due to the small sample size. Although encouraging, this strategy cannot be recommended for routine management of AMI.

There is also emerging data regarding the safety of performing PTCA (both elective and emergent) in centers without on-site cardiac surgery back-up [97]. The PAMI NoSOS (No Surgery on Site) trial documented the outcome of 492 high-risk acute MI patients (as defined in the PAMI 2 trial) presenting at 19 community hospitals performing primary PTCA without cardiac surgery available at the institution [98]. All patients underwent cardiac catheterization and 88% underwent PCI (53% received stents). Of these, TIMI 3 flow was achieved in 94% and TIMI 2 or 3 flow with < 50% residual stenosis was achieved in 97% of patients. In-hospital mortality was 2.8% and disabling stroke occurred in 0.4%. Only one patient required emergent CABG and there were no recurrent MIs. At six months, the composite end-point of death, recurrent MI or disabling stroke was 7.7%; similar to results obtained in experienced interventional laboratories with cardiovascular surgery on site.

Critics of primary percutaneous intervention argue that the procedure cannot be routinely accomplished in a timely and effective fashion. The 1999 ACC/AHA Guidelines on the

Management of Acute Myocardial Infarction [99] recommend that (A) balloon dilation occurs within 90 ± 30 minutes of the diagnosis of acute MI (increased from ≤ 90 minutes in the 1996 guidelines [100]); (B) TIMI grade 2 or 3 flow be established in > 90% of patients; (C) emergent CABG rates be < 5%; (D) PTCA be performed in > 85% of patients with acute MI brought to the catheterization laboratory, and (E) mortality be < 12%. With the exception of time delays, these goals were easily achieved in most primary PCI trials. Miller et al showed that these goals could also be obtained in the community hospital setting [101]. There is evidence that vessel patency rates and clinical outcome are not compromised by a time delay of up to 60–120 minutes [102]. Berger et all showed that in the GUSTO IIb trial, time from enrollment to first balloon inflation was an independent predictor of death and that mortality began increasing after 60 minutes [103]. Studies by Cannon et al and Liem et al suggest that mortality increases and myocardial salvage decreases after a delay of 120 minutes [104, 105].

It has been suggested that primary PCI should not be performed by low-volume operators (usually defined as less than 75 cases/year). However, an analysis of the PAMI 2 database revealed no significant differences in the rates of in-hospital death, CABG or acute PCI success [106]. Similar findings were reported in the GUSTO IIb trial [23]. A larger study by Ellis et al found that overall, high-volume operators have a lower incidence of major complications but that the difference was not consistent for all operators studied [107]. There is some evidence that institutional experience as a whole may influence procedural outcome with better results achieved in busier centers [108, 109].

PATIENT SELECTION AND PERIPROCEDURAL CARE

As previously stated, from a technical perspective primary PCI can be performed successfully in over 90% of patients. However the decision to proceed must be agreed upon by both the patient and physician. Patients with multiple co-morbidities or other advanced disease states (i.e. metastatic malignancies) may choose not to undergo the procedure. When time allows, the risks, benefits and alternatives (thrombolytic therapy or medical stabilization) should be discussed with the patient and written, informed consent obtained.

Once the decision has been made to proceed to angiography and primary PCI, if appropriate, the patient is usually given 325 mg of soluble aspirin along with some form of heparin (ACC/AHA guidelines recommend a bolus of 70 units/kg of unfractionated heparin). Oxygen, nitrates, morphine and beta-blockers are administered as needed for double-product control and pain relief. Occasionally, mechanical ventilation and/or a transvenous pacemaker is necessary. If a glycoprotein IIb/IIIa receptor antagonist is to be used, it may be started in the emergency department. However, if the patient has a significant likelihood of going to bypass surgery (for left main disease, severe three-vessel disease or mechanical complication), the administration of these drugs should be postponed until the coronary anatomy is defined. A brief checklist made available in the emergency department may help eliminate oversights during what may be a rapidly unfolding sequence of events.

Once the patient has undergone diagnostic angiography and a suitable culprit lesion identified, primary PCI is performed. If a glycoprotein IIb/IIIa receptor antagonist is to be used, it should be started prior to crossing the lesion if possible. If these agents are used, we titrate the activated clotting time (ACT) to approximately 250 seconds, otherwise we attempt to keep the ACT between 300 and 350 seconds. In general we use ionic, low osmolar contrast (such as ioxaglate) in order to avoid any possible prothrombotic tendencies [3]. We place an intra-aortic balloon pump only in patients with evidence of sustained hemodynamic compromise or intractable arrhythmias.

Most patients undergo initial PTCA often followed by placement of an intracoronary stent. As discussed above, other lesion specific modalities may be applied in select cases. Usually only the culprit lesion is intervened upon in the acute setting. Other significant stenoses may be treated with a staged procedure once the patient has recovered from the index event (although some operators may perform multi-vessel PCI in this setting).

All patients should be placed on aspirin (usually indefinitely) following PCI unless a definitive contraindication is present. Systemic heparin is generally not continued after the procedure unless balloon counterpulsation is used or the patient is at high-risk for an embolic event. Any patient receiving a stent should also be placed on a second antiplatelet agent (clopidogrel or ticlopidine), usually for four weeks. Some providers will add a second anti-platelet for two to four weeks following PTCA only but there are no randomized data to support this strategy. Beta-blockers, ace inhibitors and hypolipidemic agents should be instituted as specified in the ACC/AHA Guidelines [99].

Low-risk patients (see above) may be transferred to a step-down telemetry unit and usually do not need further risk stratification. They may be safely discharged on hospital day three if their course remains uneventful [25]. Intermediate and high-risk patients should be initially admitted to a coronary care unit and may require a staged procedure or non-invasive risk stratification prior to hospital discharge. All patients are seen in one to two weeks to insure that they continue to recover appropriately and to insure proper access site healing.

FUTURE INSIGHTS

Many dedicated investigators are working on the development of better and easier to use stents and other devices. In addition, combination drug therapy involving reduced dose thrombolytic therapy and glycoprotein IIb/IIIa receptor antagonists are being studied both as a method of improving pharmacologic reperfusion and as an adjunct to planned PCI ('facilitated angioplasty') [110]. Strategies to improve myocardial salvage such as inhibition of the sodium/hydrogen exchanger [111], filtration/ inhibition of neutrophils [112], myocardial delivery of hyperbaric oxygen [113] and hypothermic angioplasty are being studied. Methods to improve myocardial perfusion grade in addition to time flow are also being studied. In addition, the search for methods to reduce restenosis continue. Despite great progress there is still much left to do in the area of primary percutaneous intervention for acute myocardial infarction.

CONCLUSION

Primary percutaneous intervention for acute myocardial infarction is both feasible and safe. With the development of easily deployable stents as well as better adjunctive pharmacology, primary PCI can be performed in nearly all patients with acute MI. Continued advances in device and drug therapy will further expand the applicability of this strategy.

REFERENCES

1. Antman EM, Braunwald E. Acute myocardial infarction. In: Braunwald E, ed, *Heart Disease. A textbook of cardiovascular medicine* (Philadelphia, Pennsylvania: WB Saunders Company, 1997) 1184–1188.
2. Grines CL. Primary angioplasty—the strategy of choice, *N Engl J Med* 1996; **335**:1313–1316.
3. Grines CL, Browne KF, Marco J et al. A comparison of immediate angioplasty with thrombolytic therapy for acute myocardial infarction, *N Engl J Med* 1993; **328**:673–679.
4. O'Keefe JH, Bailey WL, Rutherford BD, Hartzler GO. Primary angioplasty for acute myocardial infarction in 1000 consecutive patients. Results in an unselected population and high-risk subgroups, *Am J Cardiol* 1993; **72**:107G–115G.
5. Hartzler GO, Rutherford BD, McConahay DR et al. Percutaneous transluminal coronary angioplasty with and without thrombolytic therapy for treatment of acute myocardial infarction, *Am Heart D* 1983; **106**:965–973.
6. Rothbaum DA, Linnemeier TJ, Landin RJ et al. Emergency percutaneous transluminal coronary angioplasty in acute myocardial infarction: A three year experience, *J Am Coll Cardiol* 1987; **10**:264–272.
7. Marco J, Caster L, Szatmary LJ, Fajadet J. Emergency percutaneous transluminal coronary angioplasty without thrombolysis as initial therapy in acute myocardial infarction, *Int J Cardiol* 1987; **15**:55–63.
8. Lee L, Bates ER, Pitt B, Walton JA, Laufer N, O'Neill WW. Percutaneous transluminal coronary angioplasty improves survival in acute myocardial infarction complicated by cardiogenic shock, *Circulation* 1988; **78**:1345–1351.
9. Ellis SG, O'Neill WW, Bates ER, Walton JA, Nabel EG, Topol EJ. Coronary angioplasty as primary therapy for acute myocardial infarction 6–48 hours after symptom onset: report of an initial experience, *J Am Coll Cardiol* 1989; **13**:1122–1126.
10. Veran E, Repetto S, Boscarini M, Ghezzi I, Binaghi G. Emergency coronary angioplasty in patients with severe left ventricular dysfunction or cardiogenic shock after acute myocardial infarction, *Eur Heart J* 1989; **10**:958–966.
11. Flaker GC, Webel RR, Meinhardt S et al. Emergency angioplasty in acute anterior myocardial infarction, *Am Heart J* 1989; **118**:1154–1160.
12. Kahn JK, Rutherford BD, McConahay DR et al. Catheterization laboratory events and hospital outcome with direct angioplasty for acute myocardial infarction, *Circulation* 1990; **82**:1910–1915.
13. Rogers WJ, Dean LS, Moore PB, Wool WJ, Burgard SL, Bradley EL. Comparison of primary angioplasty versus thrombolytic therapy for acute myocardial infarction, *Am J Cardiol* 1994; **74**:111–118.
14. Tiefenbrunn AJ, Chandra NC, French WJ, Gore JM, Rogers WJ. Clinical experience with primary percutaneous transluminal coronary angioplasty compared with Ateplase (recombinant tissue-type plasminogen activator) in

patients with acute myocardial infarction. A report from the second national registry of myocardial infarction (NRMI), *J Am Coll Cardiol* 1998; **31**:1240–1245.

15. Grines CL. Selection of patients for reperfusion therapy. In: Califf RM, Mark DB, Wagner GS, eds, *Acute Coronary Care* 2nd edn (St Louis, Missouri: Mosby-Year Book, Inc, 1995) 215–228.

16. Dauerman HL, Pinto DS, Ho KL et al. Acute infarct angioplasty: differential mortality of trial eligible and ineligible patients, *Circulation* 1998; **98**:1–22.

17. Brodie BR, Weintraub RA, Stuckey TD et al. Outcomes of direct coronary angioplasty for acute myocardial infarction in candidates and non-candidates for thrombolytic therapy, *Am J Cardiol* 1991; **67**:7–12.

18. Gibbons RJ, Holmes DR, Reeder GS et al. Immediate angioplasty compared with the administration of a thrombolytic agent followed by conservative treatment for myocardial infarction, *N Engl J Med* 1993; **328**:685–691.

19. Zijlstra F, De Boer MJ, Hoorntje JCA et al. A comparison of immediate coronary angioplasty with intravenous streptokinase in acute myocardial infarction, *N Engl J Med* 1993; **328**:680–684.

20. Zijlstra F, Hoorntje JC, de Boer MJ et al. Long-term benefit of primary angioplasty as compared with thrombolytic therapy for acute myocardial infarction, *N Engl J Med* 1999; **341**:1413–1419.

21. Stone GW, Grines CL, Browne KF et al. Predictors of in-hospital and six-month outcome after acute myocardial infarction in the reperfusion era: the primary angioplasty in myocardial infarction (PAMI) trial, *J Am Coll Cardiol* 1995; **25**:370–377.

22. Zijlstra F, Hoorntje JCA, De Boer MJ et al. Long-term benefit of primary angioplasty as compared with thrombolytic therapy for acute myocardial infarction, *N Engl J Med* 1999; **341**:1413–1419.

23. GUSTO IIb Angioplasty Substudy Investigators. A clinical trial comparing primary coronary angioplasty with tissue plasminogen activator for acute myocardial infarction, *N Engl J Med* 1997; **336**:1521–1528.

24. DeGeare VS, Stone GW, Grines CL. The case for primary catheter-based reperfusion in acute MI. In: Braunwald E, ed, *Heart Disease Updates* (Philadelphia: WB Saunders, 1999).

25. Stone GW, Marsalese D, Brodie BR et al. A prospective, randomized evaluation of prophylactic intra-aortic balloon counterpulsation in high-risk patients with acute myocardial infarction treated with primary angioplasty, *J Am Coll Cardiol* 1997; **29**:1459–1467.

26. Weaver WD, Simes RJ, Betriu A et al. Comparison of primary coronary angioplasty and intravenous thrombolytic therapy for acute myocardial infarction. A quantitative review, *JAMA* 1997; **278**: 2093–2098.

27. The GUSTO Investigators. An international randomized trial comparing four thrombolytic strategies for active myocardial infarction, *N Engl J Med* 1993; **329** (10): 673–682.

28. O'Neill WW, Griffen JJ, Stone GW et al. Operator and institutional volume do not affect the procedural outcome of primary angioplasty therapy, *J Am Coll Cardiol* 1996; **27**:13A.

29. Grines CL, Ellis SG, Jones M et al. Primary coronary angioplasty vs thrombolytic therapy for acute myocardial infarction: long-term follow-up of ten randomized trials, *Circulation* 1999; **100**:I-499.

30. Thiemann DR, Coresh J, Schulman SP et al. Lack of benefit for intravenous thrombolysis in patients with myocardial infarction who are older than 75 years, *Circulation* 2000; **101**:2239–2246.

31. Holmes DR, White HD, Pieper KS et al. Effect of age on outcome with primary angioplasty versus thrombolysis, *J Am Coll Cardiol* 1999; **33** (2):412–419.

32. DeGeare VS, Stone GW, Grines L et al. Angiographic and clinical characteristics associated with increased in-hospital mortality in elderly patients undergoing percutaneous intervention: a pooled analysis of the PAMI trials, *Am J Cardiol* 2000; **86**:30–34.

33. Hands ME, Rutherford JD, Muller JE et al. The in-hospital development of cardiogenic shock after myocardial infarction: predictors of occurrence, outcome and prognosis factors, *J Am Coll Cardiol* 1989; **14**:40–46.

34. Gruppo Italiano per Studio della Streptochinasi nell'Infarto Miocardio (GISSI). Effectiveness of intravenous thrombolytic treatment in acute myocardial infarction, *Lancet* 1986; **I**:397–401.

35. Kennedy JW, Gensin GG, Timmis GC et al. Acute myocardial infarction treated with streptokinase: a report of the Society for Cardiac Angiography, *Am J Cardiol* 1985; **55**:871–877.

36. The International Study Group. In-hospital mortality and clinical course of 20,891 patients with suspected acute myocardial infarction randomized between alteplase and streptokinase with or without heparin, *Lancet* 1990; **336**:71–75.

37. Gruppo Italiano per Studio della Streptochinasi nell'Infarto Miocardio (GISSI). Long-term effects of intravenous thrombolysis in acute myocardial infarction: final report of the GISSI study, *Lancet* 1987; **II**:871–874.

38. Lee L, Erbel R, Brown TM et al. Multicenter registry of angioplasty therapy of cardiogenic shock: initial and long-term survival, *J Am Coll Cardiol* 1991; **17**:599–603.

39. Bates ER, Topol EJ. Limitations of thrombolytic therapy for acute myocardial infarction complicated by congestive heart failure and cardiogenic shock, *J Am Coll Cardiol* 1991; **18**: 1077–1084.

40. Hochman JS, Sleeper LA, Webb JG et al for the SHOCK investigators. Early revascularization in acute myocardial infarction complicated by cardiogenic shock, *N Engl J Med* 1999; **341** (9):625–634.

41. DeGeare VS, Goldstein JA, Gangadharan V, Levin RN, Boura JA, Grines LL. Predictive value of the Killip classification in patients undergoing primary percutaneous intervention for acute MI: a pooled analysis of the PAMI trials, *Circulation* 1999; **100** (suppl I):I-809.

42. Kavanaugh KM, Topol EJ. Acute intervention during myocardial infarction in patients with prior coronary bypass surgery, *Am J Cardiol* 1990; **65**:924–926.

43. Grines CL, Booth DC, Nissen SE et al. Mechanism of acute myocardial infarction in patients with prior coronary artery bypass grafting and therapeutic implications, *Am J Cardiol* 1990; **65**:1292–1296.

44. The CORAMI Study Group. Outcome of attempted rescue coronary angioplasty after failed thrombolysis for acute myocardial infarction, *Am J Cardiol* 1994; **74**:172–174.

45. Ellis SG, da Silva ER, Heyndrickx G et al. Randomized comparison of rescue angioplasty with conservative management of patients with early failure of thrombolysis for acute anterior myocardial infarction, *Circulation* 1994; **90**: 2280–2284.

46. Gibson CM, Cannon CP, Greene RM for the TIMI 4 study group. Rescue angioplasty in the thrombolysis in myocardial infarction (TIMI) 4 trial, *Am J Cardiol* 1997; **80**:21–26.

47. Ross AM, Lundergran CF, Rohrbeck SC for the GUSTO I angiographic investigators. Rescue angioplasty after failed thrombolysis: technical and clinical outcomes in a large thrombolysis trial, *J Am Coll Cardiol* 1998; **31**:1511–1517.

48. Miller JM, Smalling R, Ohman EM for the GUSTO III investigators. Effectiveness of early coronary angioplasty and abciximab for failed thrombolysis (reteplase or alteplase) during acute myocardial infarction (results from the GUSTO-III trial), *Am J Cardiol* 1999; **84**:779–784.

49. Rodriguez A, Bernardi V, Fernandez M for the GRAMI investigators. In-hospital and late results of coronary stents versus conventional balloon angioplasty in acute myocardial infarction (GRAMI trial), *Am J Cardiol* 1998; **81**: 1286–1291.

50. Saito S, Hosokawa G, Suzuki S, Nakamura S for the Japanese PASTA trial study group. Primary stent implantation is superior to balloon angioplasty in acute myocardial infarction—the result of the Japanese PASTA (Primary Angioplasty Versus Stent Implantation in Acute Myocardial Infarction) Trial, *J Am Coll Cardiol* 1997; **29**:390A.

51. Antoniucci D, Santoro G, Bolognese L et al. A clinical trial comparing primary stenting of the infarct-related artery with optimal primary angioplasty for acute myocardial infarction. Results from the Florence Randomized Elective Stenting in Acute Coronary Occlusions (FRESCO) Trial, *J Am Coll Cardiol* 1998; **31**:1234–1239.

52. Stone GW, Brodie BR, Griffin JJ et al. Prospective, multicenter study of the safety and feasibility of primary stenting in acute myocardial infarction: in-hospital and 30-day results of the PAMI Stent Pilot Trial, *J Am Coll Cardiol* 1998; **31**:23–30.

53. Grines CL, Cox DA, Stone GW et al for the Stent Primary Angioplasty in Myocardial Infarction Study Group. Coronary angioplasty with or without stent implantation for acute myocardial infarction, *N Engl J Med* 1999; **341** (26): 1949–1956.

54. Grines CL, Cox DA, Stone GW et al. Stent-PAMI: 12 month results and predicators of mortality, *J Am Coll Cardiol* 2000; **35** (suppl A):402A.

55. Stone GW for the CADILLAC investigators.

Presented at the 12th Annual Transcatheter Cardiovascular Therapeutics Conference, Washington, DC, October 2000.

56. Reisman M. Procedure. In: *Guide to Rotational Atherectomy* (Birmingham, MI: Physicians' Press) 37–117.

57. Saito S, Kim K, Hosokawa G et al. Short- and long-term clinical effects of primary directional coronary atherectomy for acute myocardial infarction, *Cathet Cardiovasc Diagn* 1996; **39**:157–165.

58. Kaplan BM, Larkin T, Safian RD et al. Prospective study of extraction atherectomy in patients with acute myocardial infarction, *Am J Cardiol* 1996; **78**:383–388.

59. Kaplan BM, Larkin T, Safian RD et al. Prospective study of extraction atherectomy in patients with acute myocardial infarction, *Am J Cardiol* 1996; **78**:383–388.

60. Topol EJ. Catheter-based reperfusion for acute myocardial infarction. In: Topol EJ, ed, *Textbook of Interventional Cardiology* 3rd edn (Philadelphia, Pennsylvania: WB Saunders Company 1999) 265–279.

61. Alexander JH, Kong DF, Cantor WJ. Highlights from the 71st American Heart Association scientific sessions: November 8–11, 1998, *Am Heart J* 1999; **137** (3):555–574.

62. Estella P, Ryan TJ, Landzberg JS, Bittl JA. Excimer laser: assisted coronary angioplasty for lesions containing thrombus, *J Am Coll Cardiol* 1993; **21**:1550–1556.

63. Topaz O, Melvor M, Stone GW et al. Acute results, complications, and effect of lesion characteristics on outcome with the solid-state, pulsed-wave, mid-infrared laser angioplasty system: final multicenter registry report. Holmium: YAG Laser Multicenter Investigators, *Lasers Surg & Med* 1998; **22** (4):228–239.

64. Rosenschein U, Roth A, Rassin T et al. Analysis of coronary ultrasound thrombolysis endpoints in acute myocardial infarction (ACUTE Trial). Results of the feasibility phase, *Circulation* 1997; **95**:1411–1416.

65. Hamm CW, Steffen W, Terres W et al. Intravascular therapeutic ultrasound thrombolysis in acute myocardial infarction, *Am J Cardiol* 1997; **80**:200–204.

66. Leon MB, Safian RD, Freed M. *Interventional cardiology self-assessment and review*, Volumes I and II (Birmingham, Michigan: Physicians' Press 1999) 191.

67. Antman EM for the TIMI 9B investigators. Hirudin in acute myocardial infarction. Thrombolysis and thrombin inhibition in myocardial infarction (TIMI) 9B trial, *Circulation* 1996; **94**:911–921.

68. The global use of strategies to open occluded coronary arteries (GUSTO) IIb investigators. A comparison of recombinant hirudin with heparin for the treatment of acute coronary syndromes, *N Engl J Med* 1996; **335**:775–782.

69. Rabah MM, Premmereur J, Graham M et al. Usefulness of intravenous enoxaparin for percutaneous intervention in stable angina pectoris, *Am J Cardiol* 1999; **84**:1391–1395.

70. Hall P, Nakamura S, Maiello L. A randomized comparison of combined ticlopidine and aspirin therapy versus aspirin alone after successful intravascular ultrasound-guided stent implantation, *Circulation* 1996; **93**:215–222.

71. Schomig A, Neumann FJ, Walter H. Coronary stent placement in patients with acute myocardial infarction: comparison of clinical and angiographic outcome after randomization to antiplatelet or anticoagulant therapy, *J Am Coll Cardiol* 1997; **29** (1):28–34.

72. Bertrand ME, Legrand V, Boland J. Randomized multicenter comparison of conventional anticoagulation versus antiplatelet therapy in unplanned and elective coronary stenting. The full anticoagulation versus aspirin and ticlopidine (FANTASTIC) study, *Circulation* 1998; **98**:1597–1603.

73. Urban P, Macaya C, Rupprecht HJ for the MATTIS investigators. Randomized evaluation of anticoagulation versus antiplatelet therapy after coronary stent placement in high-risk patients. The multicenter aspirin and ticlopidine trial after intracoronary stenting (MATTIS), *Circulation* 1998; **98**:2126–2132.

74. Berger PB. Aspirin, ticlopidine and clopidogrel in and out of the catheterization laboratory, *J Inv Cardiol* 1999; **11**:20–29A.

75. Neumann FJ, Schomig A. Stent anticoagulation and technique. In: Topol EJ, ed, *Textbook of Interventional Cardiology*, 3rd edn (Cleveland, OH: WB Saunders Company 1999) 592.

76. Bennett CL, Connors JM, Carwile JM. Thrombotic thrombocytopenic purpura associated with clopidogrel, *N Engl J Med* 2000; **342**:1773–1777.

77. Bertand ME. Clopidogrel Aspirin Stent Interventional Cooperative Study. Presented at the American College of Cardiology 48th Annual Scientific Sessions. March 1999, New Orleans, LA.

78. The PURSUIT Trial Investigators. Inhibition of platelet glycoprotein IIb/IIIa with eptifibatide in patients with acute coronary syndromes, *N Engl J Med* 1998; **339**:436–443.

79. The Platelet Receptor Inhibition in Ischemic Syndrome Management (PRISM) Study Investigators. A comparison of aspirin plus tirofiban with aspirin plus heparin for unstable angina, *N Engl J Med* 1998; **338**:1498–1505.

80. The Platelet Receptor Inhibition in Ischemic Syndrome Management in Patients Limited by Unstable Signs and Symptoms (PRISM-PLUS) Study Investigators. Inhibition of the platelet glycoprotein IIb/IIIa receptor with tirofiban in unstable angina and non-Q wave myocardial infarction, *N Engl J Med* 1998; **338**:1488–1497.

81. The PARAGON Investigators. International, randomized, controlled trial of lamifiban (a platelet glycoprotein IIb/IIIa inhibitor), heparin, or both in unstable angina, *Circulation* 1998; **97**:2386–2395.

82. The CAPTURE Investigators. Randomized placebo-controlled trial of effect of abciximab before and during coronary intervention in refractory unstable angina: the CAPTURE study, *Lancet* 1997; **349**:1429–1435.

83. The EPISTENT Investigators. Randomized placebo-controlled and balloon-angioplasty controlled trial to assess safety of coronary stenting with use of platelet glycoprotein IIb/IIIa blockade, *Lancet* 1998; **352**:87–92.

84. Lefkovits J, Ivanhoe RJ, Califf RM et al for the EPIC Investigators. Effects of platelet glycoprotein IIb/IIIa receptor blockade by a chimeric monoclonal antibody (Abciximab) on acute and six-month outcomes after percutaneous transluminal coronary angioplasty for acute myocardial infarction, *Am J Cardiol* 1996; **77**:1045–1051.

85. Brener SJ, Barr LA, Burchenal JEB et al on behalf of the ReoPro and Primary PTCA Organization and Randomized Trial (RAP-PORT) Investigators. Randomized, placebo-controlled trial of platelet glycoprotein IIb/IIIa blockade with primary angioplasty for acute myocardial infarction, *Circulation* 1998; **98**: 734–741.

86. Montalescot G. Abciximab before direct angioplasty and stenting in myocardial infarction regarding acute and long term follow-up. Presented at the American College of Cardiology 48th Annual Scientific Sessions, March 1999, New Orleans, LA.

87. MERIT (Medical Education Reports, Interviews, and Testimony) Newsflash, *Health Science Communications* 2000; **1** (3):5.

88. The EPILOG Investigators. Platelet glycoprotein IIb/IIIa receptor blockade and low dose heparin during percutaneous coronary revascularization, *N Engl J Med* 1997; **336**:1689–1696.

89. Lieu TA, Lundstrom RJ, Ray GT et al. Initial cost of primary angioplasty for acute myocardial infarction, *J Am Coll Cardiol* 1996; **28**:882–889.

90. Stone GW, Grines CL, Rothbaum D et al for the PAMI Trial Investigators. Analysis of the relative costs and effectiveness of primary angioplasty versus tissue-type plasminogen activator: the primary angioplasty in myocardial infarction (PAMI) trial, *J Am Coll Cardiol* 1997; **29** (5):901–907.

91. DeBoer MJ, van Haut BA, Liem AL et al. A cost-effective analysis of primary coronary angioplasty versus thrombolysis for acute myocardial infarction, *Am J Cardiol* 1995; **76**: 830–833.

92. Solomon R, Werner C, Mann D, D'Elia J, Silva P. Effects of saline, mannitol, and furosemide on acute decreases in renal function induced by radiocontrast agents, *N Engl J Med* 1994; **331**:1416–1420.

93. Stevens MA, McCullough PA, Tobin KJ et al. A prospective randomized trial of prevention measures in patients at high risk for contrast nephropathy, *J Am Coll Cardiol* 1999; **33**:403–411.

94. Heupler FA, for the members of the laboratory performance standards committee of the society for cardiac angiography and interventions. Guidelines for performing angiography in patients taking metformin, *Cathet Cardiovasc Diagn* 1998; **43**:121–123.

95. Thomsen HS, Bush WH. Review article. Treatment of the adverse effects of contrast media, *Acta Radiologica* 1998; **39**:212–218.

96. Grines CL, Balestrini C, Westerhausen DR et al. A randomized trial of thrombolysis vs transfer for primary PTCA in high risk AMI patients: results of the AIR PAMI trial, *J Am Coll Cardiol* 2000; **35**:376A.

97. Jhangiani AH, Jorgensen MB, Kotlewski A. Community practice of primary angioplasty for myocardial infarction, *Am J Cardiol* 1997; **80**: 209–212.

98. Wharton TP, Johnston JD, Turco MA et al. Primary angioplasty for acute myocardial infarction with no surgery on site: outcomes, core angiographic analysis and six-month follow-up in the 500 patient prospective PAMI-No S.O.S. registry, *J Am Coll Cardiol* 1999; **33** (suppl A):352A.

99. Ryan TJ, Antman EM, Brooks NH et al. ACC/AHA guidelines for the management of patients with acute myocardial infarction: executive summary and recommendations. A report of the American College of Cardiology/American Heart Association task force on practice guidelines (committee on management of acute myocardial infarction), *Circulation* 1999; **100**:1016–1030.

100. Ryan TJ, Anderson JL, Antman EM et al. ACC/AHA guidelines for the management of patients with acute myocardial infarction. A report of the American College of Cardiology/American Heart Association task force on practice guidelines (committee on management of acute myocardial infarction), *J Am Coll Cardiol* 1996; **28** (5):1328–1428.

101. Miller PF, Brodie BR, Weintraub RA et al. Emergency coronary angioplasty for acute myocardial infarction. Results from a community hospital, *Arch Intern Med* 1987; **147**:1565–1570.

102. Brodie BR, Stuckey TD, Wall TC et al. Importance of time of reperfusion for hospital and long-term survival and recovery of left ventricular function after primary angioplasty for acute myocardial infarction, *Circulation* 1997; (suppl 1):I-32.

103. Berger PB, Ellis SG, Holmes DR et al. Relationship between delay in performing direct coronary angioplasty and early clinical outcome in patients with acute myocardial infarction. Results from the Global Use of Strategies to Open Occluded Arteries in Acute Coronary Syndromes (GUSTO-IIb) Trial, *Circulation* 1999; **100**:14–20.

104. Cannon CP, Gibson CB, Lambrew CT et al. Relationship of symptom-onset-to-balloon time and door-to-balloon time with mortality in patients undergoing angioplasty for acute myocardial infarction, *JAMA* 2000; **283**: 2941–2947.

105. Liem AL, Van T Hof AWJ, Hoorntje JCA. Influence of treatment delay on infarct size and clinical outcome in patients with acute myocardial infarction treated with primary angioplasty, *J Am Coll Cardiol* 1998; **32**:629–633.

106. O'Neill WW, Griffin JJ, Stone G et al. Operator and institutional volume do not affect the procedural outcome of primary angioplasty therapy, *J Am Coll Cardiol* 1996; **27**:13A.

107. Ellis SG, Weintraub W, Holmes D et al. Relation of operator volume and experience to procedural outcome of percutaneous coronary revascularization at hospitals with high interventional volumes, *Circulation* 1997; **96**: 2479–2484.

108. Caputo RP, Lopez JJ, Stoler RC et al. The effect of institutional experience on the outcome of primary angioplasty for acute MI, *J Am Coll Cardiol* 1996; **27**:13A.

109. Cannon CP, Gibson M, Lambrew CT et al. Higher institutional volume of primary angioplasty cases is associated with lower mortality in acute myocardial infarction: an analysis of 27,080 patients, *Circulation* 1999; **100** (18):I-809.

110. Giugliano RP, Antman EM, McCabe CH et al. Factors associated with major hemorrhage during reperfusion therapy in acute myocardial infarction: A TIMI 14 substudy, *J Am Coll Cardiol* 1999; **33**:398A.

111. Theroux P. Guard during ischemia against necrosis, *Clin Cardiol* 1999; **22**:369–372.

112. Patel MB, Qureshi MA, Goldstein JA, O'Neill WW. Reperfusion with leukocyte depleted blood during primary PTCA in patients with acute myocardial infarction: initial clinical experience, *Circulation* 1999; **100** (suppl I): I-358.

113. Spears JR, Henney C, Prcevshi P et al. Reperfusion microvascular ischemia attenuated with aqueous oxygen infusion in a porcine coronary occlusion model, *Circulation* 1999; **100** (suppl I):I-512.

114. GUSTO III investigators. A comparison of reteplase with alteplase for acute myocardial infarction, *N Engl J Med* 1997; **337**:1118–1123.

115. Chesebro JH, Knatterud G, Roberts R et al. Thrombolysis in myocardial infarction (TIMI) trial, Phase I: comparison between intravenous tissue plasminogen activator and intravenous streptokinase. Clinical findings through hospital discharge, *Circulation* 1987; **76** (1):142–154.

116. Cannon CP, McCabe CH, Diver DJ et al and the TIMI 4 investigators. Comparison of front-loaded recombinant tissue-type plasminogen activator, anistreplase and combination thrombolytic therapy acute myocardial infarction: results of the thrombolysis in myocardial infarction (TIMI) 4 trial, *J Am Coll Cardiol* 1994; **24** (7):1602–1610.

117. Wall TC, Califf RM, George BS et al for the TAMI-7 study group. Accelerated plasminogen activator dose regimens for coronary thrombolysis, *J Am Coll Cardiol* 1992; **19** (3):482–489.

118. ISIS-2 (Second International Study of Infarct Survival) Collaborative Group. Randomized trial of intravenous streptokinase, oral aspirin, both, or neither among 17,187 cases of suspected acute myocardial infarction: ISIS-2, *Lancet* 1988; **2**:349–360.

119. ISIS-3 (Third International Study of Infarct Survival) Collaborative Group. ISIS-3: a randomised comparison of streptokinase vs tissue plasminogen activator vs anistreplase and of aspirin plus heparin vs aspirin alone among 41,299 cases of suspected acute myocardial infarction, *Lancet* 1992; **339** (8796):753–770.

120. GISSI-2: a factorial randomised trial of alteplase versus streptokinase and heparin versus no heparin among 12,490 patients with acute myocardial infarction, *Lancet* 1990; **336**:65–71.

121. Anderson JL, Sorensen SG, Moreno FL et al and the TEAM-2 study investigators. Multicenter patency trail of intravenous anistreplase compared with streptokinase in acute myocardial infarction, *Circulation* 1991; **83**:126–140.

122. Califf RM, Topol EJ, Stack RS et al for the TAMI study group. Evaluation of combination thrombolytic therapy and timing of cardiac catheterization in acute myocardial infarction. Results of thrombolysis and angioplasty in myocardial infarction—phase 5 randomized trial, *Circulation* 1991; **83**:1543–1556.

123. Smalling RW, Bode C, Kalbfeisch J et al and the RAPID investigators. More rapid, complete, and stable coronary thrombolysis with bolus administration of reteplase compared with alteplase infusion in acute myocardial infarction, *Circulation* 1995; **91**:2725–2732.

124. Bode C, Smalling RW, Berg G et al. Randomized comparison of coronary thrombolysis achieved with double-bolus reteplase (recombinant plasminogen activator) and front-loaded, accelerated alteplase (recombinant tissue plasminogen activator) in patients with acute myocardial infarction, *Circulation* 1996; **94**:891–898.

125. Brodie BR, Grines CL, Ivanhoe R et al. Six-month clinical and angiographic follow-up after direct angioplasty for acute myocardial infarction: final results from the Primary Angioplasty Registry, *Circulation* 1994; **25**:156–162.

126. COBALT Investigators. A comparison of continuous infusion of alteplase with double bolus administration for acute myocardial infarction, *N Engl J Med* 1997; **337**:1124–1130.

127. Topol EJ, Califf RM, Vandormael M et al and the thrombolysis and angioplasty in myocardial infarction-6 study group. A randomized trial of late reperfusion therapy for acute myocardial infarction, *Circulation* 1992; **85** (6):2090–2099.

128. Veen G, Meyer A, Verheugt FW et al. Culprit lesion morphology and stenosis severity in the prediction of reocclusion after coronary thrombolysis: angiographic results of the APRICOT study. Antithrombotics in the Prevention of Reocclusion in Coronary Thrombolysis, *J Am Coll Cardiol* 1993; **22** (7):1755–1762.

129. Takens BH, Brugemann J, van der Meer J, den Heijer P, Lie KI. Reocclusion three months after successful thrombolytic treatment of acute myocardial infarction with anisoylated plasminogen streptokinase activating complex, *Am J Cardiol* 1990; **65**:1422–1424.

130. White HD, French JK, Hamer AW et al. Frequent reocclusion of patent infarct-related arteries between four weeks and one year: effects of antiplatelet therapy, *J Am Coll Cardiol* 1995; **25** (1):218–223.

131. O'Neill WW, Weintraub R, Grines CL et al. A prospective placebo-controlled randomized trial of intravenous streptokinase and angioplasty therapy of acute myocardial infarction, *Circulation* 1992; **86** (6):1710–1717.

21

Acute myocardial infarction: SMASH perspective

Jean-Christophe E Stauffer and Philip M Urban

CONTENTS • Introduction • Data from non-randomized registries • Dedicated randomized control trials • Unresolved issues • Practical recommendations: early recognition and prevention

INTRODUCTION

The single most important advance in therapy of acute myocardial infarction is the advent of strategies to rapidly reopen the totally occluded infarct-related artery with either thrombolytic agents or angioplasty. Multiple large randomized clinical trials (thrombolysis) have consistently demonstrated restoration of patency (up to 80%), preserved left ventricular function and improved survival [1–5].

Smaller randomized trials (PTCA) have confirmed a superiority of angioplasty over thrombolytic treatment with a lower rate of death or non-fatal reinfarction and a lower rate of stroke [6]. However it is noteworthy that most of these trials excluded patients presenting in cardiogenic shock.

This ominous complication still occurs in 6–10% of cases [7–9]. Historical mortality rated around 80–90% [10], and recent data reported mortality around 60–70% [8, 9]. Thus it remains the leading in-hospital cause of death of patients admitted with an acute myocardial infarction.

Two placebo-controlled trials of thrombolytic therapy demonstrated a reduction in the incidence of cardiogenic shock [11, 12]. Primary angioplasty appears to be associated with similar or possibly somewhat lower incidence of cardiogenic shock, but despite the wider use of such strategies, it was still diagnosed in seven percent of patients admitted to several hospitals during a 23-year period [13].

It is relevant to observe that most patients who develop cardiogenic shock will do so after hospital admission. In the GUSTO I trial, out of 41,000 patients with an acute myocardial infarction, 0.8% had shock on hospital admission and 5.3% developed shock thereafter [9], with approximately 50% doing so within the first 24 hours.

DATA FROM NON-RANDOMIZED REGISTRIES

In the mid 1980s, most interventional cardiologists were reluctant to undertake invasive evaluation of patients in cardiogenic shock. It all started with case reports (such as the one presented in Figures 21.1–21.4), followed by uncontrolled observational studies and registries.

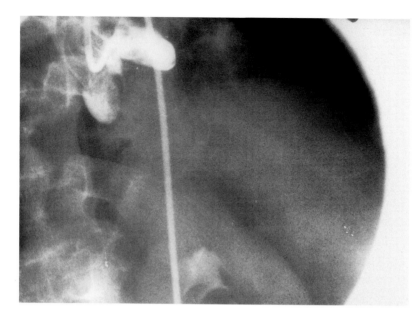

Figure 21.1
Thirty degree right anterior oblique coronary angiography of the left system demonstrating occlusion of the main stem in a patient in acute cardiogenic shock.

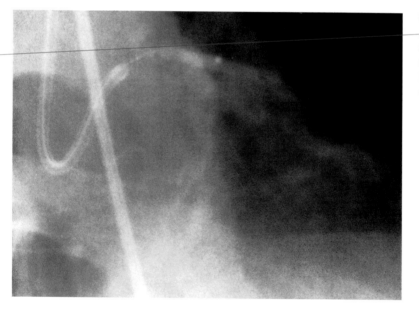

Figure 21.2
After a forceful injection of dye, recanalization of the left system angioplasty of the left main and proximal anterior descending artery.

Observational studies

More than 25 papers reported encouraging results with percutaneous intervention [14–40] with an overall mortality in the range of 40–50% but with considerable variation (14–78% mortality reported!). Bypass surgery claimed even better results overall [9, 26, 32, 36, 38, 41–64] but again with reported mortality of 0% [53] or as high as 91% [38]. Despite these encouraging data, the exact benefit of such treatment modality is difficult to assess as prob-

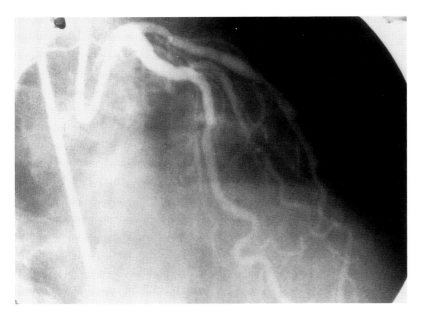

Figure 21.3
Final result after balloon
angioplasty.

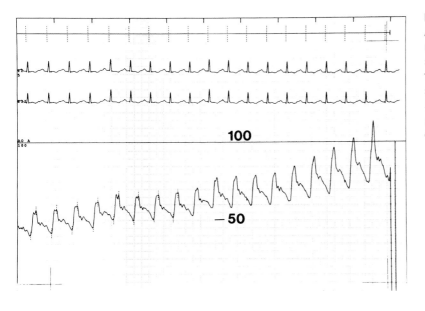

Figure 21.4
Aortic pressure measurement
recording obtained a few
seconds after recanalization of
the left coronary artery. Each
systole is associated with a
5 mmHg increase in blood
pressure, related to recruitment
of myocytes.

able selection of less ill patients (or at least de facto of patients still alive at time of cardiac catheterization and/or surgery); associated with a likely tendency to report only positive results (of the more aggressive treatment) may have both contributed to major bias.

Registries

The largest cohort of patients with cardiogenic shock in a prospective registry comes from GUSTO I trial [9]. Of the 41,021 general population selected, 7.2% (2972) developed

Table 21.1 Major inclusion and exclusion criteria

	SHOCK	SMASH
Inclusion criteria:		
Cause of cardiogenic shock	Pump failure	Pump failure
Systolic blood pressure	<90 mmHg or requiring Inotropes	<90 mmHg despite Inotropes
Maximum time from AMI to randomization	<36 + 12 hrs.	<48 hrs.
Cardiac index	<2.2 l/min/m²	<2.2 l/min/m²
Pulmonary capillary wedge pressure	>15 mmHg	>15 mmHg
Exclusion criteria:		
MR, VSD, tamponade	Yes	Yes
Severe non-cardiac disease	Yes	Yes
Unsuitable for revascularization	Yes	Yes
Age limit	No	No

Table 21.2 Baseline characteristics at inclusion

	SHOCK	SMASH
Age	66 ± 10	65 ± 9
Male sex	68%	67%
Diabetes	31%	18%
Prior heart failure	6%	25%
Anterior AMI	60%	45%
Median time (h) from chest pain	5.0 (2.2–12.0) (invasive)	2.5 (0.0–27.0 invasive)
to shock onset	6.2 (2.4–15.5) (med. treatment)	5.0 (0.0–45.0 med. treatment)
CPR, VT or VF prior to randomization	33%	28%
Heart rate (bpm)	103 ± 22 (invasive)	101 ± 30 (invasive)
	100 ± 23 (med. treatment)	105 ± 0 (med. treatment)
Systolic BP (mmHg)	89 ± 23 (invasive)	77 ± 10 (invasive)
	87 ± 17 (med. treatment)	78 ± 13 (med. treatment)

cardiogenic shock with an overall 30-day mortality of 56%. The 30-day mortality was lower in the 406 patients who underwent early catheterization (30% versus 62%). The 30-day mortality was even lower in those with successful percutaneous transluminal coronary angioplasty (PTCA) (35% versus 55%). The 36 patients for whom surgical revascularization was performed had a 30-day mortality of 44%. This survival benefit remained at one year with an odds ratio of 0.6 (95% confidence interval 0.4, 0.9) [65]. Unfortunately 606 patients who had angiograms had no angiographic data available for analysis, and a further 152 patients died within the first hour, before angiography could be performed. Despite these limitations multi-variate analysis suggested that an aggressive strategy of early catheterization followed by revascularization when appropriate was inde-pendently associated with a reduced 30-day mortality (odds ratio 0.43, 95% CI = 0.34–0.54). In a subgroup analysis, the authors concluded that the lower mortality noticed in the American patient cohort may have been due to greater use of invasive diagnostic and thera-peutic procedures [35]. This statement should be seen as only a hypothesis, clearly especially if one considers that the incidence of shock was higher in the American cohort in comparison to the non-American population (8.3% versus 6.1%). This difference corresponds to a 20% increase of diagnosis of cardiogenic shock and suggests the possibility that American doctors may have used broader criteria for diagnosing cardiogenic shock. It is also worth noticing that even non-revascularized American patients had lower mortality than their non-American coun-terparts. The same point is clearly demonstra-ted on a recent report by Menon and colleagues [66] who evaluated the outcome of patients with cardiogenic shock in the GUSTO I and GUSTO III [67] trials. They reported a dif-ference in incidence of cardiogenic shock between the two trials (7.2% GUSTO I and 5.5% GUSTO III), which is mainly due to selection. The two populations are very dissimilar, GUSTO III patients being at much higher risk than GUSTO I patients (elderly, more diabetes, more anterior infarctions and higher Killip class on admission). This certainly explains the higher 30-day mortality observed in GUSTO III, compared with GUSTO I: 62% versus 54%. These differences in outcomes suggest it is essential to rely on randomized controlled trials to truly assess the impact of any revasculariza-tion for cardiogenic shock.

The other two large registries come from the shock trial [68], presented in the following chapter.

DEDICATED RANDOMIZED CONTROL TRIALS

Despite the fact that previous commentators thought that randomized trials performed in very sick patients with cardiogenic shock were unlikely [69], two such trials have been carried out: the SMASH (Swiss Multicenter Angio-plasty for SHock) [70] and the SHOCK (SHould we emergently revascularize Occluded Coronaries for cardiogenic shocK) [71]. While the SHOCK trial will be discussed in the follow-ing chapter, we will focus here on major differ-ences and similarities between the two trials.

Design of trials

Both trials were launched in the early 1990s to evaluate the impact of emergent revasculariza-tion for cardiogenic shock. Although neither the SMASH nor the SHOCK investigators were aware that another trial was being set up, both trials address the problem in a nearly identical manner. The major inclusion and exclusion criteria are listed in Table 21.1. Only patients with primary pump failure were included. The SMASH trial was powered to detect a 30% and the SHOCK trial a 20% reduction in all-cause mortality at 30 days (primary end-point). Both trials chose to further assess one-year mortality as a secondary end-point.

Baseline characteristics

Baseline characteristics are presented in Table 21.2.

Interventions

The interventions carried out in both the SMASH and SHOCK trials are illustrated in Figures 21.5 and 21.6.

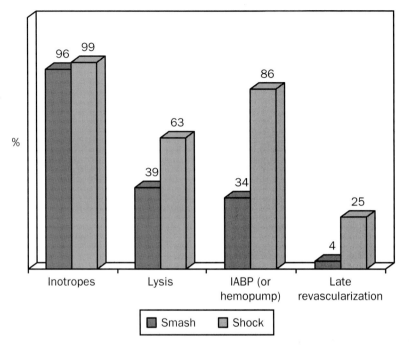

Figure 21.5
Interventions in non-invasive groups of SHOCK and SMASH (index hospital admission only).

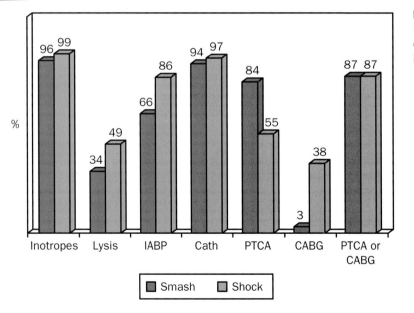

Figure 21.6
Interventions in invasive groups of SHOCK and SMASH (index hospital admission only).

Results of trials

The SMASH trial unfortunately had to be terminated early because of major problems in patient recruitment after only 55 of the planned 120 patients had been included. The results showed no significant difference in the primary end-point of 30 days mortality between the two groups (69% mortality in the invasive group versus 78% in the medically-managed group, RR = 0.88, 95% CI = 0.6–1.2, p = NS) (see Fig. 21.7).

The SHOCK trial also showed a non-significant mortality difference in the primary end-point (46.7% vs 56%, p = 0.11). However after a follow-up of one year [72], the mortality rate changed from 53% for the revascularization population vs 66% for the medically-treated group, an absolute difference of survival of 13.2% with 95% (CI of 2.2–24.1%, p = 0.025).

Interpretation of differences and similarities between SMASH and SHOCK

Strictly speaking both trials are negative concerning their primary end-point. A pessimistic interpretation of these data would consider such neutral effects irrelevant to justify a radical change in our treatment of patients with cardiogenic shock. One could argue that the six months benefit demonstrated in the SHOCK study (secondary end-point) is only due to five extra deaths in the medical treatment group compared to the revascularized group between day 30 and six months.

The optimistic view will focus on the one-year result of SHOCK, clearly indicating major benefit in terms of survival following an early invasive approach. The SMASH trial (although prematurely terminated) serves as a good confirmation of the SHOCK results.

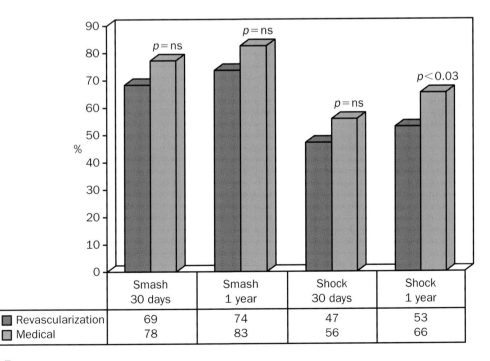

	Smash 30 days	Smash 1 year	Shock 30 days	Shock 1 year
■ Revascularization	69	74	47	53
□ Medical	78	83	56	66

Figure 21.7
All-cause mortality at 30 days (primary end-point) and at one year for SHOCK and SMASH.

- Both trials showed very similar absolute difference in mortality reduction at 30 days (9% for SMASH and 9.3% for SHOCK). Furthermore, the SMASH data would suggest that this trend persists at one-year follow-up, with a relatively low further mortality between 30 days and one year (5% mortality in both arms of SMASH, 6% and 10% respectively in the invasive and medical arms of SHOCK).
- One could hypothesize that the primary end-point was not well chosen. Thirty-day mortality may well be too soon, and just as an early hazard has been shown to be associated with thrombolytic treatment [73]; it is very likely that there is such a component of acute risk associated with early coronary angiography and revascularization.
- The higher overall mortality in the SMASH study compared to the SHOCK study reflects probably the inclusion of sicker patients, who all remain hypotensive despite inotropic support and volume replacement. This definition was felt to be necessary because invasive measurements of left heart filling pressure and cardiac output were not a prerequisite for diagnosis prior to inclusion. In retrospect, this definition was probably too strict and contributed to difficulties in patient recruitment in SMASH.

Other factors may have contributed to a higher mortality in the SMASH trial such as: lesser use of thrombolysis (34% vs 49%) and intra-aortic balloon counterpulsation (66% vs 86%) (particularly in the medical arm), as well as a markedly lower use of bypass surgery in the invasive group.

When the results of both SMASH and SHOCK are put into perspective with other randomized-controlled trials of patients with acute myocardial infarction (Fig. 21.8), a critical point becomes apparent. The relative risk reduction at 30 days is moderate 0.88 (0.60–1.20, 95% CI) for SMASH and 0.72 (0.54–0.95, 95% CI) for SHOCK; nevertheless, the absolute ben-

efit is important, with a trend suggesting nine lives saved for every 100 patients treated at 30 days, in both trials. By one year, a significant difference was seen in SHOCK, with 13.2 lives saved for every 100 patients treated.

Rather then truly assessing the isolated benefit of revascularization per se, both trials evaluated a therapeutic strategy (including inotropic agents, thrombolytic therapy, intra-aortic balloon counterpulsation, etc.), which was carried out at dedicated large-volume centers with high-volume operators [74–76].

UNRESOLVED ISSUES

Complete or target vessel revascularization

Revascularization: what is the exact mechanism of benefit? The most fundamental objective of revascularization is to relieve coronary obstruction or stenoses and in so doing, improve perfusion and function of myocardial regions in jeopardy. Echocardiography suggests that left ventricular function improves after revascularization [77]. This implies that target vessel revascularization has to be performed without delay to be most beneficial. Unfortunately cardiogenic shock often presents rather late after the onset of myocardial infarction [8, 13, 35]. For those patients, revascularization of the target vessel could still provide some benefit (long-term) through provision of collateral blood flow to another zone in the event of reinfarction or decreased arrhythmogenicity with patency of an infarct related artery [78].

In patients with more than one-vessel disease, compensatory hyperkinesis may not be possible or maintained because of energy reserve exhaustion. Initially hyperkinetic myocardium may become hypokinetic with a consequential fall in cardiac output. Therefore, in theory there is a rationale for treating severe coronary stenosis located outside the infarct area whether by percutaneous coronary intervention (PCI) or surgery.

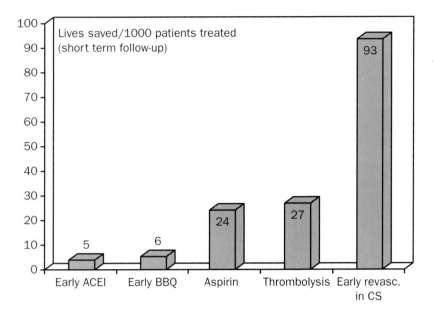

Figure 21.8
Number of lives saved for 1000 patients treated early for AMI (short-term follow-up).

Stents in all procedures?

During the last decade, there has been a major trend toward implantation of stents in most PCI; for example in Switzerland it represented 73% of the procedures [79] in 1999. In patients with an acute myocardial infarction without cardiogenic shock, stenting was initially avoided due to concern about high rates of stent thrombosis (thrombotic milieu). However high-pressure inflations and potent antiplatelet treatment have reduced the incidence of subacute stent thrombosis to less than 1%. Randomized trials, although not performed with contemporary stent designs or use of IIb/IIIa inhibitor agents, have demonstrated reduced abrupt closure and in-hospital ischemic target vessel revascularization as well as long-term event-free survival [80–83]. Registries have shown the usefulness of coronary stenting during cardiogenic shock [84] and during the last two years of the SHOCK trial, 70% of patients randomized to angioplasty had stents deployed.

As in the non-cardiogenic population, stents result in significant incremental improvements in luminal dimensions, reducing recurrent ischemic episodes and restenosis [85].

In cardiogenic shock patients, failed angioplasty carries a dim prognosis so that one would like to obtain the best result at the end of the procedure, with in particular the least chance of reocclusion. The fear of deteriorating coronary flow or increasing the propensity for clot formation seems to be now mostly under control with the introduction of platelet glycoprotein IIb/IIIa receptor antagonist (see below) and intra-aortic balloon counterpulsation (IABP).

Role of platelet glycoprotein IIb/IIIa receptor antagonist

The platelet glycoprotein IIb/IIIa inhibitors have been shown to improve the outcome of patients with unstable angina or non-ST segment elevation [86, 87]. As the ultimate goal of PCI is not only coronary reperfusion but specifically tissue (myocardial) reperfusion and considering these drugs appear to improve microvascular flow [88], their use seems rational. Small retrospective studies have shown improved clinical outcome in patients with shock [89]. In the PURSUIT trial (Platelet Glycoprotein IIb/IIIa in Unstable Angina: Receptor Suppression Using Integrelin Therapy trial) the impact of eptifibatide in patients who had cardiogenic shock was analyzed. Out of 9449 patients enrolled with non-ST elevation acute coronary syndromes, 2.5% developed cardiogenic shock [90]. Randomization to eptifibatide did not affect the incidence of shock ($p = 0.71$, OR = 0.95, 95% CI = 0.72–1.25), but did reduce the mortality at 30 days ($p = 0.03$, adjusted OR = 0.51, 95% CI = 0.23–0.94).

Surgery or PCI for left main stenosis?

For years only surgical revascularization was considered for treatment of left main coronary artery disease. More recently, with the availability of stents, many interventionalists will also consider PCI [91], especially in the subset of patients presenting ostial or mid-shaft location [91, 92]. In the cardiogenic shock patient it has been used as reported, for example in one study of 40 patients with an acute myocardial infarction, 92% in shock [93]. The rates of in-hospital death and the need for surgical revascularization for those treated by angioplasty alone were 70% and 22%, respectively, while those with stent implantation had rates of 35% and 6%. At 12 months, the survival rate with angioplasty alone or with stenting was 35% and 53% ($p = 0.18$). At present a decision to submit a patient to surgery or angioplasty with planned stenting should be based on local expertise and shared as a team approach between the cardiac surgeon and the interventional cardiologist.

Role of mechanical support device?

Intra-aortic balloon pump (IABP) is the most commonly used mechanical device. In comparison with current pharmacologic treatment it has the major advantage of increasing coronary perfusion and cardiac output while reducing myocardial ischemia and afterload [94]. In the pre-thrombolytic era and prior to the use of PCI, a non-randomized cooperative trial clearly demonstrated IABP to be extremely effective in reversing end-organ hypoperfusion in patients in cardiogenic shock, who were refractory to vasopressor therapy [95]. But there was no impact on the mortality, which remained high (83%), probably due to the inability to increase coronary flow beyond a critical stenosis [96]. Several experiments on the combined utilization of IABP and thrombolysis (so called enhanced thrombolysis), have shown dissolution of clot restored to normal levels with IABP [97]. In the GUSTO I trial out of 310 patients with cardiogenic shock receiving thrombolytic therapy, 62 were also treated with early insertion of an IABP [98]. Although they had a higher incidence of adverse events and bleeding episodes, their 30-day mortality rate was lower (47% versus 60%) even when adjusted for other clinical variables. TACTICS (Thrombolysis And Counterpulsation To Improve Cardiogenic Shock survival), and HEROICS (How Effective are Revascularization Options In Cardiogenic Shock) were designed to study these strategies, but have been stopped prematurely with negative results [99]. Other circulatory support devices are currently being investigated, these include short-term left ventricular assist devices such as the Hemopump [100] and cardiopulmonary assist devices (e.g., Bard CPS) [101].

How to treat late shock?

All currently available data address primarily patients with cardiogenic shock present on admission or developing soon after. Some patients develop shock later in the course [9]. The development of late shock can be related to reinfarction or a mechanical complication such as papillary muscle or ventricular wall rupture (so-called secondary shock for the latter). The cohort of patients with reinfarction are to be considered quickly for revascularization (whether by PCI or CABG), as most of them have already lost a large amount of myocardium and shock is then due to smaller infarcts with less sizable amount of salvageable myocardium. In this setting, an emergency echocardiography examination is extremely useful to exclude a mechanical cause of shock (tamponade, rupture of the interventricular septum or papillary muscle . . .), as in these cases emergency surgical repair is imperative.

PRACTICAL RECOMMENDATIONS: EARLY RECOGNITION AND PREVENTION

As mentioned earlier, the pooled results of SMASH and SHOCK, especially when they are put into perspective with other randomized-controlled trials of patients with acute myocardial infarction (see Figure 21.8), clearly demonstrate a major benefit of early revascularization. Nevertheless, once cardiogenic shock is present, the prognosis is dismal. At a community level, most of the myocardial infarction patients are hospitalized in an institution without cardiac catheterization facilities on site. Sensible triage and early assessment of their risk of later shock development is mandatory so that tailored treatment, recognition of pre-shock state and early transfer to tertiary centers contribute to the best management of myocardial infarction patients.

Many clinical factors predisposing to shock have been identified: they include older age, female gender, large infarction, anterior location, prior infarction, diabetes mellitus, prior hypertension and higher Killip class [102–104]. Early identification of such high-risk patients with transfer planned and made prior to the development of established shock for early revascularization would certainly make such interventions more efficient.

A period of pre-shock state with non-hypotensive peripheral hypoperfusion may precede shock (for example as in 43% of the SHOCK registry patients [105]); energetic treatment may prevent development of a vicious circle where systemic arterial hypotension leads to further coronary hypoperfusion resulting in worsening of hemodynamic condition.

Pending results of the currently conducted trials, if thrombolysis is being considered, it should be associated with vigorous vasopressor and/or IABP treatment, in an attempt to normalize coronary perfusion pressure. Tertiary centers should have the experience and the skill to perform PCI or CABG on such very sick patients. It should be recognized that treating cardiogenic shock patients is possible only as a team approach with aggressive strategy considered early on most patients. Nevertheless, evidence-based medicine is not all and clinical experience will help identify patients in whom such measures are futile (older age, co-morbidity); for them a conservative management and compassionate care may well be the best strategy [106].

REFERENCES

1. The Thrombolysis in Myocardial Infarction (TIMI) trial. Phase I findings. TIMI Study Group, *N Engl J Med* 1985; **312**:932–936.
2. Chesebro JH, Knatterud G, Roberts R et al. Thrombolysis in Myocardial Infarction (TIMI) Trial, Phase I: A comparison between intravenous tissue plasminogen activator and intravenous streptokinase. Clinical findings through hospital discharge, *Circulation* 1987; **76**:142–154.
3. Comparison of invasive and conservative strategies after treatment with intravenous tissue plasminogen activator in acute myocardial infarction. Results of the thrombolysis in myocardial infarction (TIMI) phase II trial. The TIMI Study Group, *N Engl J Med* 1989; **320**:618–627.
4. Immediate vs delayed catheterization and angioplasty following thrombolytic therapy for acute myocardial infarction. TIMI II A results. The TIMI Research Group, *JAMA* 1988; **260**:2849–2858.
5. Randomized trial of intravenous streptokinase, oral aspirin, both, or neither among 17,187 cases

of suspected acute myocardial infarction: ISIS-2. ISIS-2 (Second International Study of Infarct Survival) Collaborative Group, *Lancet* 1988; **2**:349–360.

6. Waever WD, Simes RJ, Betriu A et al. Comparison of primary coronary angioplasty and intravenous thrombolytic therapy for acute myocardial infarction: a quantitative review, *JAMA* 1997; **278**: 2093–2098.

7. Goldberg RJ, Gore JM, Alpert JS et al. Cardiogenic shock after acute myocardial infarction. Incidence and mortality from a community-wide perspective, 1975 to 1988, *N Engl J Med* 1991; **325**:1117–1122.

8. Hochman JS, Boland J, Sleeper LA et al. Current spectrum of cardiogenic shock and effect of early revascularization on mortality. Results of an International Registry. SHOCK Registry Investigators, *Circulation* 1995; **91**:873–881.

9. Holmes DR Jr, Bates ER, Kleiman NS et al. Contemporary reperfusion therapy for cardiogenic shock: the GUSTO I trial experience. The GUSTO I Investigators. Global Utilization of Streptokinase and Tissue Plasminogen Activator for Occluded Coronary Arteries, *J Am Coll Cardiol* 1995; **26**:668–674.

10. Killip T III, Kimball JT. Treatment of myocardial infarction in a coronary care unit. A two year experience with 250 patients, *Am J Cardiol* 1967; **20**:457–464.

11. Meinertz T, Kasper W, Schumacher M, Just H. The German multicenter trial of anisoylated plasminogen streptokinase activator complex versus heparin for acute myocardial infarction, *Am J Cardiol* 1988; **62**: 347–351.

12. Wilcox RG, von der Lippe G, Olsson CG et al. Trial of tissue plasminogen activator for mortality reduction in acute myocardial infarction. Anglo-Scandinavian Study of Early Thrombolysis (ASSET), *Lancet* 1988; **2**: 525–530.

13. Goldberg RJ, Samad NA, Yarzebski J et al. Temporal trends in cardiogenic shock complicating acute myocardial infarction, *N Engl J Med* 1999; **340**:1162–1168.

14. O'Neill W, Erbel R, Laufer N et al. Coronary angioplasty therapy of cardiogenic shock complicating acute myocardial infarction, *Circulation* 1985; **72**:309.

15. Brown TM Jr, Iannone LA, Gordon DF et al. Percutaneous myocardial reperfusion reduces

mortality in acute myocardial infarction (MI) complicated by cardiogenic shock, *Circulation* 1985; **72**:309.

16. Shani J, Rivera M, Greengart A et al. Percutaneous transluminal coronary angioplasty in cardiogenic shock, *J Am Coll Cardiol* 1986; **7**:149A.

17. Heuser RR, Maddoux GL, Gross JE et al. Coronary angioplasty in the treatment of cardiogenic shock: the therapy of choice, *J Am Coll Cardiol* 1986; **7**:219A.

18. Disler L, Haitas B, Benjamin J, Steingo L, McKibbin J. Cardiogenic shock in evolving myocardial infarction: treatment by angioplasty and streptokinase, *Heart Lung* 1987; **16**:649–652.

19. Landin RJ, Rothbaum DA, Linnemeier TJ, Ball MW. Hospital mortality of patients undergoing emergency angioplasty for acute myocardial infarction: relationship of mortality to cardiogenic shock and unsuccessful angioplasty. *Circulation* 1988; **78**:II–9.

20. Laramee LA, Rutherford BD, Ligon RW, McConahay DR, Hartzler GO. Coronary angioplasty for cardiogenic shock following myocardial infarction, *Circulation* 1988; **78**:II–634.

21. Lee L, Bates ER, Pitt B et al. Percutaneous transluminal coronary angioplasty improves survival in acute myocardial infarction complicated by cardiogenic shock, *Circulation* 1988; **78**:1345–1351.

22. Verna E, Repetto S, Boscarini M, Ghezzi I, Binahgi G. Emergency coronary angioplasty in patients with severe left ventricular dysfunction or cardiogenic shock after acute myocardial infarction, *Eur Heart J* 1989; **10**:958–966.

23. Shawl FA, Domanski MJ, Hernandez TJ, Punja S. Emergency percutaneous cardiopulmonary bypass support in cardiogenic shock from acute myocardial infarction, *Am J Cardiol* 1989; **64**: 967–970.

24. Meyer P, Blanc P, Baudouy M, Morand P. Treatment of primary cardiogenic shock by coronary transluminal angioplasty during the acute phase of myocardial infarction, *Arch Mal Coeur Vaiss* 1990; **83**:329–334.

25. Lee L, Erbel R, Brown TM et al. Multicenter registry of angioplasty therapy of cardiogenic shock: initial and long-term survival, *J Am Coll Cardiol* 1991; **17**:599–603.

26. Bengtson JR, Kaplan AJ, Pieper KS et al. Prognosis in cardiogenic shock after acute

myocardial infarction in the interventional era, *J Am Coll Cardiol* 1992; **20**:1482–1489.

27. Gacioch GM, Ellis SG, Lee L et al. Cardiogenic shock complicating acute myocardial infarction: the use of coronary angioplasty and the integration of the new support devices into patient management, *J Am Coll Cardiol* 1992; **19**:647–653.

28. Hibbard MD, Holmes DR Jr, Bailey KR et al. Percutaneous transluminal coronary angioplasty in patients with cardiogenic shock, *J Am Coll Cardiol* 1992; **19**: 639–646.

29. Moosvi AR, Khaja F, Villanueva L et al. Early revascularization improves survival in cardiogenic shock complicating acute myocardial infarction, *J Am Coll Cardiol* 1992; **19**:907–914.

30. Yamamoto H, Hayashi Y, Oka Y et al. Efficacy of percutaneous transluminal coronary angioplasty in patients with acute myocardial infarction complicated by cardiogenic shock, *Jpn Circ J* 1992; **56**:815–821.

31. Seydoux C, Goy JJ, Beuret P et al. Effectiveness of percutaneous transluminal coronary angioplasty in cardiogenic shock during acute myocardial infarction, *Am J Cardiol* 1992; **69**:968–969.

32. Himbert D, Juliard JM, Steg PG et al. Limits of reperfusion therapy for immediate cardiogenic shock complicating acute myocardial infarction, *Am J Cardiol* 1994; **74**:492–494.

33. Morrison D, Crowley ST, Bies R, Barbiere CC. Systolic blood pressure response to percutaneous transluminal coronary angioplasty for cardiogenic shock, *Am J Cardiol* 1995; **76**: 313–314.

34. Eltchaninoff H, Simpfendorfer C, Franco I et al. Early and one-year survival rates in acute myocardial infarction complicated by cardiogenic shock: a retrospective study comparing coronary angioplasty with medical treatment, *Am Heart J* 1995; **130**:459–464.

35. Holmes DR Jr, Califf RM, Van der Werf F et al. Difference in countries' use of resources and clinical outcome for patients with cardiogenic shock after myocardial infarction: results from the GUSTO trial, *Lancet* 1997; **349**:75–78.

36. Antoniucci D, Valenti R, Santoro GM et al. Systematic direct angioplasty and stent-supported direct angioplasty therapy for cardiogenic shock complicating acute myocardial infarction: in-hospital and long-term survival, *J Am Coll Cardiol* 1998; **31**:294–300.

37. Calton R, Jaison TM, David T. Primary angioplasty for cardiogenic shock complicating acute myocardial infarction, *Indian Heart J* 1999; **51**: 47–54.

38. Perez-Castellano N, Garcia E, Serrano JA et al. Efficacy in invasive strategy for the management of acute myocardial infarction complicated by cardiogenic shock, *Am J Cardiol* 1999; **83**:989–993.

39. Edep ME, Brown DL. Effect of early revascularization on mortality from cardiogenic shock complicating acute myocardial infarction in California, *Am J Cardiol* 2000; **85**:1185–1188.

40. Fabbiocchi F, Bartorelli AL, Montorsi P et al. Elective coronary stent implantation in cardiogenic shock complicating acute myocardial infarction: in-hospital and six-month clinical and angiographic results, *Catheter Cardiovasc Interv* 2000; **50**:384–389.

41. Mundth ED, Buckley MJ, Leinbach RC et al. Myocardial revascularization for the treatment of cardiogenic shock complicating acute myocardial infarction, *Surgery* 1971; **70**:78–87.

42. Dunkman WB, Leinbach RC, Buckley MJ et al. Clinical and hemodynamic results of intra-aortic balloon pumping and surgery for cardiogenic shock, *Circulation* 1972; **46**:465–477.

43. Miller MG, Hedley-White J, Weintraub RM, Restall DS, Alexander M. Surgery for cardiogenic shock, *Lancet* 1974; **2**:1342–1345.

44. Mills NL, Ochsner JL, Bower PJ, Patton RM, Moore CB. Coronary artery bypass for acute myocardial infarction, *South Med J* 1975; **68**:1475–1480.

45. Cascade PN, Wajszczuk WJ, Rubenfire M, Pursel SE, Kantrowitz A. Patient selection for cardiac surgery in left ventricular power failure, *Arch Surg* 1975; **110**:1363–1367.

46. Willerson JT, Curry GC, Watson JT, Leshin SJ et al. Intra-aortic balloon counterpulsation in patients in cardiogenic shock, medically refractory left ventricular failure and/or recurrent ventricular tachycardia, *Am J Med* 1975; **58**: 183–191.

47. Johnson SA, Scanlon PJ, Loeb HS et al. Treatment of cardiogenic shock in myocardial infarction by intra-aortic balloon counterpulsation surgery, *Am J Med* 1977; **62**:687–692.

48. Ehrich DA, Biddle TL, Kronenberg MW, Yu PN. The hemodynamic response to intra-aortic counterpulsation in patients with cardiogenic

shock complicating acute myocardial infarction, *Am Heart J* 1977; **93**:274–279.

49. Bardet J, Masquet C, Kahn JC, Gourgon R et al. Clinical and hemodynamic results of intra-aortic balloon counterpulsation and surgery for cardiogenic shock, *Am Heart J* 1977; **93**:280–288.

50. O'Rourke MF, Sammel N, Chang VP. Arterial counterpulsation in severe refractory heart failure complicating acute myocardial infarction, *Br Heart J* 1979; **41**:308–316.

51. Subramanian VA, Roberts AJ, Zema MJ et al. Cardiogenic shock following acute myocardial infarction; late functional results after emergency cardiac surgery, *NY State J Med* 1980; **80**:947–952.

52. DeWood MA, Notske RN, Hensley GR et al. Intra-aortic balloon counterpulsation with and without reperfusion for myocardial infarction shock, *Circulation* 1980; **61**:1105–1112.

53. Kirklin JK, Blackstone EH, Zorn GL Jr et al. Intermediate-term results of coronary artery bypass grafting for acute myocardial infarction, *Circulation* 1985; **72**:II175–II178.

54. Phillips SJ, Zeff RH, Skinner JR et al. Reperfusion protocol and results in 738 patients with evolving myocardial infarction, *Ann Thorac Surg* 1986; **41**:119–125.

55. Laks H, Rosenkranz E, Buckberg GD. Surgical treatment of cardiogenic shock after myocardial infarction, *Circulation* 1986; **74**:11–16.

56. Athanasuleas CL, Geer DA, Arciniegas JG et al. A reappraisal of surgical intervention for acute myocardial infarction, *J Thorac Cardiovasc Surg* 1987; **93**:405–414.

57. Guyton RA, Arcidi JM Jr, Langford DA et al. Emergency coronary bypass for cardiogenic shock, *Circulation* 1987; **76**:V22–V27.

58. Bolooki H. Emergency cardiac procedures in patients in cardiogenic shock due to complications of coronary artery disease, *Circulation* 1989; **79**:137–148.

59. Beyersdorf F, Sarai K, Maul FD, Wendt T, Satter P. Immediate functional benefits after controlled reperfusion during surgical revascularization for acute coronary occlusion, *J Thorac Cardiovasc Surg* 1991; **102**:856–866.

60. Allen BS, Buckberg GD, Fontan FM et al. Superiority of controlled surgical reperfusion versus percutaneous transluminal coronary angioplasty in acute coronary occlusion, *J Thorac Cardiovasc Surg* 1993; **105**:864–879.

61. Quigley RL, Milano CA, Smith LR et al. Prognosis and management of anterolateral myocardial infarction in patients with severe left main disease and cardiogenic shock. The left main shock syndrome, *Circulation* 1993; **88**:65–70.

62. Donatelli F, Benussi S, Triggiani M et al. Surgical treatment for life-threatening acute myocardial infarction: a prospective protocol, *Eur J Cardiothorac Surg* 1997; **11**:228–233.

63. Komiya T, Shiraga K, Yamazaki K, Ban K, Date O. Emergent coronary artery bypass grafting within twenty-four hours following acute myocardial infarction, *Kyobu Geka* 1999; **52(suppl 8)**: 606–610.

64. Oguma F, Kasuya S, Yamamoto K et al. Surgical results of emergent coronary artery bypass grafting, *Kyobu Geka* 1999; **52(suppl 8)**: 662–666.

65. Berger PB, Holmes DR Jr, Stebbins AL et al. Impact of an aggressive invasive catheterization and revascularization strategy on mortality in patients with cardiogenic shock in the Global Utilization of Streptokinase and Tissue Plasminogen Activator for Occluded Coronary Arteries (GUSTO I) trial. An observation study, *Circulation* 1997; **96**:122–127.

66. Menon V, Hochman JS, Stebbins A et al. Lack of progress in cardiogenic shock: lessons from the GUSTO trials, *Eur Heart J* 2000; **21**:1928–1936.

67. A comparison of reteplase with alteplase for acute myocardial infarction. The Global Use of Strategies to Open Occluded Coronary Arteries (GUSTO III) Investigators, *N Engl J Med* 1997; **337**:1118–1123.

68. Carnendran L, Abboud R, Sleeper LA et al for the SHOCK Investigators. Trends in cardiogenic shock: report from the SHOCK Study, *Eur Heart J* 2001; **22**:472–478.

69. Gunnar RM. Cardiogenic shock complicating acute myocardial infarction, *Circulation* 1988; **78**:1508–1510.

70. Urban P, Stauffer JC, Bleed D et al. A randomized evaluation of early revascularization to treat shock complicating acute myocardial infarction. The (Swiss) Multicenter Trial of Angioplasty for Shock-(S)MASH, *Eur Heart J* 1999; **20**:1030–1038.

71. Hochman JS, Sleeper LA, Webb JG et al. Early revascularization in acute myocardial infarction complicated by cardiogenic shock. SHOCK Investigators. Should we emergently revascu-

larize occluded coronaries for cardiogenic shock, *N Engl J Med* 1999; **341**:625–634.

72. Hochman JS, Sleeper LA, White HD et al. One-year survival following early revascularization for cardiogenic shock, *JAMA* 2001; **285**:190–192.

73. Fibrinolytic Therapy Triallists' (FTT) Collaborative Group. Indications for fibrinolytic therapy in suspected acute myocardial infarction: collaborative overview of early mortality and major morbidity results from all randomised trials of more than 1000 patients, *Lancet* 1994; **343**:311–322.

74. Canton JG, Every NR, Magid DJ et al. The volume of primary angioplasty procedures and survival after acute myocardial infarction. National Registry of Myocardial Infarction 2 Investigators, *N Engl J Med* 2000; **342**:1573–1580.

75. Magid DJ, Calonge BN, Rumsfeld JS et al. Relation between hospital primary angioplasty volume and mortality for patients with acute MI treated with primary angioplasty vs thrombolytic therapy, *JAMA* 2000; **84**:3131–3138.

76. McGrath PD, Wennberg DE, Dickens JD Jr et al. Relation between operator and hospital volume and outcomes following percutaneous coronary interventions in the era of the coronary stent, *JAMA* 2000; **284**:3139–3144.

77. Picard MH, Davidoff R, Mendes LA et al. Determinants of mortality from cardiogenic shock: observations from the SHOCK trial, *Circulation* 1999; **100(suppl I)**:1–19.

78. White HD, Cross DB, Elliott JM, Norris RM, Yee TW. Long-term prognostic importance of patency of the infarct-related coronary artery after thrombolytic therapy for acute myocardial infarction, *Circulation* 1994; **89**:61–67.

79. Whal A. Im Namen der Arbeitsgruppe Interventionelle Kardiologie der Schweizerischen Gesellschaft für Kardiologie. Herzeingriffe in der Schweiz 1999. *Kardiovaskuläre Medizin* 2001; **4**:268–281.

80. Suryapranata H, van't Hof AW, Hoorntje JC, de Boer MJ, Zijlstra F. Randomized comparison of coronary stenting with balloon angioplasty in selected patients with acute myocardial infarction, *Circulation* 1998; **97**:2502–2505.

81. Antoniucci D, Santoro GM, Bolognese L et al. A clinical trial comparing primary stenting of the infarct-related artery with optimal primary angioplasty for acute myocardial infarction: results from the Florence Randomized Elective Stenting in Acute Coronary Occlusions (FRESCO) trial, *J Am Coll Cardiol* 1998; **31**: 1234–1239.

82. Grines CL, Cox DA, Stone GW et al. Coronary angioplasty with or without stent implantation for acute myocardial infarction. Stent Primary Angioplasty in Myocardial Infarction Study Group, *N Engl J Med* 1999; **341**:1949–1956.

83. Maillard L, Hamon M, Khalife K et al. A comparison of systematic stenting and conventional balloon angioplasty during primary percutaneous transluminal coronary angioplasty for acute myocardial infarction. STENTIM-2 Investigators, *J Am Coll Cardiol* 2000; **35**: 1729–1736.

84. Webb JG, Carere RG, Hilton JD et al. Usefulness of coronary stenting for cardiogenic shock, *Am J Cardiol* 1997; **79**:81–84.

85. Eeckhout E, Kappenberger L, Goy JJ. Stents for intracoronary placement: current status and future directions, *J Am Coll Cardiol* 1996; **27**:757–765.

86. Randomized placebo-controlled trial of abciximab before and during coronary intervention in refractory unstable angina: the CAPTURE study, *Lancet* 1997; **349**:1429–1435.

87. The PURSUIT Trial Investigators. Inhibition of platelet glycoprotein IIb/IIIa with eptifibatide in patients with acute coronary syndromes. Platelet Glycoprotein IIb/IIIa in Unstable Angina: Receptor Suppression Using Integrilin Therapy, *N Engl J Med* 1998; **339**:436–443.

88. Choudhri TF, Hoh BL, Zerwes HG et al. Reduced microvascular thrombosis and improved outcome in acute murine stroke by inhibiting GP IIb/IIIa receptor-mediated platelet aggregation, *J Clin Invest* 1998; **102**: 1301–1310.

89. Giri S, Kernan FJ, Mitchel JF et al. Synergistic interaction between intracoronary stenting and IIA/IIB inhibition for improving clinical outcomes in primary angioplasty for cardiogenic shock, *Circulation* 1999; **100(suppl I)**:I–380.

90. Hasdai D, Harrington RA, Hochman JS et al. Platelet glycoprotein IIb/IIIa blockade and outcome of cardiogenic shock complicating acute coronary syndromes without persistent ST-segment elevation, *J Am Coll Cardiol* 2000; **36**:685–692.

91. Park SJ, Park SW, Hong MK et al. Stenting of unprotected left main coronary artery stenoses:

immediate and late outcomes, *J Am Coll Cardiol* 1998; **31**:37–42.

92. Silvestri M, Barragan P, Sainsous J et al. Unprotected left main coronary artery stenting: immediate and medium-term outcomes of 140 elective procedures, *J Am Coll Cardiol* 2000; **35**:1543–1550.

93. Marso SP, Steg G, Plokker T et al. Catheter-based reperfusion of unprotected left main stenosis during an acute myocardial infarction (the ULTIMA experience). Unprotected Left Main Trunk Intervention Multi-center Assessment, *Am J Cardiol* 1999; **83**:1513–1517.

94. Mueller H, Ayres SM, Conklin EF et al. The effects of intra-aortic counterpulsation on cardiac performance and metabolism in shock associated with acute myocardial infarction, *J Clin Invest* 1971; **50**:1885–1900.

95. Scheidt S, Wilner G, Mueller H et al. Intra-aortic balloon counterpulsation in cardiogenic shock. Report of a cooperative clinical trial, *N Engl J Med* 1973; **288**:979–984.

96. Kern MJ, Aguirre F, Bach R et al. Augmentation of coronary blood flow by intra-aortic balloon pumping in patients after coronary angioplasty, *Circulation* 1993; **87**:500–511.

97. Prewitt RM, Gu S, Garber PJ, Ducas J. Marked systemic hypotension depresses coronary thrombolysis induced by intracoronary administration of recombinant tissue-type plasminogen activator, *J Am Coll Cardiol* 1992; **20**: 1626–1633.

98. Anderson RD, Ohman EM, Holmes DR Jr et al. Use of intra-aortic balloon counterpulsation in patients presenting with cardiogenic shock: observations from the GUSTO I study. Global Utilization of Streptokinase and TPA for Occluded Coronary Arteries, *J Am Coll Cardiol* 1997; **30**:708–715.

99. Ohman EM, Nannas J, Stomel RJ et al. Thrombolysis And Counterpulsation To Improve cardiogenic shock Survival (TACTIS): results of a prospective randomized trial, *Circulation* 2000; **102**: II–600.

100. Smalling RW, Sweeney M, Lachterman B et al. Transvalvular left ventricular assistance in cardiogenic shock secondary to acute myocardial infarction. Evidence for recovery from near fatal myocardial stunning, *J Am Coll Cardiol* 1994; **23**: 637–644.

101. Shawl FA, Domanski MJ, Hernandez TP, Punja S. Emergency percutaneous cardiopulmonary bypass support in cardiogenic shock from acute myocardial infarction, *Am J Cardiol* 1989; **64**:967–970.

102. Hands ME, Rutherford JD, Muller JE et al. The in-hospital development of cardiogenic shock after myocardial infarction: incidence, predictors of occurrence, outcome and prognostic factors. The MILIS Study Group, *J Am Coll Cardiol* 1989; **14**:40–46.

103. Hasdai D, Califf RM, Thompson TD et al. Predictors of cardiogenic shock after thrombolytic therapy for acute myocardial infarction, *J Am Coll Cardiol* 2000; **35**:136–143.

104. Engelen DJ, Gorgels AP, Cheriex EC et al. Value of the electrocardiogram in localizing the occlusion site in the left anterior descending coronary artery in acute anterior myocardial infarction, *J Am Coll Cardiol* 1999; **34**:389–395.

105. Menon V, Slater JN, White HD et al. Acute myocardial infarction complicated by systemic hypoperfusion without hypotension: report of the SHOCK trial registry, *Am J Med* 2000; **108**:374–380.

106. Kubler W. Treatment of cardiac diseases: evidence based or experience based medicine? *Heart* 2000; **84**:134–136.

22

Cardiogenic shock: SHOCK trial perspective

Debabrata Mukherjee, Eric R Bates and Judith S Hochman

CONTENTS • Introduction • Design of the SHOCK trial • Results of the SHOCK trial • Results of the SHOCK registry • Lessons from the SHOCK trial and registry • Conclusions and future directions

INTRODUCTION

In the current era of infarct artery reperfusion, the leading cause of death in patients hospitalized for acute myocardial infarction is cardiogenic shock [1, 2]. Cardiogenic shock complicates 7–10% of cases of acute myocardial infarction and is associated with a > 60% mortality rate [3, 4]. Previous non-randomized studies have reported significantly lower mortality rates with emergent revascularization for cardiogenic shock [5–15], but these studies may have been limited by small sample size and selection bias [16, 17]. In these small series, mortality in patients undergoing early primary angioplasty ranged from 26–72% [15, 16]. A randomized trial comparing angioplasty with medical therapy for patients in cardiogenic shock was prematurely terminated because of poor recruitment, and the published report of the 55 patients showed no benefit of angioplasty [18]. A second prospective randomized trial comparing early revascularization with intensive medical therapy in the management of cardiogenic shock was successfully completed and is the subject of this chapter.

DESIGN OF THE SHOCK TRIAL

The 'Should We Emergently Revascularize Occluded Coronaries for Cardiogenic Shock' (SHOCK) trial [19–21] was a randomized, multicenter, international trial, which compared two treatment strategies: emergency revascularization versus initial medical stabilization. A registry of 1190 patients with cardiogenic shock was also compiled concurrently. For patients assigned to revascularization, angioplasty or coronary artery bypass graft surgery had to be performed as soon as possible and within six hours of randomization. Intra-aortic balloon counterpulsation use was recommended. For patients assigned to medical stabilization, intensive medical therapy was required. Both intra-aortic balloon counterpulsation and thrombolytic therapy were recommended. Delayed revascularization at least 54 hours after randomization was permitted in the medical arm if clinically appropriate.

The primary end-point of the study was overall 30-day mortality. Secondary end-points were overall mortality at six and 12 months after enrollment. Eligibility criteria included ST-segment elevation, Q wave infarction, new left bundle-branch block, or posterior infarction with anterior ST-segment depression, and cardiogenic shock due predominantly to left ventricular dysfunction. Cardiogenic shock was diagnosed by both clinical and hemodynamic criteria. Clinical criteria were hypotension (systolic blood pressure < 90 mmHg for at least 30 minutes or the need for supportive measures to maintain systolic blood pressure ≥ 90 mmHg) and end-organ hypoperfusion (cool extremities or a urine output < 30 ml per hour, and heart rate ≥ 60 beats per minute). The hemodynamic criteria were a cardiac index ≤ 2.2 liters/min/m² and a pulmonary-capillary wedge pressure ≥ 15 mmHg. Shock onset had to be within 36 hours of infarction, and randomization had to occur ≤ 12 hours after the diagnosis of shock. Clinical exclusion criteria included severe systemic illness, mechanical or other cause of shock, severe valvular disease, dilated cardiomyopathy, the inability of care givers to gain access for catheterization, and unsuitability for revascularization.

RESULTS OF THE SHOCK TRIAL

A total of 1492 patients with suspected shock were screened and 302 patients underwent randomization. They included 152 patients assigned to emergency revascularization and 150 assigned to initial medical treatment. The mean (± SD) age was 66 ± 10 years, 32% were women, and 55% had been transferred from another hospital. Median time from onset of myocardial infarction to shock was 5.6 hours. The patients in the two groups had similar baseline characteristics, except that more patients assigned to medical therapy had previously undergone bypass surgery (10% vs 2%, $p = 0.003$). Both groups received intensive medical therapy and 86% underwent intra-aortic balloon counterpulsation. Treatments received in both groups are summarized in Table 22.1. Seventy-one patients assigned to revascularization and 84 assigned to medical therapy died within 30 days. The 30-day mortality rates for the revascularization and medical therapy

groups were 46.7% and 56.0%, respectively (difference between the groups, −9.3%; 95% confidence interval for the difference, −20.5–1.9%; $p = 0.11$). The relative difference was 17% (relative risk, 0.83; 95% confidence interval, 0.67–1.04). Estimated 30-day survival is shown in Fig. 22.1 [20]. Patients assigned to revascularization had a higher risk of death on days one and two, whereas those assigned to medical therapy had a relatively constant risk of death over the first week. In the revascularization group, 30-day mortality was 45.3% among the 75 patients who underwent only angioplasty and 42.1% among those who underwent surgery (57 patients, including nine who underwent angioplasty before surgery). Six month overall mortality was lower in the revascularization group than in the medical therapy group (50.3% vs 63.1%; 95% confidence interval for the difference, −23.2 to −0.9%; $p = 0.027$). Between 30 days and six months after randomization, five patients assigned to revascularization and 10 assigned to medical therapy died. The one-year survival benefit was maintained in the early revascularization ($n = 152$) compared with the intensive medical therapy ($n = 149$) group (46.7% vs 33.6%, $p < 0.03$) (rela-

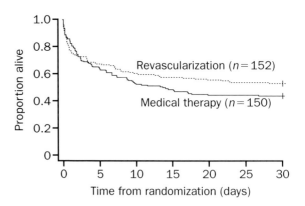

Figure 22.1 Kaplan–Meier curves showing overall 30-day survival in the SHOCK study. The 30-day survival rate was 53.3% for patients assigned to revascularization and 44.0% for those assigned to medical therapy [20].

Table 22.1 Treatment of the study patients (adapted from reference [20])

Treatment	Revascularization (n = 152)	Medical therapy (n = 150)
CPR, VT, or VF before randomization (%)	32.7	23.9
Thrombolytic therapy (%)	49.3	63.3
Inotropes or vasopressors (%)	99.3	98.6
Intra-aortic balloon counterpulsation (%)	86.2	86.0
Pulmonary-artery catheterization (%)	93.4	96.0
Left ventricular assist device (%)	3.6	0.9
Heart transplantation (%)	2.0	0.7
Coronary angiograph (%)	96.7	66.7
Angioplasty (%)	54.6	14.0
Stent placed	35.7	52.3
Platelet glycoprotein IIb/IIIa receptor antagonist	41.7	25.0
Coronary artery bypass grafting (%)	37.5	11.3
Angioplasty or coronary artery bypass grafting (%)	86.8	25.3
Median time from randomization to revascularization (hr)	1.4	102.8
	(0.6–2.8)	(79.0–162.0)

CPR denotes cardiopulmonary resuscitation, VT sustained ventricular tachycardia, and VF sustained ventricular fibrillation.

tive risk for death, 0.72; 95% CI, 0.54–0.95). The absolute difference in survival was 13.2% (95% CI, 2.2–24.1%). Figure 22.2 [21] demonstrates the incremental survival benefit of early revascularization after one month ($p = 0.04$).

Subgroup analyses

Two of the ten pre-specified subgroups had a significant interaction with treatment and 30-day mortality: age and history of myocardial infarction. Only age interacted significantly with treatment both at 30 days and at six months ($p = 0.01$ and $p = 0.003$, respectively). The relative-risk estimates and 95% confidence intervals in the 10 pre-specified subgroups are shown in Fig. 22.3 [20]. The interaction between

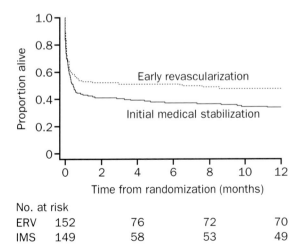

No. at risk

ERV	152	76	72	70
IMS	149	58	53	49

Figure 22.2 Kaplan–Meier survival curve one-year post-randomization. Survival estimates for early revascularization (n = 152) and initial medical stabilization (n = 149) groups. Log-rank test $p = 0.04$. ERV indicates early revascularization group; IMS, initial medical stabilization group [21].

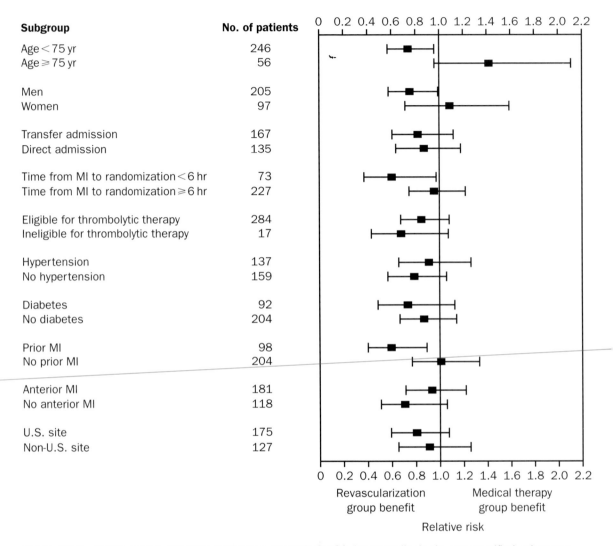

Figure 22.3 Relative risks and 95% confidence intervals for 30-day mortality in the pre-specified subgroups. Significant interaction between treatment and subgroup variables was found only for age (< 75 vs ≥ 75 years) ($p = 0.01$) and prior myocardial infarction (MI) as compared with no prior infarction ($p = 0.02$) [20].

treatment group and history of myocardial infarction was significant at 30 days ($p = 0.02$), but not at six months ($p = 0.15$).

Success of angioplasty

A successful angioplasty met three criteria in the SHOCK study. These included less than 50% post-procedure stenosis, at least 20% improvement in the degree of stenosis, and at least Thrombolysis in Myocardial Infarction (TIMI) II or III flow. The success rate was 77% for the group assigned to revascularization (81 patients) and 80% for the group assigned to medical therapy (20 patients). In the former group, successful angioplasty was associated with lower 30-day mortality (38% for patients with successful angioplasty vs 79% for those with unsuccessful angioplasty, $p = 0.003$). The use of stents and platelet glycoprotein IIb/IIIa receptor antagonists increased over time but did not result in a survival benefit in this small number of patients.

RESULTS OF THE SHOCK REGISTRY

The SHOCK registry showed a significant reduction in in-hospital mortality from January 1992 to August 1997 (71–60%) among patients with cardiogenic shock complicating acute myocardial infarction [22]. Mortality was reduced both in patients with suspected cardiogenic shock as well as in patients with shock due to left ventricular failure. Correspondingly, there was a significant increase in the proportion of patients revascularized (35.5–51%) and revascularized within two hours of the onset of shock (23.2–35.8%). These findings support the subgroup analyses in the SHOCK trial which, apart from showing patients < 75 years fared best with revascularization, also showed that the early benefits of revascularization were greatest within six hours of diagnosis [23].

LESSONS FROM THE SHOCK TRIAL AND REGISTRY

(1) There was a strong trend toward improved survival with revascularization at 30 days and significantly improved survival at six months and at one year [19–21]. (2) The similarity of the beneficial treatment effect in patients undergoing early revascularization in both the SHOCK trial registry and the SHOCK randomized trial strongly supports the generalizability of the SHOCK trial results [24]. (3) Patients with clinical signs of hypofusion (cool extremities or a urine output of < 30 ml per hour, and a heart rate of ≥ 60 beats per minute), even in the presence of normal blood pressure, have a substantial risk of in-hospital death [25]. (4) Patients without pulmonary congestion at initial clinical

evaluation may still have cardiogenic shock due to predominant left ventricular function and do not have better outcome than patients with pulmonary congestion [26]. (5) The extent of coronary artery disease, the location of the culprit lesion and the baseline coronary TIMI flow grade are correlated with in-hospital mortality. Patients with mechanical complications, three-vessel coronary artery disease, left main or saphenous vein graft lesions, and less than TIMI III flow had lower survival rates [27, 28]. (6) In patients with predominant LV failure, onset of shock after acute MI occurred within 24 hours in 74% of cases. Overall mortality was slightly higher in patients developing shock earlier [29]. (7) Patients with non-ST segment elevation MI and cardiogenic shock have a higher-risk profile than patients with ST-segment elevation MI, but similar in-hospital mortality. Patients with non-ST segment elevation MI had more recurrent ischemia and underwent angiography less often. This represents an opportunity for earlier intervention in these individuals. Early reperfusion therapy for possible circumflex artery occlusion should be considered when non-ST elevation MI causes shock [30]. (8) Diabetics with cardiogenic shock complicating AMI have a higher baseline risk profile, but after adjustment, diabetics have an in-hospital mortality that is only slightly higher than that of non-diabetics. Diabetics who undergo revascularization have a similar survival benefit as non-diabetics [31]. (9) Mitral regurgitation complicating AMI occurred more often in females, and those with non-ST elevation MI or inferoposterior MI. Most of these patients had pulmonary edema clinically. Less than half of the severe mitral regurgitation patients were selected for surgery, and in-hospital surgical mortality was 39%. Earlier recognition and surgical correction may improve prognosis in these individuals [32]. (10) Patients with cardiogenic shock as a result of ventricular septal rupture have a high (87%) in hospital-mortality rate. Ventricular septal rupture may occur early after myocardial infarction, and women and the elderly are more susceptible. Surgery remains the best therapeutic option in this setting, although overall prognosis is poor [33]. (11) Cardiac free-wall rupture and tamponade may also present as cardiogenic shock after MI. Overall survival after intervention is similar to that of the shock cohort. All patients with cardiogenic shock after MI should have echocardiography in order to detect subacute rupture or tamponade so that appropriate intervention can be initiated [34]. (12) In the registry, patients with shock due to predominant LV failure who were treated with thrombolysis, IABP and revascularization by PCI/CABG had a lower in-hospital mortality rate compared with standard medical therapy. Patients presenting to hospitals without revascularization capability should be considered for early thrombolysis and IABP followed by immediate transfer for PCI or CABG [35].

CONCLUSIONS AND FUTURE DIRECTIONS

The 9% absolute difference in 30-day mortality between the revascularization and medical therapy groups in the SHOCK trial was less than the prespecified 20% difference. However, the trial demonstrated a larger difference between the groups in mortality beyond 30 days. Six-month mortality was 13 percentage points lower for the group assigned to emergency revascularization and this benefit persisted at one year. This increase in benefit over time contrasts with the converging survival curves for patients with myocardial infarction without shock who are treated with primary angioplasty or thrombolytic therapy [36, 37]. In the Global Utilization of Streptokinase and t-PA for Occluded Coronary Arteries trial [38], a similar divergence in the two-year survival curves for patients with normal coronary flow and those with abnormal flow was noted. Considering the success rates of current care for patients with acute myocardial infarction, new interventions rarely result in more than a moderate relative reduction (i.e., 15–25%) in mortality [39]. The 17% relative reduction in overall

mortality at 30 days with revascularization found in this study is in keeping with this general observation, and is clinically relevant and therapeutically worthwhile since it represents 93 lives saved per 1000 patients treated [40]. This is more than double the number of lives saved by the administration of thrombolytic therapy within one hour after the onset of infarction [41]. The 39% relative improvement in one-year survival represents an absolute benefit of 132 lives saved for every thousand patients treated, a benefit comparable to that seen with coronary bypass graft surgery for left main disease [32, 42]. The SHOCK trial suggests that early revascularization reduces the very high mortality associated with cardiogenic shock, particularly in patients younger than 75 years of age. Based on the SHOCK trial, the ACC/AHA Task Force on Practice Guidelines made the following Class I recommendation for primary PCI for acute transmural MI: 'In patients who are within 36 h of an acute ST-elevation/Q wave or new left bundle branch block MI who develop cardiogenic shock, are < 75 years of age, and revascularization can be performed within 18 h of the onset of shock by individuals skilled in the procedure and supported by experienced personnel in an appropriate laboratory environment' [43].

Future directions for this devastating complication of myocardial infarction include studies of the metabolic state of the myocardium during cardiogenic shock [44]. The benefit of infusions of high-dose glucose–insulin–potassium solutions in patients with left ventricular pump failure after aortocoronary bypass surgery, as well as in patients who require urgent coronary-artery bypass surgery, has been reported by several investigators [45–47]. There is a large body of animal evidence to support the use of $Na^+–H^+$ exchanger inhibition in improving myocardial function [48], however clinical use has produced conflicting results [49, 50]. These and other metabolic interventions may warrant further investigation in cardiogenic shock since mortality remains high despite revascularization.

REFERENCES

1. Holmes DR, Jr, Bates ER, Kleiman NS et al. Contemporary reperfusion therapy for cardiogenic shock: the GUSTO-I trial experience, *J Am Coll Cardiol* 1995; **26**:668–674.

2. Becker RC, Gore JM, Lambrew C et al. A composite view of cardiac rupture in the United States National Registry of Myocardial Infarction, *J Am Coll Cardiol* 1996; **27**:1321–1326.

3. Kilip T III, Kimball JT. Treatment of myocardial infarction in a coronary care unit. A two year experience with 250 patients, *Am J Cardiol* 1967; **20**:457–464.

4. Goldberg RJ, Gore JM, Alpert JS et al. Cardiogenic shock after acute myocardial infarction. Incidence and mortality from a community-wide perspective, 1975 to 1988, *N Engl J Med* 1991; **325**:1117–1122.

5. Lee L, Bates ER, Pitt B et al. Percutaneous transluminal coronary angioplasty improves survival in acute myocardial infarction complicated by cardiogenic shock, *Circulation* 1988; **78**:1345–1351.

6. Verna E, Repetto S, Boscarini M, Ghezzi I, Binaghi G. Emergency coronary angioplasty in patients with severe left ventricular dysfunction or cardiogenic shock after acute myocardial infarction, *Eur Heart J* 1989; **10**:958–966.

7. Moosvi AR, Khaja F, Villanueva L et al. Early revascularization improves survival in cardiogenic shock complicating acute myocardial infarction, *J Am Coll Cardiol* 1992; **19**:907–914.

8. Yamamoto H, Hayashi Y, Oka Y et al. Efficacy of percutaneous transluminal coronary angioplasty in patients with acute myocardial infarction complicated by cardiogenic shock, *Jpn Circ J* 1992; **56**:815–821.

9. Hibbard MD, Holmes DR Jr, Bailey KR et al. Percutaneous transluminal coronary angioplasty in patients with cardiogenic shock, *J Am Coll Cardiol* 1992; **19**:639–646.

10. Guyton RA, Arcidi JM Jr, Langford DA et al. Emergency coronary bypass for cardiogenic shock, *Circulation* 1987; **76**:V22–V27.

11. Kirklin JK, Blackstone EH, Zorn GL Jr et al. Intermediate-term results of coronary artery bypass grafting for acute myocardial infarction, *Circulation* 1985; **72**:175–178.

12. Subramanian VA, Roberts AJ, Zema MJ et al. Cardiogenic shock following acute myocardial infarction; late functional results after emergency cardiac surgery, *NY State J Med* 1980; **80**:947–952.

13. DeWood MA, Notske RN, Hensley GR et al. Intra-aortic balloon counterpulsation with and without reperfusion for myocardial infarction shock, *Circulation* 1980; **61**:1105–1112.

14. Dunkman WB, Leinbach RC, Buckley MJ et al. Clinical and hemodynamic results of intra-aortic balloon pumping and surgery for cardiogenic shock, *Circulation* 1972; **46**:465–477.

15. Antoniucci D, Valenti R, Santoro GM et al. Systematic direct angioplasty and stent-supported direct angioplasty therapy for cardiogenic shock complicating acute myocardial infarction: in-hospital and long-term survival, *J Am Coll Cardiol* 1998; **31**:294–300.

16. Himbert D, Juliard JM, Steg PG et al. Limits of reperfusion therapy for immediate cardiogenic shock complicating acute myocardial infarction, *Am J Cardiol* 1994; **74**:492–494.

17. Hochman JS, Boland J, Sleeper LA et al. Current spectrum of cardiogenic shock and effect of early revascularization on mortality. Results of an International Registry, *Circulation* 1995; **91**:873–881.

18. Urban P, Stauffer JC, Bleed D et al. A randomized evaluation of early revascularization to treat shock complicating acute myocardial infarction. The (Swiss) Multicenter Trial of Angioplasty for Shock-(S)MASH, *Eur Heart J* 1999; **20**:1030–1038.

19. Hochman JS, Sleeper LA, Godfrey E et al. Should we emergently revascularize occluded coronaries for cardiogenic shock: an international randomized trial of emergency PTCA/CABG-trial design, *Am Heart J* 1999; **137**:313–321.

20. Hochman JS, Sleeper LA, Webb JG et al. Early revascularization in acute myocardial infarction complicated by cardiogenic shock. SHOCK Investigators, *N Engl J Med* 1999; **341**:625–634.

21. Hochman JS, Sleeper LA, White HD et al. One-year survival following early revascularization for cardiogenic shock, *JAMA* 2001; **285**:190–192.

22. Carnendran L, Abboud R, Sleeper LA et al. Trends in cardiogenic shock: report from the SHOCK study, *Eur Heart J* 2001; **22**:472–478.

23. Marber MS, Redwood SR. The management of cardiogenic shock: can anything be learnt from registries? *Eur Heart J* 2001; **22**:444–445.

24. Hochman JS, Buller CE, Sleeper LA et al. Cardiogenic shock complicating acute myocardial infarction—etiologies, management and

outcome: a report from the SHOCK trial registry, *J Am Coll Cardiol* 2000; **36**:1063–1070.

25. Menon V, Slater JN, White HD et al. Acute myocardial infarction complicated by systemic hypoperfusion without hypotension: report of the SHOCK trial registry, *Am J Med* 2000; **108**:374–380.

26. Menon V, White H, LeJemtel T et al. The clinical profile of patients with suspected cardiogenic shock due to predominant left ventricular failure: a report from the SHOCK trial registry, *J Am Coll Cardiol* 2000; **36**:1071–1076.

27. Wong SC, Sanborn T, Sleeper LA et al. Angiographic findings and clinical correlates in patients with cardiogenic shock complicating acute myocardial infarction: a report from the SHOCK trial registry, *J Am Coll Cardiol* 2000; **36**:1077–1083.

28. Webb JG, Sanborn TA, Sleeper LA et al. Percutaneous coronary intervention for cardiogenic shock in the SHOCK trial registry, *Am Heart J* 2001; **141**:964–970.

29. Webb JG, Sleeper LA, Buller CE et al. Implications of the timing of onset of cardiogenic shock after acute myocardial infarction: a report from the SHOCK trial registry, *J Am Coll Cardiol* 2000; **36**: 1084–1090.

30. Jacobs AK, French JK, Col J et al. Cardiogenic shock with non-ST segment elevation myocardial infarction: a report from the SHOCK trial registry, *J Am Coll Cardiol* 2000; **36**:1091–1096.

31. Shindler DM, Palmeri ST, Antonelli TA et al. Diabetes mellitus in cardiogenic shock complicating acute myocardial infarction: a report from the SHOCK trial registry, *J Am Coll Cardiol* 2000; **36**:1097–1103.

32. Thompson CR, Buller CE, Sleeper LA et al. Cardiogenic shock due to acute severe mitral regurgitation complicating acute myocardial infarction: a report from the SHOCK trial registry, *J Am Coll Cardiol* 2000; **36**:1104–1109.

33. Menon V, Webb JG, Hillis LD et al. Outcome and profile of ventricular septal rupture with cardiogenic shock after myocardial infarction: a report from the SHOCK trial registry, *J Am Coll Cardiol* 2000; **36**:1110–1116.

34. Slater J, Brown RJ, Antonelli TA et al. Cardiogenic shock due to cardiac free-wall rupture or tamponade after acute myocardial infarction: a report from the SHOCK trial registry, *J Am Coll Cardiol* 2000; **36**:1117–1122.

35. Sanborn TA, Sleeper LA, Bates ER et al. Impact of thrombolysis, intra-aortic balloon pump counterpulsation, and their combination in cardiogenic shock complicating acute myocardial infarction: a report from the SHOCK trial registry, *J Am Coll Cardiol* 2000; **36**:1123–1129.

36. Angioplasty Substudy Investigators. A clinical trial comparing primary coronary angioplasty with tissue plasminogen activator for acute myocardial infarction. The Global Use of Strategies to Open Occluded Coronary Arteries in Acute Coronary Syndromes (GUSTO IIb), *N Engl J Med* 1997; **336**:1621–1628.

37. Michels KB, Yusuf S. Does PTCA in acute myocardial infarction affect mortality and reinfarction rates? A quantitative overview (meta-analysis) of the randomized clinical trials, *Circulation* 1995; **91**:476–485.

38. Ross AM, Coyne KS, Moreyra E et al. Extended mortality benefit of early post-infarction reperfusion. GUSTO I Angiographic Investigators, *Circulation* 1998; **97**:1549–1556.

39. Yusuf S, Collins R, Peto R. Why do we need some large, simple randomized trials? *Stat Med* 1984; **3**:409–422.

40. Ryan TJ. Early revascularization in cardiogenic shock—a positive view of a negative trial, *N Engl J Med* 1999; **341**:687–688.

41. Fibrinolytic Therapy Trialists' (FTT) Collaborative Group. Indications for fibrinolytic therapy in suspected acute myocardial infarction: collaborative overview of early mortality and major morbidity results from all randomized trials of more than 1000 patients, *Lancet* 1994; **343**:311–322.

42. Varnauskas E. Twelve-year follow-up of survival in the randomized European Coronary Surgery Study, *N Engl J Med* 1988; **319**:332–337.

43. Smith SC Jr, Dove JT, Jacobs AK et al. ACC/AHA guidelines for percutaneous coronary intervention (revision of the 1993 PTCA guidelines)—executive summary: a report of the American College of Cardiology/American Heart Association task force on practice guidelines (Committee to revise the 1993 guidelines for percutaneous transluminal coronary angioplasty) endorsed by the Society for Cardiac Angiography and Interventions, *Circulation* 2001; **103**:3019–3041.

44. Hearse D. *Metabolic approaches to ischemic heart disease and its management*, (London: Science Press, 1998).

45. Coleman GM, Gradinac S, Taegtmeyer H, Sweeney M, Frazier OH. Efficacy of metabolic support with glucose-insulin-potassium for left ventricular pump failure after aortocoronary bypass surgery, *Circulation* 1989; **80**:91–96.

46. Taegtmeyer H, Goodwin GW, Doenst T, Frazier OH. Substrate metabolism as a determinant for post-ischemic functional recovery of the heart, *Am J Cardiol* 1997; **80**:3A–10A.

47. Lazar HL, Philippides G, Fitzgerald C et al. Glucose-insulin-potassium solutions enhance recovery after urgent coronary artery bypass grafting, *J Thorac Cardiovasc Surg* 1997; **113**:354–362.

48. Avkiran M. Rational basis for use of sodium-hydrogen exchange inhibitors in myocardial ischemia, *Am J Cardiol* 1999; **83**:10G–18G.

49. Buerke M, Rupprecht HJ, vom Dahl J et al. Sodium-hydrogen exchange inhibition: novel strategy to prevent myocardial injury following ischemia and reperfusion, *Am J Cardiol* 1999; **83**:19G–22G.

50. Erhardt LR. GUARD During Ischemia Against Necrosis (GUARDIAN) trial in acute coronary syndromes, *Am J Cardiol* 1999; **83**:23G–25G.

23

Cardiogenic shock: a VA perspective

Douglass A Morrison and Jerome Sacks

CONTENTS • **Introduction** • **Etiologies and mechanisms** • **Therapeutic decisions and controversies** • **Cardiogenic shock: lessons learned** • **Conclusions**

INTRODUCTION [1–10]

The mortality of myocardial infarction (MI) patients with cardiogenic shock remains high [5–7] and these patients present a very high-risk conundrum for coronary artery disease (CAD) care. Although reperfusion by thrombolytic therapy or primary angioplasty has been associated with a substantial reduction of in-hospital mortality from ST-elevation myocardial infarction (MI), it is arguable whether thrombolytic therapy has significantly reduced the mortality of MI complicated by cardiogenic shock [5, 6]. Based on case series with retrospective or literature 'control' reports, surgical or interventional revascularization appeared to reduce the high mortality of cardiogenic shock [7–11]. These results were weakened by a registry experience, which documented selection bias implicit in the decision to send a patient to diagnostic catheterization and in the decision to have a patient undergo a revascularization attempt [9]. Consequently, two international randomized trials of revascularization versus supportive therapy, SHOCK and SMASH, were initiated [7–10] and chapters 21 and 22 in this text. SHOCK did not achieve statistical significance after 30 days, but did demonstrate a

13% overall survival advantage at one year. Additionally, the subset of patients < 75 years of age appeared to derive a survival benefit from acute revascularization [7–9]. The SMASH trial was terminated because of failure to accrue adequate numbers of patients, emphasizing the difficulties inherent in performing randomized clinical trials (RCT) with critically ill patients [10, and chapter 21]. Thus, shock recommendations still engender some controversy. This chapter will review pertinent information and suggest shock guidelines based on published results. Our purpose is to synthesize the concepts one might use to decide about emergent diagnostic catheterization and the specific choice between percutaneous coronary intervention (PCI) or coronary artery bypass grafts (CABG).

ETIOLOGIES AND MECHANISMS [11–38]

By definition, cardiogenic shock is inadequate tissue perfusion, based on low cardiac output, despite adequate preload. For practical purposes, hypoperfusion may be inferred from prolonged hypotension (meaning systolic blood pressure < 90 mmHg for at least 30 minutes and usually despite inotropic infusion) accompanied by oliguria and/or clammy skin, and/or altered mental status, and/or lactic acidosis. In principle, adequate preload is established by measurement of pulmonary wedge pressure > 18 mmHg. Clinically, elevated wedge pressure is often inferred from dyspnea, tachypnea with rales and/or arterial hypoxemia, particularly in the presence of an appropriate chest x-ray pattern suggesting interstitial edema. These definitional issues are particularly important because time is of the essence in attempting to treat cardiogenic shock, and physicians must weigh the benefits obtained from a right heart catheterization with cardiac output measurements, against proceeding directly to angiography of the coronary arteries and revascularization.

Most cardiogenic shock derives from left ventricular failure. Right ventricular infarction accompanied by hypotension often carries a better prognosis, and the shock state is usually avoided with maintenance of adequate left ventricular preload, depending upon the extent of accompanying left ventricular dysfunction, as well as the presence of mechanical complications. Under the heading of mechanical complications, papillary muscle dysfunction or chordal (tendinae) rupture, interventricular septal rupture and free wall rupture are all specifically surgically correctable (albeit at significant mortality depending upon extent of infarction and ischemia). More often than not, complete papillary muscle head disruption is rapidly fatal. Similarly, although there are case reports of survival following prompt pericardiocentesis and surgical treatment of free wall rupture, most cases of cardiorhexis present as pulseless electrical activity (PEA) and are rapidly fatal.

Registry experiences suggest that ST-elevation infarcts more frequently lead to shock than non-ST elevation infarcts, but as documented in the SHOCK registry, non-ST elevation infarction can be followed by cardiogenic shock depending in part on prior infarction status and extent of coronary artery disease. Similarly, there is a reported predominance of anterior (relative to either inferior or lateral) infarcts complicated by cardiogenic shock, again depending upon prior infarction and extent of coronary disease.

THERAPEUTIC DECISIONS AND CONTROVERSIES

Stauffer and Urban have done an excellent job of summarizing the literature from the perspective they have gained in wide personal experience, as well as the SMASH trial experience (see chapter 21). Similarly, Hochman and colleagues from SHOCK have done an extraordinary job with both their randomized trial and registry [7–9, 11–17; chapter 22 by Mukherjee, Bates and Hochman).

We would like to compare their published experiences to the experience from two VA hospitals based on 45 cases of percutaneous coronary intervention for the treatment of cardiogenic shock, performed over approximately 12 years, and to data from the 16 VA sites in the AWESOME registry. Our purpose is to synthesize the concepts one might use to decide about emergent diagnostic catheterization and the choice between PCI and CABG.

Consecutive cases from two VA hospitals over 12 years [39–43]

By definition, all cases met the definition of shock given above. Of those who did not receive right heart catheterization, all were clinically in pulmonary edema (and presumably had more than adequate left ventricular preload). Most were given inotropes, starting with dopamine, titrated in an effort to achieve a mean arterial pressure of at least 60 mmHg (this usually corresponds to systolic of > 80 mmHg). All patients who had adequate ilio-femoral vasculature underwent placement of an intra-aortic balloon pump.

Variability in extent of coronary disease, prior myocardial infarction and prior CABG appear to influence whether a patient with a non-ST elevation MI, and/or inferior or lateral infarction has enough ventricular dysfunction, in aggregate, to develop cardiogenic shock. We have continued to observe that patients who failed to have an almost immediate blood pressure response to re-establishing TIMI 3 flow in the infarct-related artery, almost uniformly die within 30 days (usually within 48 hours) [39]. In two cases, when patients failed to respond to opening a single artery, PCI of a second artery was accom-

panied by the blood pressure 'jump'. Both of those patients survived to hospital discharge.

AWESOME registry revascularization experience with hypotensive patients on IABP [41–43] (Table 23.1)

Although the AWESOME study did not code explicitly for the presence of cardiogenic shock,

Table 23.1 AWESOME registry experience with emergency revascularization (based on coming to revascularization on IABP) or cardiogenic shock (based on IABP plus systolic blood pressure (SBP) < 90 at time of revascularization)

Variable	Site	Emergency and/or shock	Assigned treatment		
			CABG	PCI	Medication
IABP coming to revascularization	All 15 sites	98	40	51	7
	Sites with at least 4 IABP cases				
	1.	13	10	1	2
	2.	14	6	8	—
	3.	37	7	26	4
	4.	5	3	2	—
	5.	5	4	1	—
	6.	4	0	4	—
	Other 9 sites	20	10	9	1
	Mean of 9 low sites	2.2	1.1	1.0	0.1
IABP plus SBP < 90 at time of revascularization					
	All 15 sites	36	15	16	5
	Sites 1–6				
	1.	7	6	0	1
	2.	0	—	—	—
	3.	12	1	8	3
	4.	3	2	1	—
	5.	5	4	1	—
	6.	3	0	3	—
	Other 9 sites	6	2	3	2
	Mean of 9 low sites	0.7	0.2	0.3	0.2

Table 23.2 Three consecutive case series of cardiogenic shock treated with percutaneous coronary intervention (PCI) in two Veterans Affairs Health Care Centers

Variable	Denver VA 1988–1994	Tucson VA 1995–1998	Sept, 1999–June, 2001
Patients	17	26	12
Blood pressure < 90 mmHg	100%	100%	100%
Pressor drugs	59%	NA	75%
IABP	100%	92%	92%
PWP measured < 18 mmHg	100%	54%	83%
CI measured < 2.2 l/m²	59%	33%	75%
CAD 3-vessel	65%	73%	58%
ST-elevation MI	44%	—	83%
ST-depression MI	56%	—	17%
Prior MI	53%	—	67%
Prior CABG	44%	—	25%
Mortality			
In lab	1 (6%)	2 (8%)	3 (25%)
30 days	8 (47%)	7 (27%)	3 (25%)
Survival 30+ days	8 (47%)	17 (65%)	6 (50%)

patients can be reasonably inferred to have been in shock if they went emergently to revascularization, by either CABG or PCI, with an intra-aortic balloon pump in place and a blood pressure < 90 mmHg. Using these criteria for shock, the most impressive observation is that some centers treated patients almost exclusively by surgery, other centers treated almost exclusively by PCI, and the remaining centers treated medically or reported few to no cases of cardiogenic shock. The two centers from which we drew our experience (Table 23.2) were among the centers handling most cases which did not involve a mechanical complication (ruptured septum or free wall) with PCI.

CARDIOGENIC SHOCK: LESSONS LEARNED [1–43]

Lesson 1: Reverse the hypotension spiral

Observation from 1988–1994 VA experience: all cardiogenic shock survivors who had undergone emergent percutaneous transluminal coronary angioplasty (PTCA), had > 20 mmHg increase in systolic blood pressure within minutes of re-establishing TIMI 3 flow in 'infarct-related artery' in cardiac catheterization laboratory (CCL).

Caveat 1: Open another vessel if blood pressure does not respond to opening the presumed culprit vessel.

Caveat 2: Open everything necessary to re-establish adequate blood pressure 'the open arteries hypothesis'.

Caveat 3: Obtain TIMI-3 flow, if humanly possible: (a) through intracoronary administration of vasodilators such as adenosine ('act locally, think globally'); (b) administer drugs through the balloon catheter? ('think microvascularly'); (c) through drugs whose intracoronary administration has been accompanied by prompt improvement in TIMI flow in one or more cases of slow-flow or no-reflow: nitroglycerin, verapamil, adenosine, nitroprusside, heparin, urokinase, streptokinase, t-PA, Fluosol.

Lesson 2: Reverse the metabolic acidosis spiral by 'supporting' adequate cardiac output

Caveat 1: Intra-aortic balloon pump (IABP) if vasculature permits! Conundrum: cardiopulmonary bypass provides better support, but how do you get enough experience to be able to use it quickly and efficiently [44, 45].

Caveat 2: Pace, if heart rate is not adequate. You *may* pay a price in ventricular perforation.

Caveat 3: Intubate, if ventilation is not adequate. Delegate this task to someone experienced (an anesthetist or pulmonary fellow) who is given adequate radiation shielding, while you focus on re-establishment of TIMI-3 flow.

Caveat 4: Mechanically ventilate, if arterial oxygenation is not adequate. (You *will* pay a price in ventricular pre-load, especially if you use positive end-expiratory pressure [PEEP]).

Caveat 5: Use pressors that exact the lowest price in myocardial oxygen demand: dopamine, dobutamine; (pyrrhic vic-

tory) 'adequate' pressure but more ischemia leading to further myocardial necrosis.

Lesson 3: It isn't over when they leave the lab

Observation from the 1988–1999 VA experience: most PTCA-associated deaths did not occur in the CCL, but did occur within the first 10 days after the procedure.

Caveat 1: Treat proactively to avoid respiratory failure. This often means a Swan–Ganz catheter. To prevent post-procedural respiratory failure and death due to pulmonary edema; pulmonary hemorrhage; aspiration; barotrauma; pneumonia:
- Keep pulmonary wedge pressure < 20 mmHg.
- Monitor clotting time and platelet count.
- Intubate carefully (and like right heart cath) only if necessary.
- Do not over-PEEP.
- Use sterile technique and universal precautions.

Caveat 2: Treat proactively to avoid renal failure. Maintain cardiac output to maintain renal perfusion.

Caveat 3: Bleeding can be a catastrophe:
- Remove lines as soon as they are not needed.
- Monitor clotting tests and platelet count.
- Have only experienced people instrument heavily anticoagulated patients.

Lesson 4: It isn't over when they go home from hospital

Observation: AWESOME anecdote. Patient with one leg arrived via air ambulance in cardiogenic shock with on-going anterior MI. IABP was placed from remaining groin. Percutaneous arm approach to open and stent LAD. Blood pressure 'jump'. Ambulated and was negative for further symptoms. After one week, he was sent to the airport to fly home and he experienced sudden death at the airport.

Caveat 1: EP testing and/or ICD for survivors of cardiogenic shock? No data for this kind of emotional response to an admitted catastrophe.

Caveat 2 Aspirin or clopidogrel for life.

Caveat 3: If tolerated, beta-blocker for life.

Caveat 4: If residual LVEF < 0.40, and tolerated, ACE-I for life.

Lesson 5: Acute ST-evaluation MI treatment of choice involves a trip to the lab. An attempt at medical stabilization for non-ST elevation MI/unstable angina does not preclude urgent or emergent PCI for medically refractory subjects

Meta-analysis of all RCT data comparing thrombolytics versus PCI for ST-elevation MI, favor PCI as long as experienced lab and operator are readily available (see Chapter 20). Cardiogenic shock develops over time and most VA patients arrive after hours or days of 'chipping away' at their myocardium (see Chapter 22).

- ST-elevation MIs should undergo primary PCI if logistically feasible and transfer for rescue PCI, if persistent ischemia despite thrombolytic therapy.
- Non-ST elevation MIs should undergo cath with eye towards revascularization for recurrent or persistent ischemia (bumping troponins).

Lesson 6: If at all possible, re-establish TIMI-3 flow of the culprit vessel/cardiac catheterization laboratory in the CCL [46, 47]

Observation: AWESOME PCI in-hospital mortalities for RCT, patient refused registry and physician-directed registry of patients < seven days from MI who underwent PCI = 0%, 0%, 0%. Corresponding CABG in-hospital mortalities = 2.9%, 7.4%, 4.5%. In the last 15 years, the cardiac surgeons with whom the authors have worked have preferred to have us attempt to stabilize these patients with emergency PCI. There were some surgeons in AWESOME, who clearly preferred to take some of these acute types of patients to the operating room, and for the most part they had excellent outcomes. Nevertheless, patients need diagnostic catheterization in either case, and it is difficult to get the patient into another (operating) room, get him on bypass, harvest conduit and graft, faster than to cross with a wire and stent.

Caveat 1: For PCI Patients, stent infarct arteries whenever possible.

Caveat 2: Reopro for every acute MI with angiographic thrombus.

Lesson 7: Not everyone in shock must die in the catheterization laboratory or operating room

Among the reasons not to catheterize a patient in shock:

- Patient or family preference!
- Extreme age
- Dementia
- Life-threatening co-morbidity
- Prior congestive heart failure
- Revascularization not readily available.

Lesson 8: Everything (including high-risk cardiac revascularization) comes at a price

The price that many people try to ignore is the emotional price. Operators and crew will experience anxiety and fear. The death of these patients comes at a double toll of guilt because you 'failed' and they are 'procedural' deaths (as opposed to 'natural history of the disease'). It ought to be depressing to talk with families about the loss of a loved one and it is!

CONCLUSIONS

Cardiogenic shock is one of the most dramatic and stressful crises in medicine. As in every medical emergency, prior planning of a systematic approach is crucial. The principles on which a systematic plan for cardiogenic shock has been developed are extensions of the principles for acute myocardial infarction, acute pulmonary edema, and acute non-specific shock. They include:

- Re-establishment of TIMI 3 flow in the infarct-related artery as quickly as possible.
- Support of the blood pressure and cardiac output through mechanical and pharmacologic means.
- Identification of specifically treatable etiologies and treatment for them.
- Meticulous attention to post-procedural (PCI or CABG) details.
- Use of all long-term treatments supported by randomized clinical trials.

The more 'salvageable' the patient appears (based on age, duration of shock, level of acidosis, absence of co-morbid conditions), the more strongly an emergent revascularization effort seems to be warranted. Given that time is muscle, and muscle ultimately determines survival, decisions must be made *rapidly* or a conservative approach becomes the default 'decision'.

REFERENCES

1. Gruppo Italiano Per lo Studio Della Streptochinasi Ne'll Infarto Miocardico (GISSI). Effectiveness of intravenous thrombolytic treatment in acute myocardial infarction, *Lancet* 1986; **1**:397–401.

2. ISIS-2 (Second International Study of Infarct Survival) Collaborative Group. Randomized trial of intravenous streptokinase, oral aspirin, both, or neither among 17,187 cases of suspected acute myocardial infarction. ISIS-2, *Lancet* 1988; **2**: 349–360.

3. Fibrinolytic Therapy Trialist's (FTT) Collaborative Group. Indications for fibrinolytic therapy in suspected acute myocardial infarction: collaborative overview of early mortality and major morbidity. Results of all randomized trials of more than 1000 patients, *Lancet* 1994; **343**:311–322.

4. Levy D, Thom TJ. Death rates from coronary disease: progress and a puzzling paradox (editorial), *New Engl J Med* 1998; **339**:915–917.

5. Goldberg RJ, Gore JM, Alpert J et al. Cardiogenic shock with acute myocardial infarction. Incidence and mortality from a community wide perspective, 1975–1988, *N Engl J Med* 1991; **325**:1117–1122.

6. Goldberg RJ, Samd NA, Yarzebski J et al. Temporal trends in cardiogenic shock complicating acute myocardial infarction, *New Engl J Med* 1999; **340**:1162–1168.

7. Hochman JS, Sleeper LA, Webb JG et al. Early revascularization in acute myocardial infarction complicated by cardiogenic shock, *New Engl J Med* 1999; **341**:625–634.

8. Hochman JS, Sleeper LA, Godfrey E et al for the SHOCK Investigators. SHould we emergently revascularize Occluded Coronaries for cardiogenic shocK: an international randomized trial of emergency PTCA/CABG-trial design, *Am Heart J* 1999; **137**:313–321.

9. Hochman JS, Boland J, Sleeper LA et al and the SHOCK registry investigators. Current spectrum of cardiogenic shock and effect of early revascularization on mortality; results of an international registry, *Circulation* 1995; **91**:873–881.

10. Urban P, Stauffer JC, Bleed D et al. A randomized evaluation of early revascularization to treat shock complicating acute myocardial infarction. The (Swiss) Multicenter Trial of Angioplasty for Shock-(S)MASH, *Eur Heart J* 1999; **20**:1030–1038.

11. Hochman JS, Buller CE, Sleeper LA et al for the SHOCK Investigators. Cardiogenic shock complicating acute myocardial infarction: etiologies, management and outcome. A report from the SHOCK trial registry, *J Am Coll Cardiol* 2000; **36**:1063–1070.

12. Menon V, White H, LeJemtel T et al for the

SHOCK Investigators. The clinical profile of patients with suspected cardiogenic shock due to predominant left ventricular failure. A report from the SHOCK trial registry, *J Am Coll Cardiol* 2000; **36**:1071–1076.

13. Wong SC, Sanborn TA, Sleeper LA et al for the SHOCK Investigators. Angiographic Findings and Clinical Correlates in Patients with Cardiogenic Shock complicating acute myocardial infarction. A report from the SHOCK trial registry, *J Am Coll Cardiol* 2000; **36**:1077–1083.

14. Jacobs AK, French JK, Co J et al for the SHOCK Investigators. Cardiogenic shock with non-ST segment elevation myocardial infarction. A report from the SHOCK trial registry, *J Am Coll Cardiol* 2000; **36**:1091–1096.

15. Thompson CR, Buller CE, Sleeper LA et al for the SHOCK Investigators. Cardiogenic shock due to acute severe mitral regurgitation complicating acute myocardial infarction. A report from the SHOCK trial registry, *J Am Coll Cardiol* 2000; **36**:1104–1109.

16. Menon V, Webb JG, Hillis LD et al for the SHOCK Investigators. Outcome and profile of ventricular septal rupture with cardiogenic shock after myocardial infarction. A report from the SHOCK trial registry, *J Am Coll Cardiol* 2000; **36**:1110–1116.

17. Slater J, Brown RJ, Antonelli TA et al for the SHOCK Investigators. Cardiogenic shock due to cardiac free-wall rupture or tamponade after acute myocardial infarction. A report from the SHOCK trial registry, *J Am Coll Cardiol* 2000; **36**:1117–1122.

18. Sanborn TA, Sleeper LA, Bates ER et al for the SHOCK Investigators. Impact of thrombolysis, intra-aortic balloon counterpulsation, and their combination in cardiogenic shock complicating acute myocardial infarction. A report from the SHOCK trial registry, *J Am Coll Cardiol* 2000; **36**:1123–1129.

19. Ryan TJ. Early revascularization in cardiogenic shock: a positive view of a negative trial (editorial), *New Engl J Med* 1999; **341**:687–688.

20. Reeder GS, Gersh BJ. Modern management of acute myocardial infarction, *Current Problems in Cardiology* 2000; **25**:677–784.

21. Klein LW. Optimal therapy for cardiogenic shock: the emerging role of coronary angioplasty, *J Am Coll Cardiol* 1992; **19**:654–656.

22. Lee L, Erbel R, Brown TM et al. Multi-center registry of angioplasty therapy of cardiogenic shock: initial and long-term survival, *J Am Coll Cardiol* 1991; **17**:599–603.

23. Hibbard MD, Holmes DR Jr, Bailey KR et al. Percutaneous transluminal coronary angioplasty in patients with cardiogenic shock, *J Am Coll Cardiol* 1992; **19**:639–646.

24. Gacioch GM, Ellis SG, Lee L et al. Cardiogenic shock complicating acute myocardial infarction: the use of coronary angioplasty and the integration of the new support devices into patient management, *J Am Coll Cardiol* 1992; **19**:647–653.

25. Seydoux C, Goy JJ, Beuret P et al. Effectiveness of percutaneous transluminal coronary angioplasty in cardiogenic shock during myocardial infarction, *Am J Cardiol* 1992; **69**:968–969.

26. O'Neill WW. Angioplasty therapy of cardiogenic shock: are randomized trials necessary? *J Am Coll Cardiol* 1992; **19**:915–917.

27. Bengtson JR, Kaplan AJ, Pieper KS et al. Prognosis in cardiogenic shock after acute myocardial infarction in the interventional era, *J Am Coll Cardiol* 1992; **20**:1482–1489.

28. Holmes DR Jr, Gersh BJ, Bailey KR et al. Emergency 'rescue' percutaneous transluminal coronary angioplasty after failed thrombolysis with streptokinase: early and late results, *Circulation* 1990; **81** (suppl 3):IV 51–IV 56.

29. Lincoff AM, Popma II, Ellis SG, Vogel RA, Topol EL. Percutaneous support devices for high risk or complicated coronary angioplasty, *J Am Coll Cardiol* 1991; **17**:770–780.

30. Kahn JK, Rutherford BD, McConahay DR et al. Supported 'high risk' coronary angioplasty using intra-aortic balloon pump counterpulsation, *J Am Coll Cardiol* 1990; **15**:1151–1155.

31. Vogel RA, Shawl F, Tommaso C et al. Initial report of the National Registry of Elective Cardiopulmonary Bypass Supported Coronary Angioplasty, *J Am Coll Cardiol* 1990; **15**:23–29.

32. Overlie PA. Emergency use of portable cardiopulmonary bypass, *Cathet Cardiovasc Diagn* 1990; **20**:27–31.

33. Pavlides GS, Hauser AM, Stack RK et al. Effect of peripheral cardio-pulmonary bypass on left ventricular size, afterload and myocardial function during elective supported coronary angioplasty, *J Am Coll Cardiol* 1991; **18**:499–505.

34. Moosvi AR, Khaja F, Villanueva L et al. Early revascularization improves survival in cardio-

genic shock complicating acute myocardial infarction, *J Am Coll Cardiol* 1992; **19**:907–914.

35. Lee L, Bates ER, Pitt B et al. Percutaneous transluminal coronary angioplasty improves survival in acute myocardial infarction complicated by cardiogenic shock, *Circulation* 1988; **78**: 1345–1351.

36. ACC/AHA Task Force on Practice Guidelines. ACC/AHA Guidelines for the management of patients with acute myocardial infarction, *J Am Coll Cardiol* 1996; **28**:1332–1428.

37. ACC/AHA Task Force on Practice Guidelines: 1999 Update. ACC/AHA guidelines for the management of patients with acute myocardial infarction, *J Am Coll Cardiol* 1999; **34**:890–911.

38. ACC/AHA Task Force on Practice Guidelines. ACC/AHA guidelines for the management of patients with unstable angina and non-ST segment elevation myocardial infarction, *J Am Coll Cardiol* 2000; **36**:971–1062.

39. Morrison DA, Crowley ST, Bies R, Barbiere CC. Systolic blood pressure response to percutaneous transluminal coronary angioplasty for cardiogenic shock, *Am J Cardiol* 1995; **76**:313–314.

40. Morrison DA, Sacks J, Grover F, Hammermeister KE. Effectiveness of percutaneous transluminal coronary angioplasty for patients with medically refractory rest angina pectoris and high-risk of adverse outcomes with coronary artery bypass grafting, *Am J Cardiol* 1995; **75**:237–240.

41. Morrison DA, Sethi G, Sacks J et al. A multicenter, randomized trial of percutaneous coronary intervention versus bypass surgery in high-risk unstable angina patients, *Controlled Clin Trials* 1999; **20**:601–619.

42. Morrison DA, Sethi G, Sacks J et al for the Investigators of the Angina With Extremely Serious Operative Mortality Evaluation (AWE-SOME). Percutaneous coronary intervention versus coronary artery bypass graft surgery for patients with medically refractory myocardial ischemia and risk factors for adverse outcomes with bypass: a multicenter randomized trial, *J Am Coll Cardiol* 2001; **38**:143–149.

43. Morrison DA, Sethi G, Sacks J et al for the Investigators of the Angina With Extremely Serious Operative Mortality Evaluation (AWE-SOME). Percutaneous coronary intervention versus coronary artery bypass graft surgery for patients with medically refractory myocardial ischemia and risk factors for adverse outcomes with bypass: the VA AWESOME Multicenter Registry. Comparison with the randomized trial, *J Am Coll Cardiol* 2002; **39**:266–273.

44. DeWood MA, Notske RN, Hensley GR et al. Intraaortic balloon counterpulsation with and without reperfusion for myocardial infarction shock, *Circulation* 1980; **61**:1105–1112.

45. Brodie BR, Stuckey TD, Hansen C et al. Intra-aortic balloon counterpulsation before percutaneous transluminal coronary angioplasty reduces catheterization laboratory events in high-risk patients with acute myocardial infarction, *Am J Cardiol* 1999; **84**: 18–23.

46. Chan AW, Chew DP, Bhatt DL et al. Long-term mortality benefit with the combination of stents and abciximab for cardiogenic shock complicating acute myocardial infarction, *Am J Cardiol* 2002; **89**:132–136.

47. Giri S, Azar RR, Kiernan FJ et al. Results of primary percutaneous transluminal coronary angioplasty plus abciximab with or without stenting for acute myocardial infarction complicated by cardiogenic shock, *Am J Cardiol* 2001; **89**:126–131.

24

Chronic occlusions

Haresh Mehta and Bernhard Meier

CONTENTS • **Indications for recanalization** • **Beneficial effects of recanalization of CTO** • **Contraindications for recanalization** • **Techniques and predictors of success of PCI in CTO** • **Results of recanalization of CTO** • **Management of recurrence** • **Influence of stenting on CTO** • **Future directions** • **Subsets of patients benefiting from percutaneous or surgical therapy**

Chronic total occlusion (CTO) constitutes the main indication for approximately 10–20% of angioplasty procedures [1, 2]. Yet, it has also been one of the commonest reasons for referral for coronary artery bypass grafting surgery (CABG) rather than percutaneous coronary intervention (PCI) in spite of the reduced risk of complications with PCI. One of the primary reasons for this has generally been the lower success rate and higher recurrence rate (restenosis or reocclusions) [3, 4] associated with PCI. Although dedicated operators have reported a primary success rate close to 80% [5, 6] and the use of stents has reduced restenosis, target lesion revascularization (TLR), and reocclusion rates, no clear cut management strategy can be recommended in the absence of pertinent prospective randomized trials.

Recanalization of chronic total coronary occlusion is a low risk intervention for both the cardiac surgeons and interventionists alike. Chronically occluded arteries are usually well served by collaterals and subsequent reclosure of the vessel or closure of the graft to the vessel reliably leads to instantaneous recruitment of pre-existing collaterals. For the cardiac surgeon revascularization of a CTO is no different than performing a bypass of a non-occluded stenotic

vessel, but for an interventionist it is of a higher technical challenge to recanalize rather than to simply dilate.

Chronic total occlusion can be a manifestation of single-vessel disease or part of multivessel disease. In both situations the presence of an occluded vessel tilts the scales in favor of bypass surgery [7]. Recanalization of a CTO has been a subject of debate for the interventionist since the inception of PCI. The questions that arise are: is it beneficial to revascularize CTO? If so what are the benefits? What are the predictors of success of PCI of CTO? What subset of patients would benefit from PCI or surgical revascularization and what is the recommended therapeutic strategy? We will attempt to answer some of these questions based on reported data and our own experiences in this field.

INDICATIONS FOR RECANALIZATION

Percutaneous recanalization of CTO has unequivocally demonstrated significant relief from angina [3, 4, 8, 9] and reduction of the need for subsequent CABG. Similar studies with or without use of stents have been shown to improve left ventricular function [10–13]. Two recent reports by Noguchi et al [9] and Shizutas et al [14] comparing successful recanalization with failed recanalization attempts, showed significant reduction of cardiac mortality in the group with procedural success (75% versus 84%, $p < 0.05$). The adjusted risk increase of overall death for patients with failed recanalization was 1.8 with a 15% confidence interval (CI) of 1.2–2.6 [14]. Cardiac events occurred with similar frequency in both groups. All in all, the indication for a recanalization attempt depends on the risk benefit ratio in terms of symptom reduction, improvement of prognosis, and reduction of the need for bypass surgery versus procedural risks and costs. One of the hypotheses has been that the recanalized vessel can reduce risk by serving as a future collateral donor in case the earlier donor vessel occludes [15]. Success of attempts at percutaneous recanalization depends on the anatomical factors as well as the setting in which it is attempted. Recanalization is rarely worth the effort if a patient with no or minimal angina has to travel a distance for a procedure. On the other hand in the same patient it would make sense to attempt the procedure while the patient is undergoing a diagnostic coronary angiogram or an angioplasty for another lesion. Patients with intractable angina or a large myocardial area at stake who are even considering CABG are good candidates for an attempt at balloon recanalization— a less costly and less invasive procedure. Special mention has to be made as regards patients with multi-vessel disease and one or more CTOs. They have shown good results [16–19]. The strategy is to attempt to open the occluded vessel first, followed by the nonoccluded vessels i.e. the collateral donors. Any complication during an attempt of intervention of a donor vessel could be fatal unless the recipient vessel has been recanalized first. Further vessels should in general be attempted during the same sitting only in cases where there has been a good result with the occlusion. Bypass surgery is an option in most of these cases, but

PCI becomes more and more competitive with technical improvements. Failure to open the occluded vessel in these patients with significant angina should mandate referral for CABG. Occasionally an occluded dominant vessel is ignored and the other lesions are attempted [16–19]. This is often a high risk intervention and hence needs to be reserved for special situations. With availability of recent techniques results can be definitely improved without the need for standby bypass surgery. New percutaneous assist devices are in the investigational phase and the introduction of these devices would make high-risk PCI safer. The paradigm of intervention on chronic occlusion is that safety should not be compromised as the yield may not be worth the risk involved.

BENEFICIAL EFFECTS OF RECANALIZATION OF CTO

The natural course of CTO in the absence of interspersed acute events is benign (4% mortality in the first year) except in patients with recent occlusion of the LAD with a one year mortality of 10%. The time of the acute event to a coronary angiogram is a predictor of death ($p = 0.04$) [20]. The goal of revascularization has been either relief of angina or attenuation of requirement of subsequent coronary artery bypass graft [21–24]. However recent reports have also shown reduction in the incidence of cardiac mortality associated with successful attempts at recanalization [9, 14]. In addition improvement of regional and global left ventricular function has been reported [10–13].

CONTRAINDICATIONS FOR RECANALIZATION

Contraindications to CTO are relatively few. The only absolute contraindication to the procedure is absence of collaterals. This is a strong indicator of absence of viable myocardium worth the risk of recanalization. The absence of collaterals should be confirmed before making any such decision as collaterals can be missed due to short filming of sequences or missing a conal artery with a separate origin that collateralizes the left anterior descending coronary artery.

TECHNIQUES AND PREDICTORS OF SUCCESS OF PCI IN CTO

Multiple factors have been documented to influence attempts at recanalization. Duration of occlusion is an independent predictor of success of recanalization [4, 25–31]. Rapid decline in success rate is observed as early as during the first four weeks after the occlusion [28]. Other independent predictors having a negative influence include the presence of calcification, presence of multi-vessel disease [9], and length of the occluded segment [9, 32]. Bridging collaterals have been reported to be a strong negative predictor of success [29], but a few committed operators have obtained remarkable success rates in presence of bridging collaterals [5]. Short duration of occlusion and presence of a stump (tapered segment) exert a positive influence on the success of recanalization [21, 29]. Results of recanalization of occluded vein grafts have been dismal [33–36].

An attempt at recanalization needs careful assessment of the assumed path of the occluded artery. This can be ascertained by either review of an old angiogram or use of a still frame showing the proximal end of the collateralized artery segment filling from the donor artery or, in rare circumstances, simultaneous contrast injection into the donor coronary artery using a second arterial access to visualize the collateral artery dividing the intervention. This can be of particular help in determining the correct position of the guide wire and is most useful with use of aggressive guide wires like the stiff hydrophilic wires. They are associated with a high risk of perforations that are pertinently dangerous if they occur distal to the occlusion

in thin-walled normal arteries. This occurs after the wire has been successfully passed through the occlusion and is inadequately controlled during subsequent balloon manipulations. Using contralateral injection, Lefevre et al [37] demonstrated that the risk of perforation with the hydrophilic wire (crosswire) was smaller than previously reported [5, 38, 39].

Dedicated operators and dedicated techniques are the secret for recanalization of CTOs. Standard floppy wires may cross the CTO, but the chance is very low. Although over-the-wire systems have been largely replaced by the monorail dilatation system, this is one indication where the over-the-wire system is still a good choice, as it permits reshaping or exchange of the wire without losing the position secured in front of the occlusion with the balloon catheter. A stiff wire is generally the wire of choice as the success rate is higher than with floppy wires [5, 32, 40, 41]. The stiffness of the wire can be further augmented by using a balloon as a back-up. Some operators even inflate the balloon in the stump for optimal support to push the wire. This maneuver is fraught with an increased risk of extravascular pathways (Fig. 24.1) and may damage the otherwise healthy stump. The ball-tipped Magnum wire [42] was designed to reduce this risk. Contrast injections through the tip of the balloon catheter can be performed to check the position of the wire. In rare circumstances this or guiding catheter injections can lead to sub-intimal contrast injection with subsequent extensive dissections [43]. Contrast injection into the contralateral coronary artery which opacifies the distal segment of the occluded coronary artery via the collaterals, helps in documenting the position of the distal tip of the guide wire. An additional maneuver that helps in improving the crossing rate is to make a secondary curve 1–2 mm proximal to the wire tip of the pre-shaped conventional guide wire since the primary curve tends to straighten out on entering an occlusion or approaching the balloon to the tip for support and is no longer torquable (Fig. 24.2). Some operators utilize the parallel

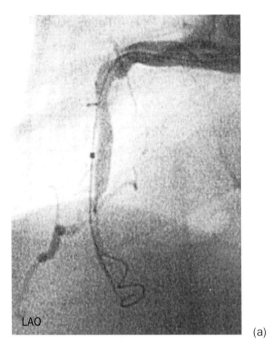

LAO

(a)

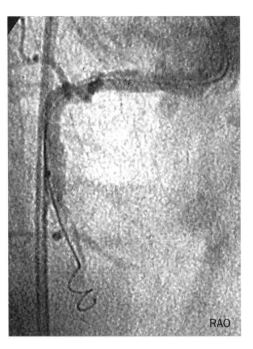

RAO

(b)

Figure 24.1 Sub-intimal passage of a hydrophilic guide wire. (a) LAO, left anterior oblique projection; (b) RAO, right anterior oblique projection.

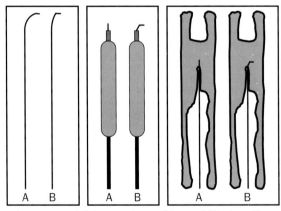

A: commercial J-curve: loss of torquability in action
B: secondary J-curve, made by thumbnail 1–2 mm proximal to wire tip

Figure 24.2 Technique of secondary curve on the guide wire.

wire approach (one wire is left in a side branch proximally and another wire is passed alongside to pierce the distal fibrous cap) to increase the crossing rate.

Successful recanalization of the CTO can be counterchecked with contrast injection in the contralateral coronary artery, to see if collaterals persist. With a good functional recanalization they disappear completely but remain recruitable in case of a later reocclusion.

Alternative techniques have been developed over the years which in some situations have led to an increased chance of recanalization of CTOs. They are briefly summarized below.

Laser (light amplification by stimulated emission of radiation)

The excimer laser wire [44–46] can be likened to a sharp needle which tends to find its way through an occluded segment. It is an expensive tool and may only be a valuable adjunctive in selected cases. In a multicenter randomized trial comparing excimer laser wire with a conventional wire (TOTAL trial) [47], no statistically significant benefit as regards crossing was observed between the two groups. A slight increased rate of crossing (50–60%) was seen only in crossover cases. Hence laser wire recanalization cannot be recommended as the approach of choice at the moment. Respective devices have disappeared from the market. A similar approach can be employed using a normal wire in an over-the-wire system. In this method the stiff end is used to cross the lesion. The wire is then reversed to normal once the lesion is crossed. The risk of perforation is as high as with the laser catheter, but almost the same result can be obtained at a lower cost. Laser debulking and other debulking devices after crossing the occlusion with the wire [47, 48] are not beneficial and hence not currently recommended on the basis of the data available. Two devices that have altered the crossing of occlusion and the subsequent long-term follow-up positively, are dedicated guide wires and stents.

Guide wires

Magnum wire
This is a specially designed guide wire for recanalization of CTO [40–42, 49]. The olive tip has the advantage of pushability and avoidance of the sub-intimal pathway. As compared to other wires, this wire needs a firm push to pass tight lesions, hence it almost always needs a balloon catheter to splint the flexible part of the wire. This can then be pushed en bloc. This technique also needs a good guide support. Primary success is increased by 10–20% compared to other conventional guide wires [41, 42, 50].

Hydrophilic wires
Glide wires (Terumo) [51, 52] have been widely used for catheterization of peripheral arteries. They are hydrophilic and very slippery when wet, but they represent an advantage in terms of lesion crossability. They have ushered in an array of hydrophilic wires to be used successfully for recanalization of CTO [38]. However this approach has been associated with a signif-

icant risk of peripheral perforation [5, 39]. In a recent randomized trial [37] comparing the glide wire (crosswire) and another conventional guide wire (ACS, Guidant), there was a significant increase in crossability in the group using the crosswire both in the randomized and the cross-over group (Fig. 24.3). No increase in complication of perforation was observed which has been attributed to repeated checks of guide wire position by injecting into the contralateral coronary artery. It has also resulted in the use of a lesser number of wires thereby reducing cost. Other stiff wires like the athlete wire (INTEC), ACS wires (Guidant) of varying stiffness (100, 200, 300, 400) have been tried to recanalize CTO, but these need highly tenacious and skilled operators to achieve high success rates [53].

RESULTS OF RECANALIZATION OF CTO

Percutaneous recanalization of CTO using standard guide wires is a relatively low-risk intervention, but plagued with low success and high recurrence rates. Success rates range from 40–80% [21–23, 25–31, 37, 42, 54–57]. On the whole the success rate was around 47% before 1990 and about 70% after 1995. This has been largely attributed to the greater experience gained in this field and improved hardware. In case of a single operator the success rate improves over time [29]. The results also depend on the indications and morphology of the vessel attempted as described earlier.

Mortality risk

Death although uncommon with this generally low-risk intervention has been reported [55]. The reason for this is generally the dissection of the left main stem while attempting a recanalization which is caused either by the wire or guiding catheter or balloon inflation. It may also be blocked due to retraction of a blood clot into the left main, while withdrawing the

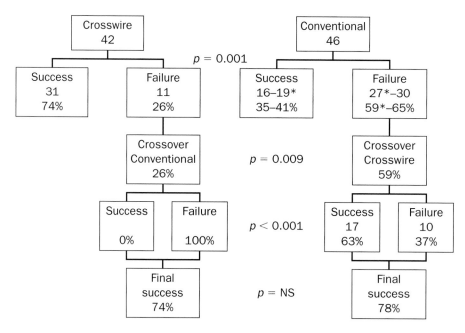

Figure 24.3 Crossability of crosswire (hydrophilic) vs conventional wire: single center randomized study. * denotes success at second attempt with the conventional guide wire (data adapted from Lefevre T et al [37]).

balloon catheter. Rare causes of death could be due to arrhythmia, accidental embolization, coronary rupture or perforation. The risk of revascularization of CTO is intermediate between diagnostic angiogram and PCI of a non-occluded vessel, but in some studies [7, 56] the mortality rate is the same or higher during follow-up. This is mainly due to the progression of the disease process and cannot be attributed to intervention on the chronic total occlusion. Chronic total occlusion on its own cannot cause unstable situations unless the donor vessel is also treated or significant collaterals are impaired. Such constellations can cause complications in this group comparable to those seen with revascularization of non-total stenosis [58]. Revascularization of CTO is not totally risk-free and this has to be taken into account for decisions about indications.

Cardiac tamponade

Tamponade secondary to perforation using aggressive wires or laser has also been reported [59, 60]. Perforations at the site of CTO are generally benign and tend to seal off [29, 61, 62]. They can be lethal if one passes through a balloon and inflates it. This leads to coronary rupture, a far more dangerous complication than coronary perforation. Tamponade should be managed by immediate balloon hemostasis, institution of rapid pericardiocentesis (with re-injection of the pericardial blood into a vein) and use of a (covered) stent, CABG, or a combination of these measures.

Emergency CABG

Emergency CABG is necessary in less than 1% of cases undergoing recanalization of chronic total occlusions [5, 21–23, 25–31, 42, 54–56]. The cause of this could be accidental damage to the left main coronary artery, occlusion of an important vessel proximal to the occlusion or impairment of collaterals perfusing the vessel to be recanalized. Infarction can occur due to the reasons mentioned above and also can be attributed to distal embolization. It is seen in 1% of successful procedures [32].

Dissections

Dissections do occur commonly in the setting of recanalization attempts of CTO, but they are usually benign and do not result in sequelae if the procedure is abandoned. Some authors have reported stenting the dissected sub-intimal path. This is possible only if the tip of the wire finds its way into the true lumen distally but this is not usually the case [63]. Rarely a long dissection can extend into and block collateral channels causing ischemia. In usual circumstances dissections tend to seal off on abandoning the procedure as the flow in the true lumen via pre-existing collaterals plasters the dissection against the wall.

Restenosis and re-occlusions

Restenosis and re-occlusions plague successful recanalization of CTOs. Recurrence rates as high as 80% have been reported [22, 23, 25, 54]. Restenosis and re-occlusion rates are more frequent with total occlusion as compared to non-total occlusion [63, 64]. Re-occlusion occurs in 10–20% of lesions [65, 66]. The remaining 30–40% constitute restenoses [4, 5, 21–23, 25–31, 42, 54, 55, 67]. Restenosis can be treated with a new percutaneous intervention.

Reocclusion

Reocclusion usually goes undetected as the vessel closure is typically silent and is accidentally picked up during routine exercise testing or reappearance of symptoms. Initial results have shown that a high coronary wedge pressure due to presence of good collaterals is a harbinger of re-occlusion due to reduced mean driving pressure across the dilated lesion leading to slow flow and thrombus formation [68]. Other factors leading to re-occlusion include unstable angina, incomplete result, occlusion of left anterior descending coronary artery (LAD) or left circumflex coronary artery (LCX), or presence of multi-vessel disease. Stent implantation reduces the risk of re-occlusion and restenosis [64–66, 69–73].

MANAGEMENT OF RECURRENCE

Symptomatic or angiographically detected restenosis and re-occlusion often need further treatment. The rate of repeat revascularization by balloon or CABG is on average 30–50% [64, 67]. The rate of repeat intervention is small in successful recanalization attempts as compared to failed attempts [21–23].

Liberal use of stents reduces the restenosis but it still persists [64, 69–70]. The rule of thumb is to redilate the restenoses group and consider CABG for symptomatic re-occlusions, but this should not be a generalization and the indications should be adapted depending on the individual situations.

INFLUENCE OF STENTING ON CTO

Stenting in native coronary artery was a blessing to prevent threatened abrupt closure and associated death or myocardial infarction leading to reduced requirement of emergency CABG. Emergency CABG is associated with increased morbidity and mortality. This is not the case in already occluded vessels which are recanalized, hence stenting was not predicted to play a dominant role in percutaneous recanalization of CTO. In addition recanalizations of CTOs cause a large area of haziness leading to the need for longer stents. This

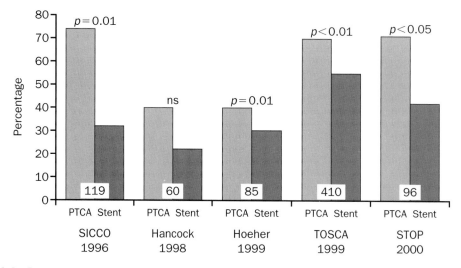

Figure 24.4   Restenosis rates: stent vs PTCA in CTOs. Results of randomized trials.

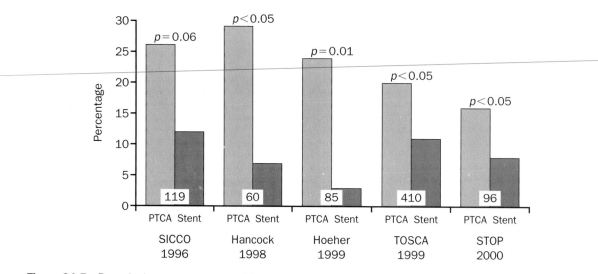

Figure 24.5   Reocclusion rates: stent vs PTCA in CTOs. Results of randomized trials.

would result in increases in restenosis and re-occlusion rates. Despite these concerns both randomized and non-randomized studies (Figs 24.4–24.6) have unequivocally demonstrated that stenting is beneficial in patients with recanalization of chronically occluded coronary vessels and helpful in significantly reducing restenosis and re-occlusion rates [65–67].

Stenting has reduced target vessel revascularization and other major cardiovascular events [65–67, 72], but there are always two sides to a coin. The reduced restenosis rate may be counterbalanced by more difficult to treat in-stent restenosis or occlusion of important side branches or collateral channels. This leads to an increased risk of infarction. Stenting helps

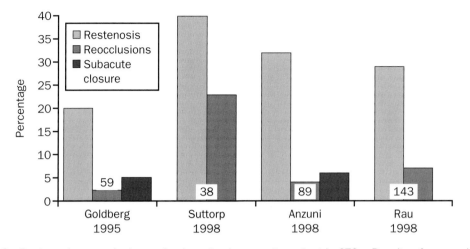

Figure 24.6 Restenosis, re-occlusion and sub-acute closure rates: stent in CTOs. Results of non-randomized trials.

about 15% of the patients with total coronary occlusion. Thus this does not warrant a 100% stenting rate. Judicious selective use of stenting should be the policy rather than the elective stenting of all cases. Re-occlusion after recanalization of CTOs are difficult to treat and long in-stent restenoses are a major problem for which no significantly beneficial option is available at the present moment and this seems a major problem on CTOs where longer stents are used to recanalize these vessels. Stenting is advisable in patients with a poor balloon result but not necessary in vessels with stent-like results, TIMI 3 flow, small calibers, or if a very long stent is required. It should be specially avoided in patients with risk of obstruction of collateral channels, which would be regrettable if needed in the future as a collateral donor.

FUTURE DIRECTIONS

Intracoronary radiation using β or γ rays is a new percutaneous treatment modality in reducing restenosis [74, 75]. It reduces neo-intimal hyperplasia [76] and causes positive vascular remodeling [74, 77]. A recent case report [57] has studied a patient with recanalization of a

CTO in the right coronary artery (RCA) with stenting and followed by intracoronary radiation. The patient was followed-up with stress tests, at six and 10 months and showed no evidence of ischemia. Follow-up angiogram at 10 months showed a patent RCA with mild intimal hyperplasia. Such a treatment strategy needs to be evaluated in clinical trials. Stents with drug eluting properties (e.g. Sirolimus-coated stents) have shown excellent initial results in small pilot studies. Randomized trials using these stents and other such prototypes are underway. If the results are confirmed in large randomized trials, this would revolutionize PCI of occlusive and non-occlusive coronary artery disease.

SUBSETS OF PATIENTS BENEFITING FROM PERCUTANEOUS OR SURGICAL THERAPY

The primary goal in patients with CTO is relief of symptoms. Recanalization of asymptomatic patients with chronic total occlusion can be justified on the basis of creating a collateral donor in the event of closure of another vessel. It could also help reactivate hibernating myocardium (Fig. 24.7). With this rather

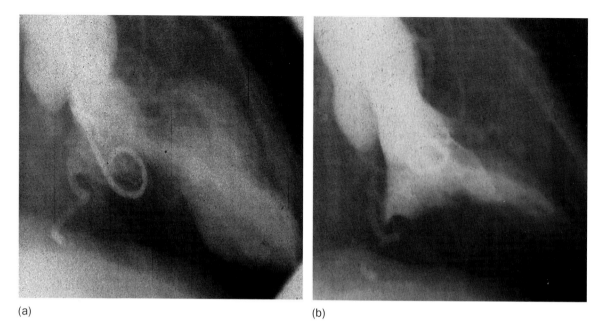

(a)

(b)

Figure 24.7 Comparative LV angiograms, (a) pre-recanalization and (b) at six-month follow-up demonstrating reversible hibernating myocardium.

hypothetical benefit, such an intervention should be attempted only if the patient is already on the catheterization table for a diagnostic study or a planned intervention on another vessel.

Restenosis and re-occlusion rates can be reduced by selective rather than elective use of stents since indiscriminate use of stents can result in important branch compromise, collateral occlusion, infarcts, or intricate in-stent restenoses.

The revascularization strategy of CTO, if justifiably indicated, should be percutaneous unless reasons like technical impossibility preclude this, or CABG is indicated due to other reasons such as multi-vessel disease that is impossible to recanalize percutaneously (more than one occluded vessel, left main disease etc.). But caution needs to be exercised even by the most experienced operator. The procedure is relatively innocuous, but not devoid of some inherent risk especially with the use of aggressive devices like hydrophilic guide wires.

REFERENCES

1. Bell MR, Berger PB, Menke KK, Holmes DR. Balloon angioplasty of chronic total coronary artery occlusions: what does it cost in radiation exposure, time, and materials? *Cathet Cardiovasc Diagn* 1992; **25**:10–15.
2. Delacretaz E, Meier B. Therapeutic strategy with total coronary artery occlusions, *Am J Cardiol* 1997; **79**:185–187.
3. Meier B. 'Occlusion angioplasty'. Light at the end of the tunnel or dead end? *Circulation* 1992; **85**:1214–1216.
4. Puma JA, Sketch MH, Tcheng JE et al. Percutaneous revascularization of chronic coronary occlusions: an overview, *J Am Coll Cardiol* 1995; **26**:1–11.
5. Kinoshita I, Katoh O, Nariyama J et al. Coronary angioplasty of chronic total occlusions with bridging collateral vessels: immediate and follow-up outcome from a large single-center experience, *J Am Coll Cardiol* 1995; **26**:409–415.
6. Bahl VK, Chandra S, Goswami KC, Manchanda SC. Crosswire for recanalization of total occlusive coronary arteries, *Cathet Cardiovasc Diagn* 1998; **45**:323–328.

7. Berger PB, Holmes DR, Ohman EM et al. Restenosis, re-occlusion and adverse cardiovascular events after successful balloon angioplasty of occluded versus non-occluded coronary arteries. Results from the Multicenter American Research Trial with Cilazapril After Angioplasty to Prevent Transluminal Coronary Obstruction and Restenosis (MARCATOR), *J Am Coll Cardiol* 1996; **27**:1–7.

8. Sathe S, Alt C, Black A et al. Initial and long-term results of percutaneous transluminal balloon angioplasty for chronic total occlusions: an analysis of 184 procedures, *Aust N Z J Med* 1994; **24**:277–281.

9. Noguchi T, Miyazaki MS, Morii I et al. Percutaneous transluminal coronary angioplasty of chronic total occlusions. Determinants of primary success and long-term clinical outcome, *Catheter Cardiovasc Interv* 2000; **49**:258–264.

10. Van Belle E, Blouard P, McFadden EP et al. Effects of stenting of recent or chronic coronary occlusions on late vessel patency and left ventricular function, *Am J Cardiol* 1997; **80**: 1150–1154.

11. Melchior JP, Doriot PA, Chatelain P et al. Improvement of left ventricular contraction and relaxation synchronism after recanalization of chronic total coronary occlusion by angioplasty, *J Am Coll Cardiol* 1987; **9**:763–768.

12. Sirnes PA, Myreng Y, Molstad P, Bonarjee V, Golf S. Improvement in left ventricular ejection fraction and wall motion after successful recanalization of chronic coronary occlusions, *Eur Heart J* 1998; **19**:273–281.

13. Danchin N, Angioi M, Cador R et al. Effect of late percutaneous angioplastic recanalization of total coronary artery occlusion on left ventricular remodeling, ejection fraction, and regional wall motion, *Am J Cardiol* 1996; **78**:729–735.

14. Shizuta SNH, Kimura T, Nakagawa Y et al. Impact of successful recanalization of chronic total occlusion on long-term survival outcome: a single center experience, *Circulation* 1999; **suppl 100**:I85 (abstract).

15. Urban P, Meier B, Finci L. Flow reversal in coronary collaterals, *Eur Heart J* 1987; **8**:1346–1350.

16. Teirstein P, Giorgi L, Johnson W et al. PTCA of the left coronary artery when the right coronary artery is chronically occluded, *Am Heart J* 1990; **119**: 479–483.

17. De Bruyne B, Renkin J, Col J, Wijns W. Percutaneous transluminal coronary angioplasty of the left coronary artery in patients with chronic occlusion of the right coronary artery: clinical and functional results, *Am Heart J* 1991; **122**:415–422.

18. Buffet P, Danchin N, Marc MO et al. Results of percutaneous transluminal coronary angioplasty of either the left anterior descending or left circumflex coronary artery in patients with chronic total occlusion of the right coronary artery, *Am J Cardiol* 1993; **71**:382–385.

19. Kishi K, Hiasa Y, Kinoshita M et al. Efficacy and safety of percutaneous transluminal coronary angioplasty of other coronary arteries in patients with chronic total occlusion of the left anterior descending artery, *J Cardiol* 1995; **25**:303–308.

20. Puma JA, Sketch MH, Tcheng JE et al. The natural history of single-vessel chronic coronary occlusion: a 25-year experience, *Am Heart J* 1997; **133**:393–399.

21. Ivanhoe RJ, Weintraub WS, Douglas JS et al. Percutaneous transluminal coronary angioplasty of chronic total occlusions. Primary success, restenosis, and long-term clinical follow-up, *Circulation* 1992; **85**:106–115.

22. Finci L, Meier B, Favre J, Righetti A, Rutishauser W. Long-term results of successful and failed angioplasty for chronic total coronary arterial occlusion, *Am J Cardiol* 1990; **66**:660–662.

23. Bell MR, Berger PB, Bresnahan JF et al. Initial and long-term outcome of 354 patients after coronary balloon angioplasty of total coronary artery occlusions, *Circulation* 1992; **85**:1003–1011.

24. Warren RJ, Black AJ, Valentine PA, Manolas EG, Hunt D. Coronary angioplasty for chronic total occlusion reduces the need for subsequent coronary bypass surgery, *Am Heart J* 1990; **120**: 270–274.

25. Melchior JP, Meier B, Urban P et al. Percutaneous transluminal coronary angioplasty for chronic total coronary arterial occlusion, *Am J Cardiol* 1987; **59**:535–583.

26. Serruys PW, Umans V, Heyndrickx GR et al. Elective PTCA of totally occluded coronary arteries not associated with acute myocardial infarction; short-term and long-term results, *Eur Heart J* 1985; **6**:2–12.

27. Dervan JP, Baim DS, Cherniles J, Grossman W. Transluminal angioplasty of occluded coronary arteries: use of a movable guide wire system, *Circulation* 1983; **68**:776–784.

28. DiSciascio G, Vetrovec GW, Cowley MJ,

Wolfgang TC. Early and late outcome of percutaneous transluminal coronary angioplasty for subacute and chronic total coronary occlusion, *Am Heart J* 1986; **111**:833–839.

29. Maiello L, Colombo A, Gianrossi R et al. Coronary angioplasty of chronic occlusions: factors predictive of procedural success, *Am Heart J* 1992; **124**: 581–584.

30. LaVeau PJ, Remetz MS, Cabin HS et al. Predictors of success in percutaneous transluminal coronary angioplasty of chronic total occlusions, *Am J Cardiol* 1989; **64**:1264–1269.

31. Jost S, Nolte CW, Simon R et al. Angioplasty of subacute and chronic total coronary occlusions: success, recurrence rate, and clinical follow-up, *Am Heart J* 1991; **122**:1509–1514.

32. Kereiakes DJ, Selmon MR, McAuley DB, Sheehan DJ, Simpson JB. Angioplasty in total coronary artery occlusion: experience in 76 consecutive patients, *J Am Coll Cardiol* 1985; **6**:526–533.

33. de Feyter PJ, Serruys P, van den Brand M et al. Percutaneous transluminal angioplasty of a totally occluded venous bypass graft: a challenge that should be resisted, *Am J Cardiol* 1989; **64**:88–90.

34. Hartmann J, McKeever L, Teran J et al. Prolonged infusion of urokinase for recanalization of chronically occluded aortocoronary bypass grafts, *Am J Cardiol* 1988; **61**:189–191.

35. Finci L, Meier B, Steffenino GD. Percutaneous angioplasty of totally occluded saphenous aortocoronary bypass graft, *Int J Cardiol* 1986; **10**: 76–79.

36. Sievert H, Kohler KP, Kaltenbach M, Kober G. Reopening of long-segment occluded aortocoronary venous bypasses. Short- and long-term results, *Dtsch Med Wochenschr* 1988; **113**:637–640.

37. Lefevre T, Louvard Y, Loubeyre C et al. A randomized study comparing two guide wire strategies for angioplasty of chronic total coronary occlusion, *Am J Cardiol* 2000; **85**:1144–1147.

38. Corcos T, Favereau X, Guerin Y et al. Recanalization of chronic coronary occlusions using a new hydrophilic guide wire, *Cathet Cardiovasc Diagn* 1998; **44**:83–90.

39. Wong CM, Kwong Mak GY, Chung DT. Distal coronary artery perforation resulting from the use of hydrophilic coated guide wire in tortuous vessels, *Cathet Cardiovasc Diagn* 1998; **44**:93–96.

40. Meier B, Carlier M, Finci L et al. Magnum wire for balloon recanalization of chronic total coronary occlusions, *Am J Cardiol* 1989; **64**:148–154.

41. Pande AK, Meier B, Urban P et al. Magnum/Magnarail versus conventional systems for recanalization of chronic total coronary occlusions: a randomized comparison, *Am Heart J* 1992; **123**:1182–1186.

42. Allemann Y, Kaufmann UP, Meyer BJ et al. Magnum wire for percutaneous coronary balloon angioplasty in 800 total chronic occlusions, *Am J Cardiol* 1997; **80**:634–637.

43. Moles VP, Chappuis F, Simonet F et al. Aortic dissection as complication of percutaneous transluminal coronary angioplasty, *Cathet Cardiovasc Diagn* 1992; **26**:8–11.

44. Sievert H, Rohde S, Ensslen R et al. Recanalization of chronic coronary occlusions using a laser wire, *Cathet Cardiovasc Diagn* 1996; **37**:220–222.

45. Hamburger JN, Gijsbers GH, Ozaki Y et al. Recanalization of chronic total coronary occlusions using a laser guide wire: a pilot study, *J Am Coll Cardiol* 1997; **30**:649–656.

46. Hamburger JN, Serruys PW, Scabra-Gomes R et al. Recanalization of total coronary occlusions using a laser guide wire (the European TOTAL Surveillance Study), *Am J Cardiol* 1997; **80**:1419–1423.

47. Serruys PW, Hamburger JN, Koolen JJ et al. Total occlusion trial with angioplasty by using laser guidewire. The TOTAL trial, *Eur Heart J* 2000; **21**:1797–1805.

48. Danchin N, Cassagnes J, Juilliere Y et al. Balloon angioplasty versus rotational angioplasty in chronic coronary occlusions (the BAROCCO STUDY), *Am J Cardiol* 1995; **75**:330–334.

49. Kitazume H, Kubo I, Iwama T. Magnum Meier wires with Crag Fx wire catheter for total occlusive coronary arteries, *Cathet Cardiovasc Diagn* 1997; **40**:198–201.

50. Seggewiss H, Fassbender D, Gleichmann U, Schmidt HK, Vogt J. Recanalization of occluded coronary arteries using the Magnum system, *Dtsch Med Wochenschr* 1992; **117**:1543–1549.

51. Freed M, Botman JE, Siegel N et al. Glide wire treatment of resistant coronary occlusions, *Cathet Cardiovasc Diagn* 1993; **30**:201–204.

52. Gray DF, Sivananthan UM, Verma SP, Michalis LK, Rees MR. Balloon angioplasty of totally and subtotally occluded coronary arteries: results using the Hydrophillic Terumo Radifocus Guide

wire M (glide wire), *Cathet Cardiovasc Diagn* 1993; **30**:293–299.

53. Reimers B, Camassa N, Di Mario C et al. Mechanical recanalization of total coronary occlusions with the use of a new guide wire, *Am Heart J* 1998; **135**:726–731.

54. Ellis SG, Shaw RE, Gershony G et al. Risk factors, time course and treatment effect for restenosis after successful percutaneous transluminal coronary angioplasty of chronic total occlusion, *Am J Cardiol* 1989; **63**:897–901.

55. Stone GW, Rutherford BD, McConahay DR et al. Procedural outcome of angioplasty for total coronary artery occlusion: an analysis of 971 lesions in 905 patients, *J Am Coll Cardiol* 1990; **15**:849–856.

56. Ruocco NA, Ring ME, Holubkov R. Results of coronary angioplasty of chronic total occlusions (the National Heart, Lung, and Blood Institute 1985–1986 Percutaneous Transluminal Angioplasty Registry), *Am J Cardiol* 1992; **69**:69–76.

57. Manginas A, Efstathopoulos E, Salvaras N et al. Intracoronary irradiation and stent placement in a chronic total coronary occlusion: long-term clinical, angiographic, and intracoronary ultrasound follow-up, *Catheter Cardiovasc Interv* 2000; **51**:199–202.

58. Plante S, Laarman G, de Feyter PJ et al. Acute complications of percutaneous transluminal coronary angioplasty for total occlusion, *Am Heart J* 1991; **121**:417–426.

59. Ellis SG, Ajluni S, Arnold AZ et al. Increased coronary perforation in the new device era. Incidence, classification, management, and outcome, *Circulation* 1994; **90**:2725–2730.

60. Ajluni SC, Glazier S, Blankenship L, O'Neill WW, Safian RD. Perforations after percutaneous coronary interventions: clinical, angiographic, and therapeutic observations, *Cathet Cardiovasc Diagn* 1994; **32**:206–212.

61. Meier B. Benign coronary perforation during percutaneous transluminal coronary angioplasty, *Br Heart J* 1985; **54**:33–35.

62. Gunnes P, Meyer BJ, Kessler B, Mulhauser B, Meier B. Magnum wire for angioplasty of total and non-total coronary lesions, *Int J Cardiol* 1997; **60**:1–6.

63. Reimers B, Di Mario C, Colombo A. Sub-intimal stent implantation for the treatment of a chronic coronary occlusion, *G Ital Cardiol* 1997; **27**:1158–1163.

64. Sirnes PA, Golf S, Myreng Y et al. Stenting in Chronic Coronary Occlusion (SICCO): a randomized, controlled trial of adding stent implantation after successful angioplasty, *J Am Coll Cardiol* 1996; **28**:1444–1451.

65. Lotan C, Rozenman Y, Hendler A et al. Stents in total occlusion for restenosis prevention. The multicentre randomized STOP study. The Israeli Working Group for Interventional Cardiology, *Eur Heart J* 2000; **21**:1960–1966.

66. Rubartelli P, Niccoli L, Verna E et al. Stent implantation versus balloon angioplasty in chronic coronary occlusions: results from the GISSOC trial. Gruppo Italiano di Studio sullo Stent nelle Occlusioni Coronariche, *J Am Coll Cardiol* 1998; **32**:90:–96.

67. Buller CE, Dzavik V, Carere RG et al. Primary stenting versus balloon angioplasty in occluded coronary arteries: the Total Occlusion Study of Canada (TOSCA), *Circulation* 1999; **100**: 236–242.

68. Urban P, Meier B, Finci L et al. Coronary wedge pressure: a predictor of restenosis after coronary balloon angioplasty, *J Am Coll Cardiol* 1987; **10**:504–509.

69. Goldberg SL, Colombo A, Maiello L et al. Intracoronary stent insertion after balloon angioplasty of chronic total occlusions, *J Am Coll Cardiol* 1995; **26**:713–719.

70. Ozaki Y, Violaris AG, Hamburger J et al. Short- and long-term clinical and quantitative angiographic results with the new, less shortening Wallstent for vessel reconstruction in chronic total occlusion: a quantitative angiographic study, *J Am Coll Cardiol* 1996; **28**:354–360.

71. Mori M, Kurogane H, Hayashi T et al. Comparison of results of intracoronary implantation of the Plamaz-Schatz stent with conventional balloon angioplasty in chronic total coronary arterial occlusion, *Am J Cardiol* 1996; **78**:985–998.

72. Hoher M, Wohrle J, Grebe OC et al. A randomized trial of elective stenting after balloon recanalization of chronic total occlusions, *J Am Coll Cardiol* 1999; **34**:722–729.

73. Sirnes PA, Golf S, Myreng Y et al. Sustained benefit of stenting chronic coronary occlusion: long-term clinical follow-up of the Stenting in Chronic Coronary Occlusion (SICCO) study, *J Am Coll Cardiol* 1998; **32**:305–310.

74. Teirstein PS, Massullo V, Jani S et al. Two-year follow-up after catheter-based radiotherapy to

inhibit coronary restenosis, *Circulation* 1999; **99**:243–247.

75. Condado JA, Waksman R, Gurdiel O et al. Long-term angiographic and clinical outcome after percutaneous transluminal coronary angioplasty and intracoronary radiation therapy in humans, *Circulation* 1997; **96**:727–732.

76. Fareh J, Martel R, Kermani P, Leclerc G. Cellular effects of beta-particle delivery on vascular smooth muscle cells and endothelial cells: a dose-response study, *Circulation* 1999; **99**: 1477–1484.

77. Meerkin D, Tardif JC, Crocker IR et al. Effects of intracoronary beta-radiation therapy after coronary angioplasty: an intravascular ultrasound study, *Circulation* 1999; **99**:1660–1665.

Section V: Comorbidity

25

Chronic pulmonary disease

Darryl Weiman, Kodangudi B Ramanathan and Douglass A Morrison

CONTENTS • Introduction • Chronic Obstructive Pulmonary Disease (COPD) and CABG risk • Preoperative evaluation • Postoperative pneumonia or mediastinal infection • Perioperative hypoventilation • Perioperative hypoxemia • Strategies to decrease the morbidity and mortality of pulmonary complications of CABG • Percutaneous coronary intervention (PCI) as an alternative to CABG • Pulmonary embolism, pulmonary hypertension and right ventricular ischemia

INTRODUCTION [1–10]

The ACC/AHA guideline on coronary artery bypass graft surgery describes the following possible mechanisms whereby coronary artery bypass graft surgery (CABG) may be associated with post-operative pulmonary insufficiency:

- Intrapulmonary shunting leading to reduced arterial oxygen tension.
- Atelectasis and alveolar collapse leading to ventilation/perfusion mismatching.
- Impaired capillary endothelial integrity leading to interstitial and alveolar edema.
- Central effects of anesthesia and narcotics leading to decreased ventilatory drive.
- Embolization of air or thrombi to the central nervous system producing both impaired ventilatory drive and neurogenic gas exchange abnormalities.
- Neuromuscular weakness contributing to hypoventilation.
- Pain from excision and chest tubes contributing to hypoventilation.
- Phrenic nerve injury from either LIMA dissection and/or ice slush, contributing to hypoventilation.

- Obesity contributing to mechanical hypoventilation, and as a risk-factor for mediastinitis [1].

Prolonged postoperative mechanical ventilation is morbidity in its own right but it also places the patient at increased risk for nosocomial pneumonia [1]. Through the combination of all of these mechanisms, CABG is frequently associated with a short-term predominantly restrictive impairment [9–11]. Nevertheless, with aggressive post-operative care, this is usually clinically mild and limited in duration.

CHRONIC OBSTRUCTIVE PULMONARY DISEASE (COPD) AND CABG RISK [1–8, 11–17] (TABLE 25.1)

The guideline stressed the role of chronic obstructive pulmonary disease (COPD) as a risk factor for perioperative (30-day) mortality. Although COPD is often defined in terms of the forced expiratory volume in one second (FEV1), a spirometric measure of pulmonary function, most authors emphasize the clinical assessment. Three particularly useful clinical

Table 25.1 COPD as a risk factor for CABG mortality

Database	Reference	Mortality in patients with COPD	Mortality in patients without COPD	Risk ratio
VA	[2]	6.4%	4.3%	1.49
STS	[3, 4]	4.1%	3.2%	1.28
New York state	[5, 6]			1.36 (1.2–1.54)
Cleveland Clinic	[7]			2.39 (1.44–3.97)
CABG database	[8]			

VA, Veterans Affairs; STS, Society of Thoracic Surgeons.

factors indicating surgical risk among patients with moderate to severe COPD (FEV1 < 50–70%) predicted are: (1) need for continuous home oxygen; (2) need for chronic corticosteroid therapy; and (3) chronic hypoventilation, defined as chronic arterial CO_2 tension > 45 mmHg. A number of studies have reported that patients with COPD undergoing CABG have more frequent atrial and ventricular arrythmias; longer intensive care unit stays; longer periods of mechanical ventilation; more reintubations and higher mortality (see below).

In the Veterans Administration study of patients undergoing CABG, FEV1 was first examined as a continuous variable comparing 414 who died during two years after surgery versus 8569 who survived for those two years [2]. The mean FEV1 was higher among the survivors (2.7 ± 0.7 vs 2.4 ± 0.7, $p = 0.001$). When patients were divided into groups of FEV1 0.25 L, there was an inverse relation with $p < 0.01$ for trend and patients with FEV1 < 1.25 L had operative mortality of 11.7% compared with 3.8% for patients with FEV1 > 1.25 L. A clinical diagnosis of COPD was among the variables to emerge from multiple logistic regression analysis as predictive of operative mortality [2].

For the Society of Thoracic Surgeons National Cardiac Surgery Database, COPD was defined as 'a patient who requires pharmacologic treatment of chronic pulmonary compromise, or a patient who has a FEV1 < 75% predicted' [3]. In the 80,881 patients included in the STS registry between 1980 and 1990, COPD was found to be a significant univariate risk factor for mortality ($p < 0.025$) with a 4.1% mortality among patients with COPD versus 3.2% among patients without COPD [4].

In the State of New York database evaluation of 7596 patients, COPD was defined as 'resulting in functional disability, hospitalization, or FEV1 < 75% predicted; or requiring bronchodilator therapy' [5]. Defined in this way, patients with COPD ($n = 504$) had a 7.9% in-hospital mortality; whereas patients without ($n = 7092$) had an in-hospital mortality of 4.6%. In a subsequent analysis of 57,187 patients, COPD was significantly associated with in-hospital mortality (OR = 1.36; 95% CI 1.20–1.54; $p < 0.001$) [6].

Higgins and colleagues reviewed 5051 consecutive patients who had undergone CABG at Cleveland Clinic. Chronic obtrusive pulmonary disease requiring medication was associated with an odds ratio (OR) of 1.71 ($p < 0.001$) for morbidity and 2.70 ($p < 0.001$) for mortality [7].

Table 25.2 Risk factors for nosocomial pneumonia or mediastinal infection

First author	Reference	Cases/total CABG	Risk factors
Milano	[18]	83/6459	Obesity ($p = 0.002$) NYHA class ($p = 0.002$) Prior heart surgery ($p = 0.008$) Duration of bypass ($p = 0.05$)
Farinas	[19]	34/3645	Smoking history History of endocarditis Emergency surgery Prolonged surgery Prolonged bypass Ventricular failure Re-operation Prolonged mechanical ventilation Prolonged ICU stay Tracheostomy
Demmy et al	[25]	31/1521	COPD Longer ICU stay Respiratory failure Connective tissue disorder
Newman et al	[26]	68/9965	COPD Prior sternotomy Low LVEF Pyuria High LV end-diastolic pressure Prolonged bypass time Aortic valve or aneurysm surgery Repeat placement on bypass Duration of surgery Surgical re-exploration Cardiopulmonary resuscitation Prolonged mechanical ventilation

In a multiple logistic regression model, COPD was significant for morbidity (OR = 1.47 95% CI 1.20–1.82; $p = 0.009$) and mortality (OR = 2.39 95% CI 1.44–3.97; $p < 0.002$).

In attempting to synthesize a single list of preoperative variables with which to risk-adjust CABG data, Jones and coworkers developed a list of seven core variables and 13 level 1 variables [8] and COPD, as defined by the State of New York, was a level 1 variable.

PREOPERATIVE EVALUATION [9–17]

There is debate as to the usefulness of routine pulmonary function testing prior to surgery. There is no debate that patients should be queried regarding smoking history, chronic cough, hemoptysis, pulmonary infection history, including pneumonia, TB and fungal infections, as well as history of pulmonary thromboembolism, airway disease, and medication use, particularly bronchodilators. Smokers should be urged and counseled to discontinue smoking.

POSTOPERATIVE PNEUMONIA OR MEDIASTINAL INFECTION [18–29]

Gaynes and coworkers reviewed the cases of CABG at the University of Michigan in 1988, identifying 18 cases of nosocomial pneumonia and then conducting a case-control evaluation. They identified COPD, duration of mechanical ventilation > 2 days and preoperative use of antacids as risk factors [22]. Milano and colleagues reviewed 6459 consecutive CABG cases from Duke University, identifying 83 cases of postoperative mediastinitis [18]. They identified obesity and duration of surgery as the most important predictors of mediastinal infection with previous heart surgery and prior heart failure also emerging from multivariable analysis as risk factors. Farinas et al reviewed 3645 cases of mediana sternotomy from Hospital Marques de Valdecilla, identifying 34 cases of suppurative mediastinitis. They found that pre-operative smoking and endocarditis, emergency surgery, prolonged pump or overall operative time, re-operation, prolonged mechanical ventilation, prolonged ICU stay or tracheostomy were all associated with this adverse outcome [19]. Newman and colleagues identified 68 cases out of 9965 consecutive CABG cases at Emory University [26]. They identified the following preoperative risk factors: COPD, prior sternotomy, low left ventricular ejection fraction (LVEF), high left ventricular

end-diastolic pressure (LVEDP), and pyuria [26]. Procedural risk factors for mediastinal infection included: aortic valve or aneurysm surgery, prolonged pump time, repeat placement on bypass, and duration of surgery [26]. Post-procedural risk factors included surgical re-exploration, cardiopulmonary resuscitation, and prolonged mechanical ventilation [26]. Their largest series seems to summarize the results of the other small series [18–29].

PERIOPERATIVE HYPOVENTILATION [30–59]

Postoperative hypoventilation can accrue from multiple factors:

- Hypothermic injury to the phrenic nerve [39–42].
- Direct injury to the phrenic nerve [36–38].
- Cardioplegic effects on diaphragmatic function [44–48].
- Anesthetic effects [49–50].
- Drug effects (other than anethestic agent) [51,52].
- Postoperative atelectasis [53–59].

Curtis and associates described an incidence of elevated left hemi-diaphragm of 26% when topical ice slush was used for myocardial preservation [39]. In their study, they noted that if the patient also had the internal mammary artery taken down for use as a bypass conduit, the incidence of hemidiaphragm paralysis increased to 39.4%. Nevertheless, by one year, 78% of patients had recovered diaphragmatic function and by two years 97% had recovered function.

Efthimiou described diaphragmatic paralysis resulting from iced slush applied directly to the phrenic nerve [40]. They emphasized the potential synergy between COPD and additional diaphragmatic paralysis.

In 1987, Esposito and Spencer studied the effect of an insulating pad placed in the pericardial cavity to protect the phrenic nerve from hypothermic injury [41]. In their study, 73% of the patients operated without the pericardial insulating pad had phrenic nerve injury. Conversely, among those patients operated with the insulating pad, only 17% had phrenic nerve injury. Cooling jackets have also been used to cool the heart to enhance myocardial protection. In a series of 750 patients reported by Bonchek, use of the cooling jacket was not accompanied by a single case of phrenic nerve injury.

During mobilization of the internal mammary artery, the phrenic nerve may be injured by clips, cautery, or unintentional transsection. The phrenic nerve lies close to the internal mammary artery above the first rib at the thoracic inlet. Electrocautery devices could injure the nerve, so it is important to mobilize the lateral aspect of the internal mammary artery above the first rib. The blood supply to the phrenic nerve may also be damaged during mobilization of the internal mammary artery.

Although it is relatively uncommon, cases of postoperative bilateral phrenic nerve injury have been reported. These patients have a far greater potential for clinically significant hypoventilation and require more aggressive management including prolonged mechanical ventilation in some cases. Abd and others have reported successful use of the rocking bed for 13 cases of postoperative diaphragmatic paralysis. This technique was initially used for the treatment of polio victims, and provided support for patients for periods up to 27 months. Curiously, six of the patients in Abd's series required the rocking bed to normalize their ventilatory status despite unilateral diaphragmatic paralysis.

Weiman and colleagues have emphasized the importance of phrenic nerve damage as a potentially avoidable cause of postoperative hypoventilation. They recommended the following steps to try to minimize this problem:

- Careful technique in taking down the left internal mammary artery in an effort to avoid injury to the phrenic nerve and its blood supply.
- Use of an insulating pad to keep cold slush

off the phrenic nerve as it crosses the pericardium.
- Avoidance of entry into the pleural cavity during internal mammary takedown.
- Scavenging cardioplegia solution as it enters the right atrium.

In addition to avoiding phrenic nerve damage, with its attendant hemidiaphragmatic paralysis, avoiding anesthesia-related problems (such as late adverse effects of high-dose fentanyl with its attendant decrease in chest wall compliance), and avoiding over use of postoperative analgesia can also decrease hypoventilation. As in all surgery, atelectasis can be important, particularly in patients with airways disease.

Studies by Wilcox and associates have demonstrated that postoperative atelectasis is multifactorial with factors such as prolonged bypass and operative times, entrance into the pleural cavity, increasing number of grafts and lower body temperature all being associated with worse atelectasis. Additionally, they documented that phrenic nerve injury and diaphragmatic paralysis was but one of multiple contributing factors. Another factor identified by Wilcox and colleagues was a result of cardioplegia entering the pulmonary circulation. When the operators removed the solution as it entered the right atrium, their patients appeared to have less postoperative atelectasis, and they surmised that the high potassium content of their cardioplegic solution was involved.

All patients receiving a general anesthetic can have a functional residual capacity decline of up to 20%. This likely occurs because of an upward shift of the diaphragm and changes in chest wall compliance resulting in changes in gas flow that are not matched with compensatory change in pulmonary blood flow. The attendant ventilation perfusion mismatch leads to an increased alveolar-arterial oxygen gradient.

A frequently used anesthetic agent, fentanyl, can be accompanied by a decrease in chest wall compliance. This is another potential cause of hypoventilation. Because fentanyl can be sequestered in adipose tissue and released slowly, this cause of hypoventilation can occur up to six hours after the operation is over. Caspi and coworkers reviewed 380 cases of cardiac surgery who had received fentanyl as part of their anesthetic regimen. They noted 29 cases of postoperative hypoventilation, 15 of whom had elevated fentanyl levels and 14 who did not. Both muscle relaxants and naloxone can be beneficial, but naloxone has vasoconstrictive properties, which can complicate its use in ischemic heart patients, particularly those who have left ventricular dysfunction.

Pleural effusion from bleeding or pleural injury can contribute to postoperative hypoventilation. Pleural injury with residual (undrained) effusion can also be accompanied by trapping of the lung by a pleural peel. This trapped lung syndrome is another cause of hypoventilation.

Iverson et al reported some degree of postoperative atelectasis in between 10 and 70% of cardiac surgery patients. Reported causes of atelectasis after surgery include:

- Low tidal volume breathing because of pain and splinting.
- Bronchospasm.
- Mucus plugging.
- Compression of lung parenchyma by hemothorax, pneumothorax or pleural effusion.

Atelectasis can lead to both hypoventilation and hypoxemia. Adequate pain medication, incentive spirometry and frequent suctioning (with pretreatment with adequate inhaled oxygen) have all been advocated to increase tidal volume. The use of intermittent positive pressure ventilation has been controversial, but likely helps patients with impaired pulmonary reserve preoperatively. Clearly, large pneumothoraces, hemothoraces and pleural effusion need to be drained.

PERIOPERATIVE HYPOXEMIA

After hypoventilation, most cases of postoperative hypoxemia relate to ventilation/perfusion mismatching. This can occur as a result of:

- Pulmonary edema.
- Pulmonary embolism.
- Aspiration and nosocomial pneumonia.
- Medications which override hypoxic vasoconstriction, among other etiologies.

Among patients undergoing CABG, pulmonary edema most often occurs as a result of left ventricular dysfunction, reflecting the sum of preoperative ventricular dysfunction plus intraoperative ischemia and/or infarction. Fluid overload may also contribute, especially among patients with preoperative diastolic dysfunction. It is unsettled as to how much cardiopulmonary bypass may contribute to non-hydrostatic pulmonary edema, but prolonged pump times are associated with prolonged postoperative mechanical ventilation.

Pulmonary embolism is relatively uncommon among CABG patients in part because of the intense anticoagulation for cardiopulmonary bypass, and platelet dysfunction associated with cardiopulmonary bypass. Nevertheless, patients with pre-existent venous disease, prolonged bed rest, low flow states, peripheral vascular disease, coagulopathy, or who required intra-aortic balloon counterpulsation, are all at increased risk.

One of the most important risk factors for aspiration is central neurologic depression, which can also contribute to hypoventilation. Pre-existent cerebrovascular disease, aortic disease, atrial fibrillation and severe ventricular dysfunction are all predispositions for additional intraoperative neurologic impairment.

A number of cardiac medications including nitroglycerin and nitroprusside can override hypoxic pulmonary vasoconstriction, which initially served to optimize ventilation/perfusion matching. Effectively, these drugs can create a shunt and thereby be associated with hypoxemia. In general, these vasodilator drugs do not effect ventilation.

STRATEGIES TO DECREASE THE MORBIDITY AND MORTALITY OF PULMONARY COMPLICATIONS OF CABG

In addition to preoperative evaluation, numerous intraoperative monitoring methods, including right heart and arterial catheters for pressure and flow, transesophageal echocardiography for biventricular function and preload assessment, blood gases and ventilatory measurements are used to optimize fluid status and ventilatory mechanics. Post-operatively, surgeons pay meticulous attention to all of the possible mechanisms of respiratory failure (both ventilation and oxygenation) elucidated in this chapter, including the following specific steps:

- Monitoring end-tidal CO_2 and adjusting the ventilator to keep CO_2 in the normal range.
- Reversing fentanyl and other sedation, if needed.
- Being aware of potential of nitroprusside or nitroglycerin to produce shunting and hypoxemia.
- Early treatment of large pleural effusions.
- Avoiding epidural anesthesia.
- Assessment of pharyngeal function and swallowing.
- Using adequate inspired oxygen prior to suctioning.
- Use of sequential pneumatic anti-embolism stockings.
- Vigorous investigation of possible pneumothorax, pericardial tamponade, pulmonary edema, and pulmonary emboli in postoperative patients who develop acute dyspnea.
- Appropriate use of positive end expiratory pressure.
- Treatment of pain, education, and incentive spirometry to encourage deep breathing (and discourage atelectasis).

Whenever possible attempts are made to decrease the duration of mechanical ventilation and intubation, moving the patient back as close as possible to his/her preoperative respiratory status.

PERCUTANEOUS CORONARY INTERVENTION (PCI) AS AN ALTERNATIVE TO CABG [60–63]

A major focus of this text is the dynamic interplay of CABG and PCI. Accordingly, it is useful to consider what preoperative variables swing the risk/benefit consideration from one option to the other. As outlined in the ACC/AHA guideline, three clinical factors associated with advanced pulmonary disease, which might make a surgeon consider palliative PCI rather than CABG are: (1) chronic home oxygen requirement; (2) chronic hypoventilation, manifested as chronic hypercapnia; (3) chronic corticosteroid use [1].

PULMONARY EMBOLISM, PULMONARY HYPERTENSION AND RIGHT VENTRICULAR ISCHEMIA [64–67]

Cardiopulmonary bypass appears to be peculiarly problematic for patients with an acute right ventricular (RV) insult, such as right ventricular infarction. This is even more the case in the face of pulmonary hypertension. This is likely the link in the clinical observation that patients on chronic home oxygen seem to pose a particularly high risk for CABG. Accordingly, RV infarction and severe pulmonary hypertension may be two additional settings where PCI might be considered as an alternative revascularization strategy.

REFERENCES

1. Eagle KA, Guyton RA, Davidoff R et al for the Committee to revise the 1991 guidelines for coronary artery bypass graft surgery. ACC/AHA

Guidelines for Coronary Artery Bypass Graft Surgery, *J Am Coll Cardiol* 199; **34**:1263–1347.

2. Grover FL, Hammermeister KE, Burchfiel C and the Cardiac Surgeons of the Department of Veterans Affairs. Initial Report of the Veterans Administration Preoperative Risk Assessment Study of Cardiac Study, *Ann Thorac Surg* 1990; **50**:12–28.

3. Clark RE for the committee: Definitions of Terms of the Society of Thoracic Surgeons National Cardiac Surgery Database, *Ann Thorac Surg* 1994; **58**:271–273.

4. Edwards FH, Clark RE, Schwartz M. Coronary Artery Bypass Grafting: The Society of Thoracic Surgeons National Database Experience, *Ann Thorac Surg* 1994; **57**:12–19.

5. Hannan EL, Kilburn H, O'Donnell JF, Lukacik G, Shields EP. Adult open heart surgery in New York State. An analysis of risk factors and hospital mortality rates, *JAMA* 1990; **264**:2768–2774.

6. Hannan EL, Kilburn H, Racz M, Shields E, Chassin MR. Improving the outcomes of coronary artery bypass surgery in New York State, *JAMA* 1994; **271**:761–766.

7. Higgins TL, Estafanous FG, Loop FD et al. Stratification of morbidity and mortality outcome by preoperative risk factors in coronary artery bypass patients. A Clinical Severity Score, *JAMA* 1992; **267**: 2344–2348.

8. Jones RH, Hannan EL, Hammermeister KE et al for the Working Group Panel on the Cooperative CABG Database Project. Identification of preoperative variables needed for adjustment of short-term mortality after coronary artery bypass graft surgery, *J Am Coll Cardiol* 1996; **28**:1478–1487.

9. Braun SR, Birnbaum MI, Chopra PS. Pre and post-operative pulmonary function abnormalities in coronary artery revascularization surgery, *Chest* 1978; **73**:318.

10. Jenkins SC, Soutar SA, Forsyth A, Keates JR, Moxham I. Lung function after coronary artery surgery using the internal mammary artery and the saphenous vein, *Thorax* 1989; **44**:209–211.

11. Shapira N, Zabatino SM, Ahmed S et al. Determinants of pulmonary function in patients undergoing coronary bypass operations, *Ann Thorac Surg* 1990; **50**:268–273.

12. Kroenke K, Lawrence VA, Theroux JF, Tuley MR. Operative risk in patients with severe obstructive pulmonary disease, *Arch Intern Med* 1992; **152**:967–971.

13. Cohen A, Katz M, Katz R, Hauptman E, Schachner A. Chronic obstructive pulmonary disease in patients undergoing coronary artery bypass grafting, *J Thorac Cardiovasc Surg* 1995; **109**:574–581.

14. Wahl GW, Swinburne AJ, Fedullo AJ, Lee DK, Shayne D. Effect of age and preoperative airway obstruction on lung function after coronary artery bypass grafting, *Ann Thorac Surg* 1993; **56**:104–107.

15. Williams CD, Brenowits JB. Prohibitive lung function and major surgical procedures, *Am J Surg* 1976; **132**:763–766.

16. Zibrak JD, O'Donnel CR, Haley K et al. Predictive factors for pulmonary complications following CABG surgery, *Chest* 1990; **98**:895.

17. Bevelaqua F, Garritau S, Hass F. Complications after cardiac operation in patients with severe pulmonary impairment, *Am Thorac Surg* 1990; **50**:602.

18. Milano CA, Kesler K, Archibald N, Sexton DJ, Jones RT. Mediastinitis after coronary artery bypass graft surgery, *Circulation* 1995; **92**: 2245–2251.

19. Farinas MC, Peralta FG, Bernal JM et al. Suppurative mediastinitis after open-heart surgery: a case-control study covering a seven-year period in Santander, Spain, *Clin Infectious Dis* 1995; **20**:272–279.

20. Loop FD, Lyde BW, Cosgrove DM et al. J. Maxwell Chamberlain memorial paper: sternal wound complications after isolated coronary artery bypass grafting: early and late mortality, morbidity, and cost of care, *Ann Thorac Surg* 1990; **49**:179–186.

21. Nagachinta T, Stephens M, Reitz B, Polk BF. Risk factors for surgical-wound infection following cardiac surgery, *J Infect Dis* 1987; **156**:967–973.

22. Risk factors for deep sternal wound infection after sternotomy: a prospective, multicenter study, *J Thorac Cardiovasc Surg* 1996; **111**: 1200–1207.

23. Grossi EA, Esposito R, Harris U et al. Sternal wound infections and use of internal mammary artery grafts, *J Thorac Cardiovasc Surg* 1991; **102**:342–347.

24. Gaynes R, Bizek B, Mowry-Hanley I, Kirsh M. Risk factors for nosocomial pneumonia after coronary artery bypass graft operations, *Ann Thorac Surg* 1991; **51**:215–218.

25. Demmy TL, Park SB, Liebler GA et al. Recent

experience with major sternal wound complications, *Ann Thorac Surg* 1990; **49**:458–462.

26. Newman LS, Szczukowski LC, Bain RP, Perlino CA. Suppurative mediastinitis after open heart surgery: a case control study of risk factors, *Chest* 1988; **94**:546–553.

27. Furnary AP, Grunkemeier GL, Floten HS et al. Continuous intravenous insulin infusion reduces the incidence of deep sternal wound infection in diabetic patients after cardiac surgical procedures, *Ann Thorac Surg* 1999; **67**:352–360.

28. Zert KJ, Furnary AP, Grunkemeier GL et al. Glucose control lowers the risk of wound infection in diabetics after open-heart operations, *Ann Thorac Surg* 1997; **63**:356–361.

29. Ottino G, De Paulis R, Pansini S et al. Major sternal wound infection after open-heart surgery: a multivariate analysis of risk factors in 2579 consecutive operative procedures, *Ann Thorac Surg* 1987; **44**:173–179.

30. Weiman DS, Ferdinand FD, Botton JWR, Brosman KM, Whitman GR. Perioperative respiratory management in cardiac surgery clinics. *Chest Medicine* 1993; **14**:283–292.

31. Nishida H, Grooters RK, Solranzadeh H et al. Discriminate use of electrocautery on the median sternotomy incision: a 0.16% wound infection rate, *J Thorac Cardiovasc Surg* 1991; **101**:488–494.

32. Mathay MA, Chatterjee K. Respiratory and hemodynamic management after cardiac surgery, *Cardiology* 1997; **3**:1–6.

33. Michel L, McMichan IC, Marsh HM, Rehder K. Measurement of ventilatory reserve as an indicator for early extubation after cardiac operation, *J Thorac Cardiovasc Surg* 1979; **78**:761–764.

34. Klineberg PL, Geer RT, Hirsh RA, Aukburg SI. Early extubation after coronary artery bypass graft surgery, *Crit Care Med* 1977; **5**:272–274.

35. Wall GW, Swinburne AJ, Fedullo A, Lee DK, Shayne D. Effect of age and preoperative airway obstruction on lung function after coronary artery bypass grafting, *Ann Thorac Surg* 1993; **56**:104–107.

36. Goyal V, Pinto RI, Mukherjee K et al. Alteration in pulmonary mechanics after coronary bypass surgery: comparison using internal mammary artery and saphenous vein grafts, *Indian Heart J* 1994; **46**:345–348.

37. Jenkins SC, Soutar SA, Forsyth A, Keates JR, Moxham I. Lung function after coronary artery surgery using the internal mammary artery and the saphenous vein, *Thorax* 1989; **44**:209–211.

38. Shapira N, Zabatino SM, Ahmed S et al. Determinants of pulmonary function in patients undergoing coronary bypass operations, *Ann Thorac Surg* 1990; **50**:268–273.

39. Curtis NJ, Nawarawong W, Walls JT et al. Elevated hemidiaphragm after cardiac operations: incidence, prognosis, and relationship to the use of topical slush, *Ann Thorac Surg* 1989; **48**:764–768.

40. Efthimiou J, Butler J, Woodham C et al. Diaphragm paralysis following cardiac surgery: role of phrenic nerve cold injury, *Ann Thorac Surg* 1991; **51**:1005–1008.

41. Esposito RA, Spencer FC. The effects of pericardial insulation on hypothermic phrenic nerve injury during open-heart surgery, *Ann Thorac Surg* 1987; **43**:303–308.

42. Bonchek LI. Myocardial protection jacket for topical hypothermia, *J Thorac Cardiovasc Surg* 1987; **94**:792–796.

43. Wilcox P, Baile EM, Hards J et al. Phrenic nerve function and its relationship to atelectasis after coronary artery bypass surgery, *Chest* 1988; **93**:693–698.

44. Wilcox PG, Pare PD, Pardy RL. Recovery after unilateral phrenic injury associated with coronary artery revascularization, *Chest* 1990; **98**:661–666.

45. Brown KA, Hoffstein V, Byrick RJ. Bedside diagnosis of bilateral diaphragmatic paralysis in a ventilator-dependent patient after open-heart surgery, *Anesth Analg* 1985; **64**:1208–1210.

46. Burgess RW, Boyd AF, Moore PG et al. Postoperative respiratory failure due to bilateral phrenic nerve palsy, *Postgrad Med* 1989; **65**:39–41.

47. Werner RA, Gelringer SR. Bilateral phrenic nerve palsy associated with open-heart surgery, *Arch Phys Med Rehabil* 1990; **71**:1000–1002.

48. Abd AG, Brawn NM, Baskin MI et al. Diaphragmatic dysfunction after open-heart surgery: treatment with a rocking bed, *Ann Intern Med* 1989; **111**:881–886.

49. Caspi J, Klausner JM, Safadi T et al. Delayed respiratory depression following fentanyl anesthesia for cardiac surgery, *Crit Care Med* 1988; **16**:238–240.

50. Sprung J, Samaan F, Hensler T et al. Excessive airway pressure due to ventilator control valve malfunction during anesthesia for open-heart surgery, *Anesthesiology* 1990; **73**:1035–1038.

51. Berthelsen P, Haxholdt O, Husum B et al. PPEP reverses nitroglycerin-induced hypoxemia following coronary artery bypass surgery, *Acta Anesthesiol Scand* 1986; **30**:243–246.

52. Robinson RJ, Brister S, Jones E et al. Epidural meperidine analgesia after cardiac surgery, *Can Anaesth Soc J* 1986; **33**:550–555.

53. Harrington OB, Duckworth JK, Starnes LC et al. Silent aspiration after coronary artery bypass grafting, *Ann Thorac Surg* 1998; **65**:1599–1603.

54. Gould FK, Freeman R, Brown MA. Respiratory complications following cardiac surgery, *Anaesthesia* 1985; **40**:1061–1064.

55. Preusser BA, Stone KS, Gonyon DS et al. Effects of two methods of pre-oxygenation on mean arterial pressure, cardiac output, peak airway pressure, and post-suctioning hypoxemia, *Heart Lung* 1988; **17**:290–299.

56. Ilabaca PA, Ochsner JL, Mills NL. Positive end-expiratory pressure in the management of the patient with a postoperative bleeding heart, *Ann Thorac Surg* 1989; **30**:281–284.

57. Iverson LIG, Ecker RR, Fox HE et al. A comparative study of IPPB, the incentive spirometer, and blow bottles: the prevention of atelectasis following cardiac surgery, *Ann Thorac Surg* 1978; **25**:197–200.

58. Pinilla JC, Oleniuk FH, Tun L et al. Use of a nasal continuous positive airway pressure mask in the treatment of postoperative atelectasis in aorto-coronary bypass surgery, *Crit Care Med* 190; **18**:836–840.

59. Ali J, Seerrette C, Wood LDH et al. Effects of postoperative positive pressure breathing on lung function, *Chest* 1984; **85**:192–196.

60. Morrison DA, Barbiere CC, Johnson R et al. Salvage angioplasty: an alternative to high-risk surgery for unstable angina, *Cathet Cardiovasc Diagn* 1992; **27**:169–178.

61. Morrison DA, Sacks J, Grover F, Hammermeister K. Effectiveness of percutaneous transluminal coronary angioplasty for patients with medically refractory rest angina pectoris and high risk of adverse outcomes with coronary artery bypass grafting, *Am J Card* 1995; **75**:237–240.

62. Morrison DA. Summary of 'high risk' and 'prohibitive risk' for surgery or angioplasty in unstable angina. In: Morrison DA, Serruys PW, eds, *Medically Refractory Rest Angina* (New York: Marcel Dekker, 1992) 385–401.

63. Grover FL, Hammermeister KE, Burchfeil C and the Veterans Affairs Surgeons. Initial report of the Veterans Administration Preoperative Risk Assessment study for cardiac surgery, *Ann Thorac Surg* 1990; **50**:12–28.

64. Fisk RL, Guilbeau EJ. Perioperative right heart failure: etiology and pathophysiology. In: Fisk RL, ed, *The Right Heart* (Philadelphia: FA Davis, Cardiovascular Clinics, 1987) 219–229.

65. Gaines WE. Perioperative right heart failure. Treatment. In: Fisk RL, ed, *The Right Heart* (Philadelphia: FA Davis, Cardiovascular Clinics, 1987) 231–238.

66. Payne DD, Cleveland RJ. Perioperative right heart dysfunction. In: Konstam MA, Isner JM, eds, *The Right Ventricle* (Boston: Kluwer Academic Publishers, 1988) 293–319.

67. Borkon AM, Reitz BA. Heart-lung transplantation. In: Konstam MA, Isner JM, eds, *The Right Ventricle* (Boston: Kluwer Academic Publishers, 1988) 321–327.

26

Cerebrovascular and peripheral vascular co-morbidity

Douglass A Morrison, Krisada Sastravaha and Gumpanart Veerakul

CONTENTS • Cerebrovascular morbidity and mortality with CABG • Cerebrovascular morbidity and mortality with PCI • Peripheral vascular disease (PVD)

CEREBROVASCULAR MORBIDITY AND MORTALITY WITH CABG [1–116]

Cerebral morbidity, consisting of (1) stroke, (2) neuropsychologic complications or decreased intellectual function, or (3) encephalopathy is one of the most prevalent and significant morbidities of coronary artery bypass graft surgery (CABG) [1–32]. It is estimated that approximately 6% of CABG patients experience some neurologic morbidity, and rates as high as 35% have been cited for deterioration of intellectual capacity, depending upon the sophistication of the pre- and postoperative testing [1–32]. The diagnosis of stroke is contingent upon focal neurologic signs such as hemipareisis or hemianopia. Abnormalities of thought processes or behavior, unaccompanied by focal neurologic or visual deficits are categorized as neuropsychologic complications. Encephalopathy is diagnosed based upon the patient's remaining obtunded or delirious.

Stroke is associated with an almost 10-fold higher perioperative mortality. Both stroke and encephalopathy are associated with increased length of stay. All three expressions of cerebral morbidity are associated with decreased quality of life [1–32].

Increased risk of adverse cerebral outcomes with CABG is seen among the following patient groups:

- Age > 70 [1–13].
- Ascending aorta calcium by either palpation, angiography, or ultrasound [22–27, 33–54].
- Prior cerebrovascular accident (stroke) [1–32].
- Atrial fibrillation [77–84].
- Left atrial and left ventricular thrombus [85–88].
- Unilateral carotid stenosis > 80% [66–71, 89–116].
- Bilateral carotid stenosis > 50% [66–71, 89–116].

All of the risk factors for cerebral morbidity with CABG are likely to increase with the progressive aging of the US and world populations. The prevalence of aortic calcification, prior cerebrovascular accident, cerebral arterial disease, atrial fibrillation, and atrial and ventricular thrombi are all greater in the elderly than among younger populations.

Recent studies suggest that cross-clamping of the aorta may cause embolization of atheromatous material leading to cerebral sequelae [12,

13, 33–50]. Avoiding the need for cross-clamping by either performing palliative percutaneous coronary intervention (PCI) alone or in combination with off-pump bypass (hybrid procedure) could potentially reduce the cerebral morbidity. Issues addressed by previous studies include the following:

- Incidence of adverse cerebral outcomes among specific patient groups.
- Problems in identifying adverse cerebral outcomes with CABG.
- Risk factors for adverse cerebral outcomes with CABG.
- Pathophysiologic mechanisms of adverse cerebral outcomes with CABG.
- Clinical approaches to reducing the adverse cerebral outcomes of CABG.

Incidence of adverse cerebral outcomes among specific patient groups

Roach and co-workers for the multicenter study of perioperative ischemia research group gathered a cohort of 2108 patients undergoing CABG in 24 US institutions [1]. They observed adverse cerebral outcomes in a total of 129 patients (6.1%). They divided these adverse outcomes into two categories: fatal and non-fatal strokes or infarction and transient ischemic attacks in 3.1% and deterioration in intellectual function or seizures in 3.0%.

Shaw and colleagues prospectively evaluated 312 patients undergoing CABG at a single center in the UK [2]. Their evaluation was more detailed and systematic, including routine evaluation by a neurologist. They identified definite stroke in 15 patients (5%), death from brain damage in one patient, prolonged encephalopathy in 10 patients (3%), ophthalmologic abnormalities in 78 patients (25%), peripheral nerve damage in 37 patients (12%) and primitive reflexes in 123 patients (39%). Although many of these findings were not considered clinically significant, they found some neurologic deficit in 61% of their patients!

John et al reported on 19,224 patients who underwent CABG in 31 hospitals in New York State [3]. This was a retrospective review and did not involve routine evaluation by a neurologist or specific intelligence testing. They reported stroke in 270 patients (1.4%). Sotaniemi and co-workers conducted a detailed neuropsychologic, cardiologic and encephalographic follow-up of 44 patients who underwent a similar surgical procedure, open-heart valve replacement [4]. They noted neurologic long-term impairment in 21% of their patients. Their study is noteworthy for its emphasis on the need to do long-term intelligence testing to really identify the most common and most important adverse neurologic outcome from open-heart surgery. Gardener et al reviewed 3279 consecutive CABG patients [5]. Their study did not include specific evaluation by a neurologist. They noted an increase in stroke incidence from 0.6% in 1979 to 2.4% in 1983.

Galloway and co-workers specifically addressed the importance of increased age by evaluating 482 patients whose age was ⩾ 70 years [6]. They reported a stroke incidence of 2.7%, obtained without specific neurologist examination. Loop and colleagues from the Cleveland Clinic reviewed 4603 patients between ages 65 and 75, noting a stroke incidence of 2.7% and 467 patients with age > 75 years, noting a stroke incidence of 2.4% [7]. This was a retrospective review without specific neurologist examination of each patient.

Problems in identifying adverse cerebral outcomes with CABG

The lessons from the above listed studies of incidence rates of adverse cerebral outcomes are put into perspective by studies of neurologic examination, intelligence testing instruments and brain imaging studies [8–10]. First, prospective studies are more accurate than retrospective reviews. This point is compounded when the retrospective review includes data from databases where the end-points were not specifically and objectively defined; this is a particular problem for neurologic outcomes such as impaired intellectual function.

It is a general truism in medicine that 'One sees what one looks for'. In the case of stroke, most physicians and surgeons are not trained or practiced in doing the type of detailed neurologic examination that neurologists perform. This helps to explain the nearly 10-fold difference in stroke rates for patients examined by a neurologist versus just picked up by the surgeon or cardiologist who follows routine post-CABG patients.

Another very important distinction, emphasized by a series of surgical studies by Kouchoukos and colleagues, is the difference in sensitivity and specificity of different methods of evaluating the same issue [11, 25, 26, 35]. These authors have compared palpation of the ascending aorta in the operating room with radiographic and ultrasound studies in identifying aortic calcification, which is a major risk factor for distal embolization during surgery. Ultrasound is significantly more sensitive and specific than either palpation or radiographic imaging [12, 24, 33, 34, 44–50, 69, 70]. Similarly, Bruggemans and co-workers have emphasized measurement error and practice effects among the methodological issues in using intelligence testing to identify deterioration in intellectual function after open-heart surgery [65, 69]. The work of Kouchoukos in identifying aortic calcification was directed at changing practice so as to improve surgical outcomes [11, 25, 35]. This emphasizes the importance of site specific factors in studies which compare incidence numbers.

Other methodological problems include the ubiquitous issue of sample size and power to detect, and the importance in postoperative studies of distinguishing transient from permanent changes.

Risk factors for adverse cerebral outcomes with CABG

The prospective and rigorously conducted studies by the Multicenter study of perioperative ischemia research group have identified eight clinical risk factors for stroke (type I neurologic adverse outcome) and six factors for impaired intellectual function (type II).

(A) risk factors for stroke:

- Proximal aortic atherosclerosis.
- History of neurologic disease.
- Use of intra-aortic balloon pumps (IABP).
- Diabetes mellitus.
- Hypertension.
- History of pulmonary disease.
- History of unstable angina.
- Age.

(B) Risk factors for decreased intellectual capacity:

- Age.
- History of pulmonary disease.
- Hypertension.
- History of excessive alcohol consumption.
- History of prior CABG.
- Dysrhythmia.

Pathophysiologic mechanisms of adverse cerebral outcomes with CABG [12–130]

The cerebral morbidity of CABG appears to derive from the following factors in decreasing order of frequency:

(A) Embolization from aortic atheroma; aortic atheromatosis is increasingly prevalent with age, reaching rates of 80% among patients over 75 years [24–50].
(B) Embolization from the left ventricle among patients with prior myocardial infarction and mural thrombi [85–88].
(C) Embolization from the left atrium among patients with atrial fibrillation [78–84].
(D) Hypoperfusion based on transient low perfusion pressure; this may be particularly

germane to patients with previous cerebral disease and/or coronary disease. One imaging study has suggested that CABG patients have a higher prevalence of cerebral structural defects than age matched controls [17, 60, 121–130].

(E) Embolization from the internal carotid artery, among patients with cerebrovascular disease [90–116].

(F) Drug effects post-operatively, especially among patients with concomitant renal or liver disorders [12, 13].

Clamping and unclamping of the aorta appears to be strongly related etiologically and temporally to (A) which is by far the most common cause of major post-CABG neurologic injury. Opening the heart, as is required in valve replacement or aneurysmectomy is associated with (B). The presence of congestive heart failure (CHF) or left ventricular dysfunction is related to (C). Heart-lung bypass is most closely related to (D). Previously a major concern, (E) cerebrovascular disease appears to be one of the lesser risk factors unless it is either severe unilateral (> 80%) or bilateral.

Clinical approaches to reducing the adverse cerebral outcomes of CABG

Percutaneous transluminal coronary angioplasty (PTCA) does not involve the major procedural factors that are associated with the neurologic complications of CABG: aortic cross-clamping, cardiac arrest, opening the heart, and heart-lung bypass. Similarly two modifications of the CABG procedure may obviate one or more factors:

- No aortic cross-clamping in some thoracotomy approaches.
- Anastomosis to beating heart (no aortic cross-clamp! No arrrest! No heart-lung bypass).

These mini-CABG strategies may not allow for complete revascularization, which has been a

weakness of percutaneous coronary intervention (PCI) (see Chapter 30). Alternatively, the mini-CABG procedure (no-cross clamp or surgery without heart–lung bypass) might be combined with PCI to allow more complete revascularization with the possibility of reduced cerebral morbidity (hybrid) [71–75]. Importantly, the long-term patency of internal mammary surgery done by one of the mini-CABG modifications is not yet known to be comparable to conventional CABG.

CEREBROVASCULAR MORBIDITY AND MORTALITY WITH PCI [131–152]

Stroke can occur as a sequela of coronary angiography or percutaneous coronary intervention [131–139]. Large prospective registry experiences (see Table 26.1) have reported rates with diagnostic catheterization between 1–2 per 1000 cases. Interventional cases are associated with comparable or slightly greater rates, depending on the population subjected to PCI. The same caveats are likely to apply to CABG, namely that none of these studies included systematic post-procedure examination by a neurologist or routine cerebral imaging studies. As such, it is only strokes large enough to be clinically obvious that are detected. The postulated mechanism for neurologic impairment after catheter procedure is distal embolization of atheromatous materia, which is dislodged by the passage of the catheter through an arterial segment with protruding atherosclerotic lesions [140–152]. It is debatable as to whether anticoagulants or antiplatelet agents lower the already low incidence of these catastrophic events.

PERIPHERAL VASCULAR DISEASE (PVD) [153–169]

It is recognized that peripheral vascular disease (PVD) and coronary artery disease (CAD) often co-exist in the same patient [153]. The preva-

Table 26.1 Studies reporting stroke rates for diagnostic catheterization and/or intervention

Study	Reference	Patients undergoing catheterization/ intervention	Reported stroke rate
Harvard 1970–71	Adams et al [131]	46,904	0.23%
Denver 1974	Schoonmaker et al [137]	6800	0.03%
Montreal 1976	Bourassa et al [136]	5250	0.13% transient
CASS 1979	Davis et al [139]	7553	2/7553
SCA 1981	Kennedy et al [135]	53,581	0.07
Beth Israel 1988	Wyman et al [134]	1609/933	0.2%/0.1%
SCA 1996	Krone et al [132]	317,592/74,963	0.1%
Montreal 2001	Chandresekar et al [138]	7953/3868	0.2%

lence of CAD among patients undergoing peripheral vascular surgery has been estimated to be between 37–78%. Coronary artery disease is the leading cause of both early and late mortality after surgery for PVD, regardless of whether the vascular surgery is for peripheral arterial disease, abdominal aortic disease or even extracranial vascular disease.

Conversely, patients with clinically significant PVD and stable angina have increased long-term mortality compared to stable angina patients who do not have PVD. Similarly, PVD is a risk factor for both short-term and long-term mortality among patients undergoing CABG. The STS database has defined PVD for these purposes as 'a history of aneurysm and/or occlusive vascular disease with or without previous extracardiac vascular surgery' [154].

In the first report of 80,881 patients undergoing CABG in the STS registry, CVA was a risk factor for surgical mortality (OR 1.59; $p = 0.0408$) but PVD was not examined [155]. In

the initial report from the VA registry, Grover and colleagues reported that among 1889 patients with PVD undergoing CABG, they observed a perioperative mortality of 7.6% [156]. Conversely, among 6128 patients without PVD who underwent CABG, a statistically significantly ($p = 0.001$) lower mortality of 3.9% was observed [156]. Similar to the early STS reports, Hannan and co-workers from the State of New York, reported CVA as a risk factor for adverse outcome with CABG, but did not report any index of PVD as predictive [157].

In the Cooperative CABG Database listing of important predictive variables, PVD, and cerebrovascular disease were given level 1 status [158]. In addition to the above-cited VA experience, this status had been supported by registry data from the Northern New England group, which also participated in the Cooperative Database [159]. Specifically, in the Northern New England experience, patients with PVD had a CABG associated mortality of 7.7% compared to 3.2% for patients without

PVD, a 2.4-fold difference, very much like the VA report [156, 159].

The usefulness of routine pre-operative cardiac evaluation, including coronary angiography, and even surgical and/or PCI revascularization prior to surgery for PVD is a complex and controversial area. Hertzer and co-workers [161] reported 1000 consecutive patients with PVD who underwent routine pre-PVD surgical evaluation with coronary angiography. They identified CABG candidates among 25% overall and 34% who had clinical angina and 14% of patients who did not appear clinically to need cardiac evaluation. The post-operative mortality for PVD surgery was lower among subjects who underwent preliminary CABG than among those who did not, but these groups were not randomly allocated so selection biases and/or confounding could have accounted for some or all of the difference. Similarly, Eagle and co-workers conducted a retrospective cohort analysis of 1834 patients with combined CAD and PVD, 986 of whom underwent preliminary CABG and 848 of whom did not [167]. In a mean follow-up of 10.4 years they noted significant survival benefits among the CABG group particularly among the subsets with three-vessel CAD and impaired LV systolic function. Again it is helpful to realize that these were not randomly allocated groups and that selection bias and confounding are not simply possible, but likely. The Veterans Affairs Cooperative Studies Program has funded the on-going CARP (Coronary Artery Revascularization in Peripheral disease) study, a nationwide prospective randomized clinical trial designed to test the hypothesis that CAD revascularization prior to PVD surgery will reduce morbidity and mortality. In the meantime, we know that peripheral vascular disease can make both diagnostic and interventional catheter cases more technically challenging. Additionally, PVD may preclude the use of support devices such as intra-aortic balloon counterpulsation for unstable patients undergoing either CABG or PCI.

REFERENCES

1. Roach GW, Kanchugar M, Mangano CM et al for the Multicenter Study of Perioperative Ischemia Research Group and the Ischemia Research and Education Foundation Investigators. Adverse cerebral outcomes after coronary bypass surgery, *N Engl J Med* 1996; **335**:1857–1863.
2. Shaw PJ, Bates D, Carthige NEF et al. Early neurological complications of coronary bypass surgery, *Brit Med J* 1985; **291**:1384–1387.
3. John R, Choudhri AF, Weinberg AD et al. Multicenter review of preoperative risk factors for stroke after coronary artery bypass grafting, *Ann Thorac Surg* 2000; **69**:30–36.
4. Sotanieni KA, Mononen H, Hokkanen TE. Long-term outcome after open-heart surgery, *Stroke* 1986; **17**:410–416.
5. Gardner TJ, Horneffer PJ, Manolio TA et al. Stroke following coronary artery bypass grafting. A ten-year study, *Ann Thorac Surg* 1985; **48**:574–581.
6. Galloway AC, Colvin SB, Grossi EA et al. Ten-year experience with aortic valve replacement in 482 patients 70 years of age or older. Operative risk and long-term results, *Ann Thorac Surg* 1990; **49**:84–93.
7. Loop FD, Lytle BW, Cosgrove DM et al. Coronary artery bypass surgery in the elderly. Indications and outcome, *Cleve Clin J Med* 1988; **55**:23–34.
8. Lyden PD, Hantson L. Assessment scales for the evaluation of stroke patients, *J Stroke Cerebrovasc Dig* 1998; **7**:113–127.
9. Schmidt R, Fazekis F, Offenbacher H et al. Brain magnetic resonance imagery in coronary artery bypass grafts: a pre- and postoperative assessment, *Neurology* 1993; **43**:775–778.
10. Gilman S. Imaging the brain, *N Engl J Med* 1998; **338**:812–820 and 889–896.
11. Davila-Roman V, Barzilai B, Wareing TH, Murphy S, Kouchoukos NT. Intraoperative ultrasonographic evaluation of the ascending aorta in 100 consecutive patients undergoing cardiac surgery, *Circulation* 1991; **84** (suppl II):III47–III53.
12. Barbut D, Caplan LR. Brain complications of cardiac surgery, *Current Problems in Cardiology* 1997; **22** (9):454–480.
13. Frishman WH, Solzol S, Aronson MK et al. Risk

factors for cardiovascular and cerebrovascular diseases and dementia in the elderly, *Curr Probl Cardiol* 1998; **23** (1):1–62.

14. Lyden PD, Hantson L. Assessment scales for the evaluation of stroke patients, *J of Stroke and Cerebrovasc Dig* 1998; **7**:113–127.

15. Frye RL, Kronmal R, Schaff HV, Myers WO, Gerib BJ. Stroke in coronary artery bypass graft surgery: an analysis of the CASS experience. The participants in the Coronary Artery Surgery Study, *Int J Cardiol* 1992; **36**:213–221.

16. Mickleborough LL, Walker PM, Takagi Y et al. Risk factors for stroke in patients undergoing coronary artery bypass grafting, *J Thorac Cardiovasc Surg* 1996; **112**:1250–1258.

17. Mora CT. The central nervous system: response to cardiopulmonary bypass. In: Mora CT, ed, *Cardiopulmonary Bypass: Principles and Techniques of Extracorporeal Circulation* (New York, NY: Springer-Verlag, 1995) 114–146.

18. Breuer AC, Furlan AJ, Hanson MR et al. Central nervous system complications of coronary artery bypass graft surgery: prospective analysis of 421 patients, *Stroke* 1983; **14**:682–687.

19. Furlan AJ, Breuer AC. Central nervous system complications of open heart surgery, *Stroke* 1984; **15**:912–915.

20. Harrison MJ. Neurologic complications of coronary artery bypass grafting: diffuse or focal ischemia? *Ann Thorac Surg* 1995; **59**:1356–1358.

21. Hornick P, Smith PL, Taylor KM. Cerebral complications after coronary bypass grafting, *Curr Opin Cardiol* 1994; **9**:670–679.

22. Lynn GM, Stefanko K, Reed JF III, Gee W, Nicholas G. Risk factors for stroke after coronary artery bypass, *J Thorac Cardiovasc Surg* 1992; **104**:1518–1523.

23. Gardner TJ, Horneffer PJ, Manolio TA et al. Stroke following coronary artery bypass grafting: a ten-year study, *Ann Thorac Surg* 1985; **40**:574–581.

24. Duda AM, Letwin LB, Sutter FP, Goldman SM. Does routine use of aortic ultrasonography decrease the stroke rate in coronary artery bypass surgery: *J Vasc Surg* 1995; **21**:98–107.

25. Kouchoukos NT, Wareing TH, Daily BB, Murphy SF. Management of the severely atherosclerotic aorta during cardiac operations, *J Card Surg* 1994; **9**:490–494.

26. Wareing TH, Davila-Roman VG, Daily BB et al. Strategy for the reduction of stroke incidence in cardiac surgical patients, *Ann Thorac Surg* 1993; **55**:1400–1407.

27. Mangano DT. Cardiovascular morbidity and CABG surgery: a perspective. Epidemiology, costs, and potential therapeutic solutions, *J Card Surg* 1995; **10**:366–368.

28. Kaste M, Fogeihoim R, Rissanen A. Economic burden of stroke and the evaluation of new therapies, *Public Health* 1998; **112**:103–112.

29. Taylor TN. The medical economics of stroke, *Drugs* 1997; **54** (suppl 3):51–57.

30. Jorgensen HS, Nakayama H, Raaschou HO, Olsen TS. Acute stroke care and rehabilitation: an analysis of the direct cost and its clinical and social determinants. The Copenhagen Stroke Study, *Stroke* 1997; **28**:1138–1141.

31. Tuman KJ, McCarthy RJ, Najafi H, Ivankovich AD. Differential effects of advanced age on neurologic and cardiac risks of coronary artery operations, *J Thorac Cardiovasc Surg* 1992; **104**:1510–1517.

32. Gardner TJ, Horeneffer PJ, Manolia TA, Hoff SJ, Pearson TA. Major stroke after coronary artery bypass surgery: changing magnitude of the problem, *J Vasc Surg* 1986; **3**:684–687.

33. Barbut D, Yao FS, Hagger DN et al. Comparison of transcranial Doppler ultrasonography and transesophageal echocardiography to monitor emboli during coronary artery bypass surgery, *Stroke* 1996; **27**:87–90.

34. Barbut D, Yao FSF, Lo YW et al. Determination of size of aortic emboli and embolic load during coronary artery bypass grafting, *Ann Thorac Surg* 1997; **63**:1262–1267.

35. Kouchoukos NT. Atherosclerosis of the ascending aorta prevalence and role as an independent predictor of cerebrovascular events in cardiac patients, *Ann Thorac Surg* 1993; **55**:1400–1408.

36. Blauth CI, Cosgrove DM, Webb BW et al. Atheroembolism from the ascending aorta: an emerging problem in cardiac surgery, *J Thorac Cardiovasc Surg* 1992; **103**:1104–1111.

37. Amarenco P, Duyckaerts C, Tzourio C et al. The prevalence of ulcerated plaques in the aortic arch in patients with stroke, *N Engl J Med* 1992; **326**:221–225.

38. Karalis DO, Chandrasekaran K, Victor MF, Ross JJ Jr, Mintz OS. Recognition and embolic potential of intra-aortic atherosclerotic debris, *J Am Coll Cardiol* 1991; **17**:73–78.

39. Toyoda K, Yasaka M, Nagata S, Yamaguchi

T. Aortogenic embolic stroke: a transesophageal echocardiographic approach, *Stroke* 1992; **23**: 1056–1061.

40. Horowitz DR, Tuhrim S, Budd J, Goldman ME. Aortic plaque in patients with brain ischemia: diagnosis by transesophageal echocardiography, *Neurology* 1992; **42**:1602–1604.

41. Atherosclerotic disease of the aortic arch as a risk factor for recurrent ischemic stroke: the French study of aortic plaques in stroke groups, *N Engl J Med* 1996; **334**:1216–1221.

42. Brennan RW, Patterson RH, Kessler J. Cerebral blood flow and metabolism during cardiopulmonary bypass: evidence of microembolic encephalopathy, *Neurology* 1971; **21**:665–672.

43. Mills NL, Everson CT. Atherosclerosis of the ascending aorta and coronary artery bypass: pathology, clinical correlates, and operative management, *J Thorac Cardiovasc Surg* 1991; **102**:546–553.

44. Tobler HG, Edwards JE. Frequency and location of atherosclerotic plaques in the ascending aorta, *J Thorac Cardiovasc Surg* 1988; **96**:304–306.

45. Ohteki H, Itoh T, Natsuaki M, Minato N, Suda H. Intraoperative ultrasonic imaging of the ascending aorta in ischemic heart disease, *Ann Thorac Surg* 1990; **50**:539–542.

46. Sylivris S, Calafiore P, Matalanis O et al. The intra-operative assessment of ascending aortic atheroma: epiaortic imaging is superior to both transesophageal echocardiography and direct palpation, *J Cardiothorac Vasc Anesth* 1997; **11**: 704–707.

47. Barbut D, La YW, Hartman OS et al. Aortic atheroma is related to outcome but not numbers of emboli during coronary bypass, *Ann Thorac Surg* 1997; **64**:454–459.

48. Katz ES, Tunick PA, Rusinek H et al. Protruding aortic atheromas predict stroke in elderly patients undergoing cardiopulmonary bypass: experience with intraoperative transesophageal echocardiography, *J Am Coll Cardiol* 1992; **20**: 70–77.

49. Marshall WO Jr, Barzilai B, Kouchoukos NT, Saffitz J. Intra-operative ultrasonic imaging of the ascending aorta, *Ann Thorac Surg* 1989; **48**:339–344.

50. Wareing TH, Davila-Roman VO, Barzilai B, Murphy SF, Kouchoukos NT. Management of the severely atherosclerotic ascending aorta during cardiac operations: a strategy for detec-

tion and treatment, *J Thorac Cardiovasc Surg* 1992; **103**:453–462.

51. Akins CW. Non-cardioplegic myocardial preservation for coronary revascularization, *J Thorac Cardiovasc Surg* 1984; **88**:174–181.

52. Culliford AT, Colvin SB, Rohrer K, Baumann FG, Spencer FC. The atherosclerotic ascending aorta and transverse arch: a new technique to prevent cerebral injury during bypass. Experience with 13 patients, *Ann Thorac Surg* 1986; **41**:27–35.

53. Pugsley W, Klinger U, Paschalis B et al. Microemboli and cerebral impairment during cardiac surgery, *Vasc Surg* 1990; **22**:34–43.

54. Stump DA, Rogers AT, Hammon JW, Newman SP. Cerebral emboli and cognitive outcome after cardiac surgery, *J Cardiothorac Vasc Anesth* 1996; **10**:113–118.

55. Stump DA, Rogers AT, Kahn ND et al. When emboli occur during coronary artery bypass graft surgery, *Anesthesiology* 1993; **79** (suppl 3A):A49.

56. Albin MS, Hamlet C, Bunegin L et al. Intracranial air embolism is detected by transcranial Doppler (TCD) during cardiopulmonary bypass procedures, *Anesthesiology* 1990; **73**:A458.

57. Moody DM, Bell MA, Chalia VR, Johnston WE, Prough DS. Brain microemboli during cardiac surgery or aortography, *Ann Neurol* 1990; **28**:477–486.

58. Pugsley W, Kinger U, Paschalis C et al. The impact of microemboli during cardiopulmonary bypass on neuropsychological functioning, *Stroke* 1994; **25**:1393–1399.

59. Padayachee TS, Parsons S, Theobold R et al. The detection of microemboli in the middle cerebral artery during cardiopulmonary bypass: a transcranial Doppler ultrasound investigation using membrane and bubble oxygenators, *Ann Thorac Surg* 1987; **44**:298–302.

60. Blauth CI, Smith PL, Arnold JV et al. Influence of oxygenator type on the prevalence and extent of microembolic retinal ischemia during cardiopulmonary bypass: assessment by digital image analysis, *J Thorac Cardiovasc Surg* 1990; **99**:61–69.

61. Arom KV, Cohen DE, Strobl FT. Effect of intraoperative intervention on neurological outcome based on electroencephalographic monitoring during cardiopulmonary bypass, *Ann Thorac Surg* 1989; **48**:476–483.

62. The Warm Heart Investigators. Randomized Trial of normothermic versus hypothermic coronary bypass surgery, *Lancet* 1994; **343**: 559–563.

63. Buffolo E, de Andrade JCS, Bramco JNR et al. Coronary artery bypass grafting without cardiopulmonary bypass, *Ann Thorac Surg* 1996; **61**:63–66.

64. Barzilot B, Kouchoukos NT. Strategy for the reduction of stroke incidence in cardiac surgical patients, *Ann Thorac Surg* 1993; **55**:1400–1408.

65. Bruggemans EF, Van de Vijver FJR, Huysmans HA. Assessment of cognitive deterioration in individual patients following cardiac surgery: correcting for measurement error and practice effects, *J Clinical Experimental Neuropsychology* 1997; **19**:543–559.

66. Schwartz LB, Bridgman AH, Keiffer RW et al. Asymptomatic carotid artery stenosis and stroke in patients undergoing cardiopulmonary bypass, *J Vas Surg* 1995; **21**:146–153.

67. Gold JP, Charlson ME, Williams-Russo P et al. Improvement of outcomes after coronary artery by-pass: a randomized trial comparing intra-operative high versus low mean arterial pressure, *J Thorac Cardiovasc Surg* 1995; **110**: 1302–1314.

68. Pugsley W, Klinger L, Paschalis C et al. Microemboli and cerebral impairment during cardiac surgery, *Vascular Surgery* 1990; **24**:34–43.

69. Doblar DD. Cerebrovascular assessment of the high risk patient: The role of transcranial Doppler ultrasound, *J Cardiothoracic Vascular Anesthesia* 1996; **10**:3–13.

70. Yao FSF, Barbut D, Hager DN, Trifiletti RR, Gold JP. Detection of aortic emboli by trans-esophageal echocardiography during coronary artery bypass surgery, *J Cardiothoracic Vascular Anesthesia* 1996; **10**:314–317.

71. Mariani MA, Boonstra PW, Grandjean JG, der Heijer P. Combining coronary angioplasty with minimally invasive coronary surgery. The 'hybrid-revascularization', *J Invasive Cardiol* 1998; **10**:233–234.

72. Lytle BW. Surgeons perspective, *J Invasive Cardiol* 1998; **10**:235.

73. King SB III. Interventionist perspective, *J Invasive Cardiol* 1998; **10**:234–236.

74. Friedrich GJ, Bonatti, Dapunt OE. Preliminary experience with minimally invasive coronary artery bypass surgery combined with coronary angioplasty. *N Engl J Med* 1997; **336**:1454–1455.

75. Benetti FJ, Mariani MA, Sani G et al. Video assisted mini-invasive coronary surgery without cardiopulmonary bypass: a multicenter study, *J Thorac Cardiovas Surg* 1996; **112**: 1478–1484.

76. D'Agostino RS, Svensson LO, Neumann DJ et al. Screening carotid ultrasonography and risk factors for stroke in coronary artery surgery patients, *Ann Thorac Surg* 1996; **62**:1714–1723.

77. Faggioli OL, Curl GR, Ricotta JJ. The role of carotid screening before coronary artery bypass, *J Vasc Surg* 1990; **12**:724–729.

78. Fuller JA, Adams GO, Buxton B. Atrial fibrillation after coronary artery bypass grafting: is it disorder of the elderly? *J Thorac Cardiovasc Surg* 1989; **97**:S21–S25.

79. Cox JL. A perspective of post-operative atrial fibrillation in cardiac patients, *Ann Thorac Surg* 1993; **56**:405–409.

80. Rubin DA, Nieminski KE, Reed GD, Herman MV. Predictors, prevention, and long-term prognosis of atrial fibrillation after coronary artery bypass graft operations, *J Thorac Cardiovasc Surg* 1987; **94**:331–335.

81. Frost L, Molgaard IL, Christiansen EH et al. Atrial fibrillation and flutter after coronary artery bypass surgery: epidemiology, risk factors and preventive trials, *Int J Cardiol* 1992; **36**:253–261.

82. Almassi GH, Schowalter T, Nicolosi AC et al. Atrial fibrillation after cardiac surgery: a major morbid event? *Ann Surg* 1997; **226**:501–511.

83. Mathew JP, Parks R, Savino JS et al. Atrial fibrillation following coronary artery bypass graft surgery: predictors, outcomes, and resource utilization: multi-center study of perioperative ischemia research group, *JAIVIA* 1996; **276**: 300–306.

84. Chauhan VS, Woodend KA, Tang AS. Lower incidence of atrial fibrillation after minimally invasive direct coronary artery bypass surgery than bypass surgery, *Circulation* 1997; **96** (suppl 1):1–263.

85. Keren A, Goldberg S, Gottlieb S et al. Natural history of left ventricular thrombi: their appearance and resolution in the posthospitalization period of acute myocardial infarction, *J Am Coll Cardiol* 1990; **15**:790–800.

86. Johannessen KA, Nordrehaug JE, von der Lippe G. Left ventricular thrombi after short-term

high-dose anticoagulants in acute myocardial infarction, *Eur Heart J* 1987; **8**:975–980.

87. Ting W, Silverman N, Levitsky S. Valve replacement in patients with endocarditis and cerebral septic emboli, *Ann Thorac Surg* 1991; **51**:18–21.

88. McKhann GM, Goldsborough MA, Borowicz LM Jr et al. Predictors of stroke risk in coronary artery bypass patients, *Ann Thorac Surg* 1997; **63**:516–521.

89. Berens ES, Kouchoukos NT, Murphy SF, Wareing TH. Preoperative carotid artery screening in elderly patients undergoing cardiac surgery, *J Vasc Surg* 1992; **15**:313–321.

90. Schwartz LB, Bridgman AH, Kieffer RW et al. Asymptomatic carotid artery stenosis and stroke in patients undergoing cardiopulmonary bypass, *J Vasc Surg* 1995; **21**:146–153.

91. Salasidis OC, Later DA, Steinmetz OK, Blair JF, Graham AM. Carotid artery duplex scanning in preoperative assessment for coronary artery revascularization: the association between peripheral vascular disease, carotid artery stenosis, and stroke, *J Vasc Surg* 1995; **21**:154–160.

92. Rizzo RJ, Whittemore AD, Couper OS et al. Combined carotid and coronary revascularization: the preferred approach to the severe vasculopath, *Ann Thorac Surg* 1992; **54**:1099–1109.

93. Brener BJ, Brief DK, Alpert J et al. A four-year experience with preoperative noninvasive carotid evaluation of two thousand twenty-six patients undergoing cardiac surgery, *J Vasc Surg* 1984; **1**:326–338.

94. Akins CW. The case for concomitant carotid and coronary artery surgery [editorial], *Br Heart J* 1995; **74**:97–98.

95. Ennix CL Jr, Lawrie GM, Morris GC Jr et al. Improved results of carotid endarterectomy in patients with symptomatic coronary disease: an analysis of 1546 consecutive carotid operations, *Stroke* 1979; **10**:122–125.

96. Hertzer NR, Lees CD. Fatal myocardial infarction following carotid endarterectomy, *Ann Surg* 1981; **194**:212–218.

97. Hertzer NR, Arison R. Cumulative stroke and survival ten years after carotid endarterectomy, *J Vasc Surg* 1985; **2**:661–668.

98. Endarterectomy for asymptomatic carotid artery stenosis. Executive committee for the asymptomatic carotid atherosclerosis study, *JAMA* 1995; **273**:1421–1428.

99. Endarterectomy for moderate symptomatic carotid stenosis. Interim results from the MRC European carotid surgery trial, *Lancet* 1996; **347**:1591–1593.

100. North American Symptomatic Carotid Endarterectomy Trial. Methods, patient characteristics, and progress, *Stroke* 1991; **22**:711–720.

101. Akins CW, Moncure AC, Daggert VIM et al. Safety and efficacy of concomitant carotid and coronary artery operations, *Ann Thorac Surg* 1995; **60**:311–317.

102. Vermeulen FE, Hamerlijnck RP, Defauw JJ, Ernst SM. Synchronous operation for ischemic cardiac and cerebrovascular disease: early results and long-term follow-up, *Ann Thorac Surg* 1992; **53**:381–389.

103. Wennberg DE, Lucas FL, Birkmeyer JD, Bredenberg CE, Fisher ES. Variation in carotid endarterectomy mortality in the Medicare population: trial hospitals, volume, and patient characteristics, *JAMA* 1998; **279**:1278–1281.

104. Cebul RD, Snow RJ, Pine R, Hertzer NR, Norris DG. Indications, outcomes, and provider volumes for carotid endarterectomy, *JAMA* 1998; **279**:1282–1287.

105. Sauve JS, Thorpe KE, Sackett DL et al. Can bruits distinguish high-grade from moderate symptomatic carotid stenosis? The North American Symptomatic Carotid Endarterectomy Trial, *Ann Intern Med* 1994; **120**:633–637.

106. Coyle KA, Gray BC, Smith RB III et al. Morbidity and mortality associated with carotid endarterectomy: effect of adjunctive coronary revascularization, *Ann Vasc Surg* 1995; **9**:21–27.

107. Prati P, Vanuzzo D, Casaroli M et al. Prevalence and determinants of carotid atherosclerosis in a general population, *Stroke* 1992; **23**:1705–1711.

108. Fabris F, Zanocchi M, Bo M et al. Carotid plaque, aging, and risk factors: a study of 457 subjects, *Stroke* 1994; **25**:1133–1140.

109. Hertzer NR, Loop FD, Beven EG, O'Hara PJ, Krajewski LP. Surgical staging for simultaneous coronary and carotid disease: a study including prospective randomization, *J Vasc Surg* 1989; **9**:455–463.

110. North American Symptomatic Carotid Endarterectomy Trial Collaborators. Beneficial effect of carotid endarterectomy in symptomatic patients with high-grade carotid stenosis, *N Engl J Med* 1991; **325**:445–453.

111. European Carotid Surgery Trialists'

Collaborative Group. MRC European Carotid Surgery Trial: interim results for symptomatic patients with severe (70–99%) or with mild (0–29%) carotid stenosis, *Lancet* 1991; **337**: 1235–1243.

112. Mayberg MR, Wilson SE, Yatsu F et al. Carotid endarterectomy and prevention of cerebral ischemia in symptomatic carotid stenosis. Veterans Affairs Cooperative Studies Program 309 Trialist Group, *JAMA* 1991; **266**:3289–3294.

113. Moore WS, Barnett HJ, Beebe HG et al. Guidelines for carotid endarterectomy: a multidisciplinary consensus statement from the ad hoc committee. American Heart Association, *Stroke* 1995; **26**:188–201.

114. Moore WS, Vescera CL, Robertson JT et al. Selection process for surgeons in the asymptomatic carotid atherosclerosis study, *Stroke* 1991; **22**:1353–1357.

115. Barnett HJ, Eliasziw M, Meldrum HE, Taylor DW. Do the facts and figures warrant a 10-fold increase in the performance of carotid endarterectomy on asymptomatic patients? *Neurology* 1996; **46**:603–608.

116. Hertzer NR. A personal view; the asymptomatic carotid atherosclerosis study results; read the label carefully, *J Vasc Surg* 1996; **23**: 167–171.

117. Murkin JM, Martzke JS, Buchan AM et al. Cognitive and neurological function after coronary artery surgery: a prospective study, *Anesth Analg* 1992; **74**:5215.

118. Smith PU. The cerebral complications of coronary artery bypass surgery, *Ann R Coll Surg Engl* 1988; **70**:212–216.

119. Hammeke TA, Hastings JE. Neuropsychologic alterations after cardiac operation. *J Thorac Cardiovasc Surg* 1988; **96**:326–331.

120. Raymond M, Conklin C, Schaeffer J et al. Coping with transient intellectual dysfunction after coronary bypass surgery, *Heart Lung* 1984; **13**:531–539.

121. Smith PL, Treasure T, Newman SP et al. Cerebral consequences of cardiopulmonary bypass, *Lancet* 1986; **1**:823–825.

122. Edmonds HL Jr, Griffiths UK, van der Laken J, Slater AD, Shields CB. Quantitative electroencephalographic monitoring during myocardial revascularization predicts postoperative disorientation and improves outcome, *J Thorac Cardiovasc Surg* 1992; **103**:555–563.

123. Murkin JM, Martzke JS, Buchan AM, Bentley C, Wong CJ. A randomized study of the influence of perfusion technique and pH management strategy in 316 patients undergoing coronary artery bypass surgery. II: neurologic and cognitive outcomes, *J Thorac Cardiovasc Surg* 1995; **110**:349–362.

124. Engelman RM, Pleer AB, Rousou JA et al. Does cardiopulmonary bypass temperature correlate with postoperative central nervous system dysfunction? *J Card Surg* 1995; **10**:493–497.

125. Nathan HJ, Munson J, Wells G et al. The management of temperature during cardiopulmonary bypass: effect on neuropsychological outcome, *J Card Surg* 1995; **10**:481–487.

126. Chrisrakis GT, Abel JG, Uichtensrein SV. Neurological outcomes and cardiopulmonary temperature: a clinical review, *J Card Surg* 1995; **10**:475–480.

127. Guyton RA, Mellirt RJ, Weintraub WS. A critical assessment of neurological risk during warm heart surgery, *J Card Surg* 1995; **10**: 488–492.

128. Harris DN, Bailey SM, Smith PU et al. Brain swelling in first hour after coronary artery bypass surgery, *Lancet* 1993; **342**:586–587.

129. Badner NH, Murkin JM, Lok P. Differences in pH management and pulsatile/non-pulsatile perfusion during cardiopulmonary bypass do not influence renal function, *Anesth Analg* 1992; **75**:696–701.

130. Henze T, Stephan H, Sonntag H. Cerebral dysfunction following extracorporeal circulation for aortocoronary bypass surgery: no differences in neuropsychological outcome after pulsatile versus nonpulsatile flow, *Thorac Cardiovasc Surg* 1990; **38**:65–68.

131. Adams DF, Fraser DB, Abrams HL. The complications of coronary arteriography, *Circulation* 1973; **48**:609–618.

132. Krone RJ, Johnson L, Noto T and the Registry Committee of the Society for Cardiac Angiography and Interventions. Five year trends in cardiac catheterization: a report from the registry of the society for cardiac angiography and interventions, *Cath and Cardiovasc Diagnosis*, 1996; **39**:31–35.

133. Vranckx P, Ysewijn T, Heidbuchel H, Herregods MC, Desmet W. Acute posterior cerebral circulation syndrome accompanied by serious cardiac rhythm disturbances: a rare but

reversible complication following bypass graft angiography, *Cath and CV Interventions* 1999; **48**:397–401.

134. Wyman M, Safian RD, Portway V et al. Current complications of diagnostic and therapeutic cardiac catheterization, *J Am Coll Cardiol* 1988; **12**:1400–1406.

135. Kennedy JW and the registry committee of the Society for Cardiac Angiography. Complications associated with cardiac catheterization and angiography, *Cath Cardiovasc Diagnosis* 1982; **8**: 5–11.

136. Bourassa MG, Noble J. Complication rates of coronary arteriography, *Circulation* 1976; **53**: 106–114.

137. Schoonmaker FW, King SB III. Coronary arteriography by the single catheter percutaneous femoral technique. Experience in 6800 cases, *Circulation* 1974; **50**:735–740.

138. Chandresekar B, Doucet S, Bilodeau L et al. Complications of cardiac catheterization in the current era: a single center experience, *Cath Cardiovasc Interventions* 2001; **52**:289–295.

139. Davis K, Kennedy JW, Kemp HG et al. Complications of coronary arteriography from the collaborative study of Coronary Artery Surgery (CASS), *Circulation* 1979; **59**: 1105–1112.

140. Kronzon I, Tunick PA. Atheromatous disease of the thoracic aorta: pathologic and clinical implications, *Ann Intern Med* 1997; **126**:629–637.

141. Bower TC, Cherry KJ, Pairolero PC. Unusual manifestations of abdominal aortic aneurysms, *Surg Clin N America* 1989; **69**:745–754.

142. Keen RR, McCarthy WJ, Shireman PK et al. Surgical management of athereoembolization, *J Vasc Surg* 1995; **21**:773–781.

143. Khatibzadeh M, Mitusch R, Stierle U, Gromoll B, Sheikhzadeh A. Aortic atherosclerotic plaques as a source of systemic embolism, *J Am Coll Cardiol* 1996; **27**:664–669.

144. Drost H, Buis B, Haan D, Hillers J. Cholesterol embolism as a complication of left heart catheterization, *Br Heart J* 1984; **52**:339–342.

145. Ricci MA, Trevisani GT, Pilcher DB. Vascular complications of cardiac catheterization, *Am J Surg* 1994; **167**:375–378.

146. Eggebrecht H, Oldenburg O, Dirsch O et al. Potential embolization by atherosclerotic debris dislodged from aortic wall during cardiac catheterization. Histologic and clinical findings in 7621 patients, *Cath Cardiovasc Interventions* 2000; **49**:389–394.

147. Kronzon I, Tunick PA. Atheromatous disease of the thoracic aorta. Pathologic and clinical implications, *Ann Int Med* 1997; **126**:629–637.

148. Keen RR, McCarthy WJ, Shireman PK et al. Surgical management of atheroembolization, *J Vasc Surg* 1995; **21**:773–781.

149. Rosman HS, Davis TP, Reddy D, Goldstein S. Cholesterol embolization: clinical findings and implications, *J Am Coll Cardiol* 1990; **15**: 1296–1299.

150. Ramirez G, O'Neill WM Jr, Lambert R, Bloomer A. Cholesterol embolization a complication of angiography, *Arch Intern Med* 1978; **138**: 1430–1432.

151. Colt HG, Begg RJ, Saporito JJ, Cooper WM, Shapiro AP. Cholesterol emboli after cardiac catheterization, *Medicine* 1988; **67**:389–400.

152. Gaines PA, Kennedy A, Moorhead P et al. Cholesterol embolism: a lethal complication of vascular catheterization, *Lancet* 1988; **1**: 168–170.

153. Eagle KA, Guyton RA, Davidoff R et al for the Committee to Revise the 1991 Guidelines for Coronary Artery Bypass Graft Surgery. ACC/AHA Guidelines for Coronary Artery Bypass Graft Surgery, *J Am Coll Cardiol* 1999; **34**:1263–1347.

154. Clark RE for the Committee to Develop a National Database for Thoracic Surgeons. Definitions of Terms of the Society of Thoracic Surgeons National Cardiac Surgery Database, *Ann Thorac Surg* 1994; **58**:271–273.

155. Edwards FH, Clark RE, Schwartz M. Coronary Artery Bypass Grafting. The Society of Thoracic Surgeons National Database Experience, *Ann Thorac Surg* 1994; **57**:12–19.

156. Grover FL, Hammermeister KE, Burchfeil C and the cardiac surgeons of the Department of Veterans Affairs. Initial Report of the Veterans Administration preoperative risk assessment study for cardiac surgery, *Ann Thorac Surg* 1990; **50**:12–28.

157. Hannan EL, Kilburn H, O'Donnell JF, Lukacik G, Shields EP. Adult open heart surgery in New York State, *JAMA* 1990; **264**:2768–2774.

158. Jones RH, Hannan EL, Hammermeister KE et al for the Cooperative CABG Database Project. Identification of preoperative variables needed for risk adjustment of short-term mortality after

coronary artery bypass graft surgery, *J Am Coll Cardiol* 1996; **28**:1478–1487.

159. Birkmeyer JD, Quinton HB, O'Connor NJ et al. The effect of peripheral vascular disease on long-term mortality after coronary artery bypass surgery. Northern New England Cardiovascular Disease Study Group, *Arch Surg* 1996; **131**:316–321.

160. Gersh BJ, Rihal CS, Rooke TW, Ballard DJ. Evaluation and management of patients with both peripheral vascular and coronary artery disease, *J Am Coll Cardiol* 1991; **18**:203–214.

161. Hertzer NR, Beven EG, Young JR et al. Coronary artery disease in peripheral vascular patients: a classification of 1000 coronary angiograms and results of surgical management, *Ann Surg* 1984; **199**:223–233.

162. Brown OW, Hollier LH, Pairolero PC, Kazmier FJ, McCready RA. Abdominal aortic aneurysm and coronary artery disease, *Arch Surg* 1981; **116**:1484–1488.

163. Jamieson WR, Janusz MT, Miyagishima RT, Gerein AN. Influence of ischemic heart disease on early and late mortality after surgery for peripheral occlusive vascular disease, *Circulation* 1982; **66** (suppl 1):92–97.

164. DeBakey ME, Crawford ES, Cooley DA et al. Cerebral arterial insufficiency: one to 11-year results following arterial reconstructive operation, *Ann Surg* 1965; **161**:921–945.

165. Crawford ES, Bomberger RA, Glaeser DH, Saleh SA, Russell WL. Aorto-iliac occlusive disease; factors influencing survival and function following reconstructive operation over a twenty-five-year period, *Surgery* 1981; **90**: 1055–1067.

166. Burnham SJ, Johnson GJ, Gurri JA. Mortality risks for survivors of vascular reconstructive procedures, *Surgery* 1982; **92**:1072–1076.

167. Eagle KA, Rihal CS, Foster ED, Mickel MC, Gersh BJ. Long-term survival in patients with coronary artery disease: importance of peripheral vascular disease: the Coronary Artery Surgery Study (CASS) Investigators, *J Am Coll Cardiol* 1994; **23**:1091–1095.

168. Lindsay J. Diagnosis and treatment of diseases of the aorta, *Current Problems in Cardiology* 1997; **22**:487–542.

169. Bajawa TK, Shalev YA, Gupta A, Khalid MA, Moussavi N. Peripheral vascular disease, *Current Problems in Cardiology* 1998; **23**:248–297.

27

Liver disease

Edmund J Bini and Chris E Lascarides

CONTENTS • Introduction • Epidemiology of liver disease and coronary artery disease in the US • Liver architecture and function • Preoperative evaluation of patients with liver disease • Estimating surgical risk • Cardiac revascularization in patients with liver disease • Preoperative management issues • Intraoperative care and cautions • Postoperative care and complications • Conclusions

INTRODUCTION

The preoperative evaluation of patients by the medical consultant has traditionally encompassed a thorough cardiovascular evaluation that was performed in order to minimize the morbidity and mortality of patients prior to surgery. Subsequently, this evaluation has been expanded to include the evaluation and management of disorders involving other organ systems, such as the hepatic, renal, and pulmonary systems.

The spectrum of patients with liver disease varies from asymptomatic individuals with abnormal liver chemistries to those with end-stage liver disease. Patients along this spectrum have different risk and management issues. Therefore, a thorough preoperative assessment is mandatory in patients with liver disease in order to minimize surgical morbidity and mortality. Patients with liver disease are at increased risk for surgery- and anesthesia-related complications compared to those with a healthy liver. In this chapter, we will provide an evidence-based approach to screening patients for liver disease, estimating the surgical risk in various subsets of individuals with hepatic dysfunction, and preoperative manage-

ment issues in these patients. Subsequently, we will discuss the intraoperative and post-operative management of patients with liver disease. This discussion will focus on patients with coronary artery disease and liver disease who need cardiac revascularization, including coronary artery bypass grafting (CABG) and percutaneous coronary interventions (PCI).

EPIDEMIOLOGY OF LIVER DISEASE AND CORONARY ARTERY DISEASE IN THE US

Liver disease is the tenth leading cause of death in the US and accounts for 25,000 deaths per year [1]. Recent data from the Centers for Disease Control and Prevention estimate that there are 23,229 cases of hepatitis A and 10,258 cases of hepatitis B reported annually [2]. The overall prevalence of hepatitis C antibody positivity in the US is 1.8%, corresponding to approximately 3.9 million persons nationwide; an estimated 2.7 million of these individuals are chronically infected with hepatitis C [3]. Population-based studies have shown that 40% of chronic liver disease is hepatitis C-related, resulting in 8000–10,000 deaths per year [1]. Medical and work-related costs of care for patients with hepatitis C are more than $600 million annually, and end-stage liver disease from hepatitis C is the most common indication for liver transplantation [1]. It is anticipated that the number of deaths related to hepatitis C-associated liver disease will increase substantially in the next 10–20 years [1, 4, 5].

In 1995, alcohol-related liver disease was associated with 101,200 hospitalizations, 13,400 deaths, and $1.8 billion in healthcare costs [6]. The number of alcohol-induced deaths was even higher (19,515 persons) in 1998 [7]. Although alcohol and viral hepatitis are the most common causes of liver disease in the US [6], other etiologies should be also considered in the differential diagnosis of acute and chronic liver disease (Table 27.1).

Cardiac disease affects 78.2 out of every 1000 persons in the US; this rate is even higher (310.7 per 1000 persons) in persons over 75 years of age [8]. An estimated 12 million persons have coronary artery disease in the US [9]. During 2001, approximately 1.1 million persons had a coronary heart disease event [9]. Coronary artery disease is the leading cause of death in the US [7]. In 1998, there were 724,859 deaths from cardiac disease and the mortality rate was 268.2 per 100,000 persons [7].

Despite the high prevalence of liver disease and coronary artery disease in the US, there are no population-based data available on the prevalence of co-existing hepatic and cardiac disease. The prevalence of coronary artery disease in asymptomatic patients with abnormal liver chemistries, acute hepatitis, or non-cirrhotic chronic liver disease has not been studied. In contrast, several small studies have investigated the prevalence of coronary artery disease in cirrhotic patients who were referred for liver transplantation [10,11]. Carey et al per-

Table 27.1 Etiology of liver disease in the US

Acute liver disease	Chronic liver disease
Alcohol-induced liver disease	Alcohol-induced liver disease
Hepatitis A, B, C, D, E	Hepatitis B, C, D
Drugs and toxins	Autoimmune hepatitis
Autoimmune hepatitis	Budd–Chiari syndrome
Budd–Chiari syndrome	Nonalcoholic steatohepatitis
Ischemic hepatitis	Primary biliary cirrhosis
Wilson's disease	Primary sclerosing cholangitis
Acute fatty liver of pregnancy	Hemochromatosis
Reye's syndrome	Alpha-1-antitrypsin deficiency
Postoperative jaundice	Cryptogenic
Cryptogenic	

formed coronary angiography on 37 patients over 50 years of age who were referred for liver transplantation and diagnosed severe coronary artery disease in 16% of patients; diabetes was significantly associated with the presence of severe coronary artery disease [10]. In this study, two patients developed renal insufficiency after angiography and three patients were denied liver transplantation because of severe coronary artery disease.

LIVER ARCHITECTURE AND FUNCTION

Because of the multiple functions of the liver, assessing the risk of patients with hepatic dysfunction prior to cardiac revascularization is a complicated endeavor. Before addressing the evaluation of patients with liver dysfunction, we will briefly review the anatomy and physiology of the liver.

The liver is composed of hexagonal lobules consisting of the portal triads centered about the hepatic venule (central vein). The components of the portal triad include an arteriole, a venule, and a bile ductule [12]. Plates of the hepatocytes radiate out from the triads to the central vein and are divided into three zones. Zone 1 encompasses the hepatocytes which are closest to the portal triad, while zone 3 contains hepatocytes closest to the central vein; zone 2 includes the remaining hepatocytes between zones 1 and 3 [12, 13]. Zone 1 hepatocytes are closest to the nutritional supply of the portal venule and hepatic arteriole and are, therefore, the most resistant to necrosis from hypoxia [14, 15]. The cells within this zone are also those that regenerate earliest. Conversely, zone 3 is most distal to the blood supply and is most susceptible to injury from hypoxia and hepatotoxins [13–16].

The liver is a unique organ in that it receives nourishment from a dual blood supply. The majority of the blood flow to the liver (66–75%) is from the oxygen poor, but nutrient rich, portal vein which drains directly from the alimentary tract [12, 17]. The remaining 25–33% of blood flow to the liver is from the oxygen rich, yet nutrient poor, hepatic artery [12, 17]. The hepatic portal flow feeding the liver is under alpha-adrenergic control and is sensitive to systemic catecholamines. Upon stimulation, the liver can deliver up to 500 ml of blood into the systemic circulation and, therefore, acts as a blood reservoir in humans [16]. Patients with liver disease have a decreased sensitivity to catecholamines, which may result in a blunted response to hypovolemia. Therefore, these patients are at increased risk of hepatic necrosis.

The functions of the liver are multiple and can be classified into the following general categories: synthetic functions, metabolic functions, excretion, storage, and immunologic functions [16]. The synthetic functions of the liver include the synthesis of plasma proteins, glucose, and cholesterol. The synthesis of the coagulation factors is perhaps the most relevant to this discussion. The liver plays an important role in the metabolism and detoxification of drugs, toxins, and endogenous waste compounds. It serves as the site where amino acids are deaminated forming urea, which is subsequently excreted in the urine, and is responsible for the excretion of bilirubin and other compounds. The liver stores nutrients, bile salts, iron, and vitamins, and helps to maintain glucose levels by storing glycogen and releasing glucose. The liver also houses a population of Kupffer cells, which act to phagocytose bacteria and other foreign matter taken up by the gastrointestinal tract and, therefore, plays an important role in the human immune response.

PREOPERATIVE EVALUATION OF PATIENTS WITH LIVER DISEASE

To illustrate the scope of this problem, consider that approximately one in 700 patients admitted for elective surgery were found to have abnormal liver function tests during routine preoperative testing [18,19]. A large number of these patients had asymptomatic viral hepatitis, most likely due to chronic hepatitis C. However, advanced liver disease must be excluded prior to surgery. On the other end of the spectrum, 10% of patients with end-stage liver disease may require surgery within the last two years of their life [20].

Patients with liver disease are at increased risk for complications during and after cardiac revascularization. The evaluation of individuals with liver disease is an inexact science, but is necessary in order to estimate the surgical risk in patients found to have liver disease, and to help manage these patients prior to, during, and after cardiac revascularization [16, 21–26]. A detailed medical history, physical examination, and laboratory testing are necessary in order to screen patients for liver disease prior to surgery.

Obtaining a detailed medical history

Screening patients for liver disease begins with a thorough medical history and a detailed physical examination [27, 28]. The medical history is the best tool to screen for the presence of liver disease in the general population prior to cardiac revascularization. The aspects of the history that are important to ascertain during this evaluation are shown in Table 27.2.

Patients should be asked about symptoms of acute hepatitis, including right upper quadrant abdominal pain, nausea, vomiting, diarrhea, fatigue, myalgias, pruritus, and jaundice. A detailed history of prior hepatitis must also be obtained.

Perhaps some of the most important information acquired during the interview is elicited during the social history. It is important to determine whether the patient has ever used intravenous drugs of abuse, such as heroin or cocaine. Specifically, it is important to ask whether the patient has used intravenous drugs even one time, as hepatitis C is a highly contagious infectious agent acquired through parenteral exposure [29, 30]. It is also necessary to quantify the amount of alcohol consumed by patients. The CAGE questionnaire or the Alcohol Use Disorders Identification Test (AUDIT) can be used to screen patients for alcohol abuse [31]. A detailed sexual history should also be obtained because of the risk of sexual transmission of viral hepatitis. The patient should also be questioned about the presence of any tattoos, because these are also a parenteral risk factor for transmission of hepatitis C [29, 30].

Patients should be questioned about prior blood transfusions (especially before 1992) and the dates when these transfusions occurred. A detailed family history concentrating on the presence of inherited liver disorders, such as hemochromatosis and alpha-1-antitrypsin deficiency, should be pursued. If the patient had prior surgery, they should be questioned about the type of anesthesia that they received and if they had any surgery- or anesthesia-related complications.

A detailed medication history should be obtained, including the names of the medications taken, dosages, and frequency. It is important to ask about the use of over-the-counter medications and herbal medications. Many over-the-counter medications contain acetaminophen, which is a hepatotoxin [32–35]. Herbal medications also may contain other hepatotoxins, which can cause a spectrum of abnormalities from asymptomatic liver enzyme elevations to acute hepatitis and fulminant hepatic failure [32, 36–40].

Physical examination

The physical examination should focus on the presence of stigmata of liver disease [27, 28]. The pertinent physical findings are shown in Table 27.2. The abdomen should be examined closely, looking for hepatomegaly, splenomegaly, ascites, and caput medusae [27]. The thorax should be inspected for spider angiomata and gynecomastia. The extremities can suggest the presence of liver disease if palmar erythema or Dupuytren's contractures are

Table 27.2 Preoperative evaluation of patients with liver disease

History	Physical examination	Laboratory testing
Intravenous drug use	Jaundice	Liver chemistries
Blood transfusions	Scleral icterus	Coagulation profile
Alcohol use	Hepatomegaly	Complete blood count
Unprotected sexual contacts	Splenomegaly	Electrolyte panel
Tattoos and body piercing	Ascites	Ammonia level
Needlestick exposure	Caput medusae	Arterial blood gas
Exposure to hepatotoxins	Abdominal collateral veins	
Medication use	Spider angiomata	
Herbal medication use	Gynecomastia	
History of jaundice or hepatitis	Palmar erythema	
Family history of liver disease	Dupuytren's contracture	
Abdominal pain	Parotid gland enlargement	
Nausea or vomiting	Testicular atrophy	
Diarrhea	Asterixis	
Fatigue	Change in mental status	
Myalgias		
Jaundice		
Pruritus		

present. Inspection and palpation of the face should be performed to exclude parotid gland enlargement. The testes in men must be evaluated for the presence of testicular atrophy. Hepatic encephalopathy should be excluded by performing a thorough mental status examination and looking for the presence of asterixis. The skin and eyes should be examined for the presence of jaundice and scleral icterus.

Laboratory testing

The use of routine blood testing to detect abnormal liver chemistries in asymptomatic patients is controversial [25, 41]. However, abnormalities are often found when laboratory testing is done for other purposes [18, 41]. Many physicians send coagulation studies and complete blood counts on their patients prior to cardiac revascularization. This is generally performed in order to determine whether the patient is at increased risk for intraoperative bleeding. A decreased platelet count may be a marker for the presence of portal hypertension and hypersplenism, while an increased prothrombin time may suggest impaired hepatic synthetic function [42].

If one chooses to send liver chemistries on asymptomatic patients, these should include aspartate aminotransferase (AST), alanine aminotransferase (ALT), alkaline phosphatase, total and direct bilirubin, and albumin [42, 43]. Additional testing may also include a coagulation profile, complete blood count, and serum electrolytes (Table 27.2). The coagulation profile may provide information regarding the risk of bleeding, the need for factor replacement, and can help to determine the degree of liver insufficiency [44]. The complete blood count will provide a baseline hemoglobin value as well as platelet count [41]. Serum electrolytes will help screen for renal insufficiency and for other electrolyte abnormalities [41]. Other tests that may be useful, but are not ordered routinely, include an ammonia level and arterial blood gas.

Other preoperative testing

Other modalities of investigation, which may be helpful in patients with known or suspected liver disease, include abdominal ultrasound and computed tomography of the abdomen [42]. These studies can help diagnose the presence of cirrhosis, ascites, and gastric or esophageal varices [42]. Percutaneous liver biopsy may be performed for tissue diagnosis or to stage the degree of liver fibrosis and determine the presence of cirrhosis [42]. An upper endoscopy can also provide information regarding the presence of gastric or esophageal varices, as well as portal hypertensive gastropathy; these lesions may bleed and increase perioperative morbidity and mortality in patients with liver disease [45–48]. Other studies that may help predict the degree of hepatic dysfunc-

tion and the risk of surgery in patients with known liver disease include galactose elimination capacity testing [49], aminopyrine breath testing [50], indocyanine green clearance testing [51], technetium-99m galactosyl human serum albumin liver scintigraphy [52–54], and the rate of metabolism of lidocaine to monoethylglycinexylidide (MEGX) [55]. These studies are not routinely used in clinical practice.

ESTIMATING SURGICAL RISK

Estimating surgical risk is a challenging science. To date, the majority of available data on the risk of surgery in patients with liver disease are from retrospective studies and case series of cirrhotic patients; these findings do not pertain to the vast majority of patients with liver disease. The available information, however, strongly suggests that the risk of morbidity and mortality is dependent upon the etiology and severity of the underlying liver disease, the extent of hepatic dysfunction, and the type of surgery being performed. Patients with liver disease can be divided into three general categories: asymptomatic patients with abnormal liver chemistries, acute liver disease, and chronic liver disease [26].

Asymptomatic patients with abnormal liver chemistries

Asymptomatic patients make up the majority of those evaluated and discovered to have abnormal liver chemistries prior to surgery [26]. These abnormalities are detected by routine preoperative laboratory testing [18, 19]. These individuals have no known underlying chronic liver disease and are most likely a subset of patients with undiagnosed chronic liver disease, such as chronic viral hepatitis, fatty liver, or undisclosed alcohol use.

The risk of perioperative morbidity and mortality in this subset of patients is generally thought to be minimal [21, 25, 26]. Elective surgical procedures should be postponed until further investigation of the liver function abnormalities can be performed [26]. Although the majority of these patients will have chronic viral hepatitis, it is possible that these patients could have acute liver disease or cirrhosis. For these reasons, the etiology and severity of hepatic dysfunction should be evaluated thoroughly prior to surgery. If the procedure is an emergency or is life threatening, surgery should be performed with extreme caution [26]. These patients should be monitored closely during surgery and in the postoperative period.

Patients with acute liver disease

This category of patients includes those with non-alcoholic acute hepatitis, alcoholic hepatitis, and fulminant hepatic failure. These three subsets of patients with acute liver disease have increasing degrees of hepatic dysfunction and increasing risks for morbidity and mortality; the risk is lowest in patients with non-alcoholic acute hepatitis and highest in those with fulminant hepatic failure.

Harville and Summerskill reported a 10% mortality rate in patients with acute viral hepatitis undergoing laparotomy and described major postoperative complications in an additional 11% of patients [56]. As with asymptomatic patients, elective surgical procedures should be postponed until patients fully recover from acute hepatitis. Emergency procedures may be performed with close monitoring and with extreme caution.

Patients with alcoholic hepatitis are at greater risk for perioperative morbidity and mortality than those with viral hepatitis. Mortality rates in this subset of patients are as high as 55–100% for open liver biopsy, exploratory laparotomy, or portosystemic shunt surgery (57–61). Greenwood et al examined patients who had a diagnosis of alcoholic hepatitis made by either open or closed biopsy and noted a five-fold increase in mortality for patients that had the diagnosis made by open

biopsy [57]. Powell-Jackson et al reported a 100% mortality rate in patients with acute alcoholic hepatitis who underwent exploratory laparotomy for extrahepatic biliary tract obstruction or intraabdominal malignancy [58]. Patients with alcoholic hepatitis should abstain from alcohol and elective procedures should be postponed at least 12 weeks or until resolution of hepatitis; repeat liver biopsy may be necessary if the possibility of persistent liver injury exists [21]. Similar to patients with acute non-alcoholic hepatitis, emergency surgical procedures should be performed cautiously and with close perioperative monitoring.

Patients with fulminant hepatic failure are very ill and are unable to withstand the stress of surgery [62, 63]. Due to the extremely small chance that these patients will survive surgery, elective and emergency procedures are contraindicated; non-surgical alternatives must be considered. Liver transplantation is the only surgical procedure that should be attempted in this subset of patients. If the patient is a candidate for liver transplantation, they should have a thorough preoperative evaluation and immediately referred to an experienced liver transplantation center [64–66].

Patients with chronic liver disease

Non-cirrhotic patients
Patients with chronic liver disease that have not developed cirrhosis are generally well compensated. They have minimal hepatic dysfunction and intact synthetic function. The majority of patients in this group have liver disease secondary to chronic viral hepatitis or alcohol; other etiologies include non-alcoholic steatohepatitis, drug-induced liver disease, primary biliary cirrhosis, primary sclerosing cholangitis, autoimmune hepatitis, hemochromatosis, and Wilson's disease. Despite the large number of patients that fall into this category, there is a surprisingly small amount of data available on the risk of surgery in these individuals.

In a retrospective study, Runyon examined

20 patients with mild to moderate asymptomatic chronic hepatitis that underwent 34 surgical procedures [67]. Two patients had elevated preoperative bilirubin levels that increased further in the postoperative period. There was no anesthesia-related liver failure, operative mortality, or major complications in any of the patients evaluated [67]. In contrast, other investigators have noted a higher morbidity and mortality in patients with chronic liver disease [68, 69]. Higashi et al reported a postoperative complication rate of 39% and mortality rate of 12% in patients with chronic viral hepatitis who underwent surgery [69]. However, these patients underwent surgery for resection of hepatocellular carcinoma and many may have had cirrhosis as well. In general, non-cirrhotic patients with well-compensated chronic liver disease tolerate surgery well. Elective or emergency surgery can be performed relatively safely after optimization of their medical condition.

Cirrhotic patients

The published literature on surgery-associated morbidity and mortality in cirrhotic patients is more extensive than for other types of liver diseases. However, these studies are predominately retrospective and have included small numbers of patients. Nonetheless, it is clear that patients with documented cirrhosis tend to have a greater risk for surgery-related morbidity and mortality than those with non-cirrhotic chronic liver disease [16, 21, 22, 25, 26]. The risk for surgery-associated morbidity or mortality is highest in those undergoing emergency surgical procedures, cardiac surgery, abdominal operations, and hepatic resection [25].

The increased risk of morbidity and mortality in cirrhotics has been shown to correlate well with the Child–Turcotte [70] or Child–Pugh classification systems [71]. In clinical practice, the Child–Pugh classification is used more often than the Child–Turcotte classification. The Child–Pugh classification system stratifies patients into class A, B, or C based on the severity of ascites, grade of hepatic encephalopathy, serum bilirubin, serum albumin, and prothrombin time [71]. This classification system is shown in Table 27.3.

In a study of 100 cirrhotic patients who underwent abdominal surgery, Garrison et al

Table 27.3 Child–Pugh classification			
	Points assigned		
	1	**2**	**3**
Ascites	Absent	Slight	Moderate
Encephalopathy	None	Grade 1–2	Grade 3–4
Bilirubin, mg/dL	< 2	2–3	> 3
Albumin, g/dL	> 3.5	2.8–3.5	< 2.8
Prothrombin time (seconds over control)	1–3	4–6	> 6

Class A, 5–6 points (well-compensated disease); B, 7–9 points (significant functional compromise); and C, 10–15 points (decompensated liver disease).

showed a strong association between Child–Pugh class and survival [72]. In this retrospective study, the mortality rates were 10% for Child–Pugh class A, 31% for B, and 76% for C. In another retrospective study of 92 cirrhotic patients who underwent abdominal surgery, Mansour et al reported similar mortality rates of 10% for Child–Pugh class A patients, 30% for class B, and 82% for class C [73]. Other studies have shown high morbidity and mortality rates in cirrhotic patients undergoing open cholecystectomy [74–76], biliary tract surgery [77–79], and other abdominal surgery [80–87]. Less invasive surgical procedures, such as laparoscopic cholecystectomy, have been associated with better outcomes in patients with cirrhosis [88–94].

Child–Pugh class A cirrhotics are generally well compensated and can be treated like patients with chronic liver disease without cirrhosis [26]. In these patients, it is safe to proceed with surgery. If necessary, surgery can be performed in Child–Pugh class B cirrhotics, but one should proceed with extreme caution [26]. Elective surgeries should be avoided in class C cirrhotics because they have decompensated liver disease and are at very high risk for morbidity and mortality [72, 73, 95]. The physician should consider alternatives to surgery in Child–Pugh class C cirrhotics, and liver transplantation should be strongly considered in this subgroup of high-risk patients [96–98].

The Acute Physiology, Age, and Chronic Health Evaluation (APACHE III) prognostic score can be used to predict survival of cirrhotic patients admitted to an intensive care unit [99]. Although the APACHE III prognostic system can accurately risk stratify critically ill patients with cirrhosis, it has not been tested as a predictor of surgical morbidity and mortality. Other models to predict mortality in patients with cirrhosis have also been developed [100, 101]. More recently, the Model for End-Stage Liver Disease (MELD) was developed by Kamath and colleagues from the Mayo Clinic [102]. The MELD score was a reliable measure of mortality risk in patients with end-stage liver disease.

The ability of these scoring systems to predict morbidity and mortality in cirrhotic patients undergoing surgery remains to be determined.

CARDIAC REVASCULARIZATION IN PATIENTS WITH LIVER DISEASE

CABG and PCI (balloon angioplasty, rotational atherectomy, or coronary artery stenting) are common cardiac revascularization procedures performed in the US. Despite the frequent use of these procedures and the high prevalence of liver disease in this country, there are very little data available on the outcomes in patients with liver disease. To date, there are no published reports on the morbidity and mortality of these procedures in asymptomatic patients with abnormal liver chemistries found on routine screening or in patients with acute or chronic non-cirrhotic liver disease. In patients with cirrhosis, cardiac surgery is associated with increased morbidity and mortality compared to patients without cirrhosis. Furthermore, cirrhotic patients undergoing cardiac surgery have worse outcomes than cirrhotic patients undergoing other non-cardiac surgical procedures. The lack of adequate data on the outcomes of patients with liver disease who need coronary interventions may be due to a reluctance to offer these procedures to patients with liver disease or failure to publish negative outcomes.

Klemperer et al reviewed the charts of 13 Child class A or B cirrhotic patients who were admitted to the cardiothoracic service between 1990 and 1996 for CABG and/or valve replacement [103]. Of these 13 patients, eight were Child class A and five were class B; 10 had cirrhosis due to alcohol. The perioperative complication rate was 25% in Child class A patients and 100% in class B. The overall mortality rate was 31%, including 0% in class A and 80% in class B patients [103].

Bizouarn et al prospectively studied 10 cirrhotic patients with Child–Pugh class A and two with class B who underwent elective cardiac surgery [104]. Seven patients (58%) experienced significant postoperative complications. Overall, three of the 12 patients (25%) died, which corresponds to a mortality rate of 20% in Child–Pugh class A and 50% in class B patients; one of the deaths occurred in the intensive care unit and the remaining two died after hospital discharge.

Risk factors for hepatic decompensation following cardiac surgery include the urgency of the procedure, the total time of cardiopulmonary bypass, the use of non-pulsatile rather than pulsatile cardiopulmonary bypass, and the need for perioperative pressor support [105]. Coagulation defects are often present in patients with liver disease [106–108], and cardiopulmonary bypass can exacerbate the underlying coagulopathy by inducing platelet dysfunction, reducing coagulation factors, activating fibrinolysis, and hypocalcemia [109, 110]. The mechanisms by which cardiopulmonary bypass can worsen coagulation dysfunction are shown in Table 27.4 [110].

Several case reports have described the technique of performing cardiac surgery before [111] or at the same time [105, 111–115] as liver transplantation. In a study of 32 patients with coronary artery disease who were managed medically ($n = 9$), by angioplasty ($n = 1$), or surgically ($n = 22$) prior to liver transplantation, Plotkin et al reported 81% morbidity and 50% mortality; these rates were equally high in medically and surgically treated patients [111]. Pollard et al described a patient who had a liver transplant followed by cardiac surgery 11 months later [110]. This latter approach is very risky because of the potential for hemodynamic instability during liver transplantation.

In asymptomatic patients with abnormal liver chemistries, cardiac revascularization should be postponed if the procedure is elective (Fig. 27.1). These patients should undergo a thorough investigation to determine the underlying cause of abnormal liver chemistries. If the procedure is an emergency or is life threatening, proceed to CABG or PCI with caution and closely monitor the patient during and after surgery (Fig. 27.1).

Table 27.4 Mechanisms of cardiopulmonary bypass-induced coagulopathy
Loss of vascular integrity required by the surgical procedure.
Qualitative and quantitative platelet dysfunction secondary to cell trauma and interaction with the synthetic surfaces, filters of the extracorporeal circuit, and hemodilution.
Reduction in coagulation factors secondary to hemodilution, cell washing, and fibrinolysis.
Primary fibrinolysis activated via the intrinsic and extrinsic pathways.
Hypocalcemia secondary to citrate-impaired liver metabolism.

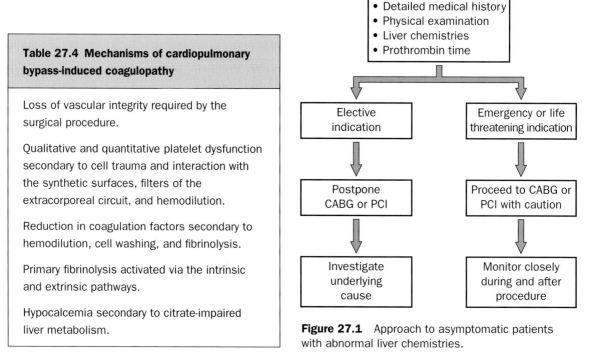

Figure 27.1 Approach to asymptomatic patients with abnormal liver chemistries.

The approach to patients with acute liver disease depends on the severity of the hepatic dysfunction (Fig. 27.2). In patients with acute hepatitis who require elective cardiac revascularization, the procedure should be postponed until the etiology of acute liver disease can be determined. In these patients, it is best to postpone the procedure until after the acute episode has resolved. In those with emergency or life-threatening indications, proceed to CABG or PCI with extreme caution and monitor the patient closely (Fig. 27.2). Cardiac revascularization should not be performed in patients with fulminant hepatic failure. These patients are at extremely high risk of procedure-related morbidity and mortality and they should be managed medically. If eligible, these patients should be referred for liver transplantation.

The approach to patients with chronic liver disease depends on whether or not cirrhosis is present (Fig. 27.3). In patients without cirrhosis, CABG or PCI are well tolerated provided the patient has compensated liver disease. In cirrhotic patients, it is important to assess the Child–Pugh class before deciding to refer the patient for cardiac revascularization. Coronary artery bypass grafts or PCI are permissible in patients with class A cirrhosis as long as they are monitored closely during and after the procedure. Patients with Child–Pugh class B cirrhosis may be able to tolerate CABG or PCI, but the patients should be medically optimized prior to proceeding with cardiac revascularization (Fig. 27.3). In these individuals, PCI may be a safer option than CABG because PCI does not require the use of cardiopulmonary bypass. Patients with Child–Pugh class C cirrhosis cannot tolerate the hemodynamic shifts associated with the use of cardiopulmonary bypass and should not undergo CABG. Although they may be able to tolerate PCI, it is probably best to manage these patients medically and consider referral for liver transplantation.

Patients who require cardiac revascularization can often be treated with either CABG or PCI. In a large meta-analysis of 3371 patients without liver disease who were randomized to CABG or angioplasty, Pocock et al reported similar outcomes after the initial revascularization procedure [116]. However, patients who were treated with angioplasty were significantly more likely to experience angina and require additional revascularization procedures than those who underwent CABG [116]. Similar findings were reported by Serruys et al, who compared CABG and coronary artery stenting [117]. Coronary artery stenting was less expensive than CABG, but it was associated with a higher incidence of angina during follow-up and a greater need for repeated revascularization [117].

The decision to perform CABG vs PCI in

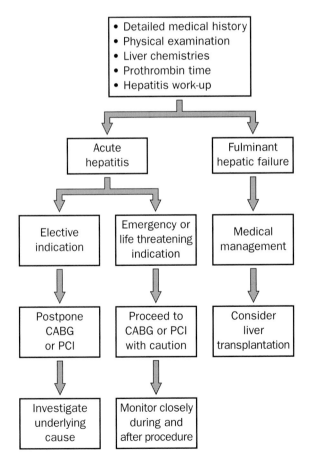

Figure 27.2 Approach to patients with acute liver disease.

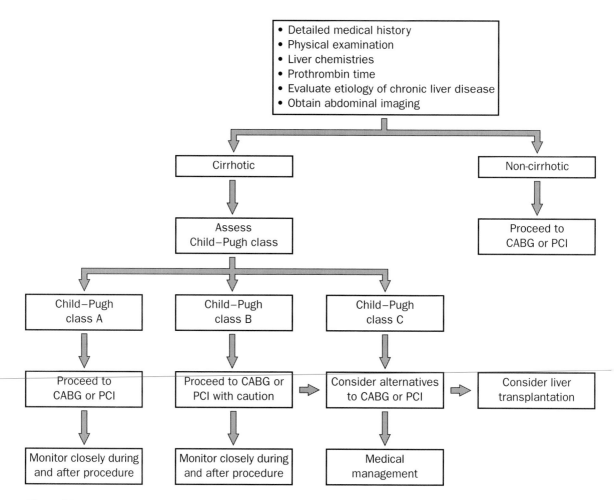

Figure 27.3 Approach to patients with chronic liver disease.

patients with liver disease must be made on a case-by-case basis. As a general rule, the least invasive options should be considered in patients with advanced liver disease. PCI is less invasive than CABG, but it is not without complications [118]. Although a detailed discussion of the complications of PCI are beyond the scope of this chapter, several complications that may occur more often in patients with liver disease warrant brief discussion. Patients with liver disease, especially those with ascites who are being treated with diuretics, may have

electrolyte abnormalities that could predispose them to cardiac arrhythmias during PCI. Peripheral vascular complications at the access site, such as bleeding, hematoma formation, and femoral artery pseudoaneurysms, may occur after PCI [118–121]. Patients with liver disease may have an underlying coagulopathy that could cause increased bleeding and access site complications after PCI. Contrast-induced nephropathy is a well-described complication of PCI, especially in patients with underlying renal disease and/or diabetes [122,123]. Since the prevalence of renal insufficiency and diabetes is higher in patients with liver disease than in the general population, these individuals may be at increased risk of developing contrast-induced nephropathy after PCI, especially in those with advanced liver disease.

In addition to CABG and PCI, minimally invasive cardiac surgery is an alternate method of cardiac revascularization. In the last several years, tremendous progress has been made in the field of minimally invasive cardiac surgery [124–130]. The invasiveness of cardiac surgery can be reduced by limiting the size of incisions and avoiding cardiopulmonary bypass [125, 126, 129]. These less invasive procedures can reduce postoperative pain and improve health-related quality of life compared with standard CABG [131]. Due to the less invasive nature of minimally invasive cardiac surgery compared with traditional CABG, the use of minimally invasive techniques may be better tolerated in patients with liver disease [132]. Evaluation of the safety and efficacy of these less invasive procedures in patients with liver disease warrants investigation.

PREOPERATIVE MANAGEMENT ISSUES

Once a decision has been made to perform cardiac revascularization in patients with liver disease, it is important to assess these individuals for the presence of coagulopathy, renal and electrolyte abnormalities, ascites, hepatic encephalopathy, esophageal varices, and malnutrition. Although a detailed discussion on the management of these problems is beyond the scope of this chapter, it is important to briefly provide some recommendations because many of these problems require treatment prior to cardiac revascularization in order to reduce intraoperative and postoperative complications.

Coagulopathy

Patients with liver disease may have a coagulopathy due to malabsorption of vitamin K or poor nutritional status [106–108]. Alternatively, coagulopathy may be due to poor hepatic synthetic function [106–108]. Correction of coagulopathy is essential, even in emergency or life-threatening situations, and is particularly important in patients undergoing cardiac revascularization. If possible, the prothrombin time should be corrected to within three seconds of control [25]. This may be accomplished by administering 10 mg of vitamin K intramuscularly for patients with malabsorption of vitamin K or poor nutritional status and by using fresh frozen plasma in those with hepatic synthetic dysfunction; a combination of vitamin K and fresh frozen plasma is often necessary [26]. If the prothrombin time does not correct to within three seconds of control, 10 U of cryoprecipitate, which contains fibrinogen and von Willebrand factor, may be given prior to cardiac revascularization [26]. Alternatively, desmopressin acetate (DDAVP) may be used [133]. In refractory cases, exchange plasmapheresis has been used to correct coagulopathy [44]. If necessary, platelet transfusions should be given to maintain a platelet count of at least $100,000/mm^3$ [16, 25].

Renal and electrolyte abnormalities

In patients with advanced liver disease, non-steroidal anti-inflammatory drugs, aminoglycosides, and other nephrotoxic drugs must be avoided [134–136]. Intravascular volume should be optimized in order to decrease the incidence of postoperative renal failure and hepatorenal syndrome [137, 138]. The use of low dose dopamine to preserve renal perfusion is of questionable benefit.

Electrolyte abnormalities are common in patients with liver disease and these should be corrected, if possible. Cirrhotic patients may have a dilutional hyponatremia; alternatively, hyponatremia, as well as hypokalemia, may be caused by diuretic use [16, 139]. Hypokalemia should be corrected prior to cardiac revascularization to minimize the risk of cardiac arrhythmias [26]. If present, alkalosis must also be corrected because this can precipitate hepatic encephalopathy [26].

Ascites

Patients with large-volume ascites require aggressive treatment with the use of diuretics, dietary sodium restriction, and, if necessary, large volume paracentesis [26]. This is important in order to prevent wound dehiscence and associated abdominal wall herniations [25,26]. In addition, large-volume ascites may also affect respiratory mechanics because of the pressure placed on the diaphragm by the ascitic fluid [26]. During diuresis, electrolytes and renal function should be monitored closely. If hyponatremia develops during diuretic therapy, restriction of free water intake may be necessary [140].

Approximately 10–27% of cirrhotic patients may have ascitic fluid infection (spontaneous bacterial peritonitis) at the time of admission to the hospital [140]. Therefore, a diagnostic paracentesis to evaluate ascitic fluid for the presence of spontaneous bacterial peritonitis should be performed in all patients with ascites upon admission to the hospital [141, 142]. Patients with spontaneous bacterial peritonitis should be treated with appropriate antibiotics prior to cardiac revascularization [26].

Hepatic encephalopathy

Lactulose should be used to treat patients with encephalopathy and the dose should be titrated to 2–3 soft bowel movements per day [47, 143]. Neomycin may be used in patients without renal dysfunction who do not respond to lactulose therapy [143, 144]. Protein restriction may be necessary in patients with hepatic encephalopathy that is refractory to medical therapy [26]. However, this should be avoided if possible because protein restriction will worsen malnutrition and, as a result, possibly increase the risk of perioperative morbidity and mortality [145]. Sedatives should be avoided in this patient population because they may precipitate or worsen hepatic encephalopathy. Preoperative recognition of hepatic encephalopathy is critical because there are many perioperative conditions that precipitate or exacerbate this disorder, including excess dietary protein, constipation, azotemia, hypokalemia, alkalosis, central nervous system depressants, infections, sepsis, dehydration, gastrointestinal bleeding, and hypoxia [25, 146].

Esophageal varices

Patients with prior bleeding from esophageal varices should be treated in the usual fashion, including non-selective beta-blockers and/or nitrates, as well as eradication of the esophageal varices using endoscopic band ligation or injection sclerotherapy [46, 47, 147]. Primary prophylactic therapy with non-selective beta-blockers and/or nitrates should be used in patients with esophageal varices who have not had a prior variceal bleed [46, 47, 147]. Several recent studies have shown that prophylactic esophageal band ligation may be efficacious in preventing variceal bleeding [148–150]. However, this is not yet considered standard of care in the US. In addition to the above measures, fluid overload should be avoided in the perioperative period because this may increase portal pressure and the risk of esophageal variceal bleeding.

Nutritional status

Malnutrition is common in patients with chronic liver disease and it can increase the risk of perioperative complications [151]. In a study of 2743 patients admitted to the intensive care unit for cardiovascular surgery, Rady et al found that preoperative hypoalbuminemia was present in 12% of patients and it was associated with an increased likelihood of postoperative organ dysfunction, nosocomial infections, prolonged mechanical ventilation, and death [152].

Preoperative nutritional support is important and may help to reduce morbidity and short-term mortality in patients with cirrhosis [153–155]. However, long-term survival in patients with hepatic resections may not be prolonged with the use of perioperative nutritional support [155].

A careful nutritional assessment is necessary in all patients with liver disease prior to cardiac revascularization. The presence of protein-calorie malnutrition can be best measured by body cell mass depletion [156]. Unfortunately, most parameters of nutritional status in patients with liver disease do not correlate with body cell mass. In this patient population, arm-muscle circumference and handgrip strength are the best predictors; combined they have a sensitivity of 94% and a negative predictive value of 97% in identifying patients with depleted body cell mass [156].

Because many patients with chronic liver disease are malnourished, protein restriction should be avoided unless refractory hepatic encephalopathy is present [26]. If oral feedings are tolerated, enteral nutrition is preferable to total parenteral nutrition. In patients with ascites or portal hypertension, placement of percutaneous endoscopic gastrostomy (PEG) feeding tubes is often not possible because of the high risk of complications.

INTRAOPERATIVE CARE AND CAUTIONS

Hemodynamic changes associated with cirrhosis

Patients with cirrhosis have baseline hemo-dynamic abnormalities that are important to understand prior to proceeding with cardiac revascularization, particularly if the use of cardiopulmonary bypass is planned. Cirrhotic patients have an increased intrahepatic vascular resistance, which leads to portal hypertension [157]. These individuals have an increased total blood volume, heart rate, and cardiac output, as well as decreased systemic vascular resistance [158–162]. Recent studies have implicated nitric oxide as the mediator responsible for the decreased vascular resistance found in cirrhotic patients [163–165]. Their plasma and non-central blood volumes are increased, but the central and arterial blood volumes are decreased [161]. These abnormalities are more pronounced in patients with ascites than in cirrhotics in the pre-ascitic phase [162, 166].

Kowalski and Abelmann studied 19 patients with alcoholic cirrhosis and three with fatty liver secondary to alcohol abuse and found that seven of these 22 patients (32%) had a high mean cardiac index [167]. The mean cardiac index of patients with liver disease was $4.3 \pm 2.7 \text{ L/min/m}^2$ compared with $3.8 \pm 0.7 \text{ L/min/m}^2$ for normal controls; one cirrhotic patient had a cardiac index as high as 11.2 L/min/m^2 [167]. In patients with ascites, the cardiac index may increase even further after large-volume paracentesis [168, 169]. Several studies have evaluated the impact of liver transplantation on cardiac output and found that these abnormalities were reversible after successful transplantation [170, 171]. In contrast, other investigators noted that these abnormalities may persist after liver transplantation [172, 173]. The reasons for these different findings are not clear.

In addition to the hemodynamic changes that are present in patients with cirrhosis, these individuals have dysregulation of the neuro-humoral system. Changes in heart rate, cardiac output and systemic vascular resistance are most prominent when patients are placed in the supine position and are likely secondary to redistribution of blood volume between the splanchnic and central circulation [158, 174]. These individuals have persistent activation of the renin–angiotensin–aldosterone system and the sympathetic nervous system and these mediators are not suppressed when patients are placed in the supine position, particularly in those with ascites [174–176]. These abnormalities are also associated with hypersecretion of arginine vasopressin [158]. As cirrhosis and portal hypertension progress, vascular resistance continues to fall, resulting in further disturbances in renal blood flow and retention of sodium and free water [163]. These hemodynamic derangements lead to increased ascites, worsening renal function, and further increases in portal pressure [158, 160].

Although this discussion on the hemodynamic derangements present in cirrhotic patients is an over-simplification of a very complex process, it is important to understand that these patients have decreased central and arterial blood volumes along with low peripheral vascular resistance and elevated cardiac output. The use of cardiopulmonary bypass is associated with a mean decrease in hepatic blood flow of 19% in non-cirrhotic patients [177]. This decrease is likely to be greater in cirrhotic patients, especially in those with decompensated liver disease.

Cirrhotic patients have a low systemic arterial pressure at baseline and this can be exacerbated by the administration of sedatives and anesthetics. More importantly, cardiopulmonary bypass may not be able to keep up with the very high cardiac outputs that are present in patients with advanced cirrhosis. Although we could not find any studies to support this hypothesis, we are aware of several cases in which cardiopulmonary bypass was unable to maintain an adequate cardiac output, resulting in severe hypotension, decreased tissue perfusion, worsening hepatic function, and even intraoperative death. For these reasons, a thorough preoperative assessment is necessary in patients with cirrhosis. In the subgroup of cirrhotic patients with severe hemodynamic derangements, less invasive options, such as PCI, should be strongly considered.

Hemodynamic effects on inhaled anesthetics

Inhaled anesthetics are commonly used during surgery, and a variety of agents are available (Table 27.5). Some of the more common agents that are used include halothane, enflurane, methoxyflurane, and isoflurane. In general, most inhaled anesthetics are associated with a reduction in hepatic blood flow and hepatic oxygen uptake [25]. In a study of 32 patients without liver disease, anesthesia resulted in a 36% decrease in hepatic blood flow during the first 30 minutes of anesthesia [178]. Anesthetics may also cause a decrease in cardiac output by exerting negative inotropic effects on the myocardium [179, 180]. This decrease in cardiac output, combined with an increase in systemic vasodilation, may result in decreased hepatic blood flow [179, 180]. Postoperative hepatic dysfunction may be a result of a decrease in blood flow or may be directly related to the hepatotoxic effects of these drugs. Although most patients can tolerate a transient decrease in hepatic blood flow, these effects may be deleterious in patients with liver disease.

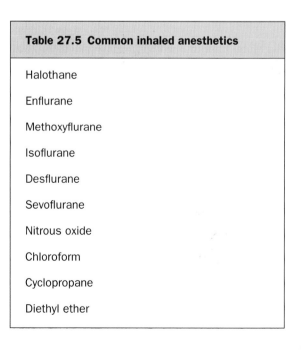

Table 27.5 Common inhaled anesthetics
Halothane
Enflurane
Methoxyflurane
Isoflurane
Desflurane
Sevoflurane
Nitrous oxide
Chloroform
Cyclopropane
Diethyl ether

The various anesthetics affect hepatic function differently [181]. Halothane and enflurane decrease hepatic blood flow to a larger degree than isoflurane [179, 180, 182]. In fact, isoflurane may actually increase hepatic blood flow and it should be considered the anesthetic agent of choice for surgical procedures in patients with liver disease [25]. In addition, isoflurane, as well as desflurane and sevoflurane, undergo less hepatic metabolism than halothane or enflurane and therefore should be associated with a lower incidence of drug-induced hepatotoxicity [25, 183, 184]. Nitrous oxide is also safe in patients with liver disease and has no known hepatotoxicity, unless used in combination with halothane [185].

Halothane is associated with significant hepatotoxicity, especially in patients with liver disease or chronic ethanol use [186]. In patients who are administered halothane, the incidence of severe hepatic dysfunction after a single exposure is one in 6000; fatal hepatic necrosis is less common and occurs in one in 35,000 patients [187, 188]. Multiple exposures to halothane, female gender, obesity, middle age, and possibly the presence of autoimmune disease have been associated with an increased risk of halothane-induced hepatotoxicity [188]. The mechanism by which halothane causes hepatic necrosis is currently unknown, but has been proposed to involve immune sensitization to metabolites of halothane in genetically predisposed individuals [183]. The clinical, biochemical, and histologic features of halothane and enflurane hepatotoxicity are similar [189]. Postoperative fever, jaundice, and liver histology revealing centrilobular necrosis associated with ballooning degeneration and fatty change were the most common findings; these abnormalities were associated with a 20% mortality [189].

In summary, halothane should be avoided in patients with liver disease in favor of the less hepatotoxic agents isoflurane and nitrous oxide. Although isoflurane decreases hepatic blood flow less than halothane and enflurane, care should be taken to avoid intraoperative hypotension, which in combination with the anesthetic-induced reduction in portal flow, can result in ischemic damage to the liver.

Risks of sedatives and analgesics

Patients with well-compensated liver disease tolerate most sedatives and analgesics well. However, these medications should be used with caution in patients with hepatic dysfunction. Since the liver plays an important role in drug metabolism and clearance, liver disease can affect plasma levels of sedatives and analgesics by several mechanisms [190]. In patients with liver disease, these abnormalities make it difficult to predict the kinetics of drug metabolism (Table 27.6). Therefore, the initial dose of sedatives and analgesics should be reduced in proportion to the severity of hepatic dysfunction.

Short acting sedatives and analgesics are the preferred agents in this patient population. Sedatives that have short half-lives include temazepam, oxazepam, and lorazepam. These

---

Table 27.6 Mechanisms of altered plasma drug levels in patients with liver disease

Reduced synthesis of albumin resulting in decreased plasma binding and increased drug levels in plasma.

Increased plasma and extracellular fluid volumes resulting in an increased volume of distribution.

Reduced hepatic clearance resulting in a prolonged half-life.

Presence of portacaval shunting which may increase the bioavailability of orally administered medications by decreasing first-pass metabolism.

agents should be administered instead of other agents with longer half-lives, such as lorazepam and diazepam [190]. Oxazepam and lorazepam are eliminated by glucuronidation without hepatic metabolism and are ideal for patients with liver dysfunction [25, 190].

Narcotics undergo a high first-pass metabolism and clearance is dependent on hepatic blood flow. Since hepatic blood flow is decreased during the intraoperative period in patients with liver disease, the half-lives of most narcotics are increased [25]. Furthermore, portosystemic shunting increases the bioavailability of orally administered narcotics. Clearance of meperidine, and morphine, which are commonly used narcotics, is decreased in this patient population and the dosing of these medications may require adjustment; fentanyl is short acting and is preferred over meperidine and morphine [16, 25].

In patients with liver disease, it is important to use sedatives and analgesics with short half-lives to avoid the risk of postoperative delirium and hepatic encephalopathy [21]. In addition to having a prolonged half-life in these patients, many of the sedatives and analgesics may be associated with hepatotoxicity [191].

Neuromuscular blocking agents can also result in decreased hepatic flow and caution must be taken when using these medications in patients with liver disease. This class of drugs poses a problem because the half-lives of these agents are prolonged in patients with liver disease because of reduced pseudocholinesterase activity, decreased biliary excretion, and increased volume of distribution [25]. If the use of neuromuscular blocking agents is necessary, atracurium is preferred because clearance is independent of renal and hepatic function [190].

Pulmonary issues

Pulmonary abnormalities are common in patients with chronic liver disease. Hourani et al screened 116 patients with advanced liver disease and found arterial blood gas abnormalities in 45% and abnormal pulmonary function tests in as many as 50% [192]. The differential diagnosis of pulmonary dysfunction in patients with liver disease includes intrinsic cardiac and pulmonary disease unrelated to liver disease, such as chronic obstructive pulmonary disease, congestive heart failure, pneumonia, and asthma. In addition, disorders specifically related to liver disease must be considered, including hepatic hydrothorax, hepatopulmonary syndrome, portopulmonary hypertension, emphysema in patients with alpha-1-antitrypsin deficiency, and fibrosing alveolitis and pulmonary granulomas in patients with primary biliary cirrhosis [193].

Hepatopulmonary syndrome is caused by intrapulmonary vascular abnormalities that include dilated precapillary and capillary beds [194]. These intrapulmonary vascular abnormalities result in a right-to-left intrapulmonary shunt, ventilation-perfusion mismatching, increased alveolar-arterial gradient while breathing room air, and moderate to severe hypoxia that is worse in the standing position [194–196]. Spider angiomata, digital clubbing, and cyanosis are common findings in patients with the hepatopulmonary syndrome [193]. Other reasons for hypoxia in patients with liver disease include hypoventilation secondary to compression of the diaphragm by ascites and increased red blood cell 2,3-DPG that shifts the oxygen dissociation curve to the right and causes hemoglobin to have a lower affinity for oxygen [193]. These pulmonary abnormalities can cause serious problems during surgery and these individuals require intensive intraoperative monitoring. Severe hypoxia with a pO_2 less than 60 mmHg is a relative contraindication to surgery, except for liver transplantation in patients with the hepatopulmonary syndrome [25].

Hypercarbia should be avoided during surgery because it results in sympathetic stimulation of the splanchnic vasculature, which leads to a decrease in hepatic blood flow. Patients with liver dysfunction also have a mild compensated respiratory alkalosis at baseline [197]. Therefore, the pCO_2 in patients with liver disease should be maintained in the range of 35–40 mmHg [25].

POSTOPERATIVE CARE AND COMPLICATIONS

Postoperative care of patients with liver disease requires careful attention to details, and many of the issues addressed in the preoperative and intraoperative period must be extended to postoperative care. The postoperative care of patients with liver disease is complex and a detailed discussion of this topic is beyond the scope of this chapter. However, several important issues merit discussion.

Close monitoring and correction of electrolyte abnormalities, fluid balance, anemia due to excessive bleeding, coagulopathy, hypoxia, and hepatic encephalopathy are critical. Fluid overload must be avoided, as this can increase ascites, hypoxemia, and the risk of variceal hemorrhage. However, dehydration must also be avoided because this may precipitate renal failure. Medications such as non-steroidal anti-inflammatory drugs, narcotics, and analgesics should be used with caution. Conditions predisposing to encephalopathy, such as constipation, alkalosis, central nervous system depressants, hypoxia, sepsis, and gastrointestinal bleeding must be addressed. Patients with liver disease may have impaired surgical wound healing due to abnormalities in protein synthesis, poor nutritional status, bleeding or infection of surgical wounds, and stress on the wound site from ascites [198–200]. Patients should be observed closely for signs of infection and, if present, antibiotics should be started promptly.

In the postoperative period, patients should be monitored for signs of hepatic dysfunction, such as jaundice, elevations of serum AST and ALT levels, worsening coagulopathy, hypoglycemia, ascites, and encephalopathy [25]. Hepatic dysfunction may range in severity from mild elevations of AST, ALT, or bilirubin levels to fulminant hepatic failure [201].

Mild elevations in liver chemistries are common after surgery, even in patients without liver disease [201, 202]. The development of postoperative jaundice occurs in less than 1% of patients without liver disease who undergo major surgery [201]. However, the presence of pre-existing liver disease is associated with an increased risk of developing postoperative hepatic dysfunction, especially after cardiac surgery [201].

In a study of 218 patients undergoing major surgery, the incidence of mild jaundice was 17% and severe jaundice was noted in 4% [203]. The majority of cases of postoperative jaundice in this study were caused by bilirubin overload from transfusions that could not be effectively excreted due to liver dysfunction. In a prospective study of 248 patients who underwent cardiopulmonary bypass, early postoperative jaundice developed in 20% [204]. In this study, development of postoperative jaundice was associated with poor outcomes; the mortality rate was 25% in jaundiced patients compared to 1% in those without jaundice [204].

The causes of postoperative jaundice are multifactorial [201, 203, 205–208], making identification of a specific etiology challenging (Table 27.7). Benign postoperative jaundice (also known as benign postoperative cholestasis) usually occurs within 10 days of surgery and often resolves spontaneously [26, 201]. However, a thorough investigation for treatable causes of jaundice must be performed before making a diagnosis of benign postoperative jaundice.

CONCLUSIONS

A detailed history and physical examination is the best way to screen patients for liver disease prior to cardiac revascularization. Routine liver chemistries are not necessary, and these tests should only be ordered if the presence of liver disease is suspected. Because cardiac

Table 27.7 Causes of jaundice in the post-operative period
Ischemic hepatitis
Anesthetic or drug-induced hepatitis
Viral hepatitis
Hemolysis from cardiopulmonary bypass
Multiple blood transfusions
Excessive bleeding and resolving hematomas
Infection and sepsis
Injury to the liver or bile ducts
Choledocholithiasis
Cholelithiasis
Pancreatitis
Total parenteral nutrition

revascularization in patients with liver disease can be associated with significant morbidity and mortality, the risks and benefits of the procedure must be considered carefully. The decision to proceed with cardiac revascularization depends on the type of procedure planned, the urgency of the procedure, the severity of the underlying liver dysfunction, and the presence of other comorbid diseases.

In patients with cirrhosis, surgical risk correlates with the Child–Pugh class. Perioperative morbidity and mortality is particularly high in patients with acute hepatitis and decompensated cirrhosis (Child–Pugh class C), especially in those undergoing cardiac surgery. In these individuals, elective cardiac surgery is contraindicated and less invasive options should be pursued. Cardiac revascularization is permissible in asymptomatic patients with abnormal liver chemistries and those with well-compensated chronic liver disease, provided a thorough preoperative risk assessment is performed. Appropriate preoperative and intraoperative management can have a significant impact on reducing postoperative morbidity and mortality. Prospective studies to determine the optimal approach to patients with liver disease who require cardiac revascularization are clearly needed.

REFERENCES

1. Anonymous. Recommendations for prevention and control of hepatitis C virus (HCV) infection and HCV-related chronic disease. Centers for Disease Control and Prevention. *Morb Mortal Wkly Rep* 1998; **47**:1–39.
2. National Center for Health Statistics. *Health, United States 2000 with Adolescent Health Chartbook*, Hyattsville, Maryland, 2000.
3. Alter MJ, Kruszon-Moran D, Nainan OV et al. The prevalence of hepatitis C virus infection in the United States, 1988 through 1994, *N Engl J Med* 1999; **341**:556–562.
4. Armstrong GL, Alter MJ, McQuillan GM, Margolis HS. The past incidence of hepatitis C virus infection: implications for the future burden of chronic liver disease in the United States, *Hepatology* 2000; **31**:777–782.
5. Wong JB, McQuillan GM, McHutchison JG, Poynard T. Estimating future hepatitis C morbidity, mortality, and costs in the United States, *Am J Public Health* 2000; **90**:1562–1569.
6. Kim WR, Gross JB Jr, Poterucha JJ, Locke GR III, Dickson ER. Outcome of hospital care of liver disease associated with hepatitis C in the United States, *Hepatology* 2001; **33**:201–206.
7. Murphy SL. Deaths: final data for 1998. *National Vital Statistics Reports*, vol 48 no. 11, (Hyattsville, Maryland: National Center for Health Statistics, 2000).
8. Adams PF, Hendershot GE, Marano MA. Current estimates from the National Health Interview Survey, 1996. National Center for Health Statistics. *Vital Health Stat* 1999; **10**:200.
9. Anonymous. Mortality from coronary heart disease and acute myocardial infarction—United States, 1998, *Morb Mortal Wkly Rep* 2001; **50**:90–93.
10. Carey WD, Dumot JA, Pimentel RR et al. The

prevalence of coronary artery disease in liver transplant candidates over age 50, *Transplantation* 1995; **59**:859–864.

11. Bayraktar Y, Bayraktar M, DeMaria N, Colantoni A, Van Thiel DH. The cardiac evaluation of liver transplant recipients: a single center's experience, *Ital J Gastroenterol Hepatol* 1997; **29**:162–167.

12. Wanless IR. Physioanatomic Considerations. In: Schiff ER, Sorrell MF, Maddrey WC, eds, *Schiff's Diseases of the Liver*, 8th edn, (Philadelphia: Lippincott Williams & Wilkins, 1999) 3–37.

13. Rappaport AM. Hepatic blood flow: morphologic aspects and physiologic regulation, *Int Rev Physiol* 1980; **21**:1–63.

14. Rappaport AM, Black RG, Lucas CC, Ridout JH, Best CH. Normal and pathologic microcirculation of the living mammalian liver, *Rev Int Hepatol* 1966; **16**:813–828.

15. Rappaport AM. Microcirculatory units in the mammalian liver. Their arterial and portal components, *Bibl Anat* 1977; **16**:116–120.

16. Conn M. Preoperative evaluation of the patient with liver disease, *Mt Sinai J Med* 1991; **58**: 75–80.

17. Karran S. Progress in the assessment of liver blood flow in health and disease, *J R Coll Surg Edinb* 1990; **35**:207–217.

18. Schemel WH. Unexpected hepatic dysfunction found by multiple laboratory screening, *Anesth Analg* 1976; **55**:810–812.

19. Wataneeyawech M, Kelly KA Jr. Hepatic diseases. Unsuspected before surgery, *NY State J Med* 1975; **75**:1278–1281.

20. Jackson FC, Christophersen EB, Peternel WW. Preoperative management of patients with liver disease, *Surg Clin North Am* 1968; **48**:907–930.

21. Friedman LS, Maddrey WC. Surgery in the patient with liver disease, *Med Clin North Am* 1987; **71**:453–476.

22. Leibowitz S. Guidelines to clearing patients with liver disease for surgery, *Mt Sinai J Med* 1977; **44**:539–543.

23. Siefkin AD, Bolt RJ. Preoperative evaluation of the patient with gastrointestinal or liver disease, *Med Clin North Am* 1979; **63**:1309–1320.

24. Gholson CF, Provenza JM, Bacon BR. Hepatologic considerations in patients with parenchymal liver disease undergoing surgery, *Am J Gastroenterol* 1990; **85**:487–496.

25. Friedman LS. The risk of surgery in patients with liver disease, *Hepatology* 1999; **29**: 1617–1623.

26. Patel T. Surgery in the patient with liver disease, *Mayo Clin Proc* 1999; **74**:593–599.

27. Naylor CD. Physical examination of the liver, *JAMA* 1994; **271**:1859–1865.

28. Greenberger N. History taking and physical examination in the patient with liver disease. In: Schiff ER, Sorrell MF, Maddrey WC, eds, *Schiff's Disease of the Liver*, 8th edn, (Philadelphia: Lippincott Williams & Wilkins, 1999) 193–203.

29. Murphy EL, Bryzman SM, Glynn SA et al. Risk factors for hepatitis C virus infection in US blood donors. NHLBI Retrovirus Epidemiology Donor Study (REDS), *Hepatology* 2000; **31**: 756–762.

30. Delage G, Infane-Rivard C, Chiavetta JA et al. Risk factors for acquisition of hepatitis C virus infection in blood donors: results of a case-control study, *Gastroenterology* 1999; **116**: 893–899.

31. Bradley KA, Bush KR, McDonell MB, Malone T, Fihn SD. Screening for problem drinking: comparison of CAGE and AUDIT. Ambulatory Care Quality Improvement Project (ACQUIP). Alcohol Use Disorders Identification Test, *J Gen Intern Med* 1998; **13**:379–388.

32. Lee WM. Review article: drug-induced hepatotoxicity, *Aliment Pharmacol Ther* 1993; **7**:477–485.

33. Zimmerman HJ, Maddrey WC. Acetaminophen (paracetamol) hepatotoxicity with regular intake of alcohol: analysis of instances of therapeutic misadventure, *Hepatology* 1995; **22**:767–773.

34. Lewis JH. Drug-induced liver disease, *Med Clin North Am* 2000; **84**:1275–1311.

35. Schiodt FV, Atillasoy E, Shakil AO et al. Etiology and outcome for 295 patients with acute liver failure in the United States, *Liver Transpl Surg* 1999; **5**:29–34.

36. Sarin SK. What should we advise about adjunctive therapies, including herbal medicines, for hepatitis C? *J Gastroenterol Hepatol* 2000; **15** (suppl):E164–E171.

37. Lee WM. Drug-induced hepatotoxicity, *N Engl J Med* 1995; **333**:1118–1127.

38. Farrell GC. Drug-induced hepatic injury, *J Gastroenterol Hepatol* 1997; **12**:S242–S250.

39. Bateman J, Chapman RD, Simpson D. Possible toxicity of herbal remedies, *Scott Med J* 1998; **43**: 7–15.

40. Stickel F, Egerer G, Seitz HK. Hepatotoxicity of botanicals, *Public Health Nutr* 2000; **3**:113–124.

41. Macpherson DS. Preoperative laboratory testing: should any tests be 'routine' before surgery? *Med Clin North Am* 1993; **77**:289–308.

42. Chopra S, Griffin PH. Laboratory tests and diagnostic procedures in evaluation of liver disease, *Am J Med* 1985; **79**:221–230.

43. King PD. Abnormal liver enzyme levels. Evaluation in asymptomatic patients, *Postgrad Med* 1991; **89**:137–141.

44. Kaul V, Munoz SJ. Coagulopathy of liver disease, *Curr Treat Options Gastroenterol* 2000; **3**: 433–438.

45. Grace ND, Groszmann RJ, Garcia-Tsao G et al. Portal hypertension and variceal bleeding: an AASLD single topic symposium, *Hepatology* 1998; **28**:868–880.

46. Roberts LR, Kamath PS. Pathophysiology and treatment of variceal hemorrhage, *Mayo Clin Proc* 1996; **71**:973–983.

47. Menon KV, Kamath PS. Managing the complications of cirrhosis, *Mayo Clin Proc* 2000; **75**:501–509.

48. Wilcox CM, Alexander LN, Straub RF, Clark WS. A prospective endoscopic evaluation of the causes of upper GI hemorrhage in alcoholics: a focus on alcoholic gastropathy, *Am J Gastroenterol* 1996; **91**:1343–1347.

49. Herold C, Heinz R, Radespiel-Troger M et al. Quantitative testing of liver function in patients with cirrhosis due to chronic hepatitis C to assess disease severity, *Liver* 2001; **21**:26–30.

50. Gill RA, Goodman MW, Golfus GR, Onstad GR, Bubrick MP. Aminopyrine breath test predicts surgical risk for patients with liver disease, *Ann Surg* 1983; **198**:701–704.

51. Watanabe Y, Kumon K. Assessment by pulse dye-densitometry indocyanine green (ICG) clearance test of hepatic function of patients before cardiac surgery: its value as a predictor of serious postoperative liver dysfunction, *J Cardiothorac Vasc Anesth* 1999; **13**:299–303.

52. Takeuchi S, Nakano H, Kim YK et al. Predicting survival and postoperative complications with Tc-GSA liver scintigraphy in hepatocellular carcinoma, *Hepatogastroenterology* 1999; **46**: 1855–1861.

53. Nakano H, Kumada K, Takekuma Y et al. Perioperative hepatic functional risk assessed with technetium-99m diethylenetriamine pen-taacetic acid-galactosyl human serum albumin liver scintigraphy in patients undergoing pancreaticoduodenectomy complicated by obstructive jaundice, *Int J Pancreatol* 1999; **25**:3–9.

54. Kim YK, Nakano H, Yamaguchi M et al. Prediction of postoperative decompensated liver function by technetium-99m galactosyl-human serum albumin liver scintigraphy in patients with hepatocellular carcinoma complicating chronic liver disease, *Br J Surg* 1997; **84**:793–796.

55. Fasoli A, Giannini E, Botta F et al. 13CO$_2$ excretion in breath of normal subjects and cirrhotic patients after 13C-aminopyrine oral load. Comparison with MEGX test in functional differentiation between chronic hepatitis and liver cirrhosis, *Hepatogastroenterology* 2000; **47**: 234–238.

56. Harville DD, Summerskill WH. Surgery in acute hepatitis: causes and effects, *JAMA* 1963; **184**:257–261.

57. Greenwood SM, Leffler CT, Minkowitz S. The increased mortality rate of open liver biopsy in alcoholic hepatitis, *Surg Gynecol Obstet* 1972; **134**:600–604.

58. Powell-Jackson P, Greenway B, Williams R. Adverse effects of exploratory laparotomy in patients with unsuspected liver disease, *Br J Surg* 1982; **69**:449–451.

59. Mikkelsen WP, Turrill FL, Kern WH. Acute hyaline necrosis of the liver. A surgical trap, *Am J Surg* 1968; **116**:266–272.

60. Mikkelsen WP, Kern WH. The influence of acute hyaline necrosis on survival after emergency and elective portacaval shunt, *Major Probl Clin Surg* 1974; **14**:233–242.

61. Mikkelsen WP. Therapeutic portacaval shunt. Preliminary data on controlled trial and morbid effects of acute hyaline necrosis, *Arch Surg* 1974; **108**:302–305.

62. Rakela J, Lange SM, Ludwig J, Baldus WP. Fulminant hepatitis: Mayo Clinic experience with 34 cases, *Mayo Clin Proc* 1985; **60**:289–292.

63. Scevola D, Barbarini G, Michelone G, Calderon W, Dughetti S. An eleven year survey (1975–1985) of fulminant hepatitis: considerations on epidemiology and pathogenesis, *Boll Ist Sieroter Milan* 1986; **65**:453–458.

64. Munoz SJ. Difficult management problems in fulminant hepatic failure, *Semin Liver Dis* 1993; **13**:395–413.

65. Sheil AG, McCaughan GW, Isai HI. Acute and subacute fulminant hepatic failure: the role of liver transplantation, *Med J Aust* 1991; **154**:724–728.

66. Atillasoy E, Berk PD. Fulminant hepatic failure: pathophysiology, treatment, and survival. *Annu Rev Med* 1995; **46**:181–191.

67. Runyon BA. Surgical procedures are well tolerated by patients with asymptomatic chronic hepatitis, *J Clin Gastroenterol* 1986; **8**: 542–544.

68. Hargrove MD Jr. Chronic active hepatitis: possible adverse effect of exploratory laparotomy, *Surgery* 1970; **68**:771–773.

69. Higashi H, Matsumata T, Adachi E. Influence of viral hepatitis status on operative morbidity and mortality in patients with primary hepatocellular carcinoma, *Br J Surg* 1994; **81**:1342–1345.

70. Child CG, Turcotte JG. Surgery and portal hypertension. In: Child CG, ed, *The liver and portal hypertension* (Philadelphia: Saunders, 1964).

71. Pugh RN, Murray-Lyon IM, Dawson JL, Pietroni MC, Williams R. Transection of the oesophagus for bleeding oesophageal varices, *Br J Surg* 1973; **60**:646–649.

72. Garrison RN, Cryer HM, Howard DA, Polk HC Jr. Clarification of risk factors for abdominal operations in patients with hepatic cirrhosis, *Ann Surg* 1984; **199**:648–655.

73. Mansour A, Watson W, Shayani V, Pickleman J. Abdominal operations in patients with cirrhosis: still a major surgical challenge, *Surgery* 1997; **122**:730–735.

74. Castaing D, Houssin D, Lemoine J, Bismuth H. Surgical management of gallstones in cirrhotic patients, *Am J Surg* 1983; **146**:310–313.

75. Aranha GV, Sontag SJ, Greenlee HB. Cholecystectomy in cirrhotic patients: a formidable operation, *Am J Surg* 1982; **143**:55–60.

76. Bloch RS, Allaben RD, Walt AJ. Cholecystectomy in patients with cirrhosis. A surgical challenge, *Arch Surg* 1985; **120**:669–672.

77. Schwartz SI. Biliary tract surgery and cirrhosis: a critical combination, *Surgery* 1981; **90**:577–583.

78. McSherry CK, Glenn F. The incidence and causes of death following surgery for nonmalignant biliary tract disease, *Ann Surg* 1980; **191**:271–275.

79. Aranha GV, Kruss D, Greenlee HB. Therapeutic options for biliary tract disease in advanced cirrhosis, *Am J Surg* 1988; **155**:374–377.

80. Doberneck RC, Sterling WA Jr, Allison DC. Morbidity and mortality after operation in non-bleeding cirrhotic patients, *Am J Surg* 1983; **146**:306–309.

81. Aranha GV, Greenlee HB. Intra-abdominal surgery in patients with advanced cirrhosis, *Arch Surg* 1986; **121**:275–277.

82. Sirinek KR, Burk RR, Brown M, Levine BA. Improving survival in patients with cirrhosis undergoing major abdominal operations, *Arch Surg* 1987; **122**:271–273.

83. Wong R, Rappaport W, Witte C et al. Risk of non-shunt abdominal operation in the patient with cirrhosis, *J Am Coll Surg* 1994; **179**:412–416.

84. Metcalf AM, Dozois RR, Wolff BG, Beart RW Jr. The surgical risk of colectomy in patients with cirrhosis, *Dis Colon Rectum* 1987; **30**:529–531.

85. Leonetti JP, Aranha GV, Wilkinson WA, Stanley M, Greenlee HB. Umbilical herniorrhaphy in cirrhotic patients, *Arch Surg* 1984; **119**:442–445.

86. Lehnert T, Herfarth C. Peptic ulcer surgery in patients with liver cirrhosis, *Ann Surg* 1993; **217**:338–346.

87. Ziser A, Plevak DJ, Wiesner RH et al. Morbidity and mortality in cirrhotic patients undergoing anesthesia and surgery, *Anesthesiology* 1999; **90**:42–53.

88. Jan YY, Chen MF. Laparoscopic cholecystectomy in cirrhotic patients. *Hepatogastroenterology* 1997; **44**:1584–1587.

89. Yerdel MA, Koksoy C, Aras N, Orita K. Laparoscopic versus open cholecystectomy in cirrhotic patients: a prospective study, *Surg Laparosc Endosc* 1997; **7**:483–486.

90. Sleeman D, Namias N, Levi D et al. Laparoscopic cholecystectomy in cirrhotic patients, *J Am Coll Surg* 1998; **187**:400–403.

91. Friel CM, Stack J, Forse A, Babineau TJ. Laparoscopic cholecystectomy in patients with hepatic cirrhosis: a five-year experience, *J Gastrointest Surg* 1999; **3**:286–291.

92. Poggio JL, Rowland CM, Gores GJ, Nagorney DM, Donohue JH. A comparison of laparoscopic and open cholecystectomy in patients with compensated cirrhosis and symptomatic gallstone disease, *Surgery* 2000; **127**:405–411.

93. Fernandes NF, Schwesinger WH, Hilsenbeck SG et al. Laparoscopic cholecystectomy and cirrhosis: a case-control study of outcomes, *Liver Transpl* 2000; **6**:340–344.

94. Morino M, Cavuoti G, Miglietta C, Giraudo G,

Simone P. Laparoscopic cholecystectomy in cirrhosis: contraindication or privileged indication? *Surg Laparosc Endosc Percutan Tech* 2000; **10**:360–363.

95. Gopalswamy N, Mehta V, Barde CJ. Risks of intra-abdominal nonshunt surgery in cirrhotics, *Dig Dis* 1998; **16**:225–231.

96. Luxon BA. Liver transplantation. Who should be referred, and when? *Postgrad Med* 1997; **102**:103–8, 113.

97. Fevery J. Liver transplantation: problems and perspectives, *Hepatogastroenterology* 1998; **45**: 1039–1044.

98. Zetterman RK. Primary care management of the liver transplant patient, *Am J Med* 1994; **96**:10S–17S.

99. Zimmerman JE, Wagner DP, Seneff MG et al. Intensive care unit admissions with cirrhosis: risk-stratifying patient groups and predicting individual survival, *Hepatology* 1996; **23**:1393–1401.

100. Cooper GS, Bellamy P, Dawson NV et al. A prognostic model for patients with end-stage liver disease, *Gastroenterology* 1997; **113**:1278–1288.

101. Rice HE, O'Keefe GE, Helton WS, Johansen K. Morbid prognostic features in patients with chronic liver failure undergoing non-hepatic surgery, *Arch Surg* 1997; **132**:880–884.

102. Kamath PS, Wiesner RH, Malinchoc M et al. A model to predict survival in patients with end-stage liver disease, *Hepatology* 2001; **33**:464–470.

103. Klemperer JD, Ko W, Krieger KH et al. Cardiac operations in patients with cirrhosis, *Ann Thorac Surg* 1998; **65**:85–87.

104. Bizouarn P, Ausseur A, Desseigne P et al. Early and late outcome after elective cardiac surgery in patients with cirrhosis, *Ann Thorac Surg* 1999; **67**:1334–1338.

105. Morris JJ, Hellman CL, Gawey BJ et al. Three patients requiring both coronary artery bypass surgery and orthotopic liver transplantation, *J Cardiothorac Vasc Anesth* 1995; **9**:322–332.

106. Mammen EF. Coagulation abnormalities in liver disease, *Hematol Oncol Clin North Am* 1992; **6**:1247–1257.

107. Mammen EF. Coagulation defects in liver disease, *Med Clin North Am* 1994; **78**:545–554.

108. Mammen EF. Coagulopathies of liver disease, *Clin Lab Med* 1994; **14**:769–780.

109. Mammen EF, Koets MH, Washington BC et al. Hemostasis changes during cardiopulmonary bypass surgery, *Semin Thromb Hemost* 1985; **11**:281–292.

110. Pollard RJ, Sidi A, Gibby GL, Lobato EB, Gabrielli A. Aortic stenosis with end-stage liver disease: prioritizing surgical and anesthetic therapies, *J Clin Anesth* 1998; **10**:253–261.

111. Plotkin JS, Scott VL, Pinna A et al. Morbidity and mortality in patients with coronary artery disease undergoing orthotopic liver transplantation, *Liver Transpl Surg* 1996; **2**:426–430.

112. Benedetti E, Massad MG, Chami Y, Wiley T, Layden TJ. Is the presence of surgically treatable coronary artery disease a contraindication to liver transplantation? *Clin Transplant* 1999; **13**:59–61.

113. Manas DM, Roberts DR, Heaviside DW et al. Sequential coronary artery bypass grafting and orthotopic liver transplantation: a case report, *Clin Transplant* 1996; **10**:320–322.

114. Massad MG, Benedetti E, Pollak R et al. Combined coronary bypass and liver transplantation: technical considerations, *Ann Thorac Surg* 1998; **65**:1130–1132.

115. Eckhoff DE, Frenette L, Sellers MT et al. Combined cardiac surgery and liver transplantation, *Liver Transpl* 2001; **7**:60–61.

116. Pocock SJ, Henderson RA, Richards AF et al. Meta-analysis of randomized trials comparing coronary angioplasty with bypass surgery, *Lancet* 1995; **346**:1184–1189.

117. Serruys PW, Unger F, Sousa JE et al. Comparison of coronary-artery bypass surgery and stenting for the treatment of multi-vessel disease, *N Engl J Med* 2001; **344**:1117–1124.

118. Landau C, Lange RA, Hillis LD. Percutaneous transluminal coronary angioplasty, *N Engl J Med* 1994; **330**:981–993.

119. O'Meara JJ, Dehmer GJ. Care of the patient and management of complications after percutaneous coronary artery interventions, *Ann Intern Med* 1997; **127**:458–471.

120. Davis C, VanRiper S, Longstreet J, Moscucci M. Vascular complications of coronary interventions, *Heart Lung* 1997; **26**:118–127.

121. Lehmann KG, Ferris ST, Heath-Lange SJ. Maintenance of hemostasis after invasive cardiac procedures: implications for outpatient catheterization, *J Am Coll Cardiol* 1997; **30**: 444–451.

122. Rich MW, Crecelius CA. Incidence, risk factors,

and clinical course of acute renal insufficiency after cardiac catheterization in patients 70 years of age or older. A prospective study, *Arch Intern Med* 1990; **150**:1237–1242.

123. Kahn JK, Rutherford BD, McConahay DR et al. High-dose contrast agent administration during complex coronary angioplasty, *Am Heart J* 1990; **120**:533–536.

124. Fontana GP. Minimally invasive cardiac surgery, *Chest Surg Clin N Am* 1998; **8**:871–890.

125. Goldstein DJ, Oz MC. Current status and future directions of minimally invasive cardiac surgery, *Curr Opin Cardiol* 1999; **14**:419–425.

126. Park JW. Interventional cardiology versus minimally invasive cardiac surgery, *Eur J Cardiothorac Surg* 1999; **16** (suppl 2):S117–S118.

127. Duhaylongsod FG. Minimally invasive cardiac surgery defined, *Arch Surg* 2000; **135**:296–301.

128. Mack MJ. Coronary surgery: off-pump and port-access, *Surg Clin North Am* 2000; **80**:1575–1591.

129. Mack M, Landreneau R. Minimally invasive cardiac surgery, *Semin Laparosc Surg* 1996; **3**:259–267.

130. Reichenspurner H, Welz A, Gulielmos V, Boehm D, Reichart B. Port-access cardiac surgery using endovascular cardiopulmonary bypass: theory, practice, and results, *J Card Surg* 1998; **13**:275–280.

131. Grossi EA, Zakow PK, Ribakove G et al. Comparison of post-operative pain, stress response, and quality of life in port access vs standard sternotomy coronary bypass patients, *Eur J Cardiothorac Surg* 1999; **16** (suppl 2): S39–S42.

132. Gaudino M, Santarelli P, Bruno P, Piancone FL, Possati G. Palliative coronary artery surgery in patients with severe non-cardiac diseases, *Am J Cardiol* 1997; **80:**1351–1352.

133. Burroughs AK, Matthews K, Qadiri M et al. Desmopressin and bleeding time in patients with cirrhosis, *Br Med J (Clin Res Ed)* 1985; **291**:1377–1381.

134. Moore RD, Smith CR, Lietman PS. Increased risk of renal dysfunction due to interaction of liver disease and aminoglycosides, *Am J Med* 1986; **80**:1093–1097.

135. Gentilini P. Cirrhosis, renal function and NSAIDs, *J Hepatol* 1993; **19**:200–203.

136. Smith CR, Moore RD, Lietman PS. Studies of risk factors for aminoglycoside nephrotoxicity, *Am J Kidney Dis* 1986; **8**:308–313.

137. Badalamenti S, Graziani G, Salerno F, Ponticelli C. Hepatorenal syndrome. New perspectives in pathogenesis and treatment, *Arch Intern Med* 1993; **153**:1957–1967.

138. Arroyo V, Gines P, Gerbes AL et al. Definition and diagnostic criteria of refractory ascites and hepatorenal syndrome in cirrhosis. International Ascites Club, *Hepatology* 196; **23**: 164–176.

139. Gines P, Berl T, Bernardi M et al. Hyponatremia in cirrhosis: from pathogenesis to treatment, *Hepatology* 1998; **28**:851–864.

140. Runyon BA. Management of adult patients with ascites caused by cirrhosis, *Hepatology* 1998; **27**:264–272.

141. Marelli A, Nardecchia L, De Gennaro F, Bodini P. Spontaneous bacterial peritonitis (SBP): prevalence and characteristics in a population of 314 cirrhotic patients evaluated at hospital admission, *Minerva Med* 1999; **90**:369–375.

142. Runyon BA. Care of patients with ascites, *N Engl J Med* 1994; **330**:337–342.

143. Fraser CL, Arieff AI. Hepatic encephalopathy, *N Engl J Med* 1985; **313**:865–873.

144. Butterworth RF. Complications of cirrhosis III. Hepatic encephalopathy, *J Hepatol* 2000; **32**:171–180.

145. Teran JC. Nutrition and liver diseases, *Curr Gastroenterol Rep* 1999; **1**:335–340.

146. Riordan SM, Williams R. Treatment of hepatic encephalopathy, *N Engl J Med* 1997; **337**: 473–479.

147. D'Amico G, Pagliaro L, Bosch J. The treatment of portal hypertension: a meta-analytic review, *Hepatology* 1995; **22**:332–354.

148. Sarin SK, Lamba GS, Kumar M, Misra A, Murthy NS. Comparison of endoscopic ligation and propranolol for the primary prevention of variceal bleeding, *N Engl J Med* 1999; **340**:988–993.

149. Lay CS, Tsai YT, Teg CY et al. Endoscopic variceal ligation in prophylaxis of first variceal bleeding in cirrhotic patients with high-risk esophageal varices, *Hepatology* 1997; **25**: 1346–1350.

150. Imperiale TF, Chalasani N. A meta-analysis of endoscopic variceal ligation for primary prophylaxis of esophageal variceal bleeding, *Hepatology* 2001; **33**:802–807.

151. DiCecco SR, Wieners EJ, Wiesner RH et al. Assessment of nutritional status of patients

with end-stage liver disease undergoing liver transplantation, *Mayo Clin Proc* 1989; **64**:95–102.

152. Rady MY, Ryan T, Starr NJ. Clinical characteristics of preoperative hypoalbuminemia predict outcome of cardiovascular surgery, *J Parenter Enteral Nutr* 1997; **21**:81–90.

153. Munoz SJ. Nutritional therapies in liver disease, *Semin Liver Dis* 1991; **11**:278–291.

154. Nompleggi DJ, Bonkovsky HL. Nutritional supplementation in chronic liver disease: an analytical review, *Hepatology* 1994; **19**:518–533.

155. Fan ST, Lo CM, Lai EC et al. Perioperative nutritional support in patients undergoing hepatectomy for hepatocellular carcinoma, *N Engl J Med* 1994; **331**:1547–1552.

156. Figueiredo FA, Dickson ER, Pasha TM et al. Utility of standard nutritional parameters in detecting body cell mass depletion in patients with end-stage liver disease, *Liver Transpl* 2000; **6**: 575–581.

157. Gupta TK, Chen L, Groszmann RJ. Pathophysiology of portal hypertension, *Baillières Clin Gastroenterol* 1997; **11**:203–219.

158. Martin PY, Gines P, Schrier RW. Nitric oxide as a mediator of hemodynamic abnormalities and sodium and water retention in cirrhosis, *N Engl J Med* 1998; **339**:533–541.

159. Mashford ML, Mahon WA, Chalmers TC. Studies of the cardiovascular system in the hypotension of liver failure, *N Engl J Med* 1962; **267**:1071–1074.

160. Bosch J, Pizcueta MP, Fernandez M et al. Hepatic, splanchnic and systemic haemodynamic abnormalities in portal hypertension, *Baillières Clin Gastroenterol* 1992; **6**:425–436.

161. Henriksen JH, Moller S. Haemodynamics and fluid retention in liver disease, *Ital J Gastroenterol Hepatol* 1998; **30**:320–332.

162. Moller S, Bendtsen F, Henriksen JH. Splanchnic and systemic hemodynamic derangement in decompensated cirrhosis, *Can J Gastroenterol* 2001; **15**:94–106.

163. Vallance P, Moncada S. Hyperdynamic circulation in cirrhosis: a role for nitric oxide? *Lancet* 1991; **337**:776–778.

164. Wiest R, Groszmann RJ. Nitric oxide and portal hypertension: its role in the regulation of intrahepatic and splanchnic vascular resistance, *Semin Liver Dis* 1999; **19**:411–426.

165. Hartleb M, Michielsen PP, Dziurkowska-Marek A. The role of nitric oxide in portal hyperten-

sive systemic and portal vascular pathology, *Acta Gastroenterol Belg* 1997; **60**:222–232.

166. Moller S, Christensen E, Henriksen JH. Continuous blood pressure monitoring in cirrhosis. Relations to splanchnic and systemic haemodynamics, *J Hepatol* 1997; **27**: 284–294.

167. Kowalski HJ, Abelmann WH. The cardiac output at rest in Laennec's cirrhosis, *J Clin Invest* 1953; **32**:1025–1033.

168. Guazzi M, Polese A, Magrini F, Fiorentini C, Olivari MT. Negative influences of ascites on the cardiac function of cirrhotic patients, *Am J Med* 1975; **59**:165–170.

169. Panos MZ, Moore K, Vlavianos P et al. Single, total paracentesis for tense ascites: sequential hemodynamic changes and right atrial size, *Hepatology* 1990; **11**:662–667.

170. Navasa M, Feu F, Garcia-Pagan JC et al. Hemodynamic and humoral changes after liver transplantation in patients with cirrhosis, *Hepatology* 1993; **17**:355–360.

171. Piscaglia F, Zironi G, Gaiani S et al. Systemic and splanchnic hemodynamic changes after liver transplantation for cirrhosis: a long-term prospective study, *Hepatology* 1999; **30**:58–64.

172. Henderson JM, Mackay GJ, Hooks M et al. High cardiac output of advanced liver disease persists after orthotopic liver transplantation, *Hepatology* 1992; **15**:258–262.

173. Hadengue A, Lebrec D, Moreau R et al. Persistence of systemic and splanchnic hyperkinetic circulation in liver transplant patients, *Hepatology* 1993; **17**:175–178.

174. Bernardi M, Fornale L, Di Marco C et al. Hyperdynamic circulation of advanced cirrhosis: a re-appraisal based on posture-induced changes in hemodynamics, *J Hepatol* 1995; **22**:309–318.

175. Bernardi M, Trevisani F, Fornale L et al. Renal sodium handling in cirrhosis with ascites: mechanisms of impaired natriuretic response to reclining, *J Hepatol* 1994; **21**:1116–1122.

176. Arroyo V, Gines P. Mechanism of sodium retention and ascites formation in cirrhosis, *J Hepatol* 1993; **17** (suppl 2):S24–S28.

177. Hampton WW, Townsend MC, Schirmer WJ, Haybron DM, Fry DE. Effective hepatic blood flow during cardiopulmonary bypass, *Arch Surg* 1989; **124**:458–459.

178. Cowan RE, Jackson BT, Grainger SL, Thompson

RP. Effects of anesthetic agents and abdominal surgery on liver blood flow, *Hepatology* 1991; **14**:1161–1166.

179. Ngai SH. Effects of anesthetics on various organs, *N Engl J Med* 1980; **302**:564–566.

180. Batchelder BM, Cooperman LH. Effects of anesthetics on splanchnic circulation and metabolism, *Surg Clin North Am* 1975; **55**:787–794.

181. Gelman S. General anesthesia and hepatic circulation, *Can J Physiol Pharmacol* 1987; **65**:1762–1779.

182. Gelman SI. Disturbances in hepatic blood flow during anesthesia and surgery, *Arch Surg* 1976; **111**:881–883.

183. Kenna JG. Immunoallergic drug-induced hepatitis: lessons from halothane, *J Hepatol* 1997; **26** (suppl 1):5–12.

184. Berghaus TM, Baron A, Geier A, Lamerz R, Paumgartner G. Hepatotoxicity following desflurane anesthesia, *Hepatology* 1999; **29**:613–614.

185. Ross JA, Monk SJ, Duffy SW. Effect of nitrous oxide on halothane-induced hepatotoxicity in hypoxic, enzyme-induced rats, *Br J Anaesth* 1984; **56**:527–533.

186. Takagi T, Ishii H, Takahashi H et al. Potentiation of halothane hepatotoxicity by chronic ethanol administration in rat: an animal model of halothane hepatitis, *Pharmacol Biochem Behav* 1983; **18** (suppl 1):461–465.

187. Gut J. Molecular basis of halothane hepatitis, *Arch Toxicol Suppl* 1998; **20**:3–17.

188. Walton B, Simpson BR, Strunin L et al. Unexplained hepatitis following halothane, *Br Med J* 1976; **1**: 1171–1176.

189. Lewis JH, Zimmerman HJ, Ishak KG, Mullick FG. Enflurane hepatotoxicity. A clinicopathologic study of 24 cases, *Ann Intern Med* 1983; **98**:984–992.

190. McEvedy BA, Shelly MP, Park GR. Anaesthesia and liver disease, *Br J Hosp Med* 1986; **36**:26–34.

191. Holt C, Csete M, Martin P. Hepatotoxicity of anesthetics and other central nervous system drugs, *Gastroenterol Clin North Am* 1995; **24**:853–874.

192. Hourani JM, Bellamy PE, Tashkin DP, Batra P, Simmons MS. Pulmonary dysfunction in advanced liver disease: frequent occurrence of an abnormal diffusing capacity, *Am J Med* 1991; **90**:693–700.

193. Fallon MB, Abrams GA. Pulmonary dysfunction in chronic liver disease, *Hepatology* 2000; **32**:859–865.

194. Castro M, Krowka MJ. Hepatopulmonary syndrome. A pulmonary vascular complication of liver disease, *Clin Chest Med* 1996; **17**:35–48.

195. Lange PA, Stoller JK. The hepatopulmonary syndrome, *Ann Intern Med* 1995; **122**:521–529.

196. King PD, Rumbaut R, Sanchez C. Pulmonary manifestations of chronic liver disease, *Dig Dis* 1996; **14**:73–82.

197. Moreau R, Hadengue A, Soupison T et al. Arterial and mixed venous acid-base status in patients with cirrhosis. Influence of liver failure, *Liver* 1993; **13**:20–24.

198. Keill RH, Keitzer WF, Nichols WK, Henzel J, DeWeese MS. Abdominal wound dehiscence, *Arch Surg* 1973; **106**:573–577.

199. Reitamo J, Moller C. Abdominal wound dehiscence, *Acta Chir Scand* 1972; **138**:170–175.

200. Irvin TT, Vassilakis JS, Chattopadhyay DK, Greaney MG. Abdominal wound healing in jaundiced patients, *Br J Surg* 1978; **65**:521–522.

201. Boyer TD. Preoperative and postoperative hepatic dysfunction. In: Zakim D, Boyer TD, eds, *Hepatology: A Textbook of Liver Disease*, 3rd edn, (Philadelphia: W. B. Saunders Company, 1996) 1912–1917.

202. Clarke RS, Doggart JR, Lavery T. Changes in liver function after different types of surgery, *Br J Anaesth* 1976; **48**:119–128.

203. Evans C, Evans M, Pollock AV. The incidence and causes of post-operative jaundice. A prospective study, *Br J Anaesth* 1974; **46**:520–525.

204. Collins JD, Bassendine MF, Ferner R et al. Incidence and prognostic importance of jaundice after cardiopulmonary bypass surgery, *Lancet* 1983; **1**:1119–1123.

205. LaMont JT, Isselbacher KJ. Post-operative jaundice, *N Engl J Med* 1973; **288**:305–307.

206. LaMont JT. Post-operative jaundice, *Surg Clin North Am* 1974; **54**:637–645.

207. Becker SD, LaMont JT. Post-operative jaundice, *Semin Liver Dis* 1988; **8**:183–190.

208. Molina EG, Reddy KR. Post-operative jaundice, *Clin Liver Dis* 1999; **3**:477–488.

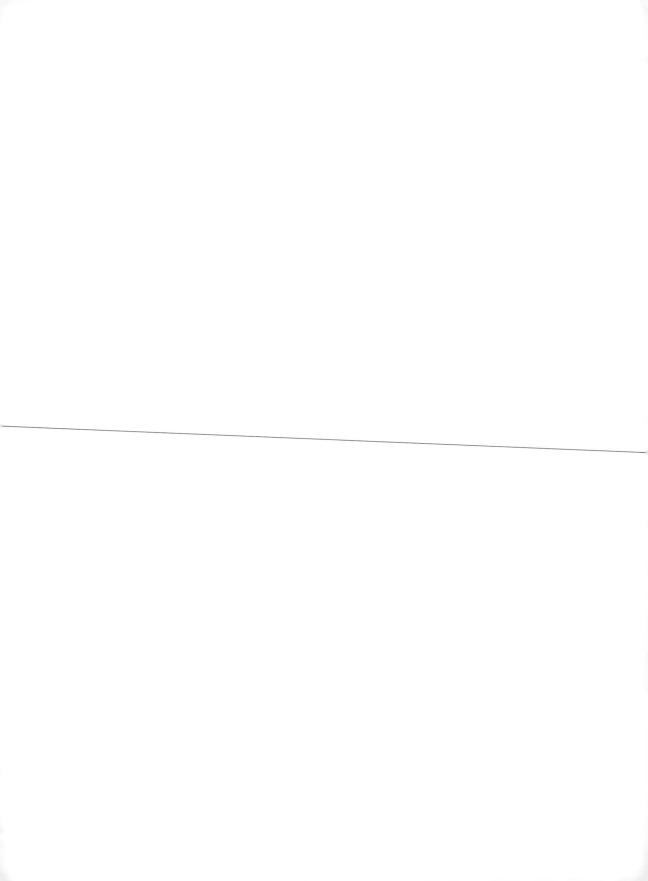

28

Renal function and high-risk coronary artery procedures

Stuart B Pett Jr

CONTENTS • Introduction • Acute renal failure • Chronic renal failure • Incidence and prevalence

INTRODUCTION

Acute and chronic renal failure are associated with a significant increase in the mortality and morbidity of myocardial infarction, catheter-based procedures and cardiac surgery. There is a high prevalence of cardiac disease in patients with chronic renal failure—particularly in those with dialysis-dependent end-stage renal disease. The number of patients with end-stage renal disease requiring revascularization is increasing. Acute renal failure can complicate any cardiac event or intervention. An understanding of the relationship between cardiac and renal function is important for those treating high-risk cardiac patients.

ACUTE RENAL FAILURE

Acute renal failure (ARF) is defined as a reversible loss of kidney function caused by some combination of pre-renal, post-renal or intrinsic renal factors. General risk factors associated with acute renal failure include pre-existing chronic renal failure, advanced age, diabetes, renal artery stenosis, atheroembolism, congestive heart failure, and hypotension [1–5].

A genetic predisposition to postoperative ARF may be present [6]. Drugs generally associated with ARF include non-steroidal anti-inflammatory drugs (NSAIDs), angiotensin-converting enzyme (ACE) inhibitors, radio-contrast agents [7, 8] aminoglycosides, or amphotericin B [9, 10].

Cardiac interventions that can cause ARF include aortic manipulation associated with cholesterol emboli [11, 12], anesthetic agents and surgical trauma. The relationship between renal function and cardiopulmonary bypass (CPB) is complex. Physiologic alterations related to the heart-lung machine include loss of pulsatile perfusion, hemolysis, hypothermia, and contact activation of several pathways including compliment, coagulation, and fibrinolysis. The net result of open heart surgery depends on the balance of factors that injure the kidney and those that improve perfusion [13–15]. The role of specific risk factors is debated. Diltiazem infusions have been reported to increase (ARDS) six-fold [16], while others have found diltiazem improves renal function [17]. Aprotinin has not been associated with significant nephrotoxicity [7]. Heparin bonded circuits may decrease renal dysfunction [18]. Although dopamine is known to increase renal blood flow, there is no evidence to support prophylactic, 'renal dose' dopamine to prevent ARF [10]. Some evidence even suggests that dopamine may actually exacerbate renal tubular injury in normal kidneys [19].

The pathophysiology of ARF usually involves the interaction of more than one risk factor. This is associated with imbalances in intra-renal flow and causes medullary hypoxia. Structural changes occur in the tubules and tubular cells slough into the lumen creating casts. This increases intra-tubular pressure and reduces glomerular filtration. Other changes include calcium leakage, release of reactive oxygen species, purine depletion, apoptosis and neutrophil infiltration [10].

ARF has been defined by any number of arbitrary parameters including absolute thresholds and relative changes in serum creatinine, alterations in creatinine clearance, and the need for dialysis (ARF-D). This lack of consensus, coupled with heterogeneous patient populations and a wide spectrum of interventions make risk stratification for the development of ARF problematic but possible [1–5]. The risk of ARF following myocardial infarction or cardiac catheterization/intervention in non-diabetic patients with normal kidney function is less than 1% [8, 20–23]. Depending on definition, the risk of ARF following coronary artery bypass grafting (CABG) ranges between 5–15% [2, 4, 5, 24, 25], and approximately 1% for ARF-D [1, 2, 4, 16, 24, 25]. The risk of postoperative ARF is dependent on the procedure and ranges from a low of 3.12% for isolated CABG to 12.75% for mitral valve-CABG combinations [24]. Counting all 230,000 cardiac procedures in the STS database, 5.31% developed ARF and 1.25% required dialysis [24]. The most critical factors in developing perioperative ARF are preoperative renal dysfunction, hypotension, duration of CPB and age [5].

ARF of any cause has a profound influence on outcome. Radiocontrast-induced ARF increases hospital mortality more than five-fold [26]. Pre-existing renal failure increases the probability of contrast-induced renal failure [27]. Patients who develop ARF following CABG have a 13.51 times greater chance of hospital mortality, and those developing ARF-D increase their odds of dying 17.35 times [24]. When all surgical procedures are considered, not just CABG, the risk of mortality from any degree of acute renal failure is 15.6% [24]. Putting ARF into perspective, the mortality odds ratio for perioperative ARF is exceeded by only the catastrophic complications of cardiac arrest, multi-system organ failure, and continuous coma [24]. The mortality odds ratio for ARF is even higher in the VA database at 27, and the morbidity odds ratio is 7.8 [28].

Management of patients with ARF begins with recognition of risk factors, prediction of individual patient risk, and prevention [29]. Modification of certain risk factors is possible, such as eliminating NSAIDs and correction of renal artery stenosis. Prehydration and the judicious use of non-ionic, iso-osmolar radiocontrast agents are important in diagnostic and catheter-based interventions—particularly in patients with CRF and diabetes [30]. Avoidance of hypotension is paramount. Prophylactic use of dopamine and aminophylline have little influence on kidney function in patients with pre-existing renal disease [27]. Initial reports suggest that pre-intervention oral administration of the antioxidant acetylcysteine (Mucomyst, AstraZeneca, Sweden) is associated with a significant reduction in the incidence of radio-contrast-induced renal failure [31].

Unproved but logical adjuncts to CPB are heparin bonded circuits [18] and pulsatile flow. Coronary artery bypass without CPB (OP-CAB) holds promise, but a clear demonstration of important clinical benefits is lacking. There is no compelling evidence that manitol, lasix, or dopamine, alone, have any role in ARF prevention [10]. Renal dose dopamine may in fact injure a normal kidney following cardiac surgery [19].

Kidney tubules, unlike cardiac or brain cells, can regenerate. The cornerstone of ARF treatment, therefore, is correction of inciting factors and physiologic support during recovery [32].

This consists of meticulous fluid and electrolyte balance, and careful titration of drugs relative to the degree of renal insufficiency [33]. Sodium bicarbonate, glucose-insulin infusions, and exchange resins are all important in maintaining homeostasis during renal healing. A systematic approach to diuretics with regard to pharmacokinetics is required [34]. Conflicting evidence exists on the individual therapeutic value of manitol, lasix, or dopamine [10], but a recent report has demonstrated significant improvement in both the intensity and duration of ARF if the three agents were infused simultaneously [35]. Promising investigational drugs include atrial naturetic peptide [29], inhibitors of endothelin, calcium channel antagonists, insulin-like growth factor I, and antibodies to ICAM-1 [10].

There is no agreement on when to start renal replacement therapy or what type to use (hemo vs peritoneal-dialysis) [36]. In the past, dialysis was avoided for a number of reasons. Fluid and electrolyte shifts were undesirable in an unstable patient and older dialysis membranes (cuprophane) were felt to exaggerate renal damage due to contact activation of neutrophils. Peritoneal dialysis and newer continuous therapies (veno-venous or veno-arterial) with more biocompatible membranes should reduce some of these concerns.

Finally, catheter-based interventions, and particularly surgical procedures should be delayed until bouts of ARF have resolved. Not infrequently, there is a moderate elevation in serum creatinine in patients following diagnostic catheterization. No study has formally addressed the question of how long to postpone further procedures. Pending definition of appropriate waiting periods, common sense dictates that adding further insult to the kidney will only complicate management and increase the risk of dialysis. There will obviously be individual situations where cardiac instability conflicts with delay, and careful analysis of risks and benefits is essential.

CHRONIC RENAL FAILURE

Chronic renal failure (CRF) and particularly dialysis-dependent end-stage renal disease (ESRD) significantly increase the risk of cardiac interventions [37]. The number of patients with ESRD requiring cardiac procedures is substantial and a large increase is anticipated during the next ten years. The National Institute of Diabetes and Digestive and Kidney Diseases projects that the annual incidence of ESRD in the US will rise from 98,952 new cases in 2000 to 176,667 by 2010 due largely to the increasing incidence of diabetes [38]. The prevalence of ESRD in the US is expected to increase from 372,407 in 2000 to 661,330 by 2010 not only because of the increase in ESRD incidence, but also from a decrease in dialysis mortality. Dialysis mortality is decreasing because of better anemia control, improved graft survival, and better dialysis techniques (switching from cuprophane to synthetic membranes). There has been a significant reduction in the overall annual mortality (first year) from 29.9% to 18.4% during the past decade. The death rate for ESRD patients over age 64, although decreasing, remains high at 28.9%. Despite improvements in mortality, the expected five-year survival of ESRD patients age 45–64 is only 40% and for those older than 64 years it drops to 15%. The average age and the prevalence of diabetes in ESRD patients is increasing. Cardiac disease accounts for nearly half of ESRD mortality, approximately three times that of infection. One in five deaths in ESRD are attributed to acute myocardial infarction. The absolute and relative numbers of ESRD patients requiring high-risk cardiac care is expected to increase dramatically during the next decade [38].

Patients undergoing coronary revascularization frequently present with some degree of renal failure, and patients with CRF frequently require coronary revascularization. Over 10,000 dialysis-dependent patients were revascularized between 1990 and 1995. The annualized revascularization rate tripled during the same period [39]. Renal failure and coronary artery disease are both associated with diabetes, hypertension, peripheral vascular disease, congestive heart failure, and advanced age. The cardiac status of patients with end-stage renal disease is further compromised by the vasculopathic state associated with dialysis. Patients with ESRD have hypertension, ventricular hypertrophy, abnormal fluid and electrolyte balance, hyperparathyroidism, dyslipidemias, hyperglycemia, hyperhomocystinuria, anemia, and abnormal vascular endothelial function [40, 41]. Coronary artery calcification is common and progressive in young adults with ESRD [42]. Clinical symptoms and cardiovascular risk profiles are not valid predictors of coronary artery disease (CAD) in diabetics with CRF [43, 44]. Renal insufficiency complicates the evaluation of diagnostic enzymes such as troponin [45, 46]. Further, the medical treatment CAD is compromised in patients with ESRD. The use of aspirin, ACE inhibitors, beta-blockers, platelet IIb/IIIa inhibitors and thrombolytics can be problematic in patients with ESRD [40, 47, 48]. Finally, nonphysiologic, three days per week dialysis intervals place greater stress on the heart, and is associated with greater fluid and electrolyte shifts than more frequent schedules [41].

The decision for cardiac intervention in dialysis patients is complex. Emergency procedures carry such a high risk that some authors deem them prohibitive. Consideration of elective interventions must be tempered by the knowledge that ESRD patients, even after revascularization, have significantly reduced life expectancy. The ability to technically achieve satisfactory revascularizations is inhibited by the magnitude and extent of coronary calcifications and the frequency of diffuse, small vessel disease. The durability of revascularization is adversely affected by the hypercoagulable state and pernicious lipid profile of ESRD patients. All considerations for revascularization must be made with the knowledge of the poor survival of ESRD patients following myocardial infarctions [41, 49].

INCIDENCE AND PREVALENCE

The prevalence of CRF in patients undergoing CABG depends on definitions—and there is no universally accepted definition of CRF. In the VA database, renal failure, as defined as serum creatinine levels of 1.5–3.0 mg/dL was noted in 13.9% of patients, but the prevalence decreased to 1.4% when the creatinine threshold for renal failure was defined as > 3.0 mg/dL. In the Society of Thoracic Surgeons (STS) database, 'renal failure' was found in 4.3% of CABG patients, with 0.94% of patients requiring preoperative dialysis. The prevalence of CRF increases in patients requiring cardiac valve surgery. In the VA database, 23.6% of valve patients have serum creatinine > 1.5 mg/dL. Around 10% of valve-CABG patients reported in the STS database have CRF [24].

Pre-existing chronic renal failure increases the risk of surgery. Mild elevations in creatinine can double and moderate to severe renal failure can more than triple hospital mortality in CABG patients [25, 50–53]. Renal failure is a significant independent mortality risk factor in patients requiring CABG following acute myocardial infarction [54]. The effect is even greater in valve patients where severe renal failure increases mortality six-fold [55]. Patients with elevated creatinine (> 3.0 mg/dL) who are not yet on dialysis appear to be at higher risk than those actually on dialysis [56]. Counting all cardiac surgery in the STS database, the univariate mortality odds ratio for CRF was 3.6 [24]. The mortality odds ratio for CRF exceeds other preoperative risk factors of reoperation, failed percutaneous coronary angioplasty (PTCA), congestive heart failure (CHF), and pulmonary hypertension. Only the ominous risk factors of early acute myocardial infarction and pre-op resuscitation have odds ratios higher than CRF [24]. In the large United States Renal Data System database, the raw in-hospital mortality for 7419 dialysis patients undergoing CABG procedures from 1978–1996 was 12.5%. A recent review of coronary bypass patients in New England also found that pre-existing CRF increases operative mortality three-fold [57].

In addition to increased mortality, morbidity and hospital stay are also increased by CRF [56, 58]. The odds ratio for any morbidity was doubled by pre-existing CRF [52, 58]. Complications include bleeding, respiratory complications, and other cardiac complications [56–59]. Surprisingly, increases in the rate of wound infections was not consistently recognized [57].

The indications for open-heart surgery in dialysis patients are uncertain. The large reference trials (VA Cooperative, CASS, European Cooperative) did not include patients with advanced renal disease. Extrapolation of indications to ESRD patients who have significantly increased operative mortality and materially decreased long-term survival is hazardous. It is simply not known whether CABG is indicated for an asymptomatic ESRD patient with triple-vessel disease and poor ventricular function. Over the past five years numerous publications from around the world document single institution experience with CABG in dialysis patients [56–82]. The futility of making clinical decisions based on isolated unadjusted death rates is amply demonstrated by the observation that hospital mortality in these 27 studies ranged from 0 to 29%! Given their personal experience, some authors concluded that the operative risk associated with CRF was insignificant or at least acceptable [40, 63, 64, 67–69, 72, 75, 83]. Others, however, felt that results were sufficiently alarming to justify a moratorium on CABG in certain subsets of kidney patients— the elderly, those requiring associated valve surgery, continued tobacco abuse, patients with functioning renal transplants or those requiring emergency procedures [66, 68, 70, 77, 78, 81, 84, 85]. Elective revascularizations of asymptomatic patients have been questioned based on the observation that long-term survival is not materially improved [70, 78]. Further, the scarcity of donor kidneys makes revascularization as a prerequisite for transplant listing uncertain [53].

If the indications for CABG are unclear, the indications for PTCA are even more uncertain [38, 39, 60, 76, 86–88]. Prior to 1995, there appeared to be a consensus that angioplasty was not warranted due to significant mortality, accelerated restenosis, and poor long-term results [87, 89–91]. Even in the new device era, the odds ratio for major adverse cardiac events (MACE) following PTCA in patients with ESRD is 3.41 [92]. Percutaneous transluminal coronary angioplasty mortality has been reported at 10.8% for CRF patients as compared to 1.8% in a matched cohort [92]. Long-term survival following PTCA is clearly compromised by CRF [61, 92]. It is unknown whether the suggestion that an increase in the utilization of coronary stents will have a material effect on results [93]. Despite publications of dismal results, more ESRD patients received PTCA during the period from 1990–1995 than CABG (5675 vs 4870) [39]. Percutaneous transluminal coronary angioplasty has also been accomplished in patients with functioning renal transplants [94]. Since 1995, several investigators attempted to compare PTCA with CABG in patients with ESRD [39, 60, 71, 74, 76, 80, 86]. Some found no hospital mortality in either group [71, 95], some with equal hospital mortalities ≤ 5% [76, 80], and others with significantly increased CABG mortality [39, 60, 74, 77]. Long-term, rather than procedural survival, however, may favor CABG over PTCA [86]. Attempts to predict the response of patients with ESRD to the various catheter-based interventions are ongoing [61, 96].

Comparisons based on comparisons of raw hospital mortality can lead to spurious conclusions. Recognized confounding co-morbidities affecting survival include older age, diabetes renal etiology, gender, ethnicity, and ESRD duration. According to the large United States Renal Data System database 7419 dialysis patients undergoing CABG between 1978 and 1995 had an unadjusted in-hospital mortality rate of 12.5% [39]. Dialysis patients undergoing PTCA during the same period had less than half the CABG mortality at 5.4%. When adjusted for co-morbidity in contemporary patients, however, the mortality odds ratio for CABG vs PTCA was 0.91 [39]. Despite a raw mortality for CABG being twice that of PTCA, when adjusted for concomitant risk factors, patients were more likely to survive CABG than PTCA.

The long-term survival and functional results of coronary revascularizations in dialysis patients are poor. Mortality at three years was between 20 and 40% [3, 63–65, 67, 69, 72, 73]. Event-free survival (freedom from death, myocardial infarction or repeat revascularization) is strikingly better for CABG than PTCA— 75% vs 20% at 12 months [76], 87% vs 40% at 18 months [80], 90% vs 18% at three years [71]. The risk of cardiac death following CABG was 85% of PTCA; in diabetic patients, the risk of death following CABG was 78% of PTCA. The risk of acute myocardial infarction following CABG was 37% of PTCA.

In summary, the procedural risk, perioperative mortality and morbidity, and long-term results following either PTCA or CABG are significantly worse in patients with ESRD. The unfavorable results have led a minority of authors to advocate significant restrictions on both procedures in ESRD patients. The majority of authors, however, suggest that the results are acceptable in many situations, particularly in view of their dismal alternatives [83, 86]. Meticulous perioperative care is required with intensive perioperative dialysis [62, 71, 97], careful attention to anticoagulation [98–100], and increased use of arterial grafts [62, 71, 73, 82]. Blunting the effects of cardiopulmonary bypass by pulsatile pumps, heparin bonded circuits [18], and off bypass procedures may be important [13, 82]. Cautious optimism exists that coronary stenting will also lead to improved results [92, 93]. Finally, it is clear that both surgeons and interventional cardiologists will be confronted with an increasing number of patients with ESRD in the future.

REFERENCES

1. Chertow GM, Lazarus JM, Christiansen CL et al. Preoperative renal risk stratification, *Circulation* 1997; **95**:878–884.
2. Conlon PJ, Stafford-Smith M, White WD et al. Acute renal failure following cardiac surgery, *Nephrology, Dialysis, Transplantation* 1999; **14**: 1158–1162.
3. Fortescue EB, Bates DW, Chertow GM. Predicting acute renal failure after coronary bypass surgery: cross-validation of two risk-stratification algorithms, *Kidney International* 2000; **57**:2594–2602.
4. Mangos GJ, Brown MA, Chan WY et al. Acute renal failure following cardiac surgery: incidence, outcomes and risk factors, *Australian & NZ J Med* 1995; **25**:284–289.
5. Suen WS, Mok CK, Chiu SW et al. Risk factors for development of acute renal failure (ARF) requiring dialysis in patients undergoing cardiac surgery, *Angiology* 1998; **49**:789–800.
6. Chew ST, Newman MF, White WD et al. Preliminary report on the association of apolipoprotein E polymorphisms, with postoperative peak serum creatinine concentrations in cardiac surgical patients, *Anesthesiology* 2000; **93**:325–331.
7. Lemmer JH Jr, Stanford W, Bonney SL et al. Aprotinin for coronary artery bypass grafting: effect on postoperative renal function, *Ann Thorac Surg* 1995; **59**:132–136.
8. Vlietstra RE, Nunn CM, Narvarte J, Browne KF. Contrast nephropathy after coronary angioplasty in chronic renal insufficiency, *Am Heart J* 1996; **132**:1049–1050.
9. Schneider M, Valentine S, Clarke GM, Newman MA, Peacock J. Acute renal failure in cardiac surgical patients, potentiated by gentamicin and calcium, *Anaesthesia & Intensive Care* 1996; **24**: 647–650.
10. Thadhani R, Pascual M, Bonventre JV. Acute renal failure, *N Engl J Med* 1996; **334**:1448–1460.
11. Otsubo H, Kaito K, Takahashi H et al. Cholesterol emboli following percutaneous transluminal coronary angioplasty as speculated by toe skin biopsy, *Internal Medicine* 1995; **34**:134–137.
12. Fraser I, Ihle B, Kincaid-Smity P. Renal failure due to cholesterol emboli, *Aust NZ J Med* 1991; **21**:418–421.

13. Ascione R, Lloyd CT, Underwood MJ, Gomes WJ, Angelini GD. On-pump versus off-pump coronary revascularization: evaluation of renal function, *Ann Thorac Surg* 1999; **68**:493–498.

14. Cartier R. Off-pump surgery and chronic renal insufficiency, *Ann Thorac Surg* 2000; **69**: 1995–1996.

15. de Moraes Lobo EM, Burdmann EA, Abdulkader RC. Renal function changes after elective cardiac surgery with cardiopulmonary bypass, *Renal Failure* 2000; **22**:487–497.

16. Young EW, Diab A, Kirsh MM. Intravenous diltiazem and acute renal failure after cardiac operations, *Ann Thorac Surg* 1998; **65**:1316–1319.

17. Amano J, Suzuki A, Sunamori M, Tofukuji M. Effect of calcium antagonist diltiazem on renal function in open heart surgery, *Chest* 1995; **107**:1260–1265.

18. Suehiro S, Shibata T, Sasaki Y et al. Heparin-coated circuits prevent renal dysfunction after open heart surgery, *Osaka City Med J* 1999; **45**:149–157.

19. Tang AT, El-Gamel A, Keevil B, Yonan N, Deiraniya AK. The effect of 'renal-dose' dopamine on renal tubular function following cardiac surgery: assessed by measuring retinol binding protein (RBP), *Eur J Cardio Thorac Surg* 1999; **15**:717–722.

20. Lepor NE. Radiocontrast nephropathy: the dye is not cast, *Rev Cardiovasc Med* 2000; **1**:43–54.

21. Lip GY, Rathore VS, Katira R, Singh SP, Won RD. Changes in renal function with percutaneous transluminal coronary angioplasty, *Int J Cardiol* 1999; **70**:127–131.

22. Malenka DJ, O'Rourke D, Miller MA et al. Cause of in-hospital death in 12,232 consecutive patients undergoing percutaneous transluminal coronary angioplasty. The Northern New England Cardiovascular Disease Study Group, *Am Heart J* 1999; **137**:632–638.

23. Rozenman Y, Gilon D, Zelingher J et al. Age- and gender-related differences in success, major and minor complication rates and the duration of hospitalization after percutaneous transluminal coronary angioplasty, *Cardiology* 1996; **87**: 396–401.

24. Data Analyses of the Society of Thoracic Surgeons National Cardiac Surgery Database. The Seventh Year—January 1998.

25. Mangano CM, Diamondstone LS, Ramsay JG et al. Renal dysfunction after myocardial revascularization: risk factors, adverse outcomes, and hospital resource utilization, *Ann Intern Med* 1998; **128**: 194–203.

26. Levy EM, Viscoli CM, Horwitz RI. The effect of acute renal failure on mortality. A cohort analysis, *JAMA* 1996; **275**:1489–1494.

27. Abizaid AS, Clark CE, Mintz GS et al. Effects of dopamine and aminophylline on contrast-induced acute renal failure after coronary angioplast in patients with preexisting renal insufficiency, *Am J Cardiol* 1999; **83**:260–263.

28. Chertow GM, Levy EM, Hammermeister KE, Grover F, Daley J. Independent association between acute renal failure and mortality following cardiac surgery, *Am J Med* 1998; **104**: 343–348.

29. Aronson S, Blumenthal R. Perioperative renal dysfunction and cardiovascular anesthesia: concerns and controversies, *J Cardiothorac Vasc Anesth* 1998; **12**:567–586.

30. Baumgart D, Haude M, George G et al. High-volume non-ionic dimeric contrast medium: first experiences during complex coronary interventions, *Catheterization & Cardiovascular Diagnosis* 1997; **40**:241–246.

31. Tepel M, van der Geit M, Schwarzfeld C, Liermann D, Zidek W. Prevention of radiographic-contrast-agent-induced reductions in renal function by acetylcysteine, *N Engl J Med* 2000; **343**:180–184.

32. Kellerman PS. Perioperative care of the renal patient, *Arch Intern Med* 1994; **154**:1674–1688.

33. Sutton RG. Renal considerations, dialysis, and ultrafiltration during CPB, *Int Anesthesiol Clin* 1996; **34**:165–176.

34. Brater DC. Diuretic therapy, *N Engl J Med* 1998; **339**:387–395.

35. Sirivella S, Gielchinsky I, Parsonnett V. Mannitol, furosemide and dopamine infusion in postoperative renal failure complicating cardiac surgery, *Ann Thorac Surg* 2000; **69**:501–506.

36. Murray P, Hall J. Renal replacement therapy for acute renal failure, *Am J Respir Crit Care Med* 2000; **162**:777–781.

37. Brooks MM, Jones RH, Bach RG et al. Predictors of mortality and mortality from cardiac causes in the bypass angioplasty revascularization investigation (BARI) randomized trial and registry. For the BARI Investigators, *Circulation* 2000; **101**: 2682–2689.

38. US Renal Data System: USRDS 2000 Annual Data Report: 2000 Atlas of ESRD in the United

States. The National Institutes of Health, National Institute of Diabetes and Digestive and Kidney Diseases, Bethesda MD, 2000.

39. Herzog CA, Ma JZ, Collins AJ. Long-term outcome of dialysis patients in the United States with coronary revascularization procedures. *Kidney Int* 1999; **56**:324–332.

40. Burke SW, Solomon AJ. Cardiac complications of end-stage renal disease, *Advances in Renal Replacement Therapy* 2000; **7**:210–219.

41. Herzog CA. Poor long-term survival of dialysis patients after acute myocardial infarction: bad treatment or bad disease? *Am J Kidney Dis* 2000; **35**:1217–1220.

42. Goodman WG, Goldin K, Kuizon BD et al. Coronary-artery calcification in young adults with end-stage renal disease who are undergoing dialysis, *N Engl J Med* 2000; **342**:1478–1483.

43. Koch M, Gradaus F, Schoebel FC, Leschke M, Grabensee B. Relevance of conventional cardiovascular risk factors for the prediction of coronary artery disease in diabetic on renal replacement therapy, *Nephrology, Dialysis, Transplantation* 1997; **12**:1187–1191.

44. Wizemann V. Coronary artery disease in dialysis patients, *Nephron* 1996; **74**:642–651.

45. Braun SL, Baum H, Neumeier D, Vogt W. Troponin T and troponin I after coronary artery bypass grafting: discordant results in patients with renal failure, *Clinical Chemistry* 1996; **42**: 781–783.

46. Ven Lente F, McErlean ES, DeLuca SA et al. Ability of troponins to predict adverse outcomes in patients with renal insufficiency and suspected acute coronary syndromes: a case-matched study, *J Am Coll Cardiol* 1999; **33**: 471–478.

47. Vaitkus PT. Current status of prevention, diagnosis, and management of coronary artery disease in patients with kidney failure, *Am Heart J* 2000; **139**:1000–1008.

48. Venkatesan J, Henrich WL. Cardiac disease in chronic uremia: management, *Advances in Renal Replacement Therapy* 1997; **4**:249–266.

49. Herzog CA, Ma JZ, Collins AJ. Poor long-term survival after acute myocardial infarction among patients on long-term dialysis, *N Engl J Med* 1998; **339**:799–805.

50. Anderson RJ, O'Brien M, MaWhinney S et al. Renal failure predisposes patients to adverse outcome after coronary artery bypass surgery,

51. Gardner TJ. Editorial Comment, *Circulation* 1997; **96**:II44–II45.

52. Grover F. Veterans Administration Continuous Improvement in Cardiac Surgery Program. August 2000, personal communication.

53. Rao SP, Lenkei S, Chu M, Bargman JM. The futility of pretransplant coronary bypass grafting in asymptomatic patients on peritoneal dialysis, *Peritoneal Dialysis International* 1998; **18**:485–488.

54. Lee JH, Murrell HK, Strony J et al. Risk analysis of coronary bypass surgery after acute myocardial infarction, *Surgery* 1997; **122**:675–681.

55. Anderson RJ, O'Brien M, MaWhinney S et al. Mild renal failure is associated with adverse outcome after cardiac valve surgery, *Am J Kidney Dis* 2000; **35**:1127–1134.

56. Durmaz I, Buket S, Atay Y et al. Cardiac surgery with cardiopulmonary bypass in patients with chronic renal failure, *J Thorac Cardiovasc Surg* 1999; **118**:306–315.

57. Liu JY, Birkmeyer NJ, Sanders JH et al. Risks of morbidity and mortality in dialysis patients undergoing coronary artery bypass surgery, *Circulation* (Online) 2000; **102**:2973–2977.

58. Hayashida N, Chihara S, Tayama E et al. Coronary artery bypass grafting in patients with mild renal insufficiency, *Japanese Circulation Journal* 2001; **65**:28–32.

59. Rao V, Weisel RD, Buth KJ et al. Coronary artery bypass grafting in patients with non-dialysis-dependent renal insufficiency, *Circulation* 1997; **96**:II38–II45.

60. Agirbasli M, Weintraub WS, Chang GL et al. Outcome of coronary revascularization in patients on renal dialysis, *Am J Cardiol* 200; **86**:395–399.

61. Asinger RW, Henry TD, Herzog CA, Paulsen PR, Kane RL. Clinical outcomes of PTCA in chronic renal failure: a case-control study for co-morbid features and evaluation of dialysis dependence, *J Invasive Cardiol* 2001; **13**:21–28.

62. Boran M, Gol MK, Sener E et al. Coronary artery bypass grafting in chronic renal dialysis patients: intensive perioperative dialysis and extensive usage of arterial grafts, *Eur J Cardio Thorac Surg* 1995; **9**:719.

63. Castelli P, Condemi AM, Munari M. Immediate and long-term results of coronary revasculariza-

tion in patients undergoing chronic hemodialysis, *Eur J Cardio Thorac Surg* 1999; **15**:51–54.

64. Christiansen S, Claus M, Philipp T, Reidemeister JC. Cardiac surgery in patients with end-stage renal failure, *Clinical Nephrology* 1997; **48**: 246–252.

65. Ferguson ER, Hudson SL, Diethelm AG et al. Outcome after myocardial revascularization and renal transplantation: a 25-year single-institution experience, *Annals of Surgery* 1999; **230**:232–241.

66. Franga DL, Kratz JM, Crumbley AJ et al. Early and long-term results of coronary artery bypass grafting in dialysis patients, *Ann Thorac Surg* 2000; **70**:813–818.

67. Frenken M, Krian A. Cardiovascular operations in patients with dialysis-dependent renal failure, *Ann Thorac Surg* 1999; **68**:887–893.

68. Horst M, Mehlhorn U, Hoerstrup SP, Suedkamp M, de Vivie ER. Cardiac surgery in patients with end-stage renal disease: 10-year experience, *Ann Thorac Surg* 2000; **69**:96–101.

69. Jahangiri M, Wright J, Edmondson S, Magee P. Coronary artery bypass graft surgery in dialysis patients, *Heart* 1997; **78**:343–345.

70. Khaitan L, Sutter FP, Goldman SM. Coronary artery bypass grafting in patients who require long-term dialysis, *Ann Thorac Surg* 2000; **69**:1135–1139.

71. Koyanagi T, Nishida H, Kitamura M et al. Comparison of clinical outcomes of coronary artery bypass grafting and percutaneous transluminal coronary angioplasty in renal dialysis patients, *Ann Thorac Surg* 1996; **61**:1793–1796.

72. Labrousse L, de Vincentiis C, Madonna F et al. Early and long-term results of coronary artery bypass grafts in patients with dialysis dependent renal failure, *Eur J Cardio Thorac Surg* 1999; **15**:691–696.

73. Nakayama Y, Sakata R, Ura M, Miyamoto TA. Coronary artery bypass grafting in dialysis patients, *Ann Thorac Surg* 1999; **68**:1257–1261.

74. Ohmoto Y, Ayabe M, Hara K et al. Long-term outcome of percutaneous transluminal coronary angioplasty and coronary artery bypass grafting in patients with end-stage renal disease, *Japanese Circulation J*, English Edition 1999; **63**:981–987.

75. Okada H, Tsukamoto I, Sugahara S et al. Does intensive perioperative dialysis improve the results of coronary artery bypass grafting in haemodialysed patients? *Nephrology, Dialysis, Transplantation* 1999; **14**:771–775.

76. Rinehart AL, Herzog CA, Collins AJ et al. A comparison of coronary angioplasty and coronary artery bypass grafting outcomes in chronic dialysis patients, *Am J Kidney Dis* 1995; **25**:281–290.

77. Rollino C, Formica M, Minelli M et al. Outcome of dialysis patients submitted to coronary revascularization, *Renal Failure* 2000; **22**: 605–611.

78. Samuels LE, Sharma S, Morris RJ et al. Coronary artery bypass grafting in patients with chronic renal failure: a reappraisal, *J Cardiac Surg* 1996; **11**:128–135.

79. Sezgin A, Mercan S, Tasdelen A, Atalay H, Aslamaci S. Open heart surgery in patients with chronic renal failure, *Transplantation Proceedings* 1998; **30**:784–785.

80. Simsir SA, Kohlman-Trigoboff D, Flood R, Lindsay J, Smith BM. A comparison of coronary artery bypass grafting and percutaneous transluminal coronary angioplasty in patients on hemodialysis, *Cardiovascular Surgery* 1998; **6**: 500–505.

81. Suehiro S, Shibata T, Sasaki Y et al. Cardiac surgery in patients with dialysis-dependent renal disease, *Ann Thorac Cardiovas Surg* 1999; **5**:376–381.

82. Tanaka H, Suzuki K, Narisawa T et al. Coronary artery bypass grafting in dialysis patients, *Jap J Thorac Cardiovas Surg* 2000; **48**: 703–707.

83. Fang LST. Commentary on 'Coronary artery bypass grafting in patients with chronic renal failure', *J Card Surg* 1996; **11**:134–135.

84. Christiansen S, Splittgerber FH, Marggraf G et al. Results of cardiac operations in five kidney transplant patients, *Thoracic & Cardiovascular Surgeon* 1997; **45**:75–77.

85. Mitruka SN, Griffith BP, Kormos RL et al. Cardiac operations in solid-organ transplant recipients, *Ann Thorac Surg* 1997; **64**:1270–1278.

86. Chertow GM, Normand SLT, Silva LR, McNeil BJ. Survival after acute myocardial infarction in patients with end-stage renal disease: results from the cooperative cardiovascular project, *Am J Kidney Dis* 2000; **35**:1044–1051.

87. Cruz DN, Bia MJ. Coronary revascularization in patients on dialysis. What treatment option should we choose: *ASAIO Journal* 1996; **42**: 139–141.

88. Herzog CA. The optimal method of coronary revascularization in dialysis patients: choosing between a rock and a hard place. *Int J Artificial Organs* 2000; **23**:215–218.

89. Ahmed WH, Shubrooks SJ, Gibson CM, Baim DS, Bittle JA. Complications and long-term outcome after percutaneous coronary angioplasty in chronic hemodialysis patients, *Am Heart J* 1994; **128**:252–255.

90. Kahn JK, Rutherford BD, McConahay DR et al. Short- and long-term outcome of percutaneous transluminal coronary angioplasty in chronic dialysis patients, *Am Heart J* 1990; **119**:484–498.

91. Reusser LM, Osborn LA, White HJ, Sexson R, Crawford MH. Increased morbidity after coronary angioplasty in patients on chronic hemodialysis, *Am J Cardiol* 1994; **73**:965–967.

92. Rubenstein MH, Harrell LC, Sheynberg BV et al. Are patients with renal failure good candidates for percutaneous coronary revascularization in the new device era? *Circulation* (Online) 2000; **102**: 2966–2972.

93. Le Feuvre C, Dambrin G, Helft G et al. Comparison of clinical outcome following coronary stenting or balloon angioplasty in dialysis versus non-dialysis patients, *Am J Cardiol* 2000; **85**:1365–1368.

94. Conte FJ, Korr KS, Katz AS, Sadaniantz A. Managing acute myocardial infarction in a renal transplant recipient, *Cardiology* 1996; **87**: 257–259.

95. Sanai T, Kimura G, Inenaga T et al. Efficacy of percutaneous transluminal coronary angioplasty for patients no hemodialysis. Comparison with those not no dialysis, *Am J Nephrol* 1999; **19**:38–44.

96. Lacson RC, Ohno-Machado L. Major complications after angioplasty in patients with chronic renal failure: a comparison of predictive models, *Proc AMIA Symp* 2000: 457–461.

97. Kubota T, Miyata A, Hirota K, Koizumi S, Ohba H. Continuous haemodiafiltration during and after CPB in renal failure patients, *Can J Anesth* 1997; **44**:1182–1186.

98. Akpek EA, Donmez A, Erol E, Sekerci S, Arslan G. Heparin and protamine requirements of patients in chronic renal failure, *Transplantation Proceedings* 1998; **30**:805–806.

99. O'Connor CJ, McCarthy R, Barnes S, Tuman KJ. The effect of chronic renal failure on plasma aprotinin levels during cardiac surgery, *Anesthesia & Analgesia* 1997; **85**:763–765.

100. Westphal K, Martens S, Strouhal U et al. Heparin-induced thrombocytopenia type II: perioperative management using danaparoid in a coronary artery bypass patients with renal failure, *Thoracic & Cardiovas Surg* 1997; **45**:318–320.

29

High-risk coronary interventions in diabetic patients

Steven P Sedlis and Jeffrey D Lorin

CONTENTS • **Introduction** • **Epidemiology** • **Outcomes in diabetics with myocardial infarction** • **Outcomes in diabetics with unstable angina** • **Pathophysiology of coronary artery disease in diabetics** • **Diabetes as a risk factor for PTCA** • **Diabetes as a risk factor for CABG** • **Randomized trials of CABG versus PTCA: relevance to high-risk diabetics** • **Insights from the AWESOME Study**

INTRODUCTION

The rising incidence of diabetes throughout the world is leading to an upsurge in coronary artery disease morbidity and mortality of epidemic proportions [1–6]. Dealing with the manifestations of coronary artery disease in diabetics poses a challenge to public health authorities and clinicians and has been the subject of numerous recent conferences, papers and reviews [4, 7]. This chapter will focus on the role of revascularization in the management of the high-risk diabetic with coronary artery disease. In particular we will address the controversy arising from the finding that diabetics with multi-vessel coronary artery disease undergoing coronary artery bypass graft surgery (CABG) in the randomized arm of the landmark NHLBI BARI study had a lower mortality than similar patients randomized to balloon angioplasty (PTCA) [8, 9] (Fig. 29.1). This finding continues to have a major impact on guidelines and recommendations for revascularization in diabetics [10–12], however the relevance of BARI to contemporary practice is now

being questioned. Current practice guidelines, based on the BARI findings, still favor CABG over PTCA for diabetics with multi-vessel disease, but revascularization techniques have changed markedly in the decade after the

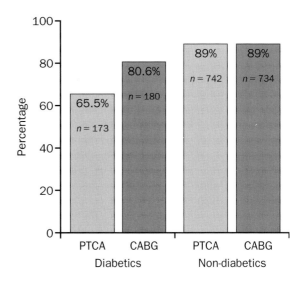

Figure 29.1 The BARI Study: 5 year survival.

completion of BARI. Furthermore, there have also been changes in the medical management of diabetic patients. In this chapter we will review recent advances in basic and clinical science and offer our opinion as to how new findings should influence rational decision-making regarding revascularization options for high-risk diabetic patients.

EPIDEMIOLOGY

The American Diabetes Association estimates that 15.7 million people in the US (5.9% of the population) have diabetes [13]. This figure includes 5.4 million people with sub-clinical diabetes who are not aware that they have the disease [13]. Nearly 95% of the diabetics in the US have type II diabetes, which is associated with obesity, sedentary lifestyle and aging [13]. Diabetes is the seventh leading cause of death (sixth-leading cause of death by disease) in the US [13]. Based on death certificate data, diabetes contributed to 198,140 deaths in 1996 [13]. The incidence of diabetes is nearly two-fold greater in certain high-risk ethnic groups including African-Americans, Latinos and Native Americans, but there is evidence that the incidence of diabetes is increasing in both high-risk and low-risk populations [3, 5, 13, 14]. This increased incidence of diabetes appears to be due to modifiable factors such as obesity and sedentary lifestyles as well as to the aging of the population [2, 4, 13, 15]. Worldwide, there were an estimated 124 million individuals with diabetes (97% type II) in 1997 and this figure is estimated to rise to 210 million by 2010 [1].

These demographic data are a source of growing concern for cardiologists, cardiac surgeons and other physicians dealing with diabetic patients since diabetics have a higher incidence of coronary artery disease than non-diabetics, and diabetics with established coronary artery disease have a far worse outcome than non-diabetics with coronary artery disease. For example, a large epidemiologic study recently conducted in Finland compared the seven-year incidence of myocardial infarction incidence among 1059 diabetic subjects with that of 1373 age-matched non-diabetic subjects. The risk of myocardial infarction (MI) among diabetics without known coronary artery disease (20.2%) was similar to the risk of myocardial infarction among non-diabetics with previous myocardial infarction (18.8%) and was far higher than the 3.5% risk of myocardial infarction among non-diabetics without known coronary artery disease [16]. Furthermore, the risk of cardiac mortality in diabetics without known cardiac disease was similar to that of non-diabetics with prior myocardial infarction even after adjusting for age, sex, total cholesterol, hypertension, and smoking [16]. Similar findings have been reported in other populations including the 3132 diabetics followed in a prospective cohort study of 91,285 US male physicians [17]. Diabetes confers an added risk in populations at high risk of myocardial infarction such as South Asians [18] and in other populations throughout the world [15, 19–21].

A recent analysis of demographic data from the US suggests that whereas mortality from coronary artery disease has dropped sharply in non-diabetics it has not changed significantly in diabetics. Representative cohorts of subjects with and without diabetes enrolled in the First National Health and Nutrition Examination Survey (NHANES I) were followed up prospectively for an average of 8 to 9 years. Outcomes were evaluated in 9639 subjects enrolled in NHANES I between 1971 and 1975 and in 8463 subjects enrolled in the NHANES I Epidemiologic Follow-up Survey between 1982 and 1984. Changes in mortality rates per 1000 person-years for all causes, heart disease, and ischemic heart disease for the 1982–1984 cohort were compared with the 1971–1975 cohort. Age-adjusted heart disease mortality fell by 36.4% in non-diabetic men and by 27% in non-diabetic women. In contrast, age-adjusted heart disease mortality in diabetic men fell only slightly (13.1%) and actually rose by 23% in diabetic women [22].

OUTCOMES IN DIABETICS WITH MYOCARDIAL INFARCTION

The major reason for the dismal prognosis of diabetics with heart disease relates to the high mortality from myocardial infarction [20, 23–30]. In the Framingham study, for example, both in-hospital mortality and one-year mortality were significantly higher in diabetics than in non-diabetics after a first myocardial infarction [23]. The reason for this disparity in outcome is still not completely understood. Hyperglycemia itself, even 'stress' hyperglycemia in patients not previously known to be diabetic worsens the short-term outcome of myocardial infarction [31, 32]. Abnormalities of autonomic function [33] and adverse effects of sulfonylurea drug therapy [34] have been associated with mortality. The increased incidence of silent ischemia in diabetics may predispose diabetics to present to the hospital later in the course of infarction and so derive less benefit from therapeutic interventions [35]. Studies from the pre-thrombolytic era suggested that diabetics have a higher incidence of left ventricular dysfunction and heart failure despite similar infarct size compared to non-diabetics [36, 37]. More recent studies suggest that an excess of heart failure remains an important cause of morbidity and mortality in diabetics following myocardial infarction even in the current era [38, 39].

Thrombolytic drugs improve the prognosis of diabetics with myocardial infarction, but mortality remains higher than in non-diabetics [40–47]. The adverse effects of diabetes are still evident in relatively recent trials of thrombolytics. In the Thrombolysis and Angioplasty in Myocardial Infarction (TAMI) trial diabetics ($n = 148$) treated with thrombolytics had an 11% mortality compared to 6% for non-diabetics ($n = 923$), but this difference was no longer significant after adjustment for baseline clinical and angiographic variables [40]. Angiographic patency rates were similar in both groups [40]. The larger and more recent Global Utilization of Streptokinase and Tissue Plasminogen Activator for Occluded Coronary Arteries (GUSTO 1) study included 5944 patients with diabetes and 34,888 patients without diabetes [44]. Mortality at 30 days was 12.5% in insulin treated diabetics, 9.7% in non-insulin treated diabetics and 6.2% in non-diabetics [44]. The effect of diabetes on mortality was independently significant after adjustment for baseline variables and remained significant at one-year follow-up [44].

Other advances in adjuvant pharmacologic therapy have also improved the outcomes of diabetics with myocardial infarction. Recent data from the GISSI-3 investigators suggests that diabetics with acute myocardial infarction derive particularly great benefit from ACE inhibition [48, 49]. A retrospective analysis of 2790 diabetics randomized to treatment with lisinopril (2.5 to 5 up to 10 mg/day) begun within 24 hours of infarction and continuing for six weeks vs placebo showed that mortality at six weeks was reduced from 12.4% to 8.7%. This treatment effect was sustained at six months (reduction in mortality from 16.1% to 12.9%) despite discontinuation of the ACE inhibitor at six weeks. The treatment effect of ACE inhibitors seen in diabetics was significantly higher than the effect seen in non-diabetics [49]. Intensive treatment with insulin may also be very beneficial for diabetics in the setting of myocardial infarction [50–52]. The Diabetes Mellitus Insulin Glucose Infusion in Acute Myocardial Infarction (DIGAMI) study compared the outcome of 306 diabetics with acute myocardial infarction treated with an intensive regimen of insulin and glucose followed by multidose insulin treatment to the outcome of 314 diabetics who received standard treatment. There was an absolute decrease in mortality of 11% in the insulin treated group that persisted for at least $3\frac{1}{2}$ years [50–52].

Primary PTCA and stenting appear to improve the prognosis for diabetic patients with acute myocardial infarction [53–55]. There is little randomized data however evaluating current interventional therapies. In the GUSTO-IIB angioplasty substudy for example, only 8.6% of diabetics and 6.7% of non-diabetics were treated with stents and glycoprotein IIb/IIIa receptor blockers were not used at all [53]. Nevertheless, at 30 days there was a trend towards a reduction in the combined end-point of death, recurrent myocardial infarction and stroke in the 81 diabetics randomized to angioplasty compared to the 96 diabetics randomized to alteplase [53]. Data from the recently completed Controlled Abciximab and Device Investigation to Lower Late Angioplasty Complications (CADILLAC) study which evaluated the effects of current design stents and glycoprotein IIb/IIIa receptor blockers for therapy of acute myocardial infarction [28] were presented in abstract form at the March 2001 Scientific Sessions of the American College of Cardiology [56]. The incidence of ischemic target vessel revascularization (TVR) and major adverse cardiac events (MACE) at six months was significantly decreased in 184 diabetics randomized to stenting with the ACS multilink stent as compared to 162 diabetics treated with balloon alone (17.3% and 20.4% vs 7.1% and 14.1% respectively) [56]. There was no significant effect on mortality and surprisingly there was no additive benefit of treatment with abciximab in this study [56].

Importantly, revascularization does seem to benefit diabetics with myocardial infarction complicated by cardiogenic shock. A recent report from the SHOCK (SHould we emergently revascularize Occluded Coronaries for cardiogenic shocK) trial registry showed that whereas overall in-hospital mortality in the setting of shock was higher for diabetics than for non-diabetics, diabetics derived a survival benefit from revascularization with either CABG or PTCA similar to that of non-diabetics [57]. Survival for diabetics in shock who underwent revascularization was 55% versus 19% without revascularization [57]. These findings support a role for percutaneous intervention in the management of the most critically ill and high-risk diabetic patients.

OUTCOMES IN DIABETICS WITH UNSTABLE ANGINA

Mortality in unstable angina is not as high as in myocardial infarction, but both short-term and long-term mortality remains higher in diabetics than in non-diabetics [26, 58, 59]. Most studies of outcomes in diabetics with unstable angina are relatively small, but the recently completed OASIS (Organization to Assess Strategies for Ischemic Syndromes) registry confirmed the adverse effect of diabetes on prognosis in a large multi-national population [26]. This study enrolled 8013 patients including 1718 diabetics. Patients with unstable angina or non-Q wave myocardial infarction hospitalized in six different countries between 1995 and 1996 were prospectively followed; mortality at two years among the diabetics (18%) was substantially higher than among non-diabetics (10%). These data may not fully reflect the outcomes achieved with current therapies since there was a low utilization of angiography (50%) in this study, and only 18% of patients underwent PTCA. More recent data from the Platelet Receptor Inhibition in Ischemic Syndrome Management in Patients Limited by Unstable Signs and Symptoms (PRISM-PLUS) study suggests that current therapies including revascularization and use of glycoprotein IIb/IIIa inhibitors are particularly beneficial for diabetics with acute coronary syndromes [60]. This study enrolled 1570 patients who were randomized to treatment with heparin plus tirofiban or heparin alone prior to angiography and definitive therapy. Approximately 23% of patients in both groups were diabetic. At 180 days the incidence of death or MI in diabetics treated with tirofiban was 11.2% versus 19.2% in diabetics treated with heparin, $p = 0.03$). Tests for quantitative interaction between tirofiban therapy and diabetic status were significant confirming that diabetic patients with unstable angina derive particular benefit from treatment with glycoprotein IIb/IIIa inhibitors.

PATHOPHYSIOLOGY OF CORONARY ARTERY DISEASE IN DIABETICS

Recent advances in basic understanding of the pathophysiology of coronary artery disease in diabetics explain some of the progress that has been made in dealing with these patients and promises to lead to more rational therapies for this high-risk population. In particular, new insights related to the pathophysiology of atherosclerosis and thrombosis in diabetics are relevant to both surgical and percutaneous coronary interventions in these patients.

The vascular biology of atherosclerosis differs in diabetic patients as compared to non-diabetic patients. Conditions commonly associated with type II diabetes, such as sedentary lifestyle, obesity, hypertension and dyslipidemia in addition to the chronic exposure of the vascular tissue to supernormal levels of glucose and insulin lead to a more diffuse and a more rapidly progressive expression of atherosclerosis and a propensity towards thrombosis. Therefore, the patient with diabetes and coronary artery disease may require a different therapeutic approach than the non-diabetic patient. Elevated levels of glucose in the blood cause alterations in the composition, size and concentration of the various lipoproteins. Hyperglycemia also leads to endothelial cell dysfunction, and a hypercoagulable state. Each stage of atherosclerosis and thrombosis is altered and enhanced by chronically elevated levels of glucose and/or insulin.

Dyslipidemia

Patients with type II diabetes are predisposed to the development of atherosclerosis despite normal levels of low density lipoprotein (LDL) due to elevated levels of triglyceride and low levels of circulating high-density lipoprotein (HDL). Patients with poorly controlled insulin-dependent diabetes often have elevated triglycerides, low HDL, and mildly elevated LDL. In the absence of other lipid disorders, tight con-trol of blood sugar in type I diabetes results in normalized lipoprotein levels [61].

Insulin resistance and insulin deficiency both result in elevated hepatic concentrations of free-fatty acids and glucose leading to increased hepatic production and secretion of athero-genic large triglyceride-rich very-low-density lipoproteins (VLDL) [62] reflected in increased concentrations of circulating triglycerides. In addition diabetes is associated with reduced activity of endothelium-bound lipoprotein lipase (LPL) and reduced peripheral metabolism of VLDL, which elevates VLDL and triglyceride levels further [63].

Elevated circulating triglyceride leads to an increased transfer of triglyceride to HDL via cholesterol ester transfer protein. Increased activity of cholesterol ester transfer protein is observed in both type I and type II diabetes [64, 65]. High-density lipoprotein enriched in triglyceride is more vulnerable to catabolism by liver enzymes [66]. Decreased LPL activity results in decreased HDL synthesis. Thus diabetics have reduced levels of HDL due to both decreased production and increased breakdown.

Elevated levels of circulating large VLDL particles are associated with higher concentrations of small dense low density lipoproteins which are linked to a high risk of myocardial infarction and coronary artery disease [67, 68].

Total cholesterol and LDL cholesterol levels are not significantly different in the type II diabetic and the non-diabetic populations [69, 70]. Although LDL levels are not elevated in diabetics, hyperglycemia leads to glycation of apolipoproteins, creating a low density lipoprotein more susceptible to oxidation [71, 72]. Glycosylation of LDL results in impaired clearance of LDL via the hepatic LDL receptor and augments uptake of LDL by monocyte-derived macrophages leading to the formation of foam cells [73, 74]. Enhanced LDL oxidation and foam cell formation are critical in the early stages of the formation of atherosclerosis.

Thus, low HDL levels, elevated levels of small dense LDL, LDL that is more vulnerable to oxidation and possibly elevated levels of triglyceride all play an important role in accelerated atherosclerosis in the diabetic patient.

Altered coagulation and hemostasis

Diabetes is associated with a hypercoagulable state. Chronically elevated glucose levels result in alterations in fibrinolysis, elevated levels of clotting factors and increased platelet activation and aggregation.

In type II diabetes, there is an increase in the plasma activity of the plasminogen activator inhibitor type 1 (PAI-1), tilting the balance of the endogenous fibrinolytic system toward thrombosis. Plasminogen activator inhibitor type 1 plays a major role in the regulation of the endogenous fibrinolysis. Increased expression of PAI-1 by cultured human umbilical vein endothelial cells has been shown to occur in response to exposure to high concentrations of glucose. This results in reduced fibrinolytic potential of endothelial cells and may predispose to coronary thrombosis and myocardial infarction [75].

Hyperinsulinemia as a result of insulin resistance is characteristic of type II diabetes. Hyperinsulinemia includes elevated levels of both insulin and insulin precursors such as proinsulin and its split products (65–66 split and 32–33 split proinsulins). Insulin precursors normally contribute 10–20% to total insulin activity [76, 77]. In hyperinsulinemia, the precursors may contribute three times as much to total insulin activity [78–80]. Proinsulin levels are increased due to increased production in the pancreas and decreased conversion of proinsulin to insulin in the patient with NIDDM. Elevated levels of insulin contribute to the prothrombotic state observed in diabetics since insulin has been shown to be an important stimulant to the synthesis of PAI-1. Insulin precursors are also important in the regulation of PAI-1 synthesis [81–83]. A clinical trial comparing proinsulin to insulin had to be discontinued when there were six myocardial infarctions

out of 73 patients in the proinsulin group. There were no myocardial infarctions in the 68 patients receiving insulin [84]. Thus elevated proinsulin, endogenous or exogenous, may lead to elevated levels of PAI-1 predisposing to myocardial infarction.

Elevated levels of fibrinogen, factor VII, von Willebrand factor, and thrombin–antithrombin III complex (TAT) have been described in diabetic patients [85–87]. These factors are also associated with a prothrombotic state.

Altered platelet function occurs in diabetic patients resulting in increased platelet adhesion and aggregation [88, 89]. Increased platelet-dependent thrombin generation, a measure of hypercoagulability, is observed in diabetics as compared to non-diabetics. Within the diabetic population there is increased platelet-dependent thrombin generation in the poorly controlled diabetics as compared to the diabetics with good glycemic control [90]. There appears to be a graded risk of enhanced platelet-mediated thrombogenesis with increasing levels of glucose in diabetics [91].

Thus the combination of impaired fibrinolysis, elevated levels of coagulation factors and increased platelet aggregation and adhesion are likely important factors explaining the increased incidence of coronary thrombosis and myocardial infarction in diabetics.

Endothelial dysfunction

Endothelial cell dysfunction plays a critical role in the pathogenesis of atherosclerosis and thrombosis. Endothelial dysfunction leads to altered vasomotor tone, impaired anticoagulation, enhanced leukocyte binding and recruitment, and increased endothelial permeability. Endothelial dysfunction in diabetics may be mediated by intracellular signaling resulting from activation of protein kinase C, oxidative stress and overproduction of certain growth factors and cytokines [92, 93].

Endothelial dysfunction can be demonstrated in diabetic animal models by an impairment of endothelium-dependent vasorelaxation [94, 95]. Hyperglycemia has been shown in animal models to cause impaired vasodilation in response to acetylcholine. Cyclo-oxygenase inhibitors restore normal vasodilation in response to acetylcholine, suggesting a vasoconstricting prostanoid such as thromboxane A_2 and prostaglandin F_2 alpha may be involved [96]. Elevated glucose acting via protein kinase C has been implicated as being at least partly responsible for the release of these prostanoids [97].

Hyperglycemia generates reactive oxygen species (ROS), which play an important role in atherosclerosis [98]. Reactive oxygen species are produced in all aerobic cells. Reactive oxygen species include free radicals (molecules with unpaired electrons including superoxide anion (O_2^-), nitric oxide (NO), and lipid radicals). Other reactive oxygen species that are not free radicals but also have oxidizing effects include molecular oxygen (O_2) and hydrogen peroxide (H_2O_2). Overproduction of ROS or underproduction of antioxidant defense mechanisms is referred to as oxidant stress and leads to the oxidation of vital macromolecules including lipids, proteins, carbohydrates and DNA. Oxidant stress has been shown to alter endothelial cell function. Nitric oxide (NO), a potent vasodilator, may be inactivated by superoxide and other reactive oxygen species leading to reduced bioavailability of nitric oxide and resulting in vasoconstriction and endothelial dysfunction. Impaired endothelium-dependent vasodilation in the coronary circulation predicts adverse cardiovascular events [99].

Under normal conditions, endothelial cells maintain fluid homeostasis in the vascular space by producing endothelial derived relaxing factor prostacyclin (PGI_2), adenosine and by maintaining a balance between production of plasminogen activator inhibitor (PAI-1) and tissue plasminogen activator (t-PA). Normal endothelium function results in attenuation of thrombin formation and inhibition of local platelet activation and aggregation. Diabetes in contrast, is characterized by a prothrombotic state due to endothelial dysfunction with decreased activity of NO, prostacyclin and increased activity of PAI-1 [75, 100, 101].

Hyperglycemia and oxidative stress result in endothelial dysfunction characterized by the appearance of cell surface adhesion molecules, enhanced adherence of monocytes, and the production of monocyte chemo-attractant protein-1 via activation of the nuclear transcription factor Kappa B (nuclear signaling) [102–104]. Enhanced monocyte-endothelial cell adherence in diabetics is reflected by an increased expression in E-Selectin (ELAM), intercellular cell adhesion molecule-1 (ICAM-1), and vascular cell adhesion molecule-1 (VCAM-1) [105]. These mechanisms create an opportunity for leukocyte adhesion and migration into the sub-endothelial space. A low-grade chronic inflammatory state persists and this may lead to progressive atherosclerosis and/or thrombosis [106].

Hyperglycemia leads to protein glycation, which alters the permeability of the endothelial basement membrane. Increased permeability of the basement membrane allows for increased lipoprotein deposition and enhanced macrophage recruitment. This expedites foam cell development in the sub-endothelial space [107]. Cultured human endothelial cells exposed to elevated levels of glucose have delayed replication and accelerated cell death [108].

Vascular remodeling

Intravascular ultrasound has shown that early atherosclerosis in coronary arteries results in a focal compensatory artery enlargement at the site of atherosclerosis. The lumen is not reduced and this cannot be detected by standard coronary angiography. It is not until the plaques grow large enough to impinge on the lumen that a reduction in lumen area occurs [109–111]. Vavuranakis and associates compared atherosclerotic coronary arteries in diabetics versus non-diabetics by intravascular ultrasound. They found that in diabetic patients the compensatory vessel enlargement to atherosclerosis was lower than in the non-diabetic patients. This impaired compensatory vessel enlargement may lead to earlier and more severe luminal stenosis for an equivalent volume of atherosclerotic plaque formed in the coronary artery in the diabetic patient [112].

Other factors leading to accelerated atherosclerosis in diabetics

Advanced glycation end products (AGEs) are a diverse group of lipids and proteins that are glycosylated via non-enzymatic pathways. They increase in settings of hyperglycemia, oxidant stress and renal failure [113]. These molecules then accumulate in the vascular tissue, a natural occurrence with aging, but a more rapid accumulation occurs in diabetes. The higher the glucose, the more rapid the accumulation of AGE [114]. Accelerated atherosclerosis occurs as a result of AGE accumulation in the vascular tissue. Glycosylated macromolecules can have atherosclerosis promoting affects directly and via receptors (RAGE).

Hyperinsulinemia was found to be an independent predictor for increased cardiovascular risk in hyperlipidemic patients [115]. Patients without diabetes, but with hyperinsulinemia detected two hours after glucose loading, had a higher severity score of stenosis and calcification on coronary angiography [116]. It is unclear whether hyperinsulinemia has direct proatherogenic effects or is only a marker for the insulin resistance syndrome. A possible mechanism explaining a direct role for insulin in the pathogenesis of atherosclerosis is that insulin potentiates the actions of platelet-derived growth factor in vascular smooth muscle increasing smooth muscle proliferation [117].

DIABETES AS A RISK FACTOR FOR PTCA

Percutaneous coronary intervention in diabetics has consistently resulted in worse long-term outcomes than in non-diabetics, despite comparable initial success rates [118, 119]. This is not due to procedural complications as procedural success in diabetics matches non-diabetics. Three possible mechanisms for poor outcomes in diabetics are stent thrombosis in the early post-procedural period, restenosis in the first six months, and progression of the underlying coronary artery disease.

Procedural success for PCI in diabetics is similar to non-diabetics both in elective cases and in patients with acute coronary syndromes. Stein et al reported angiographic success rates of 89% in 1133 diabetics and 90% success in 9300 non-diabetics undergoing elective angioplasty from 1980 to 1990 [119]. Gowda et al reported 96% PTCA success rates in diabetics versus 97% in non-diabetics in patients with non-Q wave myocardial infarction from 1992–1996 [120]. In the GUSTO-IIb angioplasty substudy, PTCA was performed in the setting of acute MI and procedural success was defined as residual stenosis < 50% and TIMI grade 3 flow. The procedural success rates were similar for the diabetics, 70.4%, and the non-diabetics 72.4% [53].

Stent thrombosis

In the first days after stent placement, the risk of stent thrombosis is approximately 1%. In the modern era of high pressure deployment and post-procedural treatment with thienopyridines and aspirin, the risk of subacute thrombosis occurs at a median of one day after implantation [121]. The evidence on the risk of subacute stent thrombosis in diabetics is mixed. There may be a trend to a higher risk in diabetic patients. Abizaid et al reported on 954 consecutive patients undergoing elective stenting and found no difference in stent thrombosis in IDDM (0.9%), vs non-IDDM (0%) and in non-diabetics (0%), $p > 0.1$ [122]. On the other hand, Silva et al reported on 104 consecutive patients undergoing primary stenting in acute myocardial infarction. Five out of 28 (18%) patients with diabetes had stent thrombosis versus 1 of 76 (1%) patients without diabetes ($p = 0.003$) [54, 123]. Elezi et al reported on 3554 consecutive patients receiving stents. There were 715 diabetic patients with 3.2% risk of subacute stent occlusion and 2.0% risk in the 2839 non-diabetic patients $p = 0.06$ [124].

In a streptozotocin treated swine model, 27 stents were placed in 11 diabetic swine and 15 stents were placed in six non-diabetic swine. There were six stent thromboses in the diabetic group and none in the non-diabetic group $p = 0.048$. The authors concluded that the hyperglycemic state predisposes stents to thrombosis [125].

Restenosis

Restenosis after PCI occurs more frequently in diabetics than non-diabetics [126–130]. Restenosis after balloon angioplasty was shown to be due to elastic recoil and neointimal hyperplasia. With coronary stents, elastic recoil is eliminated, but neointimal hyperplasia is exaggerated in diabetics as compared to non-diabetics [131, 132]. Restenosis is higher in diabetics and this response is device independent with higher rates seen after balloon angioplasty, stent implantation, directional atherectomy and rotational atherectomy [133, 134].

Increased restenosis rates after PTCA without stents has long been recognized as a significant obstacle to long-term successful treatment in the diabetic patient. The initial NHLBI Angioplasty Registry published in 1984 demonstrated a 47% restenosis rate in diabetics and 32% in non-diabetics [23]. This was confirmed by many different trials over the years [119, 128, 130, 135]. Van Belle et al reported on 300 consecutive patients from 1993–1995 treated with balloon angioplasty compared to 300 con-secutive patients from 1994–1996 undergoing stent implantation all of whom had a single-vessel native coronary artery procedure and all underwent six-month follow-up angiograms [135]. In the balloon angioplasty group, angiographic restenosis was 63% in diabetics and 36% in non-diabetics ($p = 0.0002$). Total vessel occlusion at follow-up angiography occurred at rates of 14% in the diabetic group and 3% in the non-diabetics ($p = 0.001$).

Stents have lowered restenosis rates as compared to balloon angioplasty [136, 137]. In an analysis of diabetics in the STRESS trial, patients randomized to PTCA had a 60% angiographic restenosis rate compared to 24% restenosis in the stent group $p < 0.01$. Target lesion revascularization (TLR) was 31% in diabetics and 13% in non-diabetics ($p = 0.03$) [138].

Although diabetics have a lower restenosis rate with stent implantation as compared to balloon PTCA, they have been shown to have higher restenosis rates than their non-diabetic counterparts in most trials. Elezi et al reported on stent implantation on 715 diabetic patients and 2839 non-diabetic patients from 1992–1997 [124]. Eighty percent of the patients underwent repeat angiography at six months. Angiographic restenosis was significantly higher in diabetics (37.5% vs 28.3%, $p < 0.001$). Repeat PTCA was performed more frequently in diabetics than in non-diabetics (21.1% vs 15.6%, $p < 0.001$). Restenosis was more frequent in diabetics with single-vessel disease, multi-vessel disease, small vessels (< 3 mm), large vessels, single stent lesions and multistent lesions. There were no differences in restenosis rates between insulin treated and non-insulin treated patients in this group.

Abizaid et al reported on 954 consecutive patients undergoing stent implantation with Palmaz-Schatz stents [122]. They not only compared diabetics to non-diabetics, but also compared insulin treated diabetics to non-insulin treated diabetics. They found higher rates of target lesion revascularization in the insulin treated group (28%) versus the non-insulin treated group (18%) and non-diabetics (16%), ($p < 0.05$).

Diabetics are not only at higher risk for restenosis, they are more likely to have diffuse instent restenosis as compared to focal instent restenosis [139]. Furthermore, there is evidence that restenosis in diabetics is more likely to result in total occlusion of the vessel that was intervened upon as compared to non-diabetics. Elezi et al reported a 5.3% total occlusion rate in diabetics and a 3.4% rate in non-diabetics ($p = 0.037$) [124]. Based on treatment, there was a trend to more total occlusions occurring in insulin treated diabetics (7.4%), as compared to patients receiving oral hypoglycemics (5.9%) and diet alone (3.1%) ($p = 0.194$). Van Belle et al reported a 2% rate of vessel occlusion rate in diabetics and 1% in non-diabetics (NS) at follow-up angiography after stent placement, but this was a smaller cohort of patients [135].

Kornowski et al performed serial intravascular ultrasound in 241 patients who had undergone follow-up angiography either for recurrent symptoms or as part of clinical protocols at a mean of 5.6 months after balloon angioplasty or stent intervention [131]. In the non-stented lesions, the reduction in the external elastic membrane cross-sectional area was similar in treated diabetics and non-diabetics. This indicated that elastic recoil plays a similar role in restenosis in both groups. In contrast, treated diabetics had a greater increase in plaque plus media cross-sectional area and this contributed to a greater percentage of the decrease in lumen cross-sectional area. This suggests that the increased restenosis seen in diabetics is due to an exaggerated tissue proliferation in response to balloon injury. In the stent group there was no elastic recoil. There was a 5.1 mm^2 intimal hyperplasia cross-sectional area within the lumen in diabetics and 2.1 mm^2 in non-diabetics, leading to the conclusion that exaggerated intimal hyperplasia in response to stent placement is the major mechanism of restenosis.

As pointed out above, diabetics are not only at higher risk for restenosis, they are more likely to have diffuse instent restenosis as compared to focal instent restenosis, a more difficult type of restenosis to treat [139]. The exact mechanism of increased intimal hyperplasia in diabetics is not known. Increased platelet-derived growth factor, insulin-like growth factor, and greater laying down of extracellular elements may contribute to the higher rates of restenosis [38, 140].

There is likely a link between restenosis and mortality in diabetic patients. Van Belle et al reported on 513 consecutive patients undergoing balloon angioplasty who had six-month follow-up angiography [141]. The 162 patients who had no restenosis had an actuarial 10-year mortality of 24%, the 257 patients who had non-occlusive restenosis had an actuarial 10-year mortality of 35%, and the 94 patients with coronary occlusion (defined as TIMI grade flow < 2) had an actuarial 10-year mortality of 59% ($p < 0.0001$).

Progression of disease

The risk of progression of coronary artery disease is higher in diabetics than in non-diabetics and there is an additive risk to vessels that have been instrumented. Rozenman et al reported on 353 angiograms on 248 patients who returned more than one month after successful angioplasty [142]. There was a 22% increase in new narrowings in diabetic patients (38 new and 174 pre-existing narrowings) compared with a 12% increase in non-diabetic patients (86 new and 734 pre-existing narrowings) ($p < 0.004$). There were new narrowings in diabetics in 16.9% of arteries which had undergone angioplasty, 13.2% in arteries which had not undergone angioplasty. The non-diabetics had a 12.7% rate of new narrowings in arteries which had undergone angioplasty and 7.3% in arteries which had not undergone angioplasty ($p = 0.009$). This reflects a more rapid rate of progression of atherosclerosis in the diabetic patient and suggests that damage to blood vessels during PCI predisposes to disease progression in vessels that have been instrumented.

Mortality

Despite similar procedural successes during PCI, differences in mortality between diabetics and non-diabetics can be demonstrated at each time period post-procedure. Abizaid et al reported in patients undergoing stent implantation, there was a significant increase in in-hospital mortality in insulin treated diabetics (2%) versus non-insulin treated diabetics (0%) and non-diabetics (0.3%), ($p < 0.02$) [122]. Elezi et al, reporting on patients undergoing stent implantation, found a 2.7% cardiac death rate in diabetic patients and 1.4% in non-diabetics ($p = 0.019$) at 30 days [124]. Pooled data from the EPIC, EPILOG and EPISTENT trials revealed a 3.3% one-year mortality in the diabetic patients and 2.1% mortality in the non-diabetic patients, $p = 0.012$ [143–146]. This was a relatively low risk population with two thirds of the patients enrolled in these trials having single-vessel disease. At five years, the absolute differences in mortality in diabetics with multi-vessel disease are extraordinary. In the BARI trial, at 5.4 years follow-up, cardiac mortality in the PCI-treated group with treated diabetes was 20.6% and in the non-diabetic group was 4.8% [129, 147]. Barsness et al reported on a similar cohort at Duke in patients undergoing PCI with multi-vessel disease and found a 24% mortality in diabetics and 12% mortality in non-diabetics at five years [118].

Proteinuria presents a hazard specific to the diabetic patient. Proteinuria is a major risk factor for mortality in diabetics and the higher the rate of proteinuria, the higher the mortality. Marso et al reviewed 2784 patients who underwent PCI at the Cleveland Clinic from 1993–1995 [148]. There were 2247 non-diabetics and 537 diabetics who had urinalysis performed. There were 320 diabetics without proteinuria and 217 diabetics with proteinuria. Two-year mortality was 7.3% for non-diabetics and 13.5% for diabetics ($p < 0.001$). The diabetics without proteinuria had a 9.1% two-year mortality compared to 20.3% in the diabetics with proteinuria ($p < 0.001$). The patients with

low concentration proteinuria ($n = 217$) had a two-year mortality of 16.2%; the patients with high concentration proteinuria ($n = 35$) had a 43.1% mortality ($p < 0.001$).

The poor long-term outcomes in diabetics are likely due to many factors and can be explained, at least in part, by the differences in the underlying vascular biology in diabetics. Diabetics have been shown to have more diffuse coronary artery disease, smaller coronary arteries, more calcification, a more exuberant response to trauma leading to increased restenosis, and a hypercoagulable state [131, 149–151]. Diabetics have also been shown to have a more rapidly progressive atherosclerosis leading to newer plaques and more thrombosis in untreated segments of the coronaries [142].

Future directions

There is emerging data that abciximab can decrease mortality following PCI in diabetics. In pooled data from EPIC, EPILOG and EPISTENT, there was lower one-year mortality in diabetic patients who received abciximab as compared to diabetic patients receiving placebo, 2.5% vs 4.5% ($p = 0.031$) [143–146]. The mechanism of this benefit is not well understood, but the one-time administration of an antiplatelet agent providing a long-term mortality benefit is exciting and may pave the way for newer drug therapy or newer applications of existing drugs.

Since there seems to be a link between restenosis and mortality in diabetics, perhaps reducing intimal hyperplasia with radiation therapy or coated stents that inhibit smooth muscle migration and proliferation will be especially useful in the diabetic patient [28].

DIABETES AS A RISK FACTOR FOR CABG

Diabetes has long been recognized as a risk factor for CABG [152] and remains an independent predictor of operative mortality for CABG in the current era [118, 153–157]. For example, in the latest iteration of the risk model developed by the Department of Veterans Affairs Continuous Improvement in Cardiac Surgery Program [158, 159] based on 11,636 procedures performed at VA centers from October 1997 through September 2000 the odds ratio for 30-day operative mortality was 1.2 for diabetics treated with oral hypoglycemics and 1.4 for diabetics on insulin.

The excess operative mortality for diabetes compared to non-diabetics may in part be due to the more advanced coronary artery disease in these patients, but there are other factors related to the metabolic abnormalities of diabetes that seem to play a role. Diabetes is a risk factor for the development of postoperative complications such as renal failure [160] and sternal wound infection [161–163] which are themselves associated with operative mortality. These complications of CABG in diabetics are a significant cause of increased length of hospital stay and impose major economic and social burdens on survivors, their families and on society [7, 164–167].

Diabetes is also associated with significant late morbidity and mortality following CABG. Numerous studies have shown that there is decreased survival and reduced quality of life post-CABG in diabetics [168–174]. Special mention must be made of the devastating impact of stroke following CABG. A significant correlation between diabetes and stroke was found in a landmark study conducted by the Multicenter Study of Perioperative Ischemia Research Group who analyzed the incidence of cerebral dysfunction in 2108 patients including 529 diabetics undergoing CABG between September 1991 and September 1993 [175]. The incidence of stroke (type 1 cerebral dysfunction) was 5.5% in diabetics compared to 2.4% in non-diabetics and this difference remained significant after multivariate analysis [175]. There was a trend towards more cognitive dysfunction (type 2 cerebral dysfunction) in diabetics (3.4% vs 3.0%) but this trend did not reach statistical significance [175]. It is likely that type 2

cerebral dysfunction was significantly under-reported in this study since formal neuropsychiatric testing was not done. More recent studies from Duke using careful neurocognitive testing pre-operatively and in follow-up have shown that the incidence of type 2 cerebral dysfunction is greater than 50% at the time of discharge from the hospital and is still present in 42% of patients five years after CABG [175]. It remains uncertain whether diabetics are more prone to type 2 cerebral dysfunction [176, 177].

There is little data on the outcome of CABG in high-risk diabetic subgroups. A study of 129 patients operated on in the 1980s showed that diabetes was an independent risk factor predicting perioperative myocardial infarction in patients undergoing CABG for unstable angina, but this observational study did not demonstrate any effect of diabetes on mortality [178]. Interestingly, a recent publication reporting data from the CABG Patch Trial database showed that diabetes was not a risk factor for mortality in patients with extremely poor left ventricular function undergoing CABG [179]. In this study of implantable cardiac defibrillator therapy, 900 patients with ejection fraction < 36% (including 342 diabetics) undergoing CABG from 1990–1996 were followed for a mean of nearly three years. Diabetes was not associated with long-term mortality in Cox multiple regression analyses, but was associated with increased complications and hospital re-admissions [179].

CABG remains an important revascularization option for high-risk diabetics, especially for those whose anatomy is not favorable for PCI. Better understanding of the metabolic consequences of diabetes is leading to improved outcomes with CABG and further progress promises to increase the safety of CABG in the future. For example, recognition of the association between elevated glucose levels and infection has been incorporated into current management strategies and it has been shown that improved short-term outcomes for diabetics undergoing CABG result from tight control of blood sugar by perioperative insulin infusion

[180, 181]. The importance of vigorous lipid management in diabetics post-CABG has also been recently recognized and is leading to lower rates of saphenous vein graft attrition and better long-term outcomes in diabetic patients treated with statins [182, 183]. It has been recently shown that elevated triglycerides in diabetics are associated with a higher mortality post-CABG [184] suggesting that improved metabolic control of diabetes and treatment with fibrates may be beneficial in such patients.

Coronary sinus levels of the potent vasoconstrictor endothelin-1 are significantly higher immediately after bypass grafting in diabetics than in non-diabetics [185] as are levels of the potentially injurious inflammatory cytokine interleukin-8 which is released from monocytes stimulated by endothelin-1 [186]. Thus endothelin receptor blockers are a potentially rational new therapy which may further reduce operative mortality in diabetics.

RANDOMIZED TRIALS OF CABG VERSUS PTCA: RELEVANCE TO HIGH-RISK DIABETICS

The randomized trials of CABG versus PTCA that are reviewed extensively elsewhere in this book have demonstrated comparable long-term survival in most patient populations with the important exception of diabetics [187]. The BARI study [8, 9] showed a significant and sustained survival benefit for CABG at five years in treated diabetics, and similar findings were noted in other randomized studies and large databases [188–190]. Reviewing these data in a recent editorial, Spencer King concluded that 'surgery with at least one internal mammary artery graft is superior to angioplasty in the broad population of patients with diabetes and multi-vessel disease' [191].

Despite the apparent superiority of CABG with a mammary artery graft over PCI in diabetics with multi-vessel disease a critical appraisal of data from previous trials and registries suggests that only limited conclusions can be drawn from these data regarding contemporary revascularization options for high-risk diabetics. As emphasized throughout this book, the previous randomized trials of CABG vs PTCA systematically excluded high-risk subgroups. Moreover, a number of studies including a large registry from Duke have failed to demonstrate a survival benefit for PCI over CABG in diabetics [118, 192]. Even the BARI registry showed comparable survival for diabetics who chose PCI over CABG [193].

A recent analysis of mortality in the BARI study showed that approximately 50% of the survival benefit for CABG in the diabetic patients could be explained by a lower mortality during Q wave myocardial infarction [194]. The incidence of Q wave myocardial infarction was the same among diabetics randomized to CABG or angioplasty. Although Q wave myocardial infarction was relatively rare in diabetics enrolled in the study (8% incidence in five year follow-up) the mortality rate was seven-fold higher in diabetics randomized to angioplasty compared to CABG [194]. Importantly, this survival benefit for CABG was almost entirely limited to patients who received at least one internal mammary artery graft [194]. These findings have therapeutic implications. Firstly, diabetic patients with prior CABG (especially those with durable patent internal mammary grafts) might be expected to retain a survival benefit from their first operation and so conceivably would have less benefit from a re-operation compared to the benefit of angioplasty. This hypothesis was not tested in BARI since all patients with prior CABG were excluded from the trial. Secondly, the improved outcome of myocardial infarction in diabetics discussed above would be expected to narrow the difference in survival between PCI and CABG in this population.

Another major cause of the difference between the outcomes in the BARI study and the outcomes that can be expected today with PCI in diabetics is the nearly universal use of stents and glycoprotein IIb/IIIa receptor blockers in contemporary practice. The BARI study enrolled patients between 1988 and 1991. Balloon angioplasty was the only procedure performed in patients randomized to the PCI arm of BARI [8, 9]. The high complication and restenosis rates associated with balloon angioplasty in diabetics with multi-vessel disease subsequently led to the abandonment of this technique in such patients [195]. The recognition that stents and glycoprotein IIb/IIIa receptor blockers reduce restenosis and long-term mortality in diabetics with multi-vessel disease have made this the default strategy for PCI in this challenging population [196]. Diabetic patients were a prospectively defined subset in the landmark multicenter Evaluation of Platelet IIb/IIIa Inhibitor for Stenting Trial (EPISTENT). Patients were randomized to stent-placebo (173 diabetic patients), stent-abciximab (162 diabetic patients) or balloon-abciximab (156 diabetic patients). The combined six-month rate of death, myocardial infarction (MI), or target vessel revascularization (TVR) occurred in 25.2% of stent-placebo, 23.4% of balloon-abciximab, and only 13.0% of stent-abciximab patients ($p = 0.005$). The one-year mortality rate for diabetics was 4.1% for stent-placebo and 1.2% for stent-abciximab patients ($p = 0.11$) [196] (Fig. 29.2).

INSIGHTS FROM THE AWESOME STUDY

Another reason for uncertainty over the best revascularization strategy for diabetics is that diabetic patients who are at high-risk for CABG might have equivalent or superior outcomes with a less invasive PCI procedure. This hypothesis was evaluated by analysis of outcomes in diabetics enrolled in the recently concluded, Angina With Extremely Serious Operative Mortality Evaluation (AWESOME) Study and was presented in abstract form at the March 2001 Scientific Sessions of the American College of Cardiology [197]. AWESOME was a nationwide, prospective, randomized clinical trial designed to test the hypothesis that PCI is

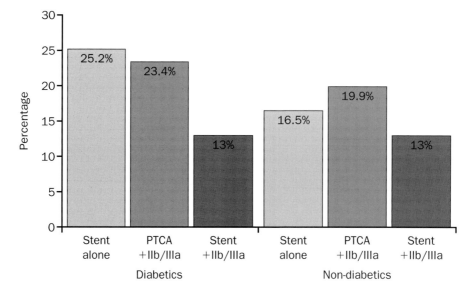

Figure 29.2 Effects of glycoprotein IIb/IIIa receptor inhibition and coronary stenting.

relatively safe and effective alternative to CABG for patients with medically refractory unstable angina and high-risk of adverse outcomes. Patients were enrolled at 16 Veterans Affairs medical centers over a five-year period (1995–2000). Patients were defined as high risk for CABG because of one or more of the following high-risk factors: prior heart surgery; myocardial infarction within seven days; left ventricular ejection fraction < 0.35; age > 70 years; intra-aortic balloon required to stabilize. In addition to the randomized trial, eligible patients, who were directed by physicians not to participate, and eligible patients who refused randomization were entered into a prospective registry. The AWESOME protocol, baseline characteristics of randomized patients, and three-year outcomes of the randomized cohort have been reported [198–200].

There were 2431 patients enrolled in AWESOME who had refractory unstable angina and at least one high risk factor for CABG. After coronary angiography had been reviewed by both interventional cardiologist and surgeon, a total of 781 (32%) were acceptable to both operators as candidates for randomization. These patients were approached for informed consent and 454 (58%) consented to a randomized choice of revascularization. The 327 patients who refused random allocation elected either PCI or CABG for themselves and are referred to as the patient choice registry. The 1650 patients for whom physician consensus would not allow random assignments constitute a prospective physician-directed registry: 651 were assigned to PCI, 692 were assigned to CABG, and 307 were assigned further medical therapy. There were a total of 758 diabetic patients in AWESOME including 144 (32%) in the randomized trial, 89 (27%) in the patient refused registry and 525 (32%) in the physician assigned registry.

The outcomes of the diabetics enrolled in AWESOME are shown in Table 29.1 and Figures 29.3–29.5. These data suggest that PCI is a safe alternative to CABG for diabetic patients with medically refractory unstable angina who are at high risk for CABG.

Table 29.1 AWESOME survival data

	6 month		36 month		Log-rank
	CABG	**PCI**	**CABG**	**PCI**	
Diabetic					
Randomized	86%	91%	73%	80%	$p > 0.40$ (ns)
Patient refused	85%	97%	85%	91%	$p > 0.35$ (ns)
Physician assignment	87%	86%	72%	73%	$p > 0.40$ (ns)
Non-diabetic					
Randomized	92%	96%	80%	79%	$p > 0.80$ (ns)
Patient refused	92%	96%	81%	88%	$p > 0.30$ (ns)
Physician assignment	90%	91%	78%	79%	$p > 0.40$ (ns)

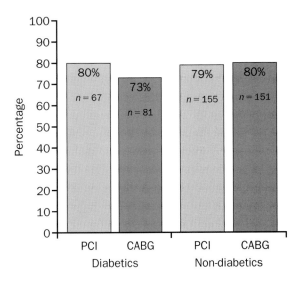

Figure 29.3 AWESOME Randomized Study: 36 month survival.

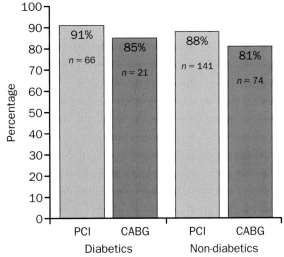

Figure 29.5 AWESOME Registry: 36 month survival; patient preference.

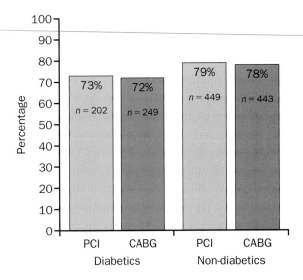

Figure 29.4 AWESOME Registry: 36 month survival; physician assigned therapy.

REFERENCES

1. Amos AF, McCarty DJ, Zimmet P. The rising global burden of diabetes and its complications: estimates and projections to the year 2010, *Diabet Med* 1997; **14** (suppl 5):S1–85.

2. Beller GA. President's page: the epidemic of type 2 diabetes and obesity in the US: cause for alarm, *J Am Coll Cardiol* 2000; **36** (7):2348–2350.

3. Burke JP, Williams K, Gaskill SP et al. Rapid rise in the incidence of type 2 diabetes from 1987 to 1996: results from the San Antonio Heart Study, *Arch Intern Med* 1999; **159** (13):1450–1456.

4. Cooper R, Cutler J, Desvigne-Nickens P et al. Trends and disparities in coronary heart disease, stroke, and other cardiovascular diseases in the United States: findings of the national conference on cardiovascular disease prevention, *Circulation* (Online) 2000; **102** (25): 3137–3147.

5. Harris MI, Flegal KM, Cowie CC et al. Prevalence of diabetes, impaired fasting glucose, and impaired glucose tolerance in US adults. The Third National Health and Nutrition Examination Survey, 1988–1994, *Diabetes Care* 1998; **21** (4):518–524.

6. Songer TJ, Zimmet PZ. Epidemiology of type II diabetes: an international perspective, *Pharmacoeconomics* 1995; **8** (suppl 1):1–11.

7. MacLeod KM, Tooke JE. Direct and indirect costs of cardiovascular and cerebrovascular complications of type II diabetes, *Pharmacoeconomics* 1995; **8** (suppl 1):46–51.

8. Comparison of coronary bypass surgery with angioplasty in patients with multi-vessel disease, *N Engl J Med* 1996; **335** (4):217–225.

9. Ferguson JJ. NHLI BARI clinical alert on diabetics treated with angioplasty, *Circulation* 1995; **92** (12):3371.

10. Braunwald E, Antman EM, Beasley JW et al. ACC/AHA guidelines for the management of patients with unstable angina and non-ST segment elevation myocardial infarction: executive summary and recommendations. A report of the American College of Cardiology/American Heart Association task force on practice guidelines (committee on the management of patients with unstable angina), *Circulation* 2000; **102** (10):1193–1209.

11. Eagle KA, Guyton RA, Davidoff R et al. ACC/AHA guidelines for coronary artery bypass graft surgery. A report of the American College of Cardiology/American Heart Association task force on practice guidelines (committee to revise the 1991 guidelines for coronary artery bypass graft surgery). American College of Cardiology/American Heart Association, *J Am Coll Cardiol* 1999; **34** (4):1262–1347.

12. Gibbons RJ, Chatterjee K, Daley J et al. ACC/AHA/ ACP-ASIM guidelines for the management of patients with chronic stable angina: a report of the American College of Cardiology/American Heart Association task force on practice guidelines (committee on management of patients with chronic stable angina), *J Am Coll Cardiol* 1999; **33** (7):2092–2197.

13. Copyright © 2000 American Diabetes Association. Diabetes Facts and Figures. Available at HTTP://www.diabetes.org/ada/facts.asp (2001).

14. Harris MI, Eastman RC, Cowie CC, Flegal KM, Eberhardt MS. Racial and ethnic differences in glycemic control of adults with type 2 diabetes, *Diabetes Care* 1999; **22** (3):403–408.

15. Harris MI. Epidemiologic studies on the pathogenesis of non-insulin-dependent diabetes mellitus (NIDDM), *Clin Invest Med* 1995; **18** (4): 231–239.

16. Haffner SM, Lehto S, Ronnemaa T, Pyorala K, Laakso M. Mortality from coronary heart disease in subjects with type 2 diabetes and in non-diabetic subjects with and without prior myocardial infarction, *N Engl J Med* 1998; **339** (4):229–234.

17. Lotufo PA, Gaziano JM, Chae CU et al. Diabetes and all-cause and coronary heart disease mortality among US male physicians, *Arch Intern Med* 2001; **161** (2):242–247.

18. Mather HM, Chaturvedi N, Fuller JH. Mortality and morbidity from diabetes in South Asians and Europeans: 11-year follow-up of the Southall Diabetes Survey, London, UK, *Diabet Med* 1998; **15** (1):53–59.

19. Casiglia E, Zanette G, Mazza A et al. Cardiovascular mortality in non-insulin-dependent diabetes mellitus. A controlled study among 683 diabetics and 683 age- and sex-matched normal subjects, *Eur J Epidemiol* 2000; **16** (7):677–684.

20. Chun BY, Dobson AJ, Heller RF. The impact of diabetes on survival among patients with first myocardial infarction, *Diabetes Care* 1997; **20** (5):704–708.

21. Torffvit O, Agardh C. The prognosis for type 2 diabetic patients with heart disease. A 10-year observation study of 385 patients, *J Diabetes Complications* 2000; **14** (6):301–306.

22. Gu K, Cowie CC, Harris MI. Diabetes and decline in heart disease mortality in US adults, *JAMA* 1999; **281** (14):1291–1297.

23. Abbott RD, Donahue RP, Kannel WB, Wilson PW. The impact of diabetes on survival following myocardial infarction in men vs women. The Framingham Study, *JAMA* 1988; **260** (23): 3456–3460.

24. Behar S, Boyko V, Reicher-Reiss H, Goldbourt U. Ten-year survival after acute myocardial infarction: comparison of patients with and without diabetes. SPRING Study Group. Secondary Prevention Reinfarction Israeli Nifedipine Trial, *Am Heart J* 1997; **133** (3):290–296.

25. Donahue RP, Goldberg RJ, Chen Z, Gore JM, Alpert JS. The influence of sex and diabetes mellitus on survival following acute myocardial infarction: a community-wide perspective, *J Clin Epidemiol* 1993; **46** (3):245–252.

26. Malmberg K, Yusuf S, Gerstein HC et al. Impact of diabetes on long-term prognosis in patients with unstable angina and non-Q wave myocardial infarction: results of the OASIS (Organization to Assess Strategies for Ischemic Syndromes) Registry, *Circulation* 2000; **102** (9):1014–1019.

27. Miettinen H, Lehto S, Salomaa V et al. Impact of

diabetes on mortality after the first myocardial infarction. The FINMONICA Myocardial Infarction Register Study Group, *Diabetes Care* 1998; **21** (1):69–75.

28. Stone GW. Stenting and IIb/IIIa receptor blockade in acute myocardial infarction: an introduction to the CADILLAC trial, *J Invasive Cardiol* 1998; **10** (suppl B):36B–47B.

29. Ulvenstam G, Aberg A, Bergstrand R et al. Long-term prognosis after myocardial infarction in men with diabetes, *Diabetes* 1985; **34** (8):787–792.

30. Vaccarino V, Parsons L, Every NR, Barron HV, Krumholz HM. Impact of history of diabetes mellitus on hospital mortality in men and women with first acute myocardial infarction. The National Registry of Myocardial Infarction 2 Participants, *Am J Cardiol* 2000; **85** (12): 1486–1489.

31. Capes SE, Hunt D, Malmberg K, Gerstein HC. Stress hyperglycaemia and increased risk of death after myocardial infarction in patients with and without diabetes: a systematic overview, *Lancet* 2000; **355** (9206):773–778.

32. Fava S, Aquilina O, Azzopardi J, Agius MH, Fenech FF. The prognostic value of blood glucose in diabetic patients with acute myocardial infarction, *Diabet Med* 1996; **13** (1):80–83.

33. Stein PK, Kleiger RE. Insights from the study of heart rate variability, *Ann Rev Med* 1999; **50**:249–261.

34. Garratt KN, Brady PA, Hassinger NL et al. Sulfonylurea drugs increase early mortality in patients with diabetes mellitus after direct angioplasty for acute myocardial infarction, *J Am Coll Cardiol* 1999; **33** (1):119–124.

35. Canto JG, Shlipak MG, Rogers WJ et al. Prevalence, clinical characteristics, and mortality among patients with myocardial infarction presenting without chest pain, *JAMA* 2000; **283** (24):3223–3229.

36. Stone PH, Muller JE, Hartwell T et al. The effect of diabetes mellitus on prognosis and serial left ventricular function after acute myocardial infarction: contribution of both coronary disease and diastolic left ventricular dysfunction to the adverse prognosis. The MILIS Study Group, *J Am Coll Cardiol* 1989; **14** (1):49–57.

37. Jaffe AS, Spadaro JJ, Schechtman K et al. Increased congestive heart failure after myocardial infarction of modest extent in patients with

diabetes mellitus, *Am Heart J* 1984; **108** (1):31–37.

38. Aronson D, Rayfield EJ, Chesebro JH. Mechanisms determining course and outcome of diabetic patients who have had acute myocardial infarction. *Ann Intern Med* 1997; **126** (4):296–306.

39. Melchior T, Rask-Madsen C, Torp-Pedersen C et al. The impact of heart failure on prognosis of diabetic and non-diabetic patients with myocardial infarction: a 15-year follow-up study, *Eur J Heart Fail* 2001; **3** (1):83–90.

40. Granger CB, Califf RM, Young S et al. Outcome of patients with diabetes mellitus and acute myocardial infarction treated with thrombolytic agents. The Thrombolysis and Angioplasty in Myocardial Infarction (TAMI) Study Group, *J Am Coll Cardiol* 1993; **21** (4):920–925.

41. Hansen HH, Kjaergaard SC, Bulow I, Fog L, Christensen PD. Thrombolytic therapy in diabetic patients with acute myocardial infarction, *Diabetes Care* 1996; **19** (10):1135–1137.

42. Kjaergaard SC, Hansen HH, Fog L, Bulow I, Christensen PD. In-hospital outcome for diabetic patients with acute myocardial infarction in the thrombolytic era, *Scand Cardiovasc J* 1999; **33** (3):166–170.

43. Lynch M, Gammage MD, Lamb P, Nattrass M, Pentecost BL. Acute myocardial infarction in diabetic patients in the thrombolytic era, *Diabet Med* 1994; **11** (2):162–165.

44. Mak KH, Moliterno DJ, Granger CB et al. Influence of diabetes mellitus on clinical outcome in the thrombolytic era of acute myocardial infarction. GUSTO-I Investigators. Global Utilization of Streptokinase and Tissue Plasminogen Activator for Occluded Coronary Arteries, *J Am Coll Cardiol* 1997; **30** (1):171–179.

45. Mak KH, Topol EJ. Emerging concepts in the management of acute myocardial infarction in patients with diabetes mellitus, *J Am Coll Cardiol* 2000; **35** (3):563–568.

46. Mueller HS, Cohen LS, Braunwald E et al. Predictors of early morbidity and mortality after thrombolytic therapy of acute myocardial infarction. Analyses of patient subgroups in the Thrombolysis in Myocardial Infarction (TIMI) trial, phase II, *Circulation* 1992; **85** (4):1254–1264.

47. Strandberg LE, Ericsson CG, O'Konor ML et al. Diabetes mellitus is a strong negative prognostic factor in patients with myocardial infarction

treated with thrombolytic therapy, *J Intern Med* 2000; **248** (2):119–125.

48. Nesto RW, Zarich S. Acute myocardial infarction in diabetes mellitus: lessons learned from ACE inhibition, *Circulation* 1998; **97** (1):12–15.

49. Zuanetti G, Latini R, Maggioni AP et al. Effect of the ACE inhibitor lisinopril on mortality in diabetic patients with acute myocardial infarction: data from the GISSI-3 study, *Circulation* 1997; **96** (12):4239–4245.

50. Malmberg K, Ryden L, Hamsten A et al. Effects of insulin treatment on cause-specific one-year mortality and morbidity in diabetic patients with acute myocardial infarction. DIGAMI Study Group. Diabetes Insulin-Glucose in Acute Myocardial Infarction, *Eur Heart J* 1996; **17** (9):1337–1344.

51. Malmberg K. Prospective randomized study of intensive insulin treatment on long term survival after acute myocardial infarction in patients with diabetes mellitus. DIGAMI (Diabetes Mellitus, Insulin Glucose Infusion in Acute Myocardial Infarction) Study Group. *BMJ* 1997; **314** (7093):1512–1515.

52. Malmberg K, Norhammar A, Wedel H, Ryden L. Glycometabolic state at admission: important risk marker of mortality in conventionally treated patients with diabetes mellitus and acute myocardial infarction: long-term results from the Diabetes and Insulin-Glucose Infusion in Acute Myocardial Infarction (DIGAMI) study, *Circulation* 1999; **99** (20):2626–2632.

53. Hasdai D, Granger CB, Srivatsa SS et al. Diabetes mellitus and outcome after primary coronary angioplasty for acute myocardial infarction: lessons from the GUSTO-IIb Angioplasty Substudy. Global Use of Strategies to Open Occluded Arteries in Acute Coronary Syndromes, *J Am Coll Cardiol* 2000; **35** (6): 1502–1512.

54. Silva JA, Ramee SR, White CJ et al. Primary stenting in acute myocardial infarction: influence of diabetes mellitus in angiographic results and clinical outcome, *Am Heart J* 1999; **138** (3 Pt 1): 446–455.

55. Waldecker B, Waas W, Haberbosch W et al. Type 2 diabetes and acute myocardial infarction. Angiographic findings and results of an invasive therapeutic approach in type 2 diabetic versus nondiabetic patients, *Diabetes Care* 1999; **22** (11):1832–1838.

56. Stuckey T, Grines CL, Cox DA et al. Does stenting and glycoprotein IIb/IIIa receptor blockade improve the prognosis of diabetics undergoing primary angioplasty in acute myocardial infarction? The CADILLAC Trial, *J Am Coll Cardiol* 2001; **37**: 1A–648A.

57. Shindler DM, Pameri ST, Antonelli TA et al. Diabetes mellitus in cardiogenic shock complicating acute myocardial infarction: a report from the SHOCK trial registry. SHould we emergently revascularize Occluded Coronaries for cardiogenic shocK? *J Am Coll Cardiol* 2000; **36** (3 Suppl A):1097–1103.

58. Calvin JE, Klein LW, VandenBerg BJ et al. Risk stratification in unstable angina. Prospective validation of the Braunwald classification, *JAMA* 1995; **273** (2):136–141.

59. Fava S, Azzopardi J, Agius-Muscat H. Outcome of unstable angina in patients with diabetes mellitus, *Diabet Med* 1997; **14** (3):209–213.

60. Theroux P, Alexander J, Pharand C et al. Glycoprotein IIb/IIIa receptor blockade improves outcomes in diabetic patients presenting with unstable angina/non-ST elevation myocardial infarction: results from the Platelet Receptor Inhibition in Ischemic Syndrome Management in Patients Limited by Unstable Signs and Symptoms (PRISM-PLUS) study, *Circulation* 2000; **102** (20):2466–2472.

61. Sosenko JM, Breslow JL, Miettinen OS, Gabbay KH. Hyperglycemia and plasma lipid levels: a prospective study of young insulin-dependent diabetic patients, *N Engl J Med* 1980; **302** (12):650–654.

62. Syvanne M, Taskinen MR. Lipids and lipoproteins as coronary risk factors in non-insulin-dependent diabetes mellitus. *Lancet* 1997; **350** (suppl 1):S120–S123.

63. Eckel RH. Lipoprotein lipase. A multifunctional enzyme relevant to common metabolic diseases, *N Engl J Med* 1989; **320** (16):1060–1068.

64. Bagdade JD, Lane JT, Subbaiah PV, Otto ME, Ritter MC. Accelerated cholesteryl ester transfer in noninsulin-dependent diabetes mellitus, *Atherosclerosis* 1993; **104** (1–2):69–77.

65. Dullaart RP, Groener JE, Dikkeschei LD, Erkelens DW, Doorenbos H. Increased cholesterylester transfer activity in complicated type 1 (insulin-dependent) diabetes mellitus—its relationship with serum lipids, *Diabetologia* 1989; **32** (1):14–19.

66. Ginsberg HN. Diabetic dyslipidemia: basic mechanisms underlying the common hyper-triglyceridemia and low HDL cholesterol levels. *Diabetes* 1996; **45** (suppl 3):S27–S30.

67. Austin MA, King MC, Vranizan KM, Krauss RM. Atherogenic lipoprotein phenotype. A proposed genetic marker for coronary heart disease risk, *Circulation* 1990; **82** (2):495–506.

68. Gardner CD, Fortmann SP, Krauss RM. Association of small low-density lipoprotein particles with the incidence of coronary artery disease in men and women, *JAMA* 1996; **276** (11):875–881.

69. Kannel WB. Lipids, diabetes, and coronary heart disease: insights from the Framingham Study, *Am Heart J* 1985; **110** (5):1100–1107.

70. Pyorala K, Pedersen TR, Kjekshus J et al. Cholesterol lowering with simvastatin improves prognosis of diabetic patients with coronary heart disease. A subgroup analysis of the Scandinavian Simvastatin Survival Study (4S), *Diabetes Care* 1997; **20** (4):614–620.

71. Creager MA, Selwyn A. When 'normal' cholesterol levels injure the endothelium, *Circulation* 1997; **96** (10):3255–3257.

72. Lopes-Virella MF, Virella G. Cytokines, modified lipoproteins, and arteriosclerosis in diabetes, *Diabetes* 1996; **45** (suppl 3):S40–S44.

73. Bucala R, Makita Z, Vega G et al. Modification of low density lipoprotein by advanced glycation end-products contributes to the dyslipidemia of diabetes and renal insufficiency, *Proc Natl Acad Sci USA* 1994; **91** (20):9441–9445.

74. Lyons TJ, Klein RL, Baynes JW, Stevenson HC, Lopes-Virella MF. Stimulation of cholesteryl ester synthesis in human monocyte-derived macrophages by low density lipoproteins from type 1 (insulin-dependent) diabetic patients: the influence of non-enzymatic glycosylation of low density lipoproteins, *Diabetologia* 1987; **30** (12): 916–923.

75. Maiello M, Boeri D, Podesta F et al. Increased expression of tissue plasminogen activator and its inhibitor and reduced fibrinolytic potential of human endothelial cells cultured in elevated glucose, *Diabetes* 1992; **41** (8):1009–1015.

76. Bowsher RR, Wolny JD, Frank BH. A rapid and sensitive radio-immunoassay for the measurement of proinsulin in human serum, *Diabetes* 1992; **41** (9):1084–1090.

77. Sobey WJ, Beer SF, Carrington CA et al. Sensitive and specific two-site immunoradiometric assays for human insulin, proinsulin, 65–66 split and 32–33 split proinsulins, *Biochem J* 1989; **260** (2): 535–541.

78. Nagi DK, Hendra TJ, Ryle AJ et al. The relationships of concentrations of insulin, intact proinsulin and 32–33 split proinsulin with cardiovascular risk factors in type 2 (non-insulin-dependent) diabetic subjects, *Diabetologia* 1990; **33** (9):532–537.

79. Nordt TK, Bode C. Impaired endogenous fibrinolysis in diabetes mellitus: mechanisms and therapeutic approaches, *Semin Thromb Hemost* 2000; **26** (5):495–501.

80. Temple RC, Clark PM, Nagi DK et al. Radioimmunoassay may over-estimate insulin in non-insulin-dependent diabetics, *Clin Endocrinol (Oxf)* 1990; **32** (6): 689–693.

81. Alessi MC, Juhan-Vague I, Kooistra T, Declerck PJ, Collen D. Insulin stimulates the synthesis of plasminogen activator inhibitor 1 by the human hepatocellular cell line Hep G_2, *Thromb Haemost* 1988; **60** (3):491–494.

82. Kooistra T, Bosma PJ, Tons HA et al. Plasminogen activator inhibitor 1: biosynthesis and mRNA level are increased by insulin in cultured human hepatocytes, *Thromb Haemost* 1989; **62** (2): 723–728.

83. Schneider DJ, Sobel BE. Augmentation of synthesis of plasminogen activator inhibitor type 1 by insulin and insulin-like growth factor type I: implications for vascular disease in hyperinsulinemic states, *Proc Natl Acad Sci USA* 1991; **88** (22):9959–9963.

84. Galloway JA, Hooper SA, Spradlin CT et al. Biosynthetic human proinsulin. Review of chemistry, in vitro and in vivo receptor binding, animal and human pharmacology studies, and clinical trial experience, *Diabetes Care* 1992; **15** (5):666–692.

85. Asakawa H, Tokunaga K, Kawakami F. Elevation of fibrinogen and thrombin–antithrombin III complex levels of type 2 diabetes mellitus patients with retinopathy and nephropathy, *J Diabetes Complications* 2000; **14** (3):121–126.

86. Ceriello A, Giugliano D, Quatraro A, Dello RP, Torella R. Blood glucose may condition factor VII levels in diabetic and normal subjects, *Diabetologia* 1988; **31** (12):889–891.

87. Ceriello A, Taboga C, Giacomello R et al.

Fibrinogen plasma levels as a marker of thrombin activation in diabetes. *Diabetes* 1994; **43** (3):430–432.

88. Tschoepe D, Roesen P, Schwippert B, Gries FA. Platelets in diabetes: the role in the hemostatic regulation in atherosclerosis, *Semin Thromb Hemost* 1993; **19** (2):122–128.

89. Winocour PD. Platelet abnormalities in diabetes mellitus, *Diabetes* 1992; **41** (suppl 2):26–31.

90. Aoki I, Shimoyama K, Aoki N et al. Platelet-dependent thrombin generation in patients with diabetes mellitus: effects of glycemic control on coagulability in diabetes, *J Am Coll Cardiol* 1996; **27** (3):560–566.

91. Shechter M, Merz CN, Paul-Labrador MJ, Kaul S. Blood glucose and platelet-dependent thrombosis in patients with coronary artery disease, *J Am Coll Cardiol* 2000; **35** (2):300–307.

92. Calles-Escandon J, Cipolla M. Diabetes and endothelial dysfunction: a clinical perspective, *Endocr Rev* 2001; **22** (1):36–52.

93. Ceolotto G, Gallo A, Miola M et al. Protein kinase C activity is acutely regulated by plasma glucose concentration in human monocytes in vivo, *Diabetes* 1999; **48** (6):1316–1322.

94. Durante W, Sen AK, Sunahara FA. Impairment of endothelium-dependent relaxation in aortae from spontaneously diabetic rats, *Br J Pharmacol* 1988; **94** (2):463–468.

95. Oyama Y, Kawasaki H, Hattori Y, Kanno M. Attenuation of endothelium-dependent relaxation in aorta from diabetic rats, *Eur J Pharmacol* 1986; **132** (1):75–78.

96. Tesfamariam B, Brown ML, Deykin D, Cohen RA. Elevated glucose promotes generation of endothelium-derived vasoconstrictor prostanoids in rabbit aorta, *J Clin Invest* 1990; **85** (3): 929–932.

97. Tesfamariam B, Brown ML, Cohen RA. Elevated glucose impairs endothelium-dependent relaxation by activating protein kinase C, *J Clin Invest* 1991; **87** (5):1643–1648.

98. Giugliano D, Ceriello A, Paolisso G. Oxidative stress and diabetic vascular complications, *Diabetes Care* 1996; **19** (3):257–267.

99. Schachinger V, Britten MB, Zeiher AM. Prognostic impact of coronary vasodilator dysfunction on adverse long-term outcome of coronary heart disease, *Circulation* 2000; **101** (16):1899–1906.

100. Johnstone MT, Creager SJ, Scales KM et al.

Impaired endothelium-dependent vasodilation in patients with insulin-dependent diabetes mellitus, *Circulation* 1993; **88** (6):2510–2516.

101. Umeda F, Inoguchi T, Nawata H. Reduced stimulatory activity on prostacyclin production by cultured endothelial cells in serum from aged and diabetic patients, *Atherosclerosis* 1989; **75** (1):61–66.

102. Morigi M, Angioletti S, Imberti B et al. Leukocyte–endothelial interaction is augmented by high glucose concentrations and hyperglycemia in a NF-kB-dependent fashion, *J Clin Invest* 1998; **101** (9):1905–1915.

103. Takahara N, Kashiwagi A, Nishio Y et al. Oxidized lipoproteins found in patients with NIDDM stimulate radical-induced monocyte chemoattractant protein-1 mRNA expression in cultured human endothelial cells, *Diabetologia* 1997; **40** (6): 662–670.

104. Yerneni KK, Bai W, Khan BV, Medford RM, Natarajan R. Hyperglycemia-induced activation of nuclear transcription factor kappa B in vascular smooth muscle cells, *Diabetes* 1999; **48** (4):855–864.

105. Baumgartner-Parzer SM, Wagner L, Pettermann M, Gessl A, Waldhausl W. Modulation by high glucose of adhesion molecule expression in cultured endothelial cells, *Diabetologia* 1995; **38** (11):1367–1370.

106. Ridker PM. Intrinsic fibrinolytic capacity and systemic inflammation: novel risk factors for arterial thrombotic disease, *Haemostasis* 1997; **27** (suppl 1):2–11.

107. King GL, Wakasaki H. Theoretical mechanisms by which hyperglycemia and insulin resistance could cause cardiovascular diseases in diabetes, *Diabetes Care* 1999; **22** (suppl 3):C31–C37.

108. Lorenzi M, Cagliero E, Toledo S. Glucose toxicity for human endothelial cells in culture. Delayed replication, disturbed cell cycle, and accelerated death, *Diabetes* 1985; **34** (7):621–627.

109. Ge J, Erbel R, Zamorano J et al. Coronary artery remodeling in atherosclerotic disease: an intravascular ultrasonic study in vivo, *Coron Artery Dis* 1993; **4** (11):981–986.

110. Nishioka T, Luo H, Eigler NL et al. Contribution of inadequate compensatory enlargement to development of human coronary artery stenosis: an in vivo intravascular ultrasound study, *J Am Coll Cardiol* 1996; **27** (7):1571–1576.

111. Stiel GM, Stiel LS, Schofer J, Donath K, Mathey DG. Impact of compensatory enlargement of atherosclerotic coronary arteries on angiographic assessment of coronary artery disease, *Circulation* 1989; **80** (6):1603–1609.

112. Vavuranakis M, Stefanadis C, Toutouzas K et al. Impaired compensatory coronary artery enlargement in atherosclerosis contributes to the development of coronary artery stenosis in diabetic patients. An in vivo intravascular ultrasound study, *Eur Heart J* 1997; **18** (7):1090–1094.

113. Reddy S, Bichler J, Wells-Knecht KJ, Thorpe SR, Baynes JW. N epsilon-(caraboxymethyl) lysine is a dominant advanced glycation end-product (AGE) antigen in tissue proteins, *Biochemistry* 1995; **34** (34):10872–10878.

114. Brownlee M, Cerami A, Vlassara H. Advanced glycosylation end-products in tissue and the biochemical basis of diabetic complications, *N Engl J Med* 1988; **318** (20):1315–1321.

115. Glueck CJ, Lang JE, Tracy T, Sieve-Smith L, Wang P. Contribution of fasting hyperinsulinemia to prediction of atherosclerotic cardiovascular disease status in 293 hyperlipidemic patients, *Metabolism* 1999; **48** (11):1437–1444.

116. Tsuchihashi K, Hikita N, Hase M et al. Role of hyperinsulinemia in atherosclerotic coronary arterial disease: studies of semi-quantitative coronary angiography, *Intern Med* 1999; **38** (9):691–697.

117. Goalstone ML, Natarajan R, Standley PR et al. Insulin potentiates platelet-derived growth factor action in vascular smooth muscle cells, *Endocrinology* 1998; **139** (10):4067–4072.

118. Barsness GW, Peterson ED, Ohman EM et al. Relationship between diabetes mellitus and long-term survival after coronary bypass and angioplasty, *Circulation* 1997; **96** (8):2551–2556.

119. Stein B, Weintraub WS, Gebhart SP et al. Influence of diabetes mellitus on early and late outcome after percutaneous transluminal coronary angioplasty, *Circulation* 1995; **91** (4):979–989.

120. Gowda MS, Vacek JL, Hallas D. One-year outcomes of diabetic versus nondiabetic patients with non-Q wave acute myocardial infarction treated with percutaneous transluminal coronary angioplasty, *Am J Cardiol* 1998; **81** (9):1067–1071.

121. Wilson SH, Rihal CS, Bell MR et al. Timing of coronary stent thrombosis in patients treated with ticlopidine and aspirin, *Am J Cardiol* 1999; **83** (7): 1006–1011.

122. Abizaid A, Kornowski R, Mintz GS et al. The influence of diabetes mellitus on acute and late clinical outcomes following coronary stent implantation, *J Am Coll Cardiol* 1998; **32** (3): 584–589.

123. Silva JA, Nunez E, White CJ et al. Predictors of stent thrombosis after primary stenting for acute myocardial infarction, *Catheter Cardiovasc Interv* 1999; **47** (4):415–422.

124. Elezi S, Kastrati A, Pache J et al. Diabetes mellitus and the clinical and angiographic outcome after coronary stent placement, *J Am Coll Cardiol* 1998; **32** (7):1866–1873.

125. Carter AJ, Bailey L, Devries J, Hubbard B. The effects of uncontrolled hyperglycemia on thrombosis and formation of neointima after coronary stent placement in a novel diabetic porcine model of restenosis, *Coron Artery Dis* 2000; **11** (6):473–479.

126. Ellis SG, Narins CR. Problem of angioplasty in diabetics, *Circulation* 1997; **96** (6):1707–1710.

127. Kastrati A, Schomig A, Elezi S et al. Predictive factors of restenosis after coronary stent placement, *J Am Coll Cardiol* 1997; **30** (6):1428–1436.

128. Kip KE, Faxon DP, Detre KM et al. Coronary angioplasty in diabetic patients. The National Heart, Lung, and Blood Institute Percutaneous Transluminal Coronary Angioplasty Registry, *Circulation* 1996; **94** (8):1818–1825.

129. The BARI investigators. Influence of diabetes on five-year mortality and morbidity comparing CABG and PTCA in patients with multivessel disease: The Bypass Angioplasty Revascularization Investigation (BARI), *Circulation* 1997; **96**:1761–1769.

130. Weintraub WS, Kosinski A, Brown CL et al. Can restenosis after coronary angioplasty be predicted from clinical variables, *J Am Coll Cardiol* 1993; **21**:6–14.

131. Kornowski R, Mintz GS, Kent KM et al. Increased restenosis in diabetes mellitus after coronary interventions is due to exaggerated intimal hyperplasia. A serial intravascular ultrasound study, *Circulation* 1997; **95** (6): 1366–1369.

132. Painter JA, Mintz GS, Wong SC et al. Serial intravascular ultrasound studies fail to show evidence of chronic Palmaz-Schatz stent recoil, *Am J Cardiol* 1995; **75** (5):398–400.

133. Levine GN, Jacobs AK, Keeler GP et al. Impact of diabetes mellitus on percutaneous revascularization (CAVEAT-I). CAVEAT-I Investigators. Coronary Angioplasty Versus Excisional Atherectomy Trial, *Am J Cardiol* 1997; **79** (6):748–755.

134. Warth DC, Leon MB, O'Neill W et al. Rotational atherectomy multicenter registry: acute results, complications and six-month angiographic follow-up in 709 patients, *J Am Coll Cardiol* 1994; **24** (3):641–648.

135. Van Belle E, Bauters C, Hubert E et al. Restenosis rates in diabetic patients: a comparison of coronary stenting and balloon angioplasty in native coronary vessels, *Circulation* 1997; **96** (5):1454–1460.

136. Fischman DL, Leon MB, Baim DS et al. A randomized comparison of coronary-stent placement and balloon angioplasty in the treatment of coronary artery disease. Stent Restenosis Study Investigators, *N Engl J Med* 1994; **331** (8):496–501.

137. Serruys PW, de Jaegere P, Kiemeneij F et al. A comparison of balloon-expandable-stent implantation with balloon angioplasty in patients with coronary artery disease. Benestent Study Group, *N Engl J Med* 1994; **331** (8):489–495.

138. Savage MP, Fischman DL, Slota P et al. Coronary intervention in the diabetic patient; improved outcome following stent implantation versus balloon angioplasty, *J Am Coll Cardiol* 1997; **29**:188A.

139. Lee SG, Lee CW, Hong MK et al. Predictors of diffuse-type in-stent restenosis after coronary stent implantation, *Catheter Cardiovasc Interv* 1999; **47** (4):406–409.

140. Bornfeldt KE, Raines EW, Nakano T et al. Insulin-like growth factor-I and platelet-derived growth factor-BB induce directed migration of human arterial smooth muscle cells via signaling pathways that are distinct from those of proliferation, *J Clin Invest* 1994; **93** (3): 1266–1274.

141. Van Belle E, Ketelers R, Bauters C et al. Patency of percutaneous transluminal coronary angioplasty sites at six-month angiographic follow-up: a key determinant of survival in diabetics after coronary balloon angioplasty, *Circulation* 2001; **103** (9):1218–1224.

142. Rozenman Y, Sapoznikov D, Mosseri M et al. Long-term angiographic follow-up of coronary balloon angioplasty in patients with diabetes mellitus: a clue to the explanation of the results of the BARI study. Balloon Angioplasty Revascularization Investigation, *J Am Coll Cardiol* 1997; **30** (6): 1420–1425.

143. Bhatt DL, Marso SP, Lincoff AM et al. Abciximab reduces mortality in diabetics following percutaneous coronary intervention, *J Am Coll Cardiol* 2000; **35** (4): 922–928.

144. The EPIC Investigators. Use of a monoclonal antibody directed against the platelet glycoprotein IIb/IIIa receptor in high-risk coronary angioplasty, *N Engl J Med* 1997; **330**:956–961.

145. The EPILOG Investigators. Platelet glycoprotein IIb/IIIa receptor blockade and low-dose heparin during percutaneous coronary revascularization, *N Engl J Med* 1997; **336**:1689–1696.

146. The EPISTENT Investigators. (Evaluation of platelet glycoprotein IIb/IIIa inhibitor for stenting). Randomized placebo-controlled and balloon-angioplasty-controlled trial to assess safety of coronary stenting with use of platelet glycoprotein IIb/IIIa blockade, *Lancet* 1998; **352**:87–92.

147. Bourassa MG, Roubin GS, Detre KM et al. Bypass Angioplasty Revascularization Investigation: patient screening, selection, and recruitment, *Am J Cardiol* 1995; **75** (9):3C–8C.

148. Marso SP, Ellis SG, Tuzcu M et al. The importance of proteinuria as a determinant of mortality following percutaneous coronary revascularization in diabetics, *J Am Coll Cardiol* 1999; **33** (5):1269–1277.

149. Melidonis A, Dimopoulos V, Lempidakis E et al. Angiographic study of coronary artery disease in diabetic patients in comparison with nondiabetic patients, *Angiology* 1999; **50** (12):997–1006.

150. Natali A, Vichi S, Landi P et al. Coronary atherosclerosis in type II diabetes: angiographic findings and clinical outcome, *Diabetologia* 2000; **43** (5):632–641.

151. Schurgin S, Rich S, Mazzone T. Increased prevalence of significant coronary artery calcification in patients with diabetes, *Diabetes Care* 2001; **24** (2):335–338.

152. Kirklin JW, Akins CW, Blackstone EH. Guidelines and indications for coronary artery bypass graft surgery: a report of the American College of Cardiology/American Heart Association task force on assessment of diag-

nostic and therapeutic cardiovascular procedures, *J Am Coll Cardiol* 1991; **17**:543–589.

153. Edwards FH, Grover FL, Shroyer AL, Schwartz M, Bero J. The Society of Thoracic Surgeons National Cardiac Surgery Database: current risk assessment, *Ann Thorac Surg* 1997; **63** (3): 903–908.

154. Hannan EL, Racz MJ, McCallister BD et al. A comparison of three-year survival after coronary artery bypass graft surgery and percutaneous transluminal coronary angioplasty, *J Am Coll Cardiol* 1999; **33** (1):63–72.

155. Higgins TL, Estafanous FG, Loop FD et al. Stratification of morbidity and mortality outcome by preoperative risk factors in coronary artery bypass patients. A clinical severity score, *JAMA* 1992; **267** (17): 2344–2348.

156. Parsonnet V, Bernstein AD, Gera M. Clinical usefulness of risk-stratified outcome analysis in cardiac surgery in New Jersey, *Ann Thorac Surg* 1996; **61** (2 Suppl):S8–S11.

157. Shroyer AL, Plomondon ME, Grover FL, Edwards FH. The 1996 coronary artery bypass risk model: the Society of Thoracic Surgeons Adult Cardiac National Database, *Ann Thorac Surg* 1999; **67** (4):1205–1208.

158. Hammermeister KE, Burchfiel C, Johnson R, Grover FL. Identification of patients at greatest risk for developing major complications at cardiac surgery, *Circulation* 1990; **82** (5 Suppl):IV380–IV389.

159. Hammermeister KE, Johnson R, Marshall G, Grover FL. Continuous assessment and improvement in quality of care. A model from the Department of Veterans Affairs Cardiac Surgery, *Ann Surg* 1994; **2319** (3):281–290.

160. Mangano CM, Diamondstone LS, Ramsay JG et al. Renal dysfunction after myocardial revascularization: risk factors, adverse outcomes, and hospital resource utilization. The multicenter study of perioperative ischemia research group, *Ann Intern Med* 1998; **128** (3):194–203.

161. Milano CA, Kesler K, Archibald N, Sexton DJ, Jones RH. Mediastinitis after coronary artery bypass graft surgery. Risk factors and long-term survival, *Circulation* 1995; **92** (8):2245–2251.

162. Slaughter MS, Olson MM, Lee JTJ, Ward HB. A fifteen-year wound surveillance study after coronary artery bypass, *Ann Thorac Surg* 2001; **56**:1063–1068.

163. Spelman DW, Russo P, Harrington G et al. Risk factors for surgical wound infection and bacteraemia following coronary artery bypass surgery, *Aust NZ J Surg* 2000; **70** (1):47–51.

164. Lazar HL, Fitzgerald C, Gross S et al. Determinants of length of stay after coronary artery bypass graft surgery. *Circulation* 1995; **92** (9 Suppl):II20–II24.

165. Mauldin PD, Becker ER, Phillips VL, Weintraub WS. Hospital resource utilization during coronary artery bypass surgery, *J Interv Cardiol* 1994; **7** (4):379–384.

166. Stewart RD, Lahey SJ, Levitsky S, Sanchez C, Campos CT. Clinical and economic impact of diabetes following coronary artery bypass, *J Surg Res* 1998; **76** (2):124–130.

167. Stewart RD, Campos CT, Jennings B et al. Predictors of 30-day hospital readmission after coronary artery bypass, *Ann Thorac Surg* 2000; **70** (1):169–174.

168. Herlitz J, Brandrup-Wognsen G, Haglid M et al. Predictors of death during five years after coronary artery bypass grafting, *Int J Cardiol* 1998; **64** (1):15–23.

169. Herlitz J, Wiklund I, Caidahl K et al. Determinants of an impaired quality of life five years after coronary artery bypass surgery, *Heart* 1999; **81** (4): 342–346.

170. Herlitz J, Wognsen GB, Karlson BW et al. Mortality, mode of death and risk indicators for death during five years after coronary artery bypass grafting among patients with and without a history of diabetes mellitus, *Coron Artery Dis* 2000; **11** (4):339–346.

171. Herlitz J, Caidahl K, Wiklund I et al. Impact of a history of diabetes on the improvement of symptoms and quality of life during five years after coronary artery bypass grafting, *J Diabetes Complications* 2000; **14** (6):314–321.

172. Myers WO, Blackstone EH, Davis K, Foster ED, Kaiser GC. CASS Registry long term surgical survival. Coronary Artery Surgery Study, *J Am Coll Cardiol* 1999; **33** (2):488–498.

173. Sprecher DL, Pearce GL. How deadly is the 'deadly quartet'? A post-CABG evaluation, *J Am Coll Cardiol* 2000; **36** (4):1159–1165.

174. Thourani VH, Weintraub WS, Stein B et al. Influence of diabetes mellitus on early and late outcome after coronary artery bypass grafting, *Ann Thorac Surg* 1999; **67** (4):1045–1052.

175. Roach GW, Kanchuger M, Mangano CM et al. Adverse cerebral outcomes after coronary

bypass surgery. Multicenter study of perioperative ischemia research group and the ischemia research and education foundation investigators, *N Engl J Med* 1996; **335** (25):1857–1863.

176. Newman M, Kirchner JL, Phillips-Bute B et al. Longitudinal assessment of neurocognitive function after coronary artery bypass surgery, *N Engl J Med* 2001; **344**:395–402.

177. Nussmeier NA. Neuropsychiatric complications of cardiac surgery, *J Cardiothorac Vasc Anesth* 1994; **8** (suppl 1):13–18.

178. Naunheim KS, Fiore AC, Arango DC et al. Coronary artery bypass grafting for unstable angina pectoris: risk analysis, *Ann Thorac Surg* 1989; **47** (4):569–574.

179. Whang W, Bigger JT. Diabetes and outcomes of coronary artery bypass graft surgery in patients with severe left ventricular dysfunction: results from the CABG patch trial database. The CABG Patch Trial Investigators and Coordinators, *J Am Coll Cardiol* 2000; **36** (4):1166–1172.

180. Furnary AP, Zerr KJ, Grunkemeier GL, Starr A. Continuous intravenous insulin infusion reduces the incidence of deep sternal wound infection in diabetic patients after cardiac surgical procedures, *Ann Thorac Surg* 1999; **67** (2): 352–360.

181. Zerr KJ, Furnary AP, Grunkemeier GL et al. Glucose control lowers the risk of wound infection in diabetics after open heart operations, *Ann Thorac Surg* 1997; **63** (2):356–361.

182. Campeau L, Hunninghake DB, Knatterud GL et al. Aggressive cholesterol lowering delays saphenous vein graft atherosclerosis in women, the elderly, and patients with associated risk factors. NHLBI post coronary artery bypass graft clinical trial. Post CABG Trial Investigators, *Circulation* 1999; **99** (25):3241–3247.

183. Hoogwerf BJ, Waness A, Cressman M et al. Effects of aggressive cholesterol lowering and low-dose anticoagulation on clinical and angiographic outcomes in patients with diabetes: the post coronary artery bypass graft trial, *Diabetes* 1999; **48** (6):1289–1294.

184. Sprecher DL, Pearce GL, Park EM, Pashkow FJ, Hoogwerf BJ. Preoperative triglycerides predict post-coronary artery bypass graft survival in diabetic patients: a sex analysis, *Diabetes Care* 2000; **23** (11):1648–1653.

185. Fogelson BG, Nawas SI, Vigneswaran WT et al. Diabetic patients produce an increase in coronary sinus endothelin 1 after coronary artery bypass grafting, *Diabetes* 1998; **47** (7):1161–1163.

186. Nawas SI, Doherty JC, Vigneswaran WT et al. Cardiopulmonary bypass increases coronary IL-8 in diabetic patients without evidence of reperfusion injury, *J Surg Res* 1999; **84** (1):46–50.

187. Pocock SJ, Henderson RA, Rickards AF et al. Meta-analysis of randomized trials comparing coronary angioplasty with bypass surgery, *Lancet* 1995; **346** (8984):1184–1189.

188. CABRI Trial Participants. First Year Results of Cabri (Coronary Angioplasty vs Bypass Revascularization Investigation), *Lancet* 2001; **346**:1179–1184.

189. Weintraub WS, Stein B, Kosinski A et al. Outcome of coronary bypass surgery versus coronary angioplasty in diabetic patients with multivessel coronary artery disease, *J Am Coll Cardiol* 1998; **31** (1):10–19.

190. Niles NW, McGrath PD, Malenka D et al. Survival of patients with diabetes and multivessel coronary artery disease after surgical or percutaneous coronary revascularization: results of a large regional prospective study, *J Am Coll Cardiol* 2001; **37**:1008–1015.

191. King SB. Coronary artery bypass graft or percutaneous coronary intervention in patients with diabetes: another nail in the coffin or 'too close to call?' *J Am Coll Cardiol* 2001; **37**:1016–1018.

192. King SB, Kosinski AS, Guyton RA, Lembo NJ, Weintraub WS. Eight-year mortality in the Emory Angioplasty versus Surgery Trial (EAST), *J Am Coll Cardiol* 2000; **35** (5):1116–1121.

193. Detre KM, Guo P, Holubkov R et al. Coronary revascularization in diabetic patients: a comparison of the randomized and observational components of the Bypass Angioplasty Revascularization Investigation (BARI), *Circulation* 1999; **99** (5): 633–640.

194. Detre KM, Lombardero MS, Brooks MM et al. The effect of previous coronary-artery bypass surgery on the prognosis of patients with diabetes who have acute myocardial infarction. Bypass Angioplasty Revascularization Investigation Investigators, *N Engl J Med* 2000; **342** (14):989–997.

195. O'Neill WW. Multi-vessel balloon angioplasty should be abandoned in diabetic patients! *J Am Coll Cardiol* 1998; **31** (1):20–22.

196. Marso SP, Lincoff AM, Ellis SG et al. Optimizing the percutaneous interventional

outcomes for patients with diabetes mellitus: results of the EPISTENT (Evaluation of platelet IIb/IIIa inhibitor for stenting trial) diabetic substudy, *Circulation* 1999; **100** (25):2477–2484.

197. Sedlis SP, Morrison DA, Sethi G et al. Percutaneous coronary intervention versus coronary bypass graft surgery: outcome of diabetics in the AWESOME randomized trial and registry, *J Am Coll Cardiol* 2001; **37**:1A–648A.

198. Morrison DA, Sethi G, Sacks J et al. A multicenter, randomized trial of percutaneous coronary intervention versus bypass surgery in high-risk unstable angina patients. The AWESOME (Veterans Affairs Cooperative Study #385, angina with extremely serious operative mortality evaluation) investigators from the Cooperative Studies Program of the Department of Veterans Affairs, *Control Clin Trials* 1999; **20** (6):601–619.

199. Morrison DA, Sethi G, Sacks J et al. Percutaneous coronary intervention versus coronary artery bypass graft surgery for patients with medically refractory myocardial ischemia and risk factors for adverse outcomes with bypass: a multi-center randomized trial, *J Am Coll Cardiol* 2001; **38**:143–149.

200. Morrison DA, Sethi G, Sacks J et al. Percutaneous coronary intervention versus coronary artery bypass graft surgery for patients with medically refractory myocardial ischemia and risk factors for adverse outcomes with bypass: prospective multicenter registry comparison with the randomized trial, *J Am Coll Cardiol* 2002; **39**:266–273.

Section VI: Adding value to the revascularization option

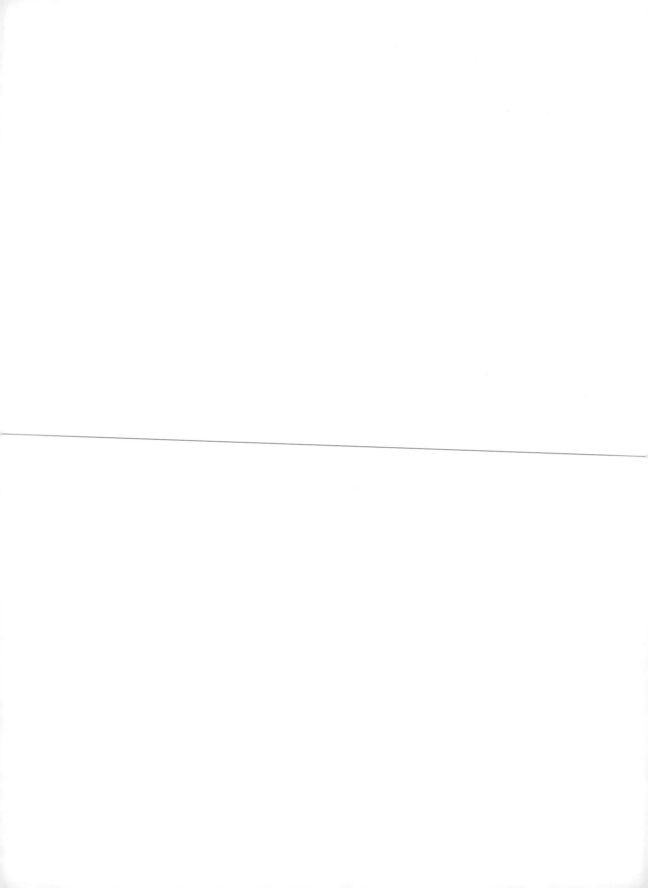

30

Off-pump coronary artery bypass in high-risk patients

Rick A Esposito

CONTENTS • Introduction • Neurological injury • Renal impairment • Acute myocardial infarction/left ventricular dysfunction • Reoperative coronary artery bypass grafting • Elderly • Limitations • Conclusion

INTRODUCTION

Coronary artery bypass surgery without the use of cardiopulmonary bypass is emerging as an important part of the strategy for surgical revascularization. By conservative estimates off-pump coronary artery bypass surgery (OPCAB) currently comprises about 15–20% of all surgical procedures for myocardial revascularization [1, 2].

The origins of off-pump surgery began with the earliest attempts at coronary revascularization. Experimental evidence for successful coronary artery bypass grafting on the beating heart was reported throughout the 1950s. Encouraged by these results, David Sabiston reported the first aortocoronary saphenous vein bypass to an obstructed right coronary artery in 1962. Although the patient expired post-operatively from a cerebral embolus, this initial report stimulated others to attempt beating heart surgery. Shortly thereafter, Debakey succeeded in grafting the left anterior descending coronary artery (LAD) on the beating heart. These early attempts would soon be overshadowed by the refinement of selective coronary angiography and the development of cardiopulmonary bypass circuitry. Working with

Sones at the Cleveland Clinic in 1966, Rene Favolaro began using saphenous vein bypass grafts to re-establish obstructed coronary artery blood flow during periods of cardiopulmonary bypass. The ability to operate on a still, bloodless field rapidly emerged as the technique of choice for coronary revascularization and by 1968 the use of cardiopulmonary bypass for coronary artery grafting became the standard approach.

Yet, there continued to be sporadic reports of beating heart surgery. In 1975, Ankeney reported his results in 175 patients undergoing direct coronary bypass without extracorporeal circulation [3]. Further published reports by Buffolo and Benetti from South America provided additional support by demonstrating the results of off-pump coronary surgery to be equivalent to coronary artery surgery with cardiopulmonary bypass [4, 5].

Despite these reports, widespread interest in beating heart surgery was not aroused until the pioneering work of Subramanian, Calafiore and Benetti. Working independently, these investigators reported success with surgical bypass of the left anterior descending artery on the beating heart using the internal mammary artery through a small left anterior thoracotomy. This procedure, minimally invasive direct coronary artery bypass (MIDCAB), was first reported as a multi-institutional experience in 188 patients at the 68th Scientific Session of the American Heart Association in November, 1995 [6].

The advent of minimally invasive coronary artery bypass surgery was met with great enthusiasm by both practitioners and the lay public. Advanced instrumentation was rapidly developed to achieve both a still surgical target and a bloodless operative field. This technology allowed for results equivalent to conventional coronary bypass surgery with cardiopulmonary bypass [7]. But regardless of these advances, the majority of patients with single-vessel LAD disease were still being treated with catheter intervention.

The next significant advance in the field was the realization that the greatest factor in minimal coronary surgery was not the incision length but the avoidance of cardiopulmonary bypass. The damaging effects of extracorporeal circulation were already well known. Some of the adverse effects included: (a) the activation of the complement system resulting in a generalized whole body inflammatory reaction; (b) the intrapulmonary sequestration of neutrophils with the release of oxygen free radicals into the pulmonary circulation; (c) systemic microembolization of gas bubbles and (d) rare macroemboli originating from the aorta and causing devastating morbidity involving the central nervous system, renal function and peripheral circulation. Additionally, the inherent need for hemodilution and anticoagulation predisposed the patient to coagulopathy and transfusion. The use of the sternotomy incision for off-pump coronary bypass grafting offered many advantages over the small anterior thoracotomy incision. These included familiarity of the approach, accessibility to the entire coronary circulation, ability to use bilateral internal mammary artery grafts and ease of conversion to cardiopulmonary bypass if necessary. The addition of new immobilizing platforms that maintained a motionless surgical field yet minimized the disturbance to the overall cardiac function made beating heart surgery applicable to most patients.

In the absence of cardiopulmonary bypass, evidence for significant improvement rapidly accumulated. Several reports were published showing significant reductions in both the levels of inflammatory cytokines generated and the amount of cardiac enzymes released with beating heart surgery [1, 8, 9]. Another advantage is the absence of hemodilution, which has resulted in a decrease in the transfusion requirements and bleeding complications [1, 10, 11]. These benefits have fostered a greater enthusiasm for the broader application of off-pump coronary artery bypass surgery.

As off-pump surgery continues to evolve and the enabling technology continues to improve, the role of OPCAB in myocardial revascularization will become more clearly defined. Perhaps off-pump surgery will be most useful in cases of expected high-risk coronary bypass surgery. There is already some evidence to suggest that this is in fact true. The following sections will review the clinical data using OPCAB for those conditions considered to be at higher risk for conventional coronary bypass surgery.

NEUROLOGICAL INJURY

Although coronary bypass surgery is successful in revascularizing the heart, it is well recognized that the procedure may have adverse effects on the brain. Concern over neurological complications has never been greater as the general population of patients undergoing coronary artery bypass surgery grows older. Attention to this important subject was recently highlighted by the study of Roach and associates. In their 1996 report including 2108 patients, they demonstrated a neurological complication rate of 6% of patients undergoing conventional coronary artery bypass surgery. The neurological morbidity was equally divided into diffuse deficits such as seizures and diminished intellectual function and the more devastating focal deficits presenting as stroke and coma [12].

Adverse neurological events following coronary bypass surgery are distinguished by three distinct clinical forms: postoperative encephalopathy, stroke and cognitive dysfunction primarily affecting memory loss. Postoperative encephalopathy appears to be multifactorial and may be more related to the reaction to anesthesia, drugs, postoperative psychosis and metabolic derangement than to the effects of cardiopulmonary bypass [13]. Stroke and coma are much more devastating complications and have been identified in 2–5% of all patients undergoing conventional coronary bypass surgery. Risk factors for stroke have been age, previous stroke, carotid artery disease and atherosclerotic aortic disease [13, 14].

Neurocognitive dysfunction

Most studies of postoperative cognitive function have shown a significant deterioration of the performance on neuropsychological tests. Depending on the tests employed, the timing of the testing and the methods used to analyze the results, cognitive disorders has been reported to occur in 11–96% of patients undergoing conventional coronary artery bypass grafting [15–19]. The cause of cognitive dysfunction has been attributed to cerebral microembolization, alteration in cerebral autoregulation, disseminated inflammatory reaction and non-physiologic perfusion [20].

If the systemic effects of cardiopulmonary bypass are the source of cognitive disorders, the elimination of the pump during coronary artery surgery should result in an improvement in cognitive performance. This premise was tested in six studies comparing cognitive performance between patients undergoing conventional coronary artery bypass surgery and those having beating heart surgery (Table 30.1). As can be seen, the results have been mixed. One half of the studies demonstrated significant improvement in cognitive testing in patients having off-pump surgery [16, 18, 19]. Two studies showed no difference in the incidence of neurocognitive disorder [17, 20]. The final study, reported by Andrew and associates showed an interesting difference. When patients undergoing OPCAB were compared to patients having single-vessel CABG, no

		Dysfunction (%)		
Study	**Type**	**CPB**	**OPCAB**	**p value**
Lloyd [17]	Randomized*	96	99	NS
Taggart [20]	Prospective[+]	–	–	NS
Diegler [16]	Randomized*	90	0	0.0001
BhaskerRao [18]	Prospective*	65	6	< 0.01
Murkin [19]	Prospective*	90	65	0.025
Andrew [15]	Prospective*	11 (scabg)	14	NS
		44 (mcabg)	14	< 0.05

Table 30.1. Neuropsychological dysfunction CPB vs OPCAB

*, Incidence analysis; [+], means analysis; scabg, single coronary artery bypass graft; mcabg, multiple coronary artery bypass graft.

difference in adverse neurologic outcomes was detected. However when compared to those patients requiring multi-vessel bypass a significant difference was found. Hence, in this study, neurocognitive dysfunction appeared to be related more to the duration of cardiopulmonary bypass than to the elimination of it [15].

Therefore, the careful evaluation of the clinical data on the effects of cardiopulmonary bypass on cognitive dysfunction does not provide a uniform consensus. Some of the ambiguous results are certainly related to the lack of standardization of neurocognitive testing and the resultant imprecision in comparing results. Equally important is the different means of analysis employed (means vs incidence) [21, 22]. Combine these factors with the likelihood that cognitive dysfunction is affected by the non-specific effects of anesthesia, associated medical conditions and duration of surgery independent of the use of CPB and a useful conclusion becomes unlikely [23].

Aside from these comparative reports, there is other clinical evidence that suggests the elimination of cardiopulmonary bypass may improve the deterioration of neurocognitive performance. Clinical reports using transcranial Doppler ultrasonography to measure cerebral microemboli have shown (a) a significantly greater number of cerebral emboli with CPB when compared to OPCAB and (b) a proportional relationship to neurocognitive dysfunction and the number of transcranial signals [18, 24, 25]. In addition, early postoperative MR scans have demonstrated marked cerebral edema in patients undergoing CPB but these changes were not found in patients undergoing OPCAB [26, 27]. Finally, biochemical markers for injury including the S-100 neuropeptide have been found to be increased ten-fold in patients undergoing CPB in comparison to those patients having OPCAB [28]. These data suggest greater brain protection with off-pump surgery.

Stroke

Despite significant advances in cardiopulmonary bypass and in coronary surgery, perioperative stroke occurs in about 3% of all patients undergoing coronary artery bypass surgery. The cumulative effect of this problem is increasing in magnitude due to a dismal outcome with an in-hospital mortality of about 30% and to the fact that the general population undergoing surgery is growing older. The incidence of neurologic complications increases markedly with age and this increase is disproportionate to the increase in the other cardiac morbidities [29]. This fact was accurately demonstrated by Gardner and associates in 1985 (Fig. 30.1). In this retrospective study from Johns Hopkins the risk of stroke in the patient group 41–50 years of age was 0.42% and increased proportionately with age so that by age greater than 75 years the risk was 7.1% [30]. This relationship continues to be true today as evidenced by the study of Roach et al showing an almost identical increase in adverse neurologic outcomes following cardiac surgery with age [12].

Why does increasing age have such a dramatic effect on the risk of stroke? Many factors have been suggested as causes of perioperative stroke during coronary artery surgery but the one that seems to have the greatest relevance is the potential for atheroemboli from a diseased aorta [31]. The risk of significant atherosclerosis of the ascending aorta parallels the risk for stroke in the elderly population. Wareing et al demonstrated the risk of atherosclerotic disease of the aorta to be 9% in the population aged 50–59 but increased to 33% in patients greater than 80 years old [32]. As with the risk of stroke, the risk of disease in the ascending aorta increases with age proportionally (Fig. 30.2). While it is certainly true that atherosclerosis of the aorta is a natural consequence of the aging process, there is little doubt that a diseased ascending and transverse aorta increases the risk of stroke during conventional coronary artery bypass surgery. By conservative estimates this risk is increased to 14–19% in patients with mod-

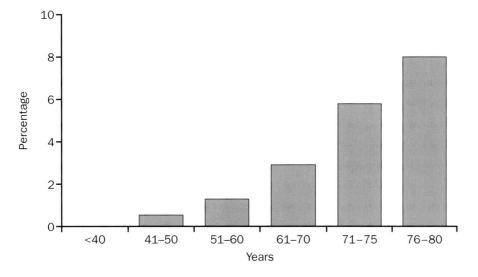

Figure 30.1 The incidence of stroke following coronary artery bypass grafting at the Johns Hopkins Hospital from 1974 through 1983. Reprinted with permission from the Society of Thoracic Surgeons. (*Ann Thorac Surg* 1985; **40**:574–581, Figure 4)

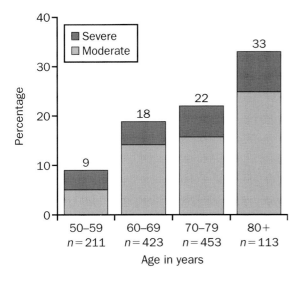

Figure 30.2 Prevalence of moderate and severe atherosclerosis of the ascending aorta to age. Reprinted with permission from the Society of Thoracic Surgeons. (*Ann Thorac Surg* 1993; **55**:1400–1408, Figure 1)

erately to severely diseased aortas [32, 33]. Two subsets of patients appear to have even a greater risk of stroke. Patients with mobile atheroma of the aortic arch have a reported intra-operative stroke rate of 25% and those with concentric ascending aortic calcification (porcelain aorta) have a reported risk of 50% after conventional bypass surgery [34–36]. The presence of severe ascending aortic and arch disease appears to be an independent risk factor for stroke in multivariate analysis increasing the risk of this complication by a factor of between 4 and 13 times over the unaffected population [12, 34, 37].

The association between atherosclerotic aortic disease and stroke has led many surgeons to alter the standard technique of coronary artery bypass. These technical changes have centred on a strategy to avoid any surgical manipulation of the diseased aorta. By selecting alternate sites for arterial cannulation such as the femoral or axillary artery and the liberal use of in situ arterial grafts for both conduits and for inflow to venous grafts, surgeons have been able to avoid clamping of the diseased aorta (no-touch technique). Several observational reports have illustrated the success of these methods with significant reduction in the perioperative stroke rates [32, 35, 36]. Despite these advances, the potential for atheroemboli generated from non-physiologic arterial perfusion still exists. This risk seems to be greatest when there is mobile atheromata of the aorta and retrograde perfusion from the femoral artery. In this situation intimal debris from the abdominal and descending thoracic aorta is at risk for embolization to the brain.

The advancement in techniques for off-pump coronary artery bypass has raised the obvious question of the role of OPCAB in decreasing the risk of perioperative stroke. From the onset, it is important to note that most if not all studies comparing the outcome following coronary surgery with and without cardiopulmonary bypass in a low-risk population show no difference in occurrence rates of stroke [19, 38]. This observation is understandable due to the low incidence of stroke in this population. However, when the subset of high-risk groups are compared there appears to be a definite trend towards better outcomes in the OPCAB group. Table 30.2 illustrates a collection of reports on high-risk patients undergoing coronary surgery with and without cardiopulmonary bypass. Before analyzing this data, two factors bear mentioning. First these four studies are retrospective, comparative analyses and therefore are limited by the constraints of that method. Second, in two studies [39, 41], the CPB group was also treated with other alternate techniques to minimize the risk of stroke including the use of cardiopulmonary bypass with the no-touch technique. Regardless of these considerations, the results appear to favor better neurologic outcomes in the OPCAB group. The observation that stroke is not completely eliminated in the OPCAB group is a consequence of the multifactorial etiology of neurologic dysfunction following cardiac surgery and to the use of partial occluding clamps on the ascending aorta in patients undergoing OPCAB. There is sufficient evidence to demonstrate that the flow disturbance caused by the application of a side-biting clamp on the ascending aorta is severe enough to result in a significant increase in cerebral embolization [42, 43]. This effect would be greatest in the presence of aortic disease.

The complete elimination of the risk of

Table 30.2. CPB vs OPCAB in patients at high-risk for intraoperative stroke					
Study	**Risk factor**	**Surgical technique (*n*)**		**Strokes (%)**	***p* value**
Trehan [39]	Mobile atheroma	No touch CPB*	(14)	7.1	NS
		OPCAB	(90)	0	
Salerno [40]	Age > 80	CPB	(172)	9.3	p < 0.0005
		OPCAB	(97)	0	
Grossi [41]	Atheromatous aorta	CPB*	(567)	6.7	NS
		OPCAB	(119)	3.4	
Yokoyama [10]	Age > 80	CPB	(58)	13.8	NS
		OPCAB	(28)	7.1	

*, Alternate technique used on CPB to minimize stroke risk.

atheroemboli during coronary bypass surgery would seem possible when OPCAB is combined with a strict no-touch technique. Figure 30.3 demonstrates the postoperative angiogram of a patient with a concentrically calcified aorta in which the left internal mammary artery was placed to the LAD and the right mammary artery served as an inflow to two marginal vein grafts. In this circumstance, the application of a vascular clamp to the ascending aorta to establish inflow to the saphenous vein grafts would have likely resulted in atheroemboli. It is probable that as experience with techniques such as these develop, the benefit of off-pump coronary bypass in avoiding adverse neurologic events will be established.

RENAL IMPAIRMENT

The effects of cardiopulmonary bypass (CPB) on renal function have been well studied. During CPB the stimulation of the renin-angiotensin-aldosterone pathway and the generation of high levels of vasopressin account for a significant increase in renal vascular resistance with a resultant diminution of renal blood flow. More than just a decrease in the net blood flow however, blood is directed away from the renal cortex towards the medulla. The absence of pulsatile flow has been implicated in this maldistribution of blood, the decrease in glomerular filtration and the loss of renal functional reserve.

In most cases of CPB, these changes to the renal blood flow do not cause a clinical deterioration in renal function. However, the loss of the functional reserve of the kidneys increases

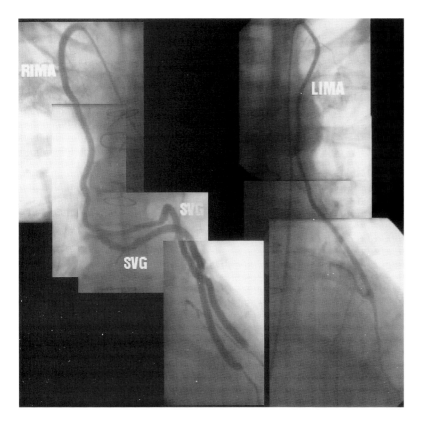

Figure 30.3 Postoperative angiogram of a patient with concentric calcification of the ascending aorta using a no-touch off-pump technique. LIMA, left internal mammary artery; RIMA, right internal mammary artery; SVG, saphenous vein graft.

the susceptibility to other adverse events such as hypotension, nephrotoxic drugs, inflammatory mediators and microemboli [44]. Sensitive assays for urinary microalbumin and tubular lysosomal enzyme, N-acetyl-D-glucosaminidase (NAG), have shown sub-clinical damage to the glomeruli and tubular functions of most patients undergoing CPB [45, 46].

Based on these results, it is not difficult to understand why renal dysfunction following coronary bypass surgery is so prevalent. In a recent, large prospective multicenter study of patients undergoing conventional coronary bypass surgery, Mangano and associates found an 8% incidence of postoperative renal dysfunction and a 1.4% chance of developing renal failure that required dialysis. Underscoring the significance of their finding, the authors also found a dramatic relationship between renal dysfunction and survival. The mortality in unaffected patients was 1% but rose to an incredible 19% if there was any renal dysfunction and 63% if dialysis was required [44]. These results were confirmed in another large prospective study from the Veterans Administration. In this study of over 42,000 patients, the chance of requiring dialysis after coronary bypass surgery was 1.1% but the mortality of this complication was 63% [47].

Fortunately, the majority of patients undergoing coronary artery surgery do not develop clinically apparent renal dysfunction. However, the combination of CPB and preoperative renal insufficiency confers a significantly greater risk of postoperative renal failure. In a study by Mangos et al the risk for postoperative renal failure was tripled if the preoperative creatinine was greater than 2.0 mmol/L [48]. Not only is the presence of reoperative renal insufficiency a predictor of postoperative renal failure but it is also a strong predictor of survival following coronary bypass surgery. In the Society of Thoracic Surgery national database the presence of a preoperative elevation of the serum creatinine increases the mortality of coronary surgery to greater than two times that of the general population [49].

The finding that CPB induces sub-clinical renal damage in most patients and the dismal outcome for patients with postoperative renal failure suggests that off-pump coronary bypass surgery may have an important role in lowering renal morbidity. Two prospective studies have shown less renal injury with OPCAB when sensitive markers of glomerular and tubular function were assayed [45, 46]. By comparing changes in serum creatinine levels before surgery to those at discharge, Bouchard was able to show significant increases in creatinine levels in patients undergoing CPB but not those having off-pump surgery [50]. It is important to note that not all studies have demonstrated improvement in renal function with OPCAB surgery. Gamoso and colleagues did not find any relationship between the creatinine clearance and the presence or absence of CPB. The result of this study must be interpreted with caution as it may have been influenced by the indiscriminate use of Lasix and Dopamine in the CPB group and the significantly greater use of perioperative angiographic dye in the OPCAB patients (25% vs 0.3%) [51].

Similar to the case of neurologic injury, the greatest potential advantage of OPCAB in preserving renal function may be in those patients with the highest risk. In a study by Yokoyama et al patients with preoperative elevation in the serum creatinine of greater than 2.0 were followed after coronary bypass surgery. Of the patients who underwent CPB, 30% developed further renal deterioration in comparison to only 15% of those undergoing OPCAB [10]. Data presented by Cartier also confirmed the apparent benefit of off-pump surgery in patients with chronic renal insufficiency. In this study postoperative serum creatinine was significantly increased in patients undergoing coronary bypass with CPB but remained unchanged in those having OPCAB [52]. The preponderance of biochemical and clinical evidence supports the beneficial effect of beating heart surgery on renal function. This benefit has the greatest significance when the preoperative renal function is abnormal.

ACUTE MYOCARDIAL INFARCTION/LEFT VENTRICULAR DYSFUNCTION

The results of coronary surgery for patients with acute myocardial infarction (MI) or with severely decreased left ventricular (LV) function using off-pump coronary bypass are similar to those obtained using conventional CPB [10, 53–56]. Although there may be a slight benefit in early survival, the predominant difference between groups has been less transfusions, less CPK release and a shorter length of stay for the off-pump patients [10, 53, 57]. Offsetting the small survival advantage is the significant trend toward fewer number of bypass grafts in the beating heart patients primarily due to less grafting of the circumflex coronary artery branches [10, 53–57, 58]. This fact probably accounts for the finding that more patients in the OPCAB group have early recurrence of symptoms (10–15%) and a greater need for additional reinterventions [55, 59]. As technology progresses and off-pump grafting of the circumflex branches becomes more accessible, the results with OPCAB in patients with acute myocardial infarction or LV dysfunction should be re-examined.

REOPERATIVE CORONARY ARTERY BYPASS GRAFTING

The proportion of reoperative coronary artery bypass procedures continues to be a growing part of most cardiac surgical programs. Similar to the risk profile of the general population undergoing coronary surgery, the risk for reoperative surgery has progressively increased [60]. As a result, it is widely acknowledged that the mortality for reoperative procedures is significantly greater. Perhaps there is no better example of this point than an analysis of the Society of Thoracic Surgeons national database. In over 13,000 reoperative procedures, the chance of not surviving surgery was a full three times greater than that observed for primary coronary bypass [49].

The sometimes dismal results with conven-tional surgery have raised questions concerning the role of off-pump surgery in reoperative coronary bypass grafting. In general, the results with reoperative OPCAB have shown either an equivalent or slightly better operative survival when compared to conventional coronary artery bypass with a range of operative mortality between 0–5.2% [10, 61–66]. On first inspection these results compare favorably to conventional reoperative surgery but the reader is reminded that the majority of the off-pump data has been collected retrospectively from primarily single-vessel bypass procedures. In fact, in the selected subset of patients needing single-vessel reoperative coronary artery bypass, the evidence supports the use of off-pump surgery (Table 30.3). In this group, there are fewer transfusions, less postoperative atrial fibrillation, shorter length of stay and improved survival [64, 66].

The analysis of the role of OPCAB in patients requiring multiple-vessel reoperative surgery is more complicated. The majority of data in this case derives from anecdotal reports of favorable outcomes. The finding that a large proportion of this patient population includes patients receiving just one bypass graft makes comparability to conventional reoperative coronary bypass patients difficult [61–63, 65]. This point also raises concerns about the completeness of revascularization in the off-pump patients. In one study by Mohr and associates, the late mortality following off-pump reoperative coronary surgery was 16% and the chance for the recurrence of angina was 12.8% [65]. On closer examination, it seems that the early benefit of off-pump reoperative surgery for multiple-vessel disease is achieved by compromising the long-term results.

There can be little doubt that as new technology emerges and technical expertise is refined, the role of off-pump surgery for reoperative coronary artery bypass will become more clearly defined. Until then there may be some clinical scenarios where OPCAB is the best approach for coronary reoperation. One example occurs when the area of myocardium in

Table 30.3. Reoperative coronary artery bypass surgery (single-vessel disease)						
				Outcome		
Study	**Procedure**	**n (number of patients)**	**Transfusion**	**Afib**	**LOS (days)**	**Mortality**
Stamos	OPCAB	91	27%*	14%*	5 ± 2*	1%*
	CABG	46	58%	29%	8 ± 4	10%
Allen	MIDCAB	23	4.3%*	0%*	3 ± 2*	4.3%
	CABG	12	8.3%	58%	7 ± 5	16.7%

( ), denotes number of patients in study; *, statistically significant differences between groups ($p < 0.05$).

need of revascularization is localized to one region of the heart. In this instance, the operative approach can be specifically tailored to that area of myocardium through a limited direct incision and the patients would therefore not be exposed to the hazards of reoperative sternotomy, dissection of the pericardial adhesions, graft embolization and cardiopulmonary bypass. Limited anterior thoracotomy and direct grafting of the left internal mammary artery to the LAD (MIDCAB) is one such example that has been demonstrated to have great success [64, 67, 68]. Another circumstance illustrating this strategy occurs when reoperative grafting is required to the lateral and posterior coronary circulation. These regions can be approached through a posterolateral thoracotomy using the descending thoracic aorta as the inflow for vein grafts. This technique may be especially suitable when there is already a patent mammary graft to the LAD as it avoids the need for mammary mobilization [63]. Finally, reoperative median sternotomy can be used for off-pump grafting to the anterior surface of the heart including the regions supplied by the LAD and right coronary arteries.

ELDERLY

As the general population ages, coronary bypass surgery of the elderly comprises one of the largest growing subsets of patients. This fact bears special significance since it is well established that advanced age is a strong, independent predictor of increased mortality and morbidity following myocardial revascularization [6, 70]. Many of these patients have significant co-morbid conditions such as previous stroke, renal insufficiency and pulmonary disease and the effect of these conditions cumulatively increases the operative risk. Despite these pre-existing risk factors, coronary bypass surgery in the elderly is currently considered routine even in patients in the ninth decade of life.

In recognition of the increased risk with conventional coronary artery bypass surgery, several studies have focused on the results with beating heart surgery in elderly patients. The majority of these studies have been retrospective and observational. In general, while the trend has been toward less neurological, renal and hemorrhagic complications and in favor of improved survival, the only statistical significant improvements have been in shorter length of hospitalization, fewer transfusions and lower costs. As is the case with the data on reoperative beating heart surgery, the inclusion of patients undergoing MIDCAB procedures and a general trend toward fewer bypass grafts in the OPCAB patients raises questions concerning the comparability of this group to those patients receiving conventional bypass surgery [10, 71–73]. Hence the perceived benefit of off-pump surgery in the elderly may simply be attributed to less extensive surgery. Clearly, additional studies are necessary before the final answer concerning the efficacy of off-pump coronary surgery in the elderly can be determined. It is possible that with a larger database or with careful prospective analysis, OPCAB will hold a greater role in the surgical revascularization of elderly patients.

LIMITATIONS

As with any emerging procedure, enthusiasm about the potential benefits must be measured against the possible limitations of the technique. In the case of off-pump surgery, the primary concerns center on the graft patency rates and on the long-term significance of incomplete revascularization.

There can be no question of a compromise in overall graft patency rates in the earliest studies of off-pump coronary surgery [74, 75]. This problem was generally attributed to both a learning curve and to the absence of adequate myocardial immobilization [74]. The development of mechanical stabilization platforms that allowed for a motionless surgical field during the construction of the anastomosis without causing an impairment of overall cardiac function has dramatically improved the success of the surgical coronary bypass. Current reports on graft patency rates are now comparable to those reported for conventional bypass surgery and are in excess of 97% graft patency [1, 76–78]. While the overall patency rate now

equals that for conventional bypass surgery, achieving an angiographic perfect anastomosis may be less [2]. The true significance of this finding can only be answered with long term patency studies.

The challenge for beating heart surgery has now shifted from improving early graft patency to obtaining complete surgical revascularization. In virtually all the published reports comparing beating heart to conventional coronary bypass surgery there has been fewer bypass grafts completed in the off-pump patients [10, 55, 57, 79–81]. The difference in the number of grafts performed has been due primarily to inaccessibility of the coronary branches to the posterior circulation. While off-pump grafting can be employed for grafts to the terminal branches of the circumflex and right coronary arteries, the necessary distraction of the heart to approach these vessels is frequently not hemodynamically tolerated. When this occurs, the options are to either abandon coronary grafting to this region or to convert to a conventional approach with cardiopulmonary bypass.

The cumulative effect of completing fewer bypass grafts is uncertain. The results in patients who had incomplete surgical revascularization was eloquently presented by Scott and associates from the Cleveland Clinic. Long-term follow-up of patients with multi-vessel disease who underwent primary grafting to only the LAD revealed an increased chance of late death when lateral wall branches were not grafted and an increased likelihood of reinterventions when diseased branches of the right coronary were not grafted [82]. The significance of incomplete revascularization in patients undergoing beating heart surgery is further underscored by mid-term results that have shown an increase in both the recurrence of angina and in the need for additional coronary interventions in OPCAB patients when compared to conventional coronary bypass patients [58, 75, 79].

Recognition of the consequences of incomplete revascularization has led some to explore alternative approaches such as procedures involving off-pump coronary bypass of the LAD and right coronary arteries and catheter-based intervention to the branches of the circumflex and lateral approaches to the circumflex branches through a thoracotomy incision [83, 84]. The role of these hybrid procedures is not yet known but their application may become obsolete by the development of newer generations of immobilizing platforms, which allow for stable heart distraction and better access to the posterior circulation.

CONCLUSION

As the experience with off-pump coronary artery bypass grafting grows larger, the benefits and limitations of this method will become more clearly defined. At present, the clinical evidence has shown a favorable impact of OPCAB in selected subsets of high-risk patients. The most likely patients to benefit from this procedure are those at risk for an adverse neurologic outcome, those with underlying renal impairment and those in need of limited coronary reoperation.

REFERENCES

1. Mack MJ. Coronary surgery. Off-pump and port-access, *Surg Clinics North America* 2000; Vol. 80:1575–1591.
2. Cooley DA. Beating heart surgery for coronary revascularization: is it the most important development since the introduction of the heart-lung machine? *Ann Thorac Surg* 2000; **70**:1779–1781.
3. Ankeney JL. To use or not to use the pump oxygenator in coronary bypass operations, *Ann Thorac Surg* 1975; **19**:108–109.
4. Buffolo E, Andrade JCS, Succi J et al. Direct myocardial revascularization without cardiopulmonary bypass, *J Thorac Cardiovasc Surg* 1985; **33**:26–29.
5. Benetti FJ, Naselli G, Wood M, Geffner L. Direct myocardial revascularization without extracorporeal circulation. Experience in 700 patients, *Chest* 1991; **100**:312–316.
6. Subramanian VA, Sani G, Benetti FJ et al. Minimally invasive coronary bypass surgery: a multicenter report of preliminary clinical experience, *Circulation* 1995; **92** (suppl 1):645.
7. Mack MJ. Beating heart surgery for coronary revascularization: Is it the most important development since the introduction of the heart-lung machine? *Ann Thorac Surg* 2000; **70**:1774–1778.
8. Wan S, Izzhat MB, Lee TW et al. Avoiding cardiopulmonary bypass in multi-vessel CABG reduces cytokine response and myocardial injury, *Ann Thorac Surg* 1998; **68**:46–51.
9. Ascione R, Lloyd CT, Underwood MJ et al. Inflammatory response after coronary revascularization with and without cardiopulmonary bypass, *Ann Thorac Surg* 2000; **69**:1198–1204.
10. Yokoyama T, Baumgartner FJ, Gheissari A et al. Off-pump versus on-pump coronary bypass in high risk sub-groups, *Ann Thorac Surg* 2000; **70**: 1546–1550.
11. Arom KV, Flavin TF, Emery RW et al. Safety and efficacy of off-pump coronary artery bypass grafting, *Ann Thorac Surg* 2000; **69**:704–710.
12. Roach GW, Kanchuger M, Mora Mangano C et al. Adverse cerebral outcomes after coronary bypass surgery, *NEJM* 1996; **335**:1857–1863.
13. Furlan AJ, Breuer AC. Central nervous system complications of open heart surgery, *Stroke* 1984; **15**:912–915.
14. Davila-Roman VG, Barzilai B, Wareing T et al. Atherosclerosis of the ascending aorta. Prevalence and role as an independent predictor of cerebrovascular events in cardiac patients, *Stroke* 1994; **25**:2010–2015.
15. Andrew MJ, Baker RA, Kneebone AC, Knight JL. Neuropsychological dysfunction after minimally invasive direct coronary artery bypass grafting, *Ann Thorac Surg* 1998; **66**:1611–1617.
16. Diegeler A, Hirsch R, Schneider F et al. Neuromonitoring and neurocognitive outcome in off-pump versus conventional coronary bypass operation, *Ann Thorac Surg* 2000; **69**:1162–1166.
17. Lloyd CT, Ascione R, Underwood MJ et al. Serum S-100 protein release and neuropsychologic outcome during coronary revascularization on the beating heart: a prospective randomized study, *J Thorac Cardiovasc Surg* 2000; **119**:148–154.
18. BhaskerRao B, VanHimbergen D, Edmonds HL et al. Evidence for improved cerebral function

after minimally invasive bypass surgery. *J Card Surg* 1998; **13**:27–31.

19. Murkin JM, Boyd WD, Ganapathy S, Adams SJ, Peterson RC. Beating heart surgery: why expect less central nervous system morbidity? *Ann Thorac Surg* 1999; **68**:1498–1501.

20. Taggart DP, Browne SM, Halligan PW, Wade DT. Is cardiopulmonary bypass still the cause of cognitive dysfunction after cardiac operations? *J Thorac Cardiovasc Surg* 1999; **118**:414–421.

21. Stump DA, James RL, Murkin JM. Is the outcome different or not? The effect of experimental design and statistics on neurobehavioral outcome studies, *Ann Thorac Surg* 2000; **70**: 1782–1785.

22. Blackstone EH. Neurologic injury from cardiac surgery: an important but enormously complex phenomenon, *J Thorac Cardiovasc Surg* 2000; **120**: 629–631.

23. Selnes OA, Goldsborough MA, Borowicz LM et al. Determinants of cognitive change after coronary artery bypass surgery: a multifactorial problem, *Ann Thorac Surg* 1999; **67**:1669–1676.

24. Pugsley W, Klinger L, Paschalis C et al. The impact of microemboli during cardiopulmonary bypass on neuropsychological functioning, *Stroke* 1994; **25**: 1393–1399.

25. Watters MP, Cohen AM, Monk CR, Angelini GD, Ryder IG. Reduced cerebral embolic signals in beating heart surgery detected by transcranial Doppler ultrasound, *Br J Anaesth* 2000; **84**: 629–631.

26. Harris DNF, Oatridge A, Dob D et al. Cerebral swelling after normothermic cardiopulmonary bypass, *Anesthesiology* 1998; **88**:340–345.

27. Anderson RE, Li TQ, Hindmarsh T, Settergren G, Vaage J. Increased extracellular brain water after coronary artery bypass grafting is avoided by off-pump surgery, *J Cardiothorac Vasc Anesth* 1999; **13**:698–702.

28. Anderson RE, Hansson LO, Vaage J. Release of S-100B during coronary artery bypass grafting is reduced by off pump surgery, *Ann Thorac Surg* 1999; **67**:1721–1725.

29. Tuman KJ, McCarthy RJ, Najafi H, Ivankovich AD. Differential effects of advanced age on neurologic and cardiac risks of coronary artery operations, *J Thorac Cardiovasc Surg* 1992; **104**: 1510–1517.

30. Gardner TJ, Horneffer PJ, Manolio TA et al. Stroke following coronary artery bypass graft-ing: a ten year study, *Ann Thorac Surg* 1985; **40**:574–581.

31. Blauth CI, Cosgrove DM, Webb BW et al. Atheroembolism from the ascending aorta. An emerging problem in cardiac surgery, *J Thorac Cardiovasc Surg* 1992; **103**:1104–1112.

32. Wareing TH, Davila-Roman VG, Daily BB et al. Strategy for the reduction of stroke incidence in cardiac surgical patients, *Ann Thor Surg* 1993; **55**:1400–1408.

33. Lynn GM, Stefano K, Reed JF, Gee W, Nicholas G. Risk factors for stroke after coronary artery bypass, *J Thorac Cardiovasc Surg* 1991; **104**: 1518–1523.

34. Ribakove GH, Katz ES, Galloway AC et al. Surgical implications of transesophageal echocardiography to grade the atheromatous aortic arch, *Ann Thor Surg* 1992; **53**:758–763.

35. Katz ES, Tunick PA, Rushinek H et al. Protruding aortic atheromas predict stroke in elderly patients undergoing cardiopulmonary bypass: experience with intra-operative transesophageal echocardiography, *J Am Coll Cardiol* 1992; **20**:70–77.

36. Mills NL, Everson CT. Atherosclerosis of the ascending aorta and coronary artery bypass. Pathology, clinical correlates and operative management, *J Thorac Cardiovasc Surg* 1991; **102**: 546–553.

37. Mickleborough LL, Walker PM, Takagi Y et al. Risk factors for stroke in patients undergoing coronary artery bypass grafting, *J Thorac Cardiovasc Surg* 1996; **112**:1250–1259.

38. Malheiros SMF, Brucki SMD, Gabbai AA et al. Neurological outcome in coronary artery surgery with and without cardiopulmonary bypass, *Acta Neurol Scand* 1995; **92**:256–260.

39. Trehan N, Mishra M, Kasliwal RR, Mishra A. Reduced neurological injury during CABG in patients with mobile aortic atheroma: a five-year follow-up study, *Ann Thorac Surg* 2000; **70**:1558–1564.

40. Ricci M, Karamanoukian HL, Abraham R et al. Stroke in octogenarians undergoing coronary artery surgery with and without cardiopulmonary bypass, *Ann Thoracic Surg* 2000; **69**:1471–1475.

41. Grossi EA, Galloway AC, LaPietra A et al. Decreased stroke with routine intraoperative transesophageal echocardiography in coronary artery bypass grafting, *Circulation* 2001; **104 (suppl II)**:441.

42. Bar-el Y, Goor DA. Clamping of the athero-sclerotic ascending aorta during coronary artery bypass operations. Its cost in strokes, *J Thorac Cardiovasc Surg* 1992; **104**:469–474.

43. Barbut D, Hinton RB, Szatrowski TP et al. Cerebral emboli detected during bypass surgery are associated with clamp removal, *Stroke* 1994; **25**: 2398–2402.

44. Mora-Mangano C, Diamondstone LS, Ramsay JG et al. Renal dysfunction after myocardial revascularization: risk factors, adverse outcomes and hospital resource utilization, *Ann Int Med* 1998; **1298**:194–203.

45. Loef BG, Henning RH, Navis G, Oeveren WV, Epema AH. Beating heart coronary artery surgery avoids renal damage as compared to surgery with cardiopulmonary bypass, *Anesthesiology* 1998; **89**:A297.

46. Ascione R, Lloyd CT, Underwood MJ, Gomes WJ, Angelini GD. On-pump versus off-pump coronary revascularization: evaluation of renal function, *Ann Thorac Surg* 1999; **68**:493–498.

47. Chertow GM, Levy EM, Hammermeister KE, Grover F, Daley J. Independent association between acute renal failure and mortality following cardiac surgery, *Am J Med* 1998; **104**:343–348.

48. Mangos GJ, Brown MA, Chan WY et al. Acute renal failure following cardiac surgery: incidence, outcomes and risk factors, *Aust NZ J Med* 1995; **25**:284–289.

49. Shroyer ALW, Plomondon ME, Grover FL, Edwards FH. The 1996 coronary artery bypass risk model: the Society of Thoracic Surgeons adult cardiac national database, *Ann Thorac Surg* 1999; **67**:1205–1208.

50. Bouchard D, Cartier R. Off-pump revascularization of multi-vessel coronary artery disease has a decreased myocardial infarction rate, *Eur J Cardiothorac Surg* 1998; **14** (suppl 1):S20–S24.

51. Gamoso MG, Philips-Bute B, Landolfo KP, Newman MF, Stafford-Smith M. Off-pump versus on-pump coronary artery bypass surgery and post-operative renal dysfunction, *Anesth Analg* 2000; **91**:1080–1084.

52. Cartier R. Off-pump surgery and chronic renal insufficiency. Letter to the editor, *Ann Thor Surg* 2000; **69**:1995–1996.

53. Arom KV, Flavin TF, Emery RW et al. Is low ejection fraction safe for off-pump coronary bypass operation? *Ann Thorac Surg* 2000; **70**:1021–1025.

54. Sternik L, Moshkovitz Y, Hod H, Mohr R. Comparison of myocardial revascularization without cardiopulmonary bypass to standard open heart technique in patients with left ventricular dysfunction, *Eur J Cardiothoracic Surg* 1997; **11**:123–128.

55. Locker C, Shapira I, Paz Y et al. Emergency myocardial revascularization for acute myocardial infarction; survival benefits of avoiding cardiopulmonary bypass, *Eur J Cardiothoracic Surg* 2000; **17**: 234–238.

56. Mohr R, Moshkovitch Y, Shapira I et al. Coronary artery bypass without cardiopulmonary bypass for patients with acute myocardial infarction, *J Thoracic Cardiovasc Surg* 1999; **118**:50–56.

57. Hirose H, Amano A, Yoshida S et al. Emergency off-pump coronary artery bypass grafting under a beating heart. *Ann Thorac Cardiovasc Surg* 1999; **5**:304–309.

58. Moshkovitz Y, Sternik L, Paz Y et al. Primary coronary artery bypass grafting without cardiopulmonary bypass in impaired left ventricular function, *Ann Thorac Surg* 1997; **63**:544–547.

59. Tugtekin SM, Gulielmos V, Cichon R et al. Off-pump surgery for anterior vessels in patients with severe dysfunction of the left ventricle, *Ann Thorac Surg* 2000; **70**:1034–1036.

60. Yau TM, Borger MA, Weisel RD, Ivanov J. The changing pattern of reoperative coronary surgery: trends in 1230 consecutive reoperation, *J Thorac Cardiovasc Surg* 2000; **120**:156–163.

61. Pfister AJ, Zaki S, Garcia JM et al. Coronary artery bypass without cardiopulmonary bypass, *Ann Thor Surg* 1992; **54**:1085–1092.

62. Fanning WJ, Kakos GS, Williams TE. Reoperative coronary artery bypass grafting without cardiopulmonary bypass, *Ann Thorac Surg* 193; **55**:486–489.

63. Trehan N, Mishra YK, Malhotra R et al. Off-pump redo coronary artery bypass grafting, *Ann Thorac Surg* 2000; **70**:1026–1029.

64. Allen KB, Matheny RG, Robison RJ, Heimansohn DA, Shaar CJ. Minimally invasive versus conventional reoperative coronary artery bypass, *Ann Thorac Surg* 1997; **64**:616–622.

65. Mohr R, Moshkovitz Y, Gurevitch J, Benetti FJ. Reoperative coronary artery bypass without cardiopulmonary bypass, *Ann Thorac Surg* 1997; **63**:S40–S43.

66. Stamou SC, Pfister AJ, Dangas G et al. Beating

heart versus conventional single-vessel reoperative coronary artery bypass, *Ann Thorac Surg* 2000; **69**: 1383–1387.

67. Miyaji K, Wolf RK, Flege JB. Minimally invasive direct coronary artery bypass for redo patients, *Ann Thorac Surg* 1999; **67**:1677–1681.

68. Boonstra PW, Grandjean JG, Mariani MA. Reoperative coronary bypass grafting without cardiopulmonary bypass through a small thoracotomy, *Ann Thorac Surg* 1997; **63**:405–407.

69. Mullany CJ, Mock MB, Brooks MM et al for the BARI Investigators. Effect of age in the Bypass Angioplasty Revascularization Investigation (BARI) randomized trial, *Ann Thorac Surg* 1999; **67**:396–403.

70. Craver JM, Puskas JD, Weintraub WW et al. 601 Octogenarians undergoing cardiac surgery: outcome and comparison with younger age groups, *Ann Thorac Surg* 1999; **67**:1104–1110.

71. Stamou SC, Dangas G, Dullum MKC et al. Beating heart surgery in octogenarians: perioperative outcome and comparisons with younger age groups, *Ann Thorac Surg* 2000; **69**:1140–1145.

72. Boyd WD, Desai ND, Del Rizzo DF et al. Off-pump surgery decreases post-operative complications and resource utilization in the elderly, *Ann Thorac Surg* 1999; **68**:1490–1493.

73. Koutlas TC, Elbeery JR, Williams JM et al. Myocardial revascularization in the elderly using beating heart coronary artery bypass surgery, *Ann Thorac Surg* 2000; **69**:1042–1047.

74. Pagni S, Qaquish NK, Senior DG, Spence PA. Anastomotic complications in minimally invasive coronary bypass grafting, *Ann Thorac Surg* 1997; **63**:S64–S67.

75. Gundry SR, Romano MA, Shattuck OH, Razzouk AJ, Bailey LL. Seven-year follow-up of coronary artery bypasses performed with and without cardiopulmonary bypass, *J Thorac Cardiovasc Surg* 1998; **115**:1273–1278.

76. Mack MJ, Osborne JA, Shennib H. Arterial graft patency in coronary artery bypass grafting: what do we really know? *Ann Thorac Surg* 1998; **66**:1055–1059.

77. Mack MJ. Is there a future for minimally invasive cardiac surgery: *Eur J Cardoiothorac Surg* 1999; **16** (suppl 2):S119–S125.

78. Omeroglu SN, Kirali K, Guler M et al. Mid-term angiographic assessment of coronary artery bypass grafting without cardiopulmonary bypass, *Ann Thorac Surg* 2000; **70**:844–849.

79. Arom KV, Flavin TF, Emery RW et al. Safety and efficacy of off-pump coronary artery bypass grafting, *Ann Thorac Surg* 2000; **69**:704–710.

80. Kshettry VR, Flavin TF, Emery RW et al. Does multi-vessel off-pump coronary artery bypass reduce post-operative morbidity? *Ann Thorac Surg* 2000; **69**:1725–1731.

81. Iaco AL, Contini M, Teodori G et al. Off- or on-bypass: what is the safety threshold? *Ann Thorac Surg* 1999; **68**:1486–1489.

82. Scott R, Blackstone EH, McCarthy PM et al. Isolated bypass grafting of the left internal thoracic artery to the left anterior descending coronary artery: late consequences of incomplete revascularization, *J Thorac Cardiovasc Surg* 2000; **120**:173–184.

83. Lloyd CT, Calafiore AM, Wilde P et al. Integrated left anterior small thoracotomy and angioplasty for coronary artery revascularization, *Ann Thorac Surg* 1999; **68**:908–912.

84. Stamou SC, Bafi AS, Boyce SW et al. Coronary revascularization of the circumflex system: different approaches and long-term outcome. *Ann Thorac Surg* 2000; **70**:1371–1377.

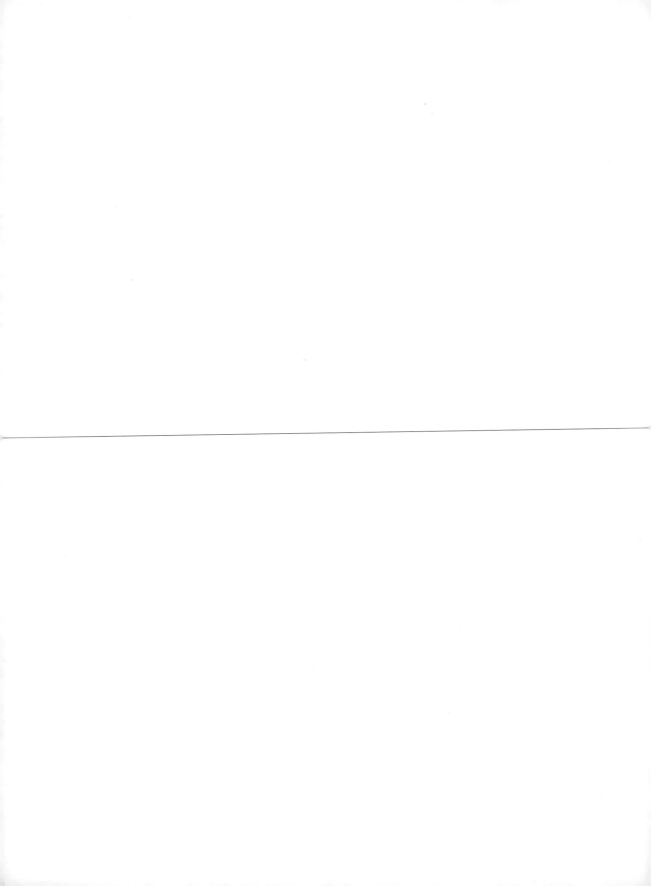

31

Support for percutaneous coronary interventions: IABP, CPS and beyond

Carl L Tommaso

CONTENTS • **Intra-aortic balloon pump** • **Cardiopulmonary support** • **Supported PCI (IABP)** • **Supported PCI (CPS)** • **IABP vs CPS comparison trials** • **Conclusion**

Since the advent of percutaneous transluminal balloon coronary angioplasty (PTCA) in 1978 [1], the application of percutaneous coronary intervention (PCI) has broadened significantly. Originally envisioned as treatment for discreet lesions in a single coronary vessel in patients with good ventricular function, new advances (more recently stents and glycoprotein IIa/IIIb inhibitors), have made many more coronary lesions and patients candidates for percutaneous techniques. These advances have also reduced the morbidity and complication rate of PCI and encouraged the expansion of indications. Additionally, many patients with severe left ventricular dysfunction, some felt not to be candidates for surgery, are being treated with PCI.

The purpose of this chapter is to discuss the clinical application of cardiac support technologies in the management of patients undergoing PCI, particularly those patients with medically refractory unstable angina. Specifically, this chapter will be devoted to a description of the tools that are available to the interventionalist to support the systemic circulation during PCI when the anatomy is so threatening that any compromise such as acute closure or even myocardial ischemia during coronary inter-

vention may threaten the survival of the patient. Similarly, support devices are also employed during a procedure, when unexpected untoward events occur necessitating mechanical circulatory support to successfully complete a procedure.

Of the devices available to the interventionalist for the support of the systemic circulation there are two, intra-aortic balloon counterpulsation (IABP) and percutaneously inserted cardiopulmonary bypass (PCPS), of which IABP is the most commonly used. The use of circulatory support devices are to stabilize the unstable patient prior to PCI and to prophylactically provide circulatory support in high-risk procedures.

The factors determining the risk of coronary angioplasty [2] can be divided into: (a) technical/anatomic or (b) clinical parameters. Technical/anatomic risk is a function of the morphology of the target lesion. The factors determining the likelihood of procedural success include lesion severity, length, calcification, vessel tortuosity, duration of total occlusion, and branching. Although these factors were crucial for the early PTCA success their significance has become less important in the stent era.

It appears that patient procedural mortality is determined by more general clinical features. Hartzler et al [3] have described the clinical parameters defining low- and high-risk patients. The two most important factors determining procedural mortality are amount of left ventricular myocardium perfused by the target lesion and overall left ventricular function. Factors such as multi-vessel angioplasty, recent myocardial infarction and patient age greater than 70 years also appear to increase risk. In addition to procedural mortality, dilatation of vessels perfusing large amounts of myocardium exposes patients to higher subsequent mortality due to acute occlusion or restenosis.

Therefore, it appears that the major factors that determine procedural risk include the amount of viable myocardium tended by the 'culprit vessel' and the pre-existing left ventricular function. Other factors such as age and proximity to acute myocardial infarction are also important factors though not as critical as the amount of viable myocardium and left ventricular (LV) function.

INTRA-AORTIC BALLOON PUMP

The IABP is a helium filled balloon placed in the descending thoracic aorta which inflates and deflates timed to the EKG, or blood pressure tracing. By inflating at the end of systole (dicrotic notch) and deflating at the onset of systole it acts as a volume displacement pump. Additionally, by elevating systemic diastolic pressure it may contribute to increased coronary perfusion pressure during diastole in some instances.

By displacing blood from the aorta, there is reduction in aortic impedance (afterload) allowing for improved emptying of the left ventricle. This results in reduction of ventricular size and diastolic pressures (preload).

In low cardiac output state there is a 20–30% improvement in cardiac output. Because of multiple factors (increased coronary perfusion, reduction in afterload, and reduction in LV size) there is improvement in the coronary supply:demand ratio. However, animal and human studies have not demonstrated global improvement in myocardial blood flow in the absence of cardiogenic shock because of autoregulatory compensation. However, in the presence of hypotension there is enhancement of proximal coronary blood flow.

The indications for IABP are due to hemodynamic situations that call for support of the systemic circulation such as cardiogenic shock, refractory ischemic situations such as unstable angina refractory to pharmacologic management, or in prophylactic situations such as high-risk PCI.

CARDIOPULMONARY SUPPORT

Percutaneously inserted cardiopulmonary bypass is a right atrium to femoral artery bypass circuit. Large bore cannulae (16–22 French) are inserted percutaneously and blood is actively withdrawn and returned to the patient by means of a centrifugal pump. Blood is passed through a heat exchanger and membrane oxygenator, before being returned to the femoral artery.

The cardiopulmonary support (CPS) can provide in excess of 5 L/min of cardiopulmonary bypass which under the circumstances of 'normal metabolic state' should be adequate to perfuse all organ systems. Notable exceptions may be where this system is being used in situations of increased metabolic demand (trauma, anemia, sepsis) where usual flow may not be adequate. During bypass because of non-pulsatile flow, vasodilation occurs which may yield hypotension. Due to the unloading nature of the pump and the vasodilation, pulmonary artery, pulmonary capillary wedge and systemic pressures may drop markedly. It is not uncommon to be able to unload the heart sufficiently to reduce the pulmonary capillary wedge from 30 mmHg to 5 mmHg. Maintenance of mean systemic pressures in the range of 60–70 mmHg may be necessary to maintain coronary perfusion and perfusion of other organ systems where atherosclerosis may be present.

This system also has the capability of cooling (or warming) a patient. Though cooling may sound attractive to reduce myocardial metabolism, it may lead to ventricular fibrillation in the unvented ventricle and it should be avoided. Because there remains some return of blood to the left ventricle, LV dilatation can occur leading to myocardial ischemia. Venting the ventricle via a catheter across the aortic valve can be done to reduce LV dilatation.

Because of the limited time of use due to the membrane oxygenator, indications for the use of PCPS are catastrophic situations where definitive therapy will be able to be administered in a short period of time. Such examples are unexpected catheterization laboratory 'crashes' where with support of the circulation definitive revascularization can be performed, or other severe hemodynamic situations where the IABP is not adequate (papillary muscle rupture) or where rhythm abnormalities preclude the use of IABP.

Other cardiac support devices such as devices designed for coronary sinus retroperfusion [4] and the Hemopump [5] have been used in some centers. However, these devices have seen limited use and acceptance.

SUPPORTED PCI (IABP)

The use of a systemic support device in conjunction with PCI has been termed 'supported angioplasty.' Because the IABP preceded PTCA and was well established prior to the widespread use of PCI, there have never been any large randomized trials or database collections of the use of the IABP in conjunction with PCI to establish its effectiveness, synergy or indications.

Hemodynamic support may be desirable for selected patients with high-risk characteristics undergoing elective coronary angioplasty.

Table 31.1 Indications for IABP

Hemodynamic
    Cardiogenic shock secondary to AMI
    Complications of AMI
        VSD
        Papillary muscle dysfunction—MR
    Cardiogenic shock due to reversible
      causes—sepsis, overdose
    Inability to wean from cardiopulmonary
      bypass
    CHF in potential transplant patients

Ischemic
    Unstable angina refractory to medical
      management awaiting intervention
    Unstable angina with LMCA or equivalent
      awaiting CABG

Prophylactic
    High-risk angioplasty
    LV dysfunction
    Large at risk territory
    Acute myocardial infarction
    Severe CAD in patient for non-cardiac
      surgery

Kahn et al [6] were the first to publish a series of non-randomized patients who underwent PTCA with IABP support. Their study included 28 patients with high-risk characteristics including: class III or IV angina in 82%, mean left ventricular ejection fraction of 24%, three-vessel disease in 93% and significant left main coronary artery disease in 25%. Ninety-six percent of attempted lesions were successful including five left main coronary artery dilations. No deaths or myocardial infarctions occurred within 72 hours of coronary angioplasty. They concluded that IABP support in patients with high-risk features undergoing elective coronary angioplasty appears effective and relatively benign.

Table 31.2 Contraindications and complications of IABP

Contraindications
    Aortic insufficiency
    Uncorrectable severe peripheral vascular disease
    Abdominal aortic aneurysm
    Aortic dissection
    Bleeding diathesis

Complications
    Limb ischemia
    Arterial (aortic and ilio-femoral) dissection
    Embolization (cholesterol or platelet/fibrin)
    Thrombocytopenia
    CVA
    Sepsis
    Balloon rupture

O'Murchu et al [7] performed a retrospective review of 159 consecutive high-risk patients who underwent rotational atherectomy, of whom 28 had an intra-aortic balloon pump placed electively before the procedure. The patients receiving IABP were older and more likely to have multi-vessel disease and left ventricular dysfunction. Significant procedure-related hypotension was encountered in nine patients, who initially did not have IABP in place and five required an emergency intra-aortic balloon pump. Procedural success was achieved in all 28 patients in the IABP patients and in only 91% of those without IABP. No reflow occurred in 18% and 17% of the IABP and non-IABP patients, respectively. Among patients with no re-flow, non-Q wave myocardial infarction occurred only in non-IABP patients (0% vs 27%). On multivariate analysis, elective intra-aortic balloon pump placement was the only variable to correlate with a successful procedure uncomplicated by hypotension. Hospital stay and vascular complications were similar in both groups.

The use of IABP during PTCA for acute myocardial infarction has been looked at prospectively. Prophylactic (IABP) counterpulsation following primary percutaneous transluminal coronary angioplasty (PTCA) in acute myocardial infarction (AMI) has been the subject of two large studies.

The Randomized IABP Study Group noted that patients randomized to aortic counterpulsation had significantly less reocclusion of the infarct-related artery during follow-up compared with control patients (8% versus 21%). In addition, there was a significantly lower event rate in patients assigned to aortic counterpulsation in terms of a composite clinical end-point (death, stroke, reinfarction, need for emergency revascularization with angioplasty or bypass surgery, or recurrent ischemia): 13% versus 24% [8].

Although the PAMI-II Trial Investigators, noted no significant difference in the predefined primary combined end-point of death, reinfarction, infarct-related artery reocclusion, stroke, new-onset heart failure or sustained hypotension in patients treated with an IABP versus those treated conservatively (28.9% vs 29.2%). The IABP strategy conferred modest benefits in reduction of recurrent ischemia (13.3% vs 19.6%) and subsequent unscheduled repeat catheterization (7.6% vs 13.3%) but did not reduce the rate of infarct-related artery reocclusion (6.7% vs 5.5%), reinfarction (6.2% vs 8.0%) or mortality (4.3% vs 3.1%) [9].

In patients with cardiogenic shock due to myocardial infarction who come to PCI, there is convincing data of the effectiveness of IABP. Of 46 patients who underwent thrombolysis within 12 hours of acute infarction with confirmed cardiogenic shock, 27 underwent IABP and 19 did not. Age, systolic blood pressure with shock, pulmonary artery catheter use, pulmonary capillary wedge pressure and the incidence of diabetes mellitus and anterior MI did not differ between groups. Patients treated with IABP had a significantly higher rate of hospital survival (93% vs 37%) [10].

In another study, the benefit of intra-aortic balloon counterpulsation before primary percutaneous transluminal coronary angioplasty (PTCA) for acute myocardial infarction in high-risk patients was associated with fewer catheterization laboratory events in patients with cardiogenic shock, patients with congestive heart failure or low ejection fraction and in all high-risk patients combined. Intra-aortic balloon pump was a significant independent predictor of freedom from catheterization laboratory events and supports the use of IAPB before primary PTCA for acute myocardial infarction in all patients with cardiogenic shock, and suggests that prophylactic IABP may also be beneficial in patients with congestive heart failure (CHF) or depressed left ventricular function [11].

SUPPORTED PCI (CPS)

Shortly after the introduction of the PCPS system, cardiologists began performing CPS-supported angioplasty. A registry was developed which was used to assess the utility of this procedure. The characteristics of the patients that underwent CPS-supported angioplasty and were entered into the registry were rather routine interventions by today's standards, however, at the time they were considered very high risk and would otherwise not have been offered PTCA except for CPS-support. One of the main contributions of the registry to the practice of PCI was demonstrating that PTCA could successfully treat patients that were of high risk without the predicted untoward consequences.

During 1988, the data from the initial 105 patients (mean age 62 years) undergoing supported angioplasty were entered into the registry [12]. This group included 20 patients whose disease was deemed too severe to permit bypass surgery and 30 patients who had dilation of their only patent coronary vessel. Seventeen patients had stenosis of the left main coronary artery and 15 underwent dilation of

Table 31.3 Indications for percutaneously inserted cardiopulmonary bypass

Indications
    Transient, reversible, cardiac or pulmonary dysfunction
    CPR failure
    Supported angioplasty
    Supported valvuloplasty (aortic)
    Post-op cardiac dysfunction
    Unexpected hemodynamic crisis during catheterization
    Failed PTCA (hemodynamically unstable)
    Mechanical complications of myocardial infarction
    Cardiogenic shock
    Hemodynamic support during other interventional procedure(s), etc.

that vessel. Chest pain and electrocardiographic changes occurred uncommonly despite prolonged balloon inflations. During the trial, there was a progressive change from cutdown insertion to percutaneous insertion of the circulatory support cannulas. The angioplasty success rate was 95% for the 105 patients, who underwent an average of 1.7 dilations per patient. Morbidity was frequent (41 patients), in most cases due to arterial, venous or nerve injury associated with cannula insertion or removal.

Data [13] from a National Registry of 23 centers using cardiopulmonary support (CPS) were analyzed to compare the risks and benefits of prophylactic CPS versus standby CPS for patients undergoing high-risk coronary angioplasty. Patients in the prophylactic CPS group had 18F or 20F venous and arterial cannulas inserted and cardiopulmonary bypass initiated. Patients in the standby CPS group were prepared for institution of cardiopulmonary bypass, but bypass was not actually initiated unless the patient sustained irreversible hemodynamic compromise. There were 389 patients in the prophylactic CPS group and 180 in the standby CPS group. The groups were comparable with respect to most baseline characteristics, except that left ventricular ejection fraction was lower in the prophylactic CPS group. Thirteen of the 180 patients in the standby CPS group sustained irreversible hemodynamic compromise during the angioplasty procedure. Emergency institution of CPS was successfully initiated in 12 of these 13 patients in < 5 minutes. Procedural success was 88.7% for the prophylactic group and 84.4% for the standby CPS group. Major complications did not differ between groups. However, 42% of patients in the prophylactic CPS group sustained femoral access site complications or required blood transfusions, compared with only 11.7% of patients in the standby CPS group. Among patients with an ejection fraction ⩽ 20%, procedural morbidity remained significantly higher in the prophylactic CPS group (41% vs 9.4%), but procedural mortality was higher in the standby group (4.8% vs 18.8%). Patients in the standby and prophylactic CPS groups had comparable success and major complication rates, but procedural morbidity was higher in the prophylactic group. When required, standby CPS established immediate hemodynamic support during most angioplasty complications. For most patients, standby CPS was preferable to prophylactic CPS during high-risk coronary angioplasty. However, patients with extremely depressed left ventricular function (ejection fraction < 20%) may benefit from institution of prophylactic CPS.

In a study of 2850 patients undergoing interventional procedures, 11 patients (0.4%) required emergency CPS [14]. None of these patients fell into a high-risk category for PTCA (i.e., sole circulation, ejection fraction > 20%, unprotected left main). Eight of these (73%) had completion of their coronary intervention while on CPS in the catheterization laboratory. Three patients were sustained on CPS until an operating room became available. All patients required blood transfusions and sustained non-Q wave myocardial infarctions. Two late in-

Table 31.4 Contraindications and complications of percutaneously inserted cardiopulmonary bypass

Contraindication
  Aortic insufficiency
  Uncorrectable severe peripheral vascular
    disease
  Abdominal aortic aneurysm
  Aortic dissection
  Bleeding diathesis

Complications
  Vascular injury or perforation
  Thrombosis
  Bleeding
  Thrombophlebitis
  A-V fistula
  Pseudo aneurysm
  Air embolism
  Hypotension
  GI bleeding/GI ischemia
  Acute renal failure
  Transient cerebral ischemia
  Transfusion
  Infection
  Skin necrosis
  Femoral nerve palsy

hospital deaths occurred. Nine patients (82%) were successfully discharged. Standby CPS provides hemodynamic support for patients who sustain a potentially catastrophic event during coronary intervention suggesting that this modality should not be limited to high-risk patients.

Little data exist regarding the effect of CPS on left ventricular function during PCI [15]. In a study of 20 patients undergoing CPS supported PTCA, changes in left ventricular size, afterload and myocardial function were assessed by continuous hemodynamic monitoring and simultaneous two-dimensional echocardiography. The cross-sectional left ventricular area during bypass support remained unchanged during diastole, whereas during systole it decreased. Global left ventricular function remained unchanged from baseline CPS but decreased during balloon inflation. The end-systolic wall stress decreased during bypass support. Left ventricular regions supplied by a vessel with ≥ 50% diameter stenosis deteriorated during bypass support, whereas regions supplied by a non-stenotic vessel did not. Regions supplied by the target vessel deteriorated further during balloon inflation. Thus, although left ventricular size and global function remain unchanged and afterload decreases during bypass support, myocardial dysfunction in regions supplied by a stenotic vessel may occur. Furthermore, regional and global left ventricular dysfunction still occur with angioplasty balloon inflation during cardiopulmonary bypass support.

IABP VS CPS COMPARISON TRIALS

In a retrospective trial over a four-year period, 149 patients underwent high-risk coronary angioplasty, using elective placement of sup-port devices. Based on physician preference, 58 patients underwent CPS and 91 underwent IABP support prior to the angioplasty [16]. Patients selected for CPS-assisted angioplasty were more likely to be males, and to have a history of chronic angina, congestive heart failure, and lower ejection fraction. Multi-vessel disease was present in 95% of CPS patients and 89% of IABP patients. Multi-vessel angioplasty was performed more frequently in the CPS group, and angioplasty success was higher in the CPS groups. Major cardiac events such as myocardial infarction, bypass surgery, stroke, and death did not differ between the groups. Peripheral vascular complications such as hematomas, vascular repair, and transfusions were higher in the CPS group. Cardiopulmonary support allowed longer balloon inflations and higher PTCA success rates compared to IABP. However, peripheral vascular complications were higher in the CPS group, and major cardiac events were similar to those in IABP-treated patients. These data suggest that either method of support may be acceptable during high-risk intervention.

In another study, 40 patients undergoing PTCA who had severely impaired left ventricular

	Intra-aortic balloon-pump	Cardiopulmonary bypass
Table 31.5 Comparison of intra-aortic balloon pump with percutaneously inserted cardiopulmonary bypass		
Arterial access	10–12 F	16–20 F
Venous access	None	18–20 F
Augmentation of cardiac output	20–30%	4–6 L/min
Rhythm dependent	Yes	No
Duration of support	Days	Hours
Ventricular unloading	Yes	Yes

ejection fraction (LVEF < 30%) were randomized between prophylactic IABP support and CPS support [17]. The indications for both groups were left ventricular dysfunction and a large area of myocardium perfused by the target vessel. The IABP and CPS supported groups were comparable in LVEF, mean pulmonary artery pressure, number of vessels dilated, mean inflation time and post-procedural hospital stay. The primary success rate and in-hospital mortality were identical in the two groups. Two patients required surgical exploration of the femoral artery and eight patients required blood transfusion in the CPS group. Intra-aortic balloon pump patients had no vascular complications and did not require blood transfusion. The authors concluded that high-risk PTCA is equally effective whether using prophylactic IABP or CPS support. However, CPS support has a higher rate of vascular complications and need for blood transfusions.

CONCLUSION

Several mechanical devices for the support of the circulation during high-risk PCI have been developed. The IABP and CPS have been used successfully under many circumstances. Other devices such as the Hemopump and coronary sinus retroperfusion have not gained acceptance. Intra-aortic balloon pump has an advantage over CPS in that there are less vascular complications, it is more familiar to the interventionalist, and can be used for an extended period of time if necessary. Cardiopulmonary support, however, can be effective where the IABP fails or is inadequate to support the circulation.

REFERENCES

1. Gruentzig AR, Senning A, Seigenthaler WE. Non-operative dilatation of coronary artery site: percutaneous transluminal coronary angio-plasty, *NEJM* 1979; **301**:61–68.
2. Tommaso CL. Management of high-risk coronary angioplasty, *Am J Cardiol* 1989; **64**:33E–37E.
3. Hartzler GO, Rutherford BD, McConahay DR, Johnson WL, Giorgi LV. 'High-risk' percutaneous transluminal coronary angioplasty, *Am J Cardiol* 1988; **61**:33G–37G.
4. Yamazaki S, Drury K, Meerbaum S, Corday E. Synchronized coronary venous retroperfusion: prompt improvement of left ventricular function in experimental myocardial ischemia, *J Am Coll Cardiol* 1985; **5**:655–636.
5. Loisance D, Dubois-Rande JL, Deleuze P et al. Prophylactic use of hemopump in high-risk coronary angioplasty, *J Am Coll Cardiol* 1990; **15**:249A.
6. Kahn J, Rutherford BD, McConahay DR et al. Supported 'high-risk' coronary angioplasty using intra-aortic balloon pump counterpulsation, *J Am Coll Cardiol* 1990; **15**:1151–1155.
7. O'Murchu B, Foreman RD, Shaw RE et al. Role of intra-aortic balloon pump counterpulsation in high-risk coronary rotational atherectomy, *J Am Coll Cardiol* 1995; **26**:1270–1275.
8. Ohman EM, George BS, White CJ et al. Use of aortic counterpulsation to improve sustained coronary artery patency during acute myocardial infarction. Results of a randomized trial. The Randomized IABP Study Group, *Circulation* 1994; **90**:792–799.
9. Stone GW, Marsalese D, Brodie BR et al. A prospective, randomized evaluation of prophylactic intra-aortic balloon counterpulsation in high-risk patients with acute myocardial infarction treated with primary angioplasty. Second Primary Angioplasty in Myocardial Infarction (PAMI-II) Trial Investigators, *J Am Coll Cardiol* 1997; **29**: 1459–1467.
10. Kovack PJ, Rasak MA, Bates ER, Ohman EM, Stomel RJ. Thrombolysis plus aortic counterpulsation: improved survival in patients who present to community hospitals with cardiogenic shock, *J Am Coll Cardiol* 1997; **29**:1454–1458.
11. Brodie BR, Stuckey TD, Hansen C, Muncy D. Intra-aortic balloon counterpulsation before primary percutaneous transluminal coronary angioplasty reduces catheterization laboratory events in high-risk patients with acute myocardial infarction, *Am J Cardiol* 1999; **84**:18–23.
12. Vogel RA, Shawl F, Tommaso C et al. Initial report of the National Registry of Elective

Cardiopulmonary Bypass Supported Coronary Angioplasty, *J Am Coll Cardiol* 1990; **15**:23–29.

13. Teirstein PS, Vogel RA, Dorros G et al. Prophylactic versus standby cardiopulmonary support for high-risk percutaneous transluminal coronary angioplasty, *J Am Coll Cardiol* 1993; **21**:590–596.

14. Guarneri EM, Califano JR, Schatz RA, Morris NB, Teirstein PS. Utility of standby cardiopulmonary support for elective coronary interventions, *Cath Cardiovasc Interv* 1999; **46**:32–35.

15. Pavlides T, Hauser AM, Stack RK et al. Effect of peripheral cardiopulmonary bypass on left ventricular size, afterload and myocardial function during elective supported coronary angioplasty, *J Am Coll Cardiol* 1991; **18**:499–505.

16. Schreiber TL, Kodali UR, O'Neill WW et al. Comparison of acute results of prophylactic intra-aortic balloon pumping with cardiopulmonary support for percutaneous transluminal coronary angioplasty (PCTA), *Cath Cardiovasc Diagn* 1998; **45**:115–119.

17. Kaul U, Sahay S, Bahl VK et al. Coronary angioplasty in high-risk patients: comparison of elective intra-aortic balloon pump and percutaneous cardiopulmonary bypass support—a randomized study, *J Interv Cardiol* 1995; **8**:199–205.

32

Stents and high-risk cardiac revascularization

David R Holmes Jr and Douglass A Morrison

CONTENTS • The role of stents in contemporary percutaneous coronary intervention • High-risk clinical settings and stent implantation • Stents to prevent or treat acute occlusion with PCI: prevention and treatment of flow-limiting dissection • Thrombus: the intersection of clinical and angiographic risk • Stent use in anatomically unfavorable settings • Stents reduce adverse outcomes (MI or death) in specific clinical settings • LV dysfunction • Use of stents among these high-risk cohorts in the AWESOME trial • Stent use among specific co-morbid populations • Practical issues in the application of stents to high-risk intervention • Summary

THE ROLE OF STENTS IN CONTEMPORARY PERCUTANEOUS CORONARY INTERVENTION [1–20]

Stents have become the dominant catheter-based revascularization strategy, being used in 80–90% of all coronary interventional procedures [1, 2]. The dramatic shift from conventional balloon angioplasty to stent-based procedures has occurred for several reasons. These include:

- Ability of stenting to yield a stable initial angiographic result, almost irrespective of the complexity of the lesion [1, 2].
- Documented efficiency of stents to treat acute or threatened closure following conventional coronary intervention [1–5].
- Decreased sub-acute closure following stent implantation related to improved operator technique and better adjunctive therapy, such as a thienopyridine and IIb/IIIa receptor inhibitors [3–12].

- Improved restenosis rates using stents in selected patient and angiographic subsets [1, 2, 6, 7].
- Decreased bleeding and shorter length of stay with stents combined with the current dual antiplatelet therapy approach relying on aspirin (ASA) and a thienopyridine [3, 8–12].
- Technological improvements with current stents, which are smaller, more trackable, and flexible; with current stents, direct stenting without predilatation can be achieved in the majority of patients [4, 5, 12, 13].
- Increased operator experience has led to increased comfort with the technology [1, 2].

Early in the development of percutaneous coronary intervention (PCI), emergency or urgent coronary artery bypass grafting (CABG) was required relatively frequently. The use of stents has dramatically reduced the need for urgent or emergent bypass surgery following percutaneous coronary intervention. The changes in complications in the field were tracked in the NHLBI percutaneous transluminal coronary angioplasty (PTCA) Registry [15]. In the initial 1977–1981 experience, of 1155 patients undergoing PTCA, death occurred in 1%, non-fatal myocardial infarction (MI) in 5% and emergency CABG in 6%. The combined end-point of death/MI or CABG occurred in 9%. By the 1985–1986 series from the NHLBI PTCA Registry, in 1801 patients mortality was not significantly changed at 1.0%, non-fatal MI was similar at 4%, but emergency CABG was significantly less at 3.5% ($p < 0.01$). In recent multicenter series, urgent or emergent surgery was required in only 0.5% of patients [16–19]. In the most recent NHLBI Dynamic Wave Registry, of 2106 patients treated during 1999, the need for emergent surgery was only 0.4% [16]. These background issues make stent implantation a very attractive therapeutic option for high-risk patients and high-risk lesions, particularly when combined with other adjunctive therapies such as IIb/IIIa agents, an intra-aortic balloon pump and a variety of left ventricular assist devices [10, 11, 16–18].

High-risk settings must take into account clinical characteristics such as co-morbid conditions, hemodynamic state, vascular abnormalities, left ventricular function, shock and acute infarction, as well as high-risk angiographic characteristics such as difficult bifurcation lesions, presence of a left main stenosis, diffuse disease or small vessels, or lesion calcification. Stents can be used to improve initial and sometimes longer-term outcomes in many of these settings. Stenting strategy however will vary considerably depending on the specific clinical setting and operator experience.

HIGH-RISK CLINICAL SETTINGS AND STENT IMPLANTATION [21–47]

There is increasing information on the outcome of stent implantation in a wide variety of higher risk clinical settings. In some of these settings, randomized trial results are available; in other settings, only single or multicenter observational data is available. In considering risk, it is useful to distinguish (a) risk of acute occlusion and myocardial infarction with or without emergency CABG [22–29], from (b) risk of hemodynamic compromise, shock and death [15–21]. For the most part, the risk of acute occlusion is determined by coronary anatomic considerations, whereas, risk of death relates to left ventricular function, clinical state (on-going ischemia, electrical storm, shock, etc., versus stable), and co-morbidity. Thrombus, particularly as a result of plaque rupture, represents a mechanistic link between several anatomic settings of risk (such as total occlusion and saphenous vein graft lesion) and several clinical settings of risk (nearly all acute coronary syndromes including both ST-elevation and non-ST elevation myocardial infarction, and unstable angina) [30–44]. It is useful to distinguish:

- Anatomic subsets where stent use has been associated with decreased acute occlusion and/or more durable long-term results [33–47].
- Clinical settings in which even minor procedural incidents can lead to fatality [21].
- Settings where both angiographic and clinical factors may make PCI favorable or unfavorable, but co-morbidity makes CABG prohibitive (Section V Co-morbidity: Chapters 25–29 in this text).

STENTS TO PREVENT OR TREAT ACUTE OCCLUSION WITH PCI: PREVENTION AND TREATMENT OF FLOW-LIMITING DISSECTION [22–29]

Both lesion anatomic characteristics and clinical parameters can predict acute occlusion after PCI. The most common cause of acute occlusion in PCI is coronary dissection. Stents are the only adjunctive device, which have been associated with a reduced incidence of coronary dissection, relative to balloon angioplasty. In the STRESS and BENESTENT trials, angiographic dissection was not specifically noted, but acute closure was reduced to < 1% [8, 9]. Although the event rates trended lower than with balloon angioplasty, given the low event rates in the two groups, neither study achieved statistical significance for acute event rates [8, 9].

Stents are the preferred means of treating flow-limiting coronary dissection, which accrues, from balloon angioplasty or atherectomy [1, 2].

THROMBUS: THE INTERSECTION OF CLINICAL AND ANGIOGRAPHIC RISK [3–5, 9–44]

Thrombotic occlusion is the second most common cause of PCI associated occlusion [3–6, 22–32]. Plaque rupture with attendant intravascular thrombosis is an important part of the pathophysiology of most de novo acute coronary syndromes. Partial coronary occlusion is seen in most unstable angina and non-ST elevation acute MI patients. Total thrombotic occlusion is seen in > 90% of early coronary angiograms from patients with ST-elevation MI [39–44].

Initially, the presence of angiographically visible thrombus was thought to be a contraindication to stent use, particularly with the early experience with subacute stent thrombosis [30–32]. As stated previously, the development of better antiplatelet regimens, and especially the use of platelet glycoprotein IIb/IIIa receptor blocking agents has revolutionized the application of stents to PCI [9–13]. In particular, data has accumulated to suggest that several settings where thrombus is an issue, have been better treated with stenting than balloon alone. Examples include: acute myocardial infarction, unstable angina, total occlusions, and saphenous vein graft lesions [33–47].

STENT USE IN ANATOMICALLY UNFAVORABLE SETTINGS [33–50]

Anatomic subsets for which either prospective registry experiences, and/or randomized trial data support the application of stents include:

- Total occlusions [33–38].
- Osteal lesions, including left main lesions [48–50].
- Saphenous vein graft lesions [45–47].

STENTS REDUCE ADVERSE OUTCOMES (MI OR DEATH) IN SPECIFIC CLINICAL SETTINGS [39–44, 51–54]

In a number of clinical settings an acute occlusion of even a relatively small arterial territory may be accompanied by hemodynamic compromise, shock or death. These include patients with:

- Low left ventricular ejection fraction (LVEF) or congestive heart failure [51, 52].
- Acute myocardial infarction [39–41].
- On-going hemodynamic compromise or shock [43, 44].
- Very elderly or frail [53, 54].

A substantial literature (mostly retrospective and prospective case series) of the application of various stent designs to different anatomies, such as small diameter vessels, long lesions, bifurcation lesions, calcified vessels, vessels with sharp angulations, total occlusions, and saphenous vein grafts shows stent use is associated with a more predictably favorable angiographic result in each of these settings. This more favorable angiographic result is also associated with decreased acute occlusions and, therefore, emergency CABG. Unfortunately, no randomized clinical trial data is available to demonstrate that long-term outcome has been improved in these anatomic subsets. The clinical predictors of acute occlusion are primarily related to acute coronary syndromes (acute ST-elevation or non-ST elevation myocardial infarction and unstable angina including early post-MI angina), where plaque rupture and thrombosis are usually part of the pathophysiology. In each of these settings, stent use, especially when accompanied by glycoprotein IIb/IIIa administration has reduced acute occlusion as manifested by acute infarction and/or emergency CABG.

LV DYSFUNCTION [51–57]

Patients with abnormal LV function are clearly at higher risk [51, 52]. In the pre-stent era, multiple studies documented that in patients with left ventricular dysfunction treated with conventional PTCA, the outcome was worse than in patients without LV dysfunction. The impact of current technology and practice on outcome of patients with LV dysfunction was assessed in the NHLBI Dynamic Wave Registry of 1159 patients undergoing percutaneous coronary intervention between 1997 and 1998 [16]. Patients were divided into three groups according to ejection fraction: Group 1, EF 40%; Group 2, EF 41–49%; Group 3, and EF 50%. The mean ejection fractions were 32, 45, and 62% respectively. Stent use differed among the groups and was highest in patients with the lowest EF (73.5% Group 1, 59.5% Group 2, 67.4% Group 3, $p = 0.04$). There was a clear impact of EF on in-hospital mortality. In Group 1 patients, the in-hospital mortality was 3.0% compared with Group 2 (1.6%) and Group 3 (1%) ($p < 0.001$). Other in-hospital adverse events did not differ significantly among the three groups. At one year, there was also a significant difference in mortality which was 11.0% Group 1, 4.5% Group 2, and 1.9% Group 3. With multivariate analysis, EF 40% was an independent predictor of mortality. Although in the current era, patients with LV dysfunction continue to have worse outcomes compared with patients with normal LV function, the results of acute intervention in these patients is still improved compared to the pre-stent era. It is, however, of interest that although procedural success rates

with current stent practice are high in the patients with LV dysfunction, and improved compared with the pre-stent era, this has not resulted in improved long-term outcomes. In the current NHLBI Dynamic Wave Registry, Kaplan–Meier estimates for one-year mortality in patients with EF 40% was 11.0%. In the 1985–86 NHLBI PTCA Registry, the four-year Kaplan–Meier estimate of mortality was 13% [17]. This relatively high mortality despite high initial procedural success may reflect the extent of coronary disease or the often severe comorbid conditions or irreversible compromise of ventricular function.

USE OF STENTS AMONG THESE HIGH-RISK COHORTS IN THE AWESOME TRIAL [53–60]

The AWESOME study (Chapter 16) evaluated another higher risk population in the setting of a randomized trial [54–57]. High-risk features required for AWESOME enrollment included one or more of 5 risk factors:

- LVEF < 35%.
- Myocardial infarction within seven days.
- Requirement for IABP.
- Age > 70 years.
- Prior CABG.

The first four risk factors correspond roughly to the first four categories of patients for whom acute occlusion is likely to be accompanied by hemodynamic compromise, pulmonary edema, refractory arrythmias, shock, or death. Over the course of the five-year study, stent use increased from 26% in 1995 to 88% in 1999/2000 accompanied by an increase in IIb/IIIa use from 1% to 52% over the same time. Of the patients randomized to a percutaneous coronary intervention, 99.5% were revascularized. In-hospital mortality was 1% and 30-day mortality was 3%. The six- and 36-month PCI survival rates (94% and 80% respectively) were not different from the patients randomized to CABG.

The AWESOME trial included a registry of

patients who fulfilled the same entrance criteria but did not undergo randomization [56, 57]. Of the 1977 patients in this registry, 1645 were assigned for revascularization (83%) and a slight majority (52%) was treated by percutaneous coronary intervention. As in the randomized portion, stent use increased dramatically from 26% to 89% over the five-year study. Among patients assigned to PCI, 93% received only PCI, and in-hospital mortality was 0.4% and 30-day mortality was 4%. These excellent results were obtained despite the high-risk nature of the patient population. The 36-month CABG survival was somewhat lower than the PCI survival (79% versus 80% among randomized patients; 77% versus 79% among registry patients) but the differences are not statistically significant. The AWESOME trial and registry support the concept that PCI, which includes stents, is a reasonable therapeutic alternative to CABG in patients with medically refractory ischemia and one or more of the risk factors of prior CABG, left ventricular dysfunction, age > 70 years, MI < seven days, or hemodynamic instability necessitating IABP.

Several lessons can be learned from randomized trials and registry experiences of clinically and angiographically high-risk patients undergoing percutaneous coronary intervention with stents. These include:

- Success rates with current technology including primary emphasis on stent implantation have improved significantly over the past 10–15 years [15–19].
- In-hospital mortality rates remain higher in these high-risk patients, but are also improved compared with the historical past [15–20].
- Intermediate and longer-term outcome is still characterized by more adverse events with increased mortality, which may be due to co-morbid conditions or the advanced disease, which is present [56, 57] (see Chapter 16).

STENT USE AMONG SPECIFIC CO-MORBID POPULATIONS [54, 58–60]

Several co-morbidities (as outlined in Section VI of this text) make patients particularly vulnerable to CABG morbidity and mortality [54, 58]. Stent use in even complicated anatomy (by reducing acute occlusion) may be clinically worthwhile! Examples include:

- Diabetes [59] (Chapter 29).
- COPD (Chapter 25).
- Renal failure (Chapter 28).
- Metastatic cancer (where intervention is purely a pain relieving procedure).
- Liver failure (Chapter 27).
- Cerebrovascular disease (Chapter 26).

PRACTICAL ISSUES IN THE APPLICATION OF STENTS TO HIGH-RISK INTERVENTION [1, 2, 20, 61, 62]

The next issues deal with how stents can and should be used and how procedures should be performed. There is limited scientifically controlled data on this, but it remains essential for the performance of the procedure.

Stent selection
Stent technology has advanced greatly. Current stents are more flexible and can be delivered more reliably and easily. Head-to-head comparison of stent performance has in general documented equivalent acute outcome performance [2, 20, 61, 62]. The operator should match the specific stent to the specific lesion to be treated. Individual features such as the presence of a large branch vessel or ostial location may mandate specific design and specific features such as side branch access or enhanced radiopacity.

Procedural performance
This is a crucial aspect. High-risk procedures should be well planned. Careful evaluation of the lesions to be treated and the relative merits of alternative procedures such as CABG should

be considered prior to any high-risk procedures. This may discourage the use of ad hoc interventions at the time of the diagnostic angiogram if the clinical setting affords that luxury—for example, if the patient is not hemodynamically compromised with ongoing ischemia.

The target lesion or lesions should be identified. We usually approach the most important lesion first, identified by an active lesion or a lesion supplying the largest amount of viable myocardium either directly or via collaterals. In the setting of multi-vessel disease, the issue of completeness of revascularization is very important. This is most relevant in patients with abnormal LV function in whom complete revascularization appears to result in improved outcome. If the primary lesion is treated with an excellent result, and if clinical conditions are favorable (including hemodynamic status, renal function, and amount of contrast used, among others), then other lesions should be treated if possible, particularly if they supply a significant amount of viable myocardium.

Stents are the preferred treatment strategy because of their excellent early safety profile and the potential to improve subsequent restenosis. In general, the stent length should be as short as possible and the stent size should be matched as well as possible to the vessel size to decrease the chance of restenosis. It is also important to avoid trapping large side branches or covering so much vessel that subsequent surgery becomes impossible. The latter is of particular concern for treating mid- and distal LAD disease. In the latter setting, placement of a stent which is too distal may rule out any subsequent surgical option for revascularizing that segment.

Stent positioning is very important. Although current stent technology is markedly improved compared with first generations, these devices are still not as deliverable as angioplasty balloons. There is increased enthusiasm for direct stenting as a means to improve efficiency. If it can be performed, it is excellent, however there are some lesion subsets in which

it is very difficult—ostial disease, very tortuous vessels and vessel calcification among others. In these settings, pre-stent dilation is very important. If direct stenting is attempted, but is not successful, the operator should not persist because this can create arterial damage which may be poorly tolerated in high-risk patients; instead, the stent should be withdrawn and predilation performed. As is true with all stent implantation procedures, the stent should be optimally matched to the lesion to be treated and optimally deployed to prevent the occurrence of subacute closure which can have a disastrous outcome in high-risk patients and lesions. In patients in whom the only remaining arterial supply to viable myocardium is treated with a stent, consideration should be given to the use of intravascular ultrasound (IVUS) to make certain that deployment is optimal.

Adjunctive therapy

Adjunctive therapy, both mechanical with IABP or a variety of assist devices and pharmacologic therapy with IIb/IIIa agents is discussed elsewhere in this book. In our practice, higher risk patients and lesions are treated more aggressively. If hemodynamic compromise is present or appears likely, then at the very least, a small sheath is placed in the femoral artery to allow for IABP if needed. The majority of patients who are high risk or have high-risk lesions are treated with a IIb/IIIa receptor inhibitor.

The trade off of restenosis versus acute outcome

Stents do nothing to prevent neointimal hyperplasia—indeed, neointimal hyperplasia is increased with stent placement. Restenosis rates are decreased within stents because of the large acute gain and the lack of acute or chronic recoil or constrictive remodeling. Restenosis, when it occurs, usually presents with recurrent angina, not with sudden cardiac death or acute myocardial infarction. Accordingly, in high-risk patients, a strategy is used to optimize the acute outcome leaving restenosis to be treated later if it occurs.

SUMMARY

Treatment of high-risk patients and high-risk lesions is complex. Angiographic risk factors are most important in predicting an acute occlusion. Clinical factors, as well as extent of coronary disease, determine how well or poorly an acute occlusion will be tolerated. Co-morbidity can make CABG prohibitively unfavorable, even in patients who are not at high risk on an angiographic or ischemia tolerance perspective. The risks and benefits of revascularization by CABG, PCI or other approaches must be very carefully considered. Stents have become a PCI mainstay because of their enhanced ability to yield an excellent initial result as well as an improved longer-term outcome. There are settings where slightly worse long-term outcome can be accepted for a better short-term survival.

REFERENCES

1. Al Suwaidi J, Berger PB, Holmes DR Jr. Coronary artery stents, *JAMA* 2000; **284** (14): 1828–1836.
2. Holmes DR Jr, Hirshfeld J, Faxon D et al. ACC consensus document on coronary artery stents, *J Am Coll Cardiol* 1998; **32**:1471–1482.
3. George BS, Voorhees WD III, Roubin GS et al. Multicenter investigation of coronary stenting to treat acute or threatened closure after percutaneous transluminal coronary angioplasty: clinical and angiographic outcomes, *J Am Coll Cardiol* 1993; **22**:135–143.
4. Schomig A, Kastrati A, Mudra H et al. Four-year experience with Palmaz-Schatz stenting in coronary angioplasty complicated by dissection with threatened or present vessel closure, *Circulation* 1994; **90**:2716–2724.
5. Lincoff AM, Topol EJ, Chapekis AT et al. Intracoronary stenting compared with conventional therapy for abrupt vessel closure complicating coronary angioplasty: a matched case-control study, *J Am Coll Cardiol* 1993; **21**:866–875.
6. Cutlip DE, Baim DS, Hok KL et al. Stent thrombosis in the modern era: a pooled analysis of multicenter coronary stent clinical trials, *Circulation* 2001; **103**:1967–1971.
7. Fischman DL, Leon MB, Baim DS et al for the Stent Restenosis Study Investigators. A randomized comparison of coronary-stent placement and balloon angioplasty in the treatment of coronary artery disease, *N Engl J Med* 1994; **331**:496–501.
8. Serruys PW, deJaegere P, Kiemeneij F et al for the BENESTENT Study Group. A comparison of balloon-expendable-stent implantation with balloon angioplasty in patients with coronary artery disease, *N Engl J Med* 1994; **331**:489–495.
9. Schomig A, Neumann F-J, Kastrati A et al. A randomized comparison of antiplatelet and anticoagulant therapy after the placement of coronary artery stents, *N Engl J Med* 1996; **334**:1084–1089.
10. Leon MB, Baim DS, Popma JJ et al. A clinical trial comparing three antithrombotic regimens after coronary artery stenting, *N Engl J Med* 1998; **339**:1665–1671.
11. The EPISTENT Investigators. Randomized placebo-controlled and balloon angioplasty controlled trial to assess safety of coronary stenting with use of platelet glycoprotein IIb/IIIa blockade, *Lancet* 1998; **352**:87–92.
12. Lincoff AM, Califf RM, Moliterno AJ et al. Complementary clinical benefits of coronary-artery stenting and blockade of platelet glycoprotein IIb/IIIa receptors, *N Engl J Med* 1999; **341**:319–327.
13. Colombo A, Hall P, Nakamura S et al. Intracoronary stenting without anticoagulation accomplished with ultrasound guidance, *Circulation* 1995; **91**:1676–1688.
14. Wilson SH, Berger PB, Mathew V et al. Immediate and late outcomes after direct stent implantation without balloon predilatation, *JACC* 2000; **35**:937–943.
15. Holmes DR Jr, Holubkov R, Vlietstra RE et al. Comparison of complications during percutaneous transluminal coronary angioplasty from 1977 to 1981 and from 1985 to 1986: The National Heart Lung and Blood Institute, Percutaneous Transluminal Coronary Angioplasty Registry, *JACC* 1988; **12**:1149–1155.
16. Faxon DP, Williams DO, Yeh W et al. Improved in-hospital outcome with expanded use of coronary stents: results from the NHLBI Dynamic Registry, *J Am Coll Cardiol* 1999; **33** (suppl A): 91A.

17. Rankin JM, Spinelli JJ, Carere RG et al. Improved clinical outcome after widespread use of coronary-artery stenting in Canada, *N Engl J Med* 1999; **341**:1957–1965.

18. Kimmel SE, Localio AR, Krone RJ et al. The effects of contemporary use of coronary stents on in-hospital mortality, *J Am Coll Cardiol* 2001; **37**:499–504.

19. Hong MK, Popma JJ, Baim DS et al. Frequency and predictors of major in-hospital ischemic complications after planned and unplanned new-device angioplasty from the New Approaches to Coronary Intervention (NACI) registry, *Am J Cardiol* 1997; **80**:40K–49K.

20. Kastrati A, Dirschinger J, Boekstegers P et al. Influence of stent design on one-year outcome after coronary stent placement: a randomized comparison of five stent types in 1147 unselected patients, *Cath CV Interventions* 2000; **50**:290–297.

21. Block PC, Peterson EC, Krone R et al. Identification of variables needed to risk adjust outcomes of coronary interventions: evidence-based guidelines for efficient data collection, *J Am Coll Cardiol* 1998; **32**:275–282.

22. Ellis SG, Roubin GS, King SB III et al. Angiographic and clinical predictors of acute closure after native vessel coronary angioplasty, *Circulation* 1988; **77**:372–379.

23. Moushmoush B, Kramer B, Hsieh AM, Klein LW. Does the AHA/ACC task force grading system predict outcome in multi-vessel coronary angioplasty, *Cath Cardiovasc Diag* 1992; **27**:97–105.

24. Tenaglia AN, Fortin DF, Califf RM et al. Predicting the risk of abrupt vessel closure after angioplasty, results of a prospective, randomized trial, *Circulation* 1994; ;**90**:2258–2266.

25. DeFeyter PJ, van den Brand M, Jaarman G et al. Acute coronary occlusion during and after percutaneous transluminal coronary angioplasty; frequency, prediction, clinical course, management and follow-up, *Circulation* 1991; **83**:927–936.

26. Sigwart U, Urban P, Golf S et al. Emergency stenting for acute occlusion after coronary balloon angioplasty, *Circulation* 1988; **78**:1121–1127.

27. Lincoff MA, Topol EJ, Chapekis MW et al. Intracoronary stenting for acute and threatened closure complicating coronary angioplasty: a matched case-control study, *J Am Coll Cardiol* 1993; **21**:866–875.

28. Ozaki Y, Keane D, Ruygrok P et al. Acute clinical and angiographic results with the new AVE micro coronary stent in bailout management, *Am J Cardiol* 1995; **76**:112–116.

29. Goy JJ, Eeckhout E, Stauffer JC et al. Emergency endoluminal stenting for abrupt vessel closure following coronary angioplasty: a randomized comparison of the Wiktor and Palmaz-Schatz stents, *Cathet Cardiovasc Diagn* 1995; **34**:1128–1132.

30. Tierstein PS, Schatz RA, DeNardo SJ et al. Angioscopic versus angiographic detection of thrombus during coronary interventional procedures, *Am J Cardiol* 1995; **75**:1083–1087.

31. Nath FC, Muller DWM, Ellis SG et al. Thrombosis of a flexible coil coronary stent: frequency, predictors, and clinical outcome, *J Am Coll Cardiol* 1993; **21**:622–627.

32. Haude M, Erbel R, Issa H et al. Subacute thrombotic complications after intracoronary implantations of Palmaz-Schatz stent, *Am Heart J* 1993; **126**:15–22.

33. Sato Y, Kimwa T, Nosaka H, Nobuyoshi M. Randomized comparison of balloon angioplasty versus coronary stent implantation for total occlusion: preliminary results, *Circulation* 1995; **92** (suppl):I-475.

34. Goldberg SL, Colombo A, Maiello L et al. Intracoronary stent insertion after balloon angioplasty of chronic total occlusions, *J Am Coll Cardiol* 1995; **26**:713–719.

35. Sines PA, Golf S, Myreng Y et al. Stenting in chronic coronary occlusion (SICCO): a randomized, controlled trial of adding stent implantation after successful angioplasty, *J Am Coll Cardiol* 1996; **28**:1444–1451.

36. Sievert H, Rohde S, Schulze R et al. Stent or angioplasty after recanalization of chronic coronary occlusions? (The SARECCO Trial), *Am J Cardiol* 1999; **84**:386–390.

37. Rubartelli P, Niccoli L, Verna E et al. Stent implantation versus balloon angioplasty in chronic coronary occlusions: results from the GISSOC trial, *J Am Coll Cardiol* 1998; **32**:90–96.

38. Buller CE, Dzavik V, Carere RG et al. Primary stenting versus balloon angioplasty in occluded coronary arteries: the Total Occlusion Study of Canada (TOSCA), *Circulation* 1999; **100**:236–242.

39. Grines CL, Cox DA, Stone GW et al. Coronary angioplasty with or without stent implantation for acute myocardial infarction, *N Engl J Med* 1999; **341**:1949–1956.

40. Antoniucci D, Santoro GM, Bolognese L et al. A clinical trial comparing primary stenting of the infarct-related artery with optimal primary angioplasty for acute myocardial infarction. Results from the Florence Randomized Elective Stenting in Acute Coronary Occlusions (FRESCO) trial, *J Am Coll Cardiol* 1998; **31**: 1234–1239.

41. Saito S, Hosokawa G, Tanaka S, Nakamura S for the PASTA trial investigators. Primary stent implantation is superior to balloon angioplasty in acute myocardial infarction; final results of the Primary Angioplasty Versus Stent Implantation in Acute Myocardial Infarction (PASTA) trial, *Cathet Cardiovasc Intervent* 1999; **48**:262–268.

42. Fabbiocchi F, Bartorelli AL, Montorsi P et al. Elective coronary stent implantation in cardiogenic shock complicating acute myocardial infarction, *Cathet Cardiovasc Intervent* 2000; **50**: 384–389.

43. Quigley RL, Milano CA, Smith R et al. Prognosis and management of anterolateral myocardial infarction in patients with severe left main disease and cardiogenic shock; the left main shock syndrome, *Circulation* 1993; **88**:65–70.

44. Spiecker M, Erbel R, Rupprecht HJ, Meyer J. Emergency angioplasty of totally occluded left main coronary artery in acute myocardial infarction and unstable angina pectoris. Institutional experience and literature review, *Eur Heart J* 1994; **15**:602–607.

45. Savage MP, Douglas JS Jr, Fischman DL et al. Stent placement compared with balloon angioplasty for obstructed coronary bypass grafts, *N Engl J Med* 1997; **337**:740–747.

46. Wong SC, Baim DS, Schatz RA et al. Immediate and late outcomes after stent implantation in saphenous vein graft lesions: the multicenter US Palmaz-Schatz stent experience, *J Am Coll Cardiol* 1995; **26**:704–712.

47. Piana RN, Moscucci M, Cohen DJ et al. Palmaz-Schatz stenting for treatment of focal vein graft stenosis: immediate results and long-term outcome, *J Am Coll Cardiol* 1994; **23**:1296–1304.

48. Zampieri P, Colombo A, Almagor Y et al. Results of coronary stenting of ostial lesions, *Am J Cardiol* 1994; **73**:901–903.

49. Park SJ, Park SW, Hong MK et al. Stenting of unprotected left main coronary stenoses: immediate and late outcomes, *J Am Coll Cardiol* 1998; **31**:37–42.

50. Lefevre T, Louvard Y, Morice MC. Indexed management of bifurcation stenting, *Stent* 1999; **2**:34–44.

51. Holmes DR Jr, Detre KM, Williams DO et al. Long-term outcome of patients with depressed left ventricular function undergoing percutaneous transluminal coronary angioplasty. The NHLBI PTCA Registry. *Circulation* 1993; **87**: 21–29.

52. Keelan PC, Koru-Sengul T, Johnston JM et al. In-hospital and one-year outcomes in patient with impaired left ventricular function undergoing contemporary percutaneous coronary revascularization. 2002, in press.

53. Morrison DA, Bies R, Sacks J. Coronary angioplasty for elderly patients with 'High-risk' unstable angina: short-term outcomes and long-term survival, *J Am Coll Cardiol* 1997; **29**:339–344.

54. Morrison DA. Summary of 'high-risk' and 'prohibitive-risk' for surgery or angioplasty in unstable angina. In: Morrison DA, Serruys PW, eds, *Medically Refractory Rest Angina* (New York: Marcel Dekker Inc, 1992) 385–401.

55. Morrison DA, Sethi G, Sacks J et al for the AWESOME Investigators. A multicenter, randomized trial of percutaneous coronary intervention versus bypass surgery in high-risk unstable angina patients, *Controlled Clin Trials* 1999; **20**:601–619.

56. Morrison DA, Sethi G, Sacks J et al for the AWESOME Investigators. Percutaneous coronary intervention versus coronary artery bypass graft surgery for patients with medically refractory myocardial ischemia and risk factors for adverse outcomes with bypass: a multicenter randomized trial, *J Am Coll Cardiol* 2001; **38**:143–149.

57. Morrison DA, Sethi G, Sacks J et al for the AWESOME investigators. Percutaneous coronary intervention versus coronary artery bypass graft surgery for patients with medically refractory myocardial ischemia and risk factors for adverse outcomes with bypass. The VA AWESOME multicenter registry: comparison with the randomized clinical trial, *J Am Coll Cardiol* 2002; **39**:266–273.

58. Grover FL, Johnson RR, Marshall G, Hammermeister KE and the Department of Veterans Affairs cardiac surgeons. Factors predictive of operative mortality among coronary artery bypass subsets, *Ann Thorac Surg* 1993; **56**:1296–1307.

59. Kornowski R, Lansky AJ. Current perspectives

on interventional treatment strategies in diabetic patients with coronary artery disease, *Cathet Cardiovasc Intervent* 2000; **50**:245–254.

60. Azar RR, Prpic R, Ho KKL et al. Impact of end-stage renal disease on clinical and angiographic outcomes after coronary stenting, *Am J Cardiol* 2000; **86**:485–489.

61. Phillips PS, Kern MJ, Serruys PW. *The Stenter's Notebook* (Birmingham, MI: Physician's Press, 1998).

62. Serruys PW, Kutryk MJB. *Handbook of Coronary Stents* (London: Martin Dunitz Ltd, 1998).

33

Pharmacologic support for PCI: glycoprotein IIb/IIIa receptor blockers

Douglass A Morrison

CONTENTS • **Biology of arterial thrombosis and acute coronary syndromes** • **Glycoprotein IIb/IIIa receptor blockade: overall picture** • **Glycoprotein IIb/IIIa receptor blockade as an adjunct to intervention** • **Glycoprotein IIb/IIIa receptor blockade for the treatment of unstable angina/non-Q MI, whether PCI is or is not planned** • **Glycoprotein IIb/IIIa receptor blockade in the treatment of acute MI (including as adjunct to primary PCI)** • **Bleeding** • **Summary**

BIOLOGY OF ARTERIAL THROMBOSIS AND ACUTE CORONARY SYNDROMES

One of the extraordinary breakthroughs of the past three decades has finally enabled clinicians to explain to patients how a 'progressive disease of aging' (atherosclerosis) can present as an acute myocardial infarction or episode of unstable angina or sudden death. Basic science and clinical data have led to the realization that plaque erosion or rupture culminates in thrombus formation [1–10]. Whether the thrombus completely, partially or intermittently obstructs an artery for a critical period may determine ST elevation versus depression or non-specific change on the surface electrocardiogram, but all acute coronary syndromes (ACS) share this common pathophysiologic link, in which the thrombus is central. In the description that follows, the platelet glycoprotein IIb/IIIa receptor is the final link in platelet aggregation with adhesive molecules, such as fibrin. Accordingly, regardless of initial stimuli, blocking that receptor blocks platelet aggregation. As previously stated in the chapter on stents, thrombus is the 'intersection' of clinical risk (all acute coronary syndromes share the pathophysiology of plaque erosion/rupture leading to acute thrombosis) and angiographic risk (morphologic patterns which predict acute occlusive syndromes). Therefore, interference with thrombosis, and particularly platelet thrombosis, has revolutionized PCI, particularly with stents, by both reducing thrombotic adverse outcomes and allowing less hemorrhagic post-stent regimens.

In normal arteries, platelets within the blood do not come into contact with collagen from within the arterial wall because of the presence of endothelial cells. Additionally, the normal endothelial cells do not interact with platelets. The first step in the atherosclerotic process is injury to the endothelial cell. Endothelial cell dysfunction can occur in response to a variety of insults including several risk factors for atherosclerosis, such as oxidized low density lipoprotein (LDL). Regardless of etiology, endothelial dysfunction can result in the following:

- Vasoconstriction; this is usually a balance between nitric oxide (NO) on the vaso-dilatation side and angiotensin II and endothelin on the vasoconstriction side.
- Platelet adhesion; Ia/Ib receptor for collagen–platelet and IIb/IIIa receptor for platelet–platelet by way of platelet–fibrinogen.
- Platelet aggregation.
- Platelet activation.
- Leukocyte adhesion.

For thrombosis to occur, injury to the endothelial cell is accompanied by denudation, which exposes platelets to collagen. Using the Ia/Ib receptor, platelets adhere to collagen. The Ia/Ib receptor starts the formation of a platelet plug to prevent bleeding. The platelet plug grows by platelet to platelet binding with fibrinogen as a bridge, using the IIb/IIIa receptor. The formation of fibrin from fibrinogen is also important because it stabilizes the plug, serving as a kind of glue. The fibrin is formed from fibrinogen by thrombin. In turn, thrombin was formed from prothrombin, by the action of tissue factor, which was released from the damaged arterial wall.

During adhesion of platelets, Von Willebrand factor also binds with the Ia/Ib receptor causing platelet activation. Platelet activation is accompanied by a shape change from smooth to spiculated, which increases the surface area upon which thrombin generation can occur. Thromboxane A_2, serotonin and other aggregatory and chemo-attractant molecules are released by the degranulation of alpha and dense granules, and an increased number of glycoprotein IIb/IIIa receptors are expressed for fibrinogen binding.

Acute coronary syndromes are intimately connected with the biology of the fundamental atherosclerotic lesion, the plaque. Initially, plasma LDL cholesterol enters the arterial intima and functions like an inflammatory mediator. Monocyte adhesion and migration through the endothelial surface occur in response to LDL. Monocytes take up the oxi-dized LDL, becoming foam cells. The collection of lipid-laden foam cells beneath the surface causes the development of the raised fatty streak, the first lesion of atherosclerosis. At this point, endothelial cell function may not be normal.

Plaques evolve to a more advanced form by recruitment of more macrophages and the formation of a central necrotic lipid core. At the same time, smooth muscle cells proliferate and wall off the core. With further evolution, endothelial denudation can occur and be accompanied by platelet adhesion. Platelet deposition can contribute to plaque growth, not only by the mass of platelets themselves, but also the release of platelet derived growth factor (PDGF), a stimulant of smooth muscle proliferation. The inflammatory motif is further supported by macrophages, which express cytokines such as tumor necrosis factor alpha and interleukin-1. Free radicals and metallo-proteinases, enzymes that can erode basement membranes and connective tissue leading to plaque rupture, are also produced. Macrophages can also produce tissue factor, contributing to thrombin and fibrin production.

Injury to the endothelium can occur to several different depths or levels and this has clinical implications. With a level 1 injury, although denudation may be widespread, it is superficial and, accordingly, thrombus forms only over the surface of the plaque. Level 2 injury involves a tear in the plaque, thereby exposing the highly thrombogenic lipid core to the blood. Level 3 injury is seen with percutaneous coronary interventions, which create tears all the way into the media; it is ordinarily not a natural cause of arterial thrombosis.

It is considered likely that most cases of either erosion (level 1) or plaque rupture (level 2) are subclinical. Although acute syndromes are not produced by these events, they can stimulate smooth muscle proliferation and/or collagen synthesis, thereby contributing to development of 'new' angiographic lesions and the growth of old ones. Alternatively, both level 1 and 2 injuries can be dynamic, leading to expanding thrombi. The sequelae include: (a) embolization of platelet clumps which can occlude small vessels; (b) partially occlusive thrombi which, especially with superimposed vasospasm, cause unstable angina; and (c) occlusive thrombi which lead to ST-elevation necrosis.

GLYCOPROTEIN IIB/IIIA RECEPTOR BLOCKADE: OVERALL PICTURE

There are 3 approved GP IIb/IIIa receptor blocking agents for parenteral use: abciximab (reopro) is a 'non-selective', longer duration, monoclonal antibody; eptifibatide (integrilin) is 'selective' for the receptor, of shorter duration, and a peptide; tirofiban (aggrastat) is 'selective' for the receptor, of shorter duration, and a non-peptide.

- Most of the randomized clinical trial (RCT) data for abciximab involves its use as an adjunct for percutaneous coronary intervention (PCI), and that is its 'approved' use.
- Most of the RCT data for eptifibatide and tirofiban involve their use in stabilizing patients with ACS and they are both 'approved' for that use (eptifibatide is also approved for PCI).
- Most of the RCT's endpoints are combinations of death, myocardial infarction (MI) and revascularization (either 'emergent' or overall), and the statistics are driven by small enzyme releases (defined as MI) and/or revascularizations, which are not blindly adjudicated.
- Nonetheless more than 30,000 patients have been randomly allocated between GP IIb/IIIa blockers and 'conventional' forms of therapy for PCI and/or ACS. Based largely on the results of these RCTs, lots of patients are receiving these expensive drugs, some of them experiencing bleeding or changes in therapy (such as surgical revascularization) that they would not otherwise.
- Why?

GLYCOPROTEIN IIB/IIIA RECEPTOR BLOCKADE AS AN ADJUNCT TO INTERVENTION (TABLE 33.1) [11–39]

Glycoprotein IIb/IIIa platelet receptor blockers have become as revolutionary to PCI as stents because:

- They block the final common pathway in platelet aggregation with adhesion molecules.
- This pharmacologic mechanism involves clinically significant interference with platelet thrombus formation, which is at the intersection of clinical risk and angiographic risk.
- They are associated with decreased acute

Table 33.1. Randomized trials of glycoprotein IIb/IIIa receptor blockade as an adjunct to intervention

Trial name	Drug	Reference	Subjects (n)
1. EPIC	Abciximab	15, 21, 22, 25	2099
2. EPILOG	Abciximab	16, 21, 22, 32	2792
3. EPISTENT	Abciximab	17, 21–23	2399
4. CAPTURE	Abciximab	20	1265
5. RAPPORT	Abciximab	54	483
6. IMPACT II	Eptifibatide	18	4010
7. RESTORE	Tirofiban	19	2139

thrombotic occlusion. They largely eliminate subacute stent thrombosis.

- They are associated with reduced distal embolization, which results in less periprocedural infarction and/or 'no-reflow'.
- They appear to have particular impact on diabetic patients, which are a high-risk subset for either PCI or CABG revascularization.
- They largely eliminate the need for anticoagulant pretreatment of PCI candidates with a 'thrombus burden'.
- They are part of the 'platelet revolution' which made the early stent regimens of dextran and warfarin obsolete, thereby facilitating the widespread use of stents in even the most 'thrombotic' subsets (totals, acute MI and vein graft interventions). They can be associated with only minimal bleeding, if one learns the lessons of EPILOG (weight-adjusted or reduced heparin and exquisite attention to sheaths).

The EPIC trial evaluated the use of the chimeric monoclonal-antibody Fab fragment (c7e3 Fab) directed against the platelet IIb/IIIa receptor, abciximab, in patients who were felt to have high risk of acute vessel closure (acute evolving myocardial infarction within 12 hours necessitating rescue angioplasty; early post-infarction angina with at least two episodes of rest angina accompanied by ECG changes; clinical or angiographic harbingers of risk). All patients received aspirin and heparin and 2099 were randomized between placebo, bolus of 0.25 mg/kg alone, or bolus plus 12 hour infusion at 10 µg/minute. The primary end-point was a prespecified composite of death from any cause, non-fatal, myocardial infarction (MI), coronary artery bypass grafts (CABG), repeat percutaneous coronary intervention (PCI), insertion of a coronary stent because of procedural failure or placement of intra-aortic balloon pump because of refractory ischemia. Bolus plus infusion was associated with a 35% relative reduction in the composite (12.8% vs 8.3%; $p = 0.008$). Bolus alone was associated

with a 10% reduction (12.8% vs 11.5%; $p = 0.43$). Conversely, there was an increase in bleeding with abciximab, larger with bolus plus infusion than bolus alone.

EPILOG extended the results of EPIC to patients undergoing urgent or elective percutaneous transluminal coronary angioplasty (PTCA), without the high-risk factors for acute occlusion that were entrance requirements in EPIC. Additionally, EPILOG tested the hypothesis that reducing the initial dose of heparin on a weight adjusted basis, might allow for the added benefits of the bolus plus infusion dosing of abciximab, while reducing the rate of bleeding complications. A total of 2792 of a planned 4800 patients were enrolled because the first interim analysis showed such a strong effect of abciximab (11.7% composite event in the placebo arm versus 5.2% in the abciximab/low-dose heparin arm for a risk ratio = 0.43, 95% CI 0.32–0.63). There was a reduction in minor bleeding comparing the high- to low-dose of heparin.

CAPTURE extended these observations by including patients who were medically refractory and awaiting planned angioplasty. This trial was also terminated early because of having reached the prespecified stopping point after 1050 patients had undergone randomization. At that point, data from 1265 patients were analyzed and there were 16.4% composite end-points (death, non-fatal MI, urgent intervention) in the placebo group vs 10.8% in the abciximab group ($p = 0.0064$). For all three of these trials, patients with planned stenting were not included, and stenting as 'bail-out' was considered among the composite outcome.

EPISTENT was designed to investigate the potentially complementary roles of stenting and abciximab. A total of 2399 were randomly allocated between stent plus placebo, stent plus abciximab, or balloon angioplasty plus abciximab. Considering the composite end-point of death and MI, stent alone was 11.4%, abciximab alone was 7.8%, and the combination of stent and abciximab was associated with a rate of 5.6%. Similarly, repeat revascularization rates were 15.4% for abciximab plus balloon, 106 for stent alone, and 8.7% for stent plus abciximab. These data suggested complementary benefits from the use of stenting with abciximab.

RAPPORT was a trial of patients undergoing direct angioplasty for ST-segment elevation acute MI. A total of 483 patients were randomized between placebo and abciximab. Abciximab was associated with a significant 62% reduction in the composite end-point of death, reinfarction, or urgent revascularization, (12.0% vs 4.6% $p = 0.005$).

The results of these individual studies were extended by either prolonged observation or by pooling the results of several studies, in order to have a larger sample within which to look at subsets [21–25]. Bhatt and co-workers pooled results from EPIC, EPILOG, and EPISTENT in order to look specifically at the 1462/6534 who had a clinical diagnosis of diabetes. Mortality in diabetics who underwent multi-vessel intervention was reduced from 7.7% to 0.9% ($p = 0.018$) with abciximab. Cho and colleagues pooled data from the same three primary studies in order to consider the role of gender. The reductions in primary end-point with abciximab were comparable for men and women. Cura and collaborators looked at data from EPILOG and EPISTENT, considering the relative roles of stenting and abciximab in various complex anatomic lesion categories (long, tandem, severely calcified, restenotic, thrombotic, osteal, occlusions, bifurcations, saphenous vein grafts, and multi-vessel). Using a combined end-point of death or myocardial infarction, Cura and coworkers demonstrated that stents and abciximab had additive benefits in complex anatomic subsets. Bhatt and colleagues combined data from EPIC, CAPTURE, EPILOG, RAPPORT, and EPISTENT, so as to consider the usefulness of abciximab as an adjunct to various devices. They found decreases in death and myocardial infarction regardless of whether the additions to balloon angioplasty only were elective stenting, bail-out stenting, or directional atherectomy. Topol and co-workers reported sustained benefits in the high-risk EPIC population out to three years. Conversely in an observational

study, workers from the Mayo clinic compared 210 patients undergoing vein graft interventions without abciximab versus 133 patients undergoing vein graft interventions with abciximab; they could not demonstrate an advantage among the non-randomly allocated cohorts.

RESTORE compared placebo with a bolus plus 36-hour infusion of tirofiban randomly allocated to 2212 patients undergoing PCI within 72 hours of admission with an unstable coronary syndrome. The composite end-point of the study included death from any cause, non-fatal MI, CABG for failed PTCA, stent for threatened or abrupt closure or repeat target vessel angioplasty for recurrent ischemia. Composite end-points were reduced at two and seven days by 38% and 27% respectively. When only urgent or emergent CABG or PCI were included, the 30-day reduction of 24% also achieved statistical significance ($p = 0.052$).

IMPACT-II randomized 4010 patients between placebo and a bolus of 135 μg/kg of eptifibatide plus one of 24-hour infusions. Patients were undergoing elective, urgent or emergent PCI and a composite end-point of death, myocardial infarction, unplanned surgical or repeat PCI, or stent for threatened or abrupt closure, was evaluated. Although the difference in primary end-point event rates between placebo and treatment arms did not achieve statistical significance, there were consistent trends, and the authors concluded that they were at the low-end of dose for efficacy.

Taken together, these studies raise the possibility of a class effect for glycoprotein IIb/IIIa receptor blocking agents as adjuncts to PCI, particularly among high-risk cohorts. Nonetheless, not only is the far largest experience available with abciximab (Reopro), but the most impressive risk reductions have been noted with this agent. These factors, coupled with the theoretic advantage of a non-specific agent, make abciximab the current favorite PCI adjunct.

The first report of direct comparison of agents was the presentation of TARGET at the American Heart Association 73rd Scientific

Session in November 2000. A total of 4812 patients undergoing primary stenting and pretreated with heparin and clopidogrel were randomly allocated between abciximab and tirofiban. The composite end-point of death, non-fatal MI, and repeat revascularization at 30 days was 20% lower in the abciximab treated cohort (6.01% vs 7.55%; $p = 0.037$).

GLYCOPROTEIN IIB/IIIA RECEPTOR BLOCKADE FOR THE TREATMENT OF UNSTABLE ANGINA/NON-Q MI, WHETHER PCI IS OR IS NOT PLANNED (TABLE 33.2) [40–46]

The largest unstable angina trial testing glycoprotein IIb/IIIa receptor blockade was PURSUIT. In this trial, 10,948 patients who had ischemic chest pain within 24 hours and either ischemic electrocardiographic changes or elevated serum CPK-MB isoenzymes were randomly assigned to either placebo or bolus plus infusion of eptifibatide (180 μg/kg bolus and 2 μg/kg infusion for 72 hours). The primary efficacy end-point was death from any cause or non-fatal MI and it was reduced from 15.7% to 14.2% by eptifibatide ($p = 0.04$). All patients received heparin and aspirin.

PRISM-PLUS began with a three-way randomization of unstable angina patients between heparin, tirofiban or the combination of heparin and tirofiban. All patients received aspirin and the study drugs were infused for 72 hours. The tirofiban only arm was stopped

early because of an excess of mortality at seven days. The composite end-point of death, MI or recurrent ischemia was seen less frequently among patients receiving heparin plus tirofiban than heparin alone (18.5% vs 22.3%; $p = 0.03$). Similarly, the composite of death or infarction was also reduced at 30 days by the combination versus heparin alone (8.7% vs 11.9%; $p = 0.03$).

PRISM randomized 3232 patients with unstable angina between heparin versus tirofiban for 48 hours. All patients received aspirin. The composite end-point of death, MI, or recurrent ischemia was reduced at 48 hours in the tirofiban group (3.8% vs 5.6%; risk ratio = 0.67, 95% CI 0.48–0.92; $p = 0.01$), but not at 30 days. Alternatively, mortality at 30 days was reduced by tirofiban (2.3% vs 3.6%; $p = 0.02$)!

Several oral agents have been evaluated with uniformly disappointing results. Accordingly, they are not currently recommended.

GLYCOPROTEIN IIB/IIIA RECEPTOR BLOCKADE IN THE TREATMENT OF ACUTE MI (INCLUDING AS ADJUNCT TO PRIMARY PCI) [47–72]

There are a number of mechanisms whereby inhibition of platelet aggregation by means of the glycoprotein IIb/IIIa receptor blockade might improve patient outcomes in acute myocardial infarction:

- Improved early reperfusion, even prior to or independent of PCI.

Table 33.2. Randomized trials of glycoprotein IIb/IIIa receptor blockade for the treatment of unstable angina/non-Q MI

Trial name	Drug	Reference	Subjects (*n*)
1. PURSUIT	Eptifibatide	42	10,948
2. PRISM	Tirofiban	44	3232
3. PRISM PLUS	Tirofiban	43	1915
4. PARAGON	Lamifiban	45	2282

Table 33.3. Randomized trials of glycoprotein IIb/IIIa receptor blockade in the treatment of acute MI

Trial name	Reference	Subjects (n)	Drug
1. RAPPORT	54	483	Abciximab
2. TAMI-8	55	70	M7e3
3. IMPACT-AMI	56	180	Eptifibatide
4. Integrilin/SK	58	181	Eptifibatide
5. TIMI-14A	59	450	Abciximab
6. SPEED		350	Abciximab
7. GUSTO-III	68, 69	392	Abciximab
8. EPIC substudy	67	64	Abciximab
9. StopAMI	70	63	Abciximab
10. ADMIRAL	81	300	Abciximab
Adjunct to direct PCI			
1. CADILLAC	52, 72	2000	Abciximab
2. RAPPORT	54	483	Abciximab
3. GRAPE	60	41	Abciximab
4. ISAR-II	71	401	Abciximab

- Adjunctive to primary angioplasty, so as to improve outcome.
- Enhanced TIMI-3 flow rates.
- Improved left ventricular function (likely as a result of improved flow).
- Reduce mortality and morbidity, both acute and chronic.

In a post hoc subset study of the EPIC trial, patients with acute MI undergoing either direct or rescue PCI were evaluated. By six months, abciximab bolus plus infusion was associated with a reduction in ischemic events from 47.8% to 4.5% ($p = 0.002$) compared with placebo. Both repeat revascularization ($p = 0.002$) and reinfarction ($p = 0.05$) were reduced by abciximab relative to placebo.

Abciximab as an adjunct to primary angioplasty was evaluated in RAPPORT, a substudy of EPIC, a post hoc subgroup of GUSTO-III, ISAR-II, and CADILLAC [26, 68–72]. In RAPPORT, abciximab was associated with a reduc-

tion in 30-day composite death, recurrent MI or repeat target vessel revascularization) from 11.2% to 5.8% ($p = 0.03$). Among the 64 patients in EPIC who underwent primary or rescue PCI, abciximab bolus plus infusion was associated with a reduction in composite 30-day end-point from 26.1% as compared to 4.5% in the placebo group ($p = 0.06$). Among the 392 GUSTO-III patients who underwent infarct artery PCI within 24 hours, and after adjustment for baseline differences, patients receiving abciximab had a 30-day mortality of 3.6% versus 9.7% among those who received placebo ($p = 0.042$). In CADILLAC, patients were randomized between stenting versus PTCA, and with or without abciximab. Target vessel revascularization was reduced with stenting, and major adverse cardiac events were reduced in both stent and PTCA arms by abciximab. Similarly, stent plus abciximab was associated with no subacute stent thrombosis!

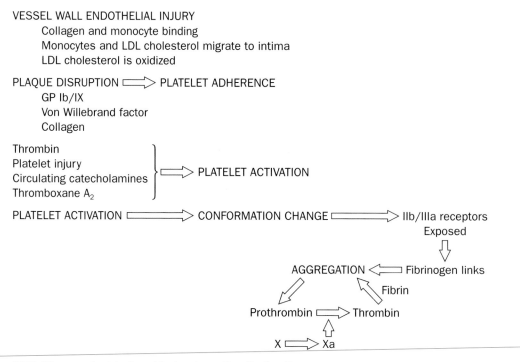

Figure 33.1 Schematic of the central role of the IIb/IIIa receptor in adhesive molecule linkage and platelet activation.

BLEEDING [73–80]

As stated previously, the EPIC trial demonstrated both a stepwise increase in bleeding as well as a reduction in the primary endpoint of abciximab from placebo, to bolus only, to bolus plus infusion. The subsequent EPILOG trial made the important contribution (besides perhaps extending the eligible population of benefit) of reducing heparin dose and paying exquisite attention to sheath detail, with the result that one could obtain the primary benefit without major bleeding increase. As an antibody, abciximab has also been associated with decreased platelet counts, but some of these derive from clumping (paseduothrombocytopenia diagnosed by sending non-citrate containing sample to the lab), and most of the real declines correct quickly after cessation of the drug. Bleeding associated with abciximab use can be treated with platelet infusion, whereas with the small molecules, stopping the infusion is adequate most of the time.

SUMMARY

Glycoprotein IIb/IIIa receptor blocking drugs, given as intravenous bolus and infusion have been demonstrated to reduce the acute complications of PCI, particularly among patients with unstable coronary syndromes, and further among unstable patients at high-risk, including acute infarction [81]. The most experience, the largest benefit, and the only winner in a head-to-head comparison is abciximab. If it is truly superior to the more specific, small molecules, it is likely due to abciximab's ability to block several different components of the platelet thrombogenic model. The use of infusions of any of the three approved agents (abciximab; eptifibatide; tirofiban) for patients with unstable angina who are not necessarily being directed toward intervention is also supported by RCT data. Both of the selective, small molecule agents, eptifibatide and tirofiban, are better studied with specific regard to stabilization of ACS patients. There are good data, consistent with a fundamental theme of this book, that patients at higher risk, as determined by biomarkers and ECG changes, are most likely to benefit. The selective agents are also less expensive and allow for more rapid return of coagulant function after they are discontinued, so that if CABG is anticipated there is less need for either delay or platelet transfusion prior to revascularization.

REFERENCES

1. Fuster V, Badimon L, Badimon JJ, Chesebro JH. The pathogenesis of coronary artery disease and the acute coronary syndromes (part I), *N Engl J Med* 1992; **326**:242–250.
2. Fuster V, Badimon L, Badimon JJ, Chesebro JH. The pathogenesis of coronary artery disease and the acute coronary syndromes (part II), *N Engl J Med* 1992; **326**:310–318.
3. Rauch U, Osende JI, Fuster V et al. Thrombus formation on atherosclerotic plaques: pathogenesis and clinical consequences, *Ann Intern Med* 2001; **134**: 224–238.
4. Becker RC. Thrombosis and the role of the platelet, *Am J Cardiol* 1999; **83** (9A):3E–6E.
5. Phillips DR, Charo IF, Parise LV, Fitzgerald LA. The platelet membrane glycoprotein IIb/IIIa complex, *Blood* 1988; **71**:831–843.
6. Lefkovits J, Plow EF, Topol EJ. Platelet glycoprotein IIb/IIIa receptors in cardiovascular medicine, *N Engl J Med* 1995; **332**:1553–1559.
7. Coller BS. Blockade of platelet GPIIb/IIIa receptors as an antithrombotic strategy, *Circulation* 1995; **92**:2373–2380.
8. Tcheng JE, Ellis SG, George BS et al. Pharmacodynamics of chimeric glycoprotein IIb/IIIa intergrin antiplatet antibody Fab 7E3 in high-risk coronary angioplasty, *Circulation* 1994; **90**:1757–1764.
9. Kleiman NS, Raizner AE, Jordan R et al. Differential inhibition of platelet aggregation induced by adenosine diphosphate or a thrombin receptor-activating peptide in patients treated with bolus chimeric 7E3 Fab: implications for inhibition of the internal pool of GPIIb/IIIa receptors, *J Am Col Cardiol* 1995; **26**: 1665–1671.
10. Mascelli MA, Lance ET, Damaraju L et al. Pharmacodynamic profile of short-term abciximab treatment demonstrated prolonged platelet inhibition with gradual recovery from GP IIb/IIIa receptor blockade, *Circulation* 1998; **97**:1680–1688.
11. Steele PM, Chesebro JH, Stanson AW et al. Balloon angioplasty. Natural history of the pathophysiological response to injury in a pig model, *Circulation Res* 1985; **57**:105–112.
12. Uchida Y, Hasegawa K, Kawamura K, Shibuya I. Angioscopic observation of the coronary luminal changes induced by percutaneous transluminal coronary angioplasty, *Am Heart J* 1989; **117**: 769–776.
13. Harrington RA, Kleiman NS, Kottke-Marchant K et al. Immediate and reversible platelet inhibition after intravenous administration of a peptide glycoprotein IIb/IIIa inhibitor during percutaneous coronary intervention, *Am J Cardiol* 1995; **76**:1222–1227.
14. Kereiakes DJ, Kleiman NS, Ambrose J et al. Randomized, double-blind, placebo-controlled dose-ranging study of tirofiban (MK-383) platelet IIb/IIIa blockade in high risk patients undergoing coronary angioplasty, *J Am Coll Cardiol* 1996; **27**:536–542.
15. EPIC Investigators. Use of a monoclonal antibody directed against the platelet glycoprotein IIb/IIIa receptor in high-risk coronary angioplasty, *N Engl J Med* 1994; **330**:956–961.
16. EPILOG Investigators. Platelet glycoprotein IIb/IIIa blockade with abciximab with low-dose heparin during percutaneous coronary revascularization, *N Engl J Med* 1997; **336**:1689–1696.
17. EPISTENT Investigators. Randomized placebo-controlled and balloon-angioplasty controlled trial to assess safety of coronary stenting with use of platelet glycoprotein IIb/IIIa blockade, *Lancet* 1998; **352**:87–92.

18. Tcheng JE, Lincoff AM, Sigmon KN et al for the IMPACT II Investigators. Randomized placebo-controlled trial of effect of eptifibatide on complications of percutaneous coronary intervention: IMPACT II, *Lancet* 1997; **349**:1422–1428.

19. RESTORE Investigators. Effects of platelet glycoprotein IIb/IIIa blockade with tirofiban on adverse cardiac events in patients with unstable angina or acute myocardial infarction undergoing coronary angioplasty, *Circulation* 1997; **96**:1445–1453.

20. CAPTURE Investigators. Randomized placebo-controlled trial of abciximab before and during coronary intervention in refractory unstable angina: the CAPTURE study, *Lancet* 1997; **349**: 1429–1435.

21. Bhatt DL, Marso SP, Lincoff AM et al. Abciximab reduces mortality in diabetics following percutaneous coronary intervention, *J Am Coll Cardiol* 2000; **35**:922–928.

22. Cho L, Topol EJ, Balog C et al. Clinical benefit of glycoprotein IIb/IIIa blockade with abciximab is independent of gender. Pooled analysis from EPIC, EPILOG, and EPISTENT trials, *J Am Coll Cardiol* 2000; **36**:381–386.

23. Cura FA, Bhatt DL, Lincoff AM et al. Pronounced benefit of coronary stenting and adjunctive glucoprotein IIb/IIIa inhibition in complex atherosclerotic lesions, *Circulation* 2000; **102**:28–34.

24. Bhatt DL, Lincoff AM, Califf RM et al. The benefit of abciximab in percutaneous coronary revascularization is not device-specific, *Am J Cardiol* 2000; **85**:1060–1064.

25. Topol EJ, Ferguson JJ, Weisman HF et al for the EPIC Investigator. Long-term protection from myocardial ischemic events in a randomized trial of brief integrin beta 3 blockade with percutaneous coronary intervention, *JAMA* 1997; **278**: 479–484.

26. Verghese M, Grill DE, Scott CG et al. The influence of abciximab use on clinical outcome after aortocoronary vein graft interventions, *J Am Coll Cardiol* 1999; **34**:1163–1169.

27. Lincoff AM, Tcheng JE, Califf RM et al. Standard versus low dose weight adjusted heparin in patients treated with the platelet glycoprotein IIb/IIIa receptor antibody fragment abciximab (c7E3 Fab) during percutaneous coronary revascularization, *Am J Cardiol* 1997; **79**:286–291.

28. Ghaffari S, Kereiakes DJ, Lincoff AM et al. Platelet glycoprotein IIb/IIIa receptor blockade with abciximab reduces ischemic complications in patients undergoing directional coronary atherectomy, *Am J Cardiol* 1998; **82**:7–12.

29. Lincoff AM, Califf RM, Anderson KM et al. Evidence for prevention of death and myocardial infarction with platelet membrane glycoprotein IIb/IIIa receptor blockade by c7E3 Fab (abciximab) among patients with unstable angina undergoing percutaneous coronary revascularization, *J Am Coll Cardiol* 1997; **30**: 149–156.

30. Topol EJ, Califf RM, Weisman HS et al. Reduction of clinical restenosis following coronary intervention with early administration of platelet IIb/IIIa integrin blocking antibody, *Lancet* 1994; **343**:881–886.

31. Topol EJ, Ferguson JJ, Weisman HF et al. Long-term protection from myocardial ischemic events in a randomized trial of brief integrin beta 3 blockade with percutaneous coronary intervention, *JAMA* 1997; **278**:479–484.

32. Lincoff AM, Tcheng JE, Califf RM et al. Sustained suppression of ischemic complications of coronary intervention by platelet GP IIb/IIIa blockage with abciximab: one year outcome in the EPILOG trial, *Circulation* 1999; **99**:1951–1958.

33. Lincoff AM, Califf RM, Moliterno DJ et al. Complementary clinical benefits of coronary artery stenting and blockade of platelet glycoprotein IIb/IIIa receptors, *New Engl J Med* 1999; **341**:319–327.

34. Topol EJ, Mark DB, Lincoff AM et al. Enhanced survival with platelet glycoprotein IIb/IIIa blockade in patients undergoing coronary stenting: one year outcomes and health care economic implications from a multicenter, randomized trial, *Lancet* 1999; **354**:2019–2024.

35. Carozza JP, Kintz RE, Fishman RF, Baim DS. Restenosis after arterial injury caused by coronary stenting in patients with diabetes mellitus, *Ann Int Med* 1993; **118**:344–349.

36. Popma JJ, Weitz J, Bittl JA et al. Antithrombotic therapy in patients undergoing coronary angioplasty, *Chest* 1998; **114**:7288–7418.

37. Garbarz E, Farah B, Vuillemenot A et al. 'Rescue' abciximab for complicated percutaneous transluminal coronary angioplasty, *Am J Cardiol* 1998; **82**:800–803.

38. Ellis SG, Vandormael MG, Cowley MJ et al. Coronary morphologic and clinical determinants of procedural outcome with angioplasty

for multi-vessel coronary disease. Implications for patient selection, *Circulation* 1990; **82**: 1193–1202.

39. Tcheng JE. Differences among the parenteral platelet glycoprotein IIb/IIIa inhibitors and implications for treatment, *Am J Cardiol* 1999; **83** (9A):7E–11E.

40. Braunwald E, Mark DB, Jones RH et al. *Unstable angina: diagnosis and management.* Clinical Practice Guideline Number 10. AHCPR Publication No. 94-0602. Rockville, MD: Agency for Health Care Policy and Research and the National Heart, Lung and Blood Institute, Public Health Service, US Department of Health and Human Services, 1994.

41. Ohman EM, Armstrong PW, Christenson RH et al. Cardiac troponin T levels for risk stratification in acute myocardial ischemia, *N Engl J Med* 1996; **335**:1333–1431.

42. PURSUIT Trial Investigators. Inhibition of platelet glycoprotein IIb/IIIa with eptifibatide in patients with acute coronary syndromes, *N Engl J Med* 1998; **339**:436–443.

43. PRISM Plus Study Investigators. Inhibition of the platelet glycoprotein IIb/IIIa receptor with tirofiban in unstable angina and non-Q wave myocardial infarction, *N Engl J Med* 1998; **338**:1488–1497.

44. PRISM Study Investigators. A comparison of aspirin plus tirofiban with aspirin plus heparin for unstable angina, *N Engl J Med* 1998; **338**: 1498–1505.

45. PARAGON Investigators. International, randomized, controlled trial of lamifiban (a platelet glycoprotein IIb/IIIa inhibitor), heparin or both in unstable angina, *Circulation* 1998; **97**: 2386–2395.

46. Harrington RA, Lincoff AM, Berdan LG et al. Maintenance of clinical benefit at six months in patients treated with platelet glycoprotein IIb/IIIa inhibitor eptifbatide versus placebo during an acute ischemic coronary event, *Circulation* 1998; **98**:I-359.

47. Van de Werf F, Topol EJ, Lee KL et al. Variations in patient management and outcomes for acute myocardial infarction in the United States and other countries, *JAMA* 1995; **273**:1586–1591.

48. Rao AK, Pratt C, Berke A et al. Thrombolysis in myocardial infarction (TIMI) trial—phase I: hemorrhagic manifestations and changes in plasma fibrinogen and the fibrinolytic system in patients treated with recombinant tissue plasminogen activator and streptokinase, *J Am Coll Cardiol* 1988; **11**:1–11.

49. O'Shea C, Tcheng JE. Platelet glycoprotein IIb/IIIa integrin inhibition in acute myocardial infarction, *J Invas Cardiol* 1999; **11**:494–499.

50. O'Neill WW. The evolution of primary PTCA therapy of acute myocardial infarction: a personal perspective, *J Invasiv Card* 1995; **7**:2F–10F.

51. Stone GW. Primary PTCA in high risk patients with acute myocardial infarction, *J Invasiv Card* 1995; **7**:12F–21F.

52. Stone GW. Stenting and IIb/IIIa receptor blockade in acute myocardial infarction: an introduction to the CADILLAC trial, *J Invasiv Cardiol* 1995; **10**:36B–47B.

53. Schultz RD, Heuser RR, Hatler C, Frey D. Use of c7E3 Fab in conjunction with primary coronary stenting for acute myocardial infarctions complicated by cardiogenic shock, *Cath and CV Diag* 1996; **39**:143–148.

54. Brener SJ, Barr LA, Burchenal JEB et al. A randomized, placebo-controlled trial of platelet glycoprotein IIb/IIIa blockade with primary angioplasty for acute myocardial infarction, *Circulation* 1998; **98**:734–741.

55. Kleiman NS, Ohman EM, Califf RM et al. Profound inhibition of platelet aggregation with monoclonal antibody 7E3 Fab after thrombolytic therapy. Results of the Thrombolysis and Angioplasty in Myocardial Infarction (TAMI) 8 Pilot Study, *J Am Coll Cardiol* 1993; **22**:381–389.

56. Ohman EM, Kleiman NS, Gacioch G et al for the IMPACT-AMI Investigators. Combined accelerated tissue-plasminogen activator and glycoprotein IIb/IIIa integrin receptor blockade with Integrilin in acute myocardial infarction: results of a randomized, placebo-controlled dose ranging trial, *Circulation* 1997; **95**:846–854.

57. Moliterno DJ, Harrington RA, Krucoff ME et al for the PARIDIGM Investigators. Randomized, placebo-controlled study of Lamifiban with thrombolytic therapy for the treatment of acute myocardial infarction: rationale and design for the Platelet Aggregation Receptor antagonist Dose Investigation and reperfusion Gain in Myocardial infarction (PARIDIGM) study, *J Throm Thrombol* 1995; **2**:165–169.

58. Ronner E, Van Kerteren HA, Zinjnen P et al. Combined therapy with Streptokinase and Integrilin, *J Am Coll Cardiol* 1998; **31** (suppl):

191A.

59. Antman EM, Giugliano RP, McCabe CH et al for the TIMI Investigators. Abciximab (REOPRO) potentiates thrombolysis in ST-elevation myocardial infarction: results of the TIMI 14 trial, *J Am Coll Cardiol* 1998; **31** (suppl):191A.

60. Merkhof-Van Den L, Liem A, Zijlstra F et al. Early coronary patency evaluation of a glycoprotein receptor antagonist (abciximab) in primary PTCA: the GRAPE pilot study, *Circulation* 1997; **96** (suppl):I-474.

61 Stone G. Stenting in acute myocardial infarction: observation studies and randomized trials—1998, *J Invas Cardiol* 1998; **10** (suppl):16A–26A.

62. Gibson CM, Goel M, Cohen DJ et al. Six-month angiographic and clinical follow-up of patients prospectively randomized to receive either triofiban or placebo during angioplasty in the RESTORE trial, *J Am Coll Cardiol* 198; **32**:28–34.

63. Colombo A, Briguori C. Primary stenting and glycoprotein IIb/IIIa inhibitors in acute myocardial infarction, *Am Heart J* 1999; **138**:S153–S157.

64. Ferguson JJ, Taqi K. IIb/IIIa receptor blockade in acute myocardial infarction, *Am Heart J* 1999; **138**:S164–S170.

65. Gensini GF, Falai M. Advances in antithrombotic therapy of acute myocardial infarction, *Am Heart J* 1999; **138**:S171–S176.

66. Hermann HC. Triple therapy for acute myocardial infarction: combining fibrinolysis, platelet IIb/IIIa inhibition, and percutaneous coronary intervention, *Am J Cardiol* 2000; **85**:10C–16C.

67. Lefkovits J, Ivanhoe RJ, Califf RM et al for the EPIC Investigators. Effects of platelet glycoprotein IIb/IIIa receptor blockade by chimeric monoclonal antibody (abciximab) on acute and six-month outcomes after percutaneous transluminal coronary angioplasty for acute myocardial infarction, *Am J Cardiol* 1996; **77**:1045–1051.

68. The GUSTO-III Investigators. A comparison of reteplase with alteplase for acute myocardial infarction, *N Engl J Med* 1997; **337**:1118–1123.

69. Miller JM, Smalling R, Ohman EM et al for the GUSTO-IIII Investigators. Effectiveness of early coronary angiography and abciximab for failed fibrinolysis (reteplase or alteplase) during acute myocardial infarction (results from GUSTO-III trial), *Am J Cardiol* 1999; **84**:779–784.

70. Schomig A, Kastrati A, Dirschinger J et al. Coronary stenting plus glucoprotein IIb/IIIa blockade compared with tissue plasminogen activator in acute myocardial infarction, *N Engl J Med* 2000; **343**:385–391.

71. Neumann FJ, Kastrati A, Schmitt C et al. Effect of glycoprotein IIb/IIIa receptor blockade with abciximab on clinical and angiographic restenosis rate after the placement of coronary stents following acute myocardial infarction, *J Am Coll Cardiol* 2000; **35**:915–921.

72. Stone GW. Results of the CADILLAC trial. Presented at Transcatheter Cardiovascular Therapeutics (TCT) XI: Frontiers in Interventional Cardiology; Washington, DC; Oct 18–22, 2000.

73. Berkowitz SD, Sane DC, Sigmon KN et al for the EPIC study group. Occurrence and clinical significance of thrombocytopenia in a population undergoing high-risk percutaneous coronary revascularization, *J Am Coll Cardiol* 1998; **32**: 311–319.

74. Aguirre FV, Topol EJ, Ferguson JJ et al for the EPIC Investigators. Bleeding complications with the chimeric antibody to platelet glycoprotein IIb/IIIa integrin in patients undergoing percutaneous coronary intervention, *Circulation* 1995; **91**: 2882–2890.

75. Sane DC, Damaraju LV, Topol EJ et al. Occurrence and clinical significance of pseudothrombocytopenia during abciximab therapy, *J Am Coll Cardiol* 2000; **36**:75–83.

76. Phillips DR, Teng W, Arfstent A et al. Effect of Ca^{2+} on GP IIb-IIIa interactions with integrilin. Enhanced GP IIb-IIIa binding and inhibition of platelet aggregation by reductions in the concentration of ionized calcium in plasma anticoagulated with citrate, *Circulation* 1997; **96**:1488–1494.

77. Juergens CP, Yeung AC, Oesterle SN. Routine platelet transfusion in patients undergoing emergency coronary bypass surgery after receiving abciximab, *Am J Cardiol* 1997; **80**:74–75.

78. Boehrer JD, Kereikes DJ, Navetta FI, Califf RM, Topol EJ for the EPIC Investigators. Effects of profound platelet inhibition with c7E3 before coronary angioplasty on complications of coronary bypass surgery, *Am J Cardiol* 1994; **74**: 1166–1170.

79. Booth J, Patel V, Balog C et al. Is bleeding risk increased in patients undergoing urgent bypass surgery following abciximab, *Circulation* 1998; **98**:I-845.

80. Tcheng JE, Keriakes DJ, Braden GA et al. Safety of abciximab retreatments. Final clinical report

of the ReoPro Readministration Registry (R3), *Circulation* 1998; **98**:I-17.

81. Monalescot G, Barragen P, Wittenberg O et al. Platelet glycoprotein IIb/IIIa inhibition with coronary stenting for acute myocardial infarction, *N Engl J Med* 2001; **344**:1895–1903.

Myocardial protection for high-risk coronary surgery

Vladimir Birjiniuk and Diane Panton Lapsley

CONTENTS • Introduction • Cardioplegia • Non-cardioplegic protection • Off-pump coronary surgery (OPCAB) • The AWESOME study: our experience at the Boston VA Medical Center, West Roxbury campus • Conclusions

INTRODUCTION

Myocardial preservation is a highly controversial topic. There have been more than 1000 publications, describing different methods of mycocardial protection, in the cardiac surgery literature since 1995. The objectives of myocardial protection are:

- to minimize the myocardial damage before surgery;
- to minimize damage during the ischemic time of the operation;
- to maximize the amount of myocardial recovery following the procedure.

CARDIOPLEGIA

The first description of use of hyperkalemic myocardial arrest for cardiac surgery was by Melrose et al in 1955 [1]. This method was soon abandoned because of significant inflammatory myocardial damage, thought to be secondary to the high potassium concentration which was used. Later, cardioplegic arrest was again tried by Buckberg et al. They showed that by arresting the heart, there was significant reduction in the myocardial oxygen consumption; lowering myocardial temperature reduced oxygen consumption even further [2].

Subsequent studies demonstrated that blood cardioplegia was superior to crystalloid and antegrade–retrograde delivery was superior to antegrade or retrograde alone [3–6]. Currently the golden standard of the cardioplegia delivery and myocardial protection may be the Buckberg method, which is practiced in about 60% of the cardiac surgery centers in the US [6].

Different additives are used in different centers to enhance the cardioplegic performance such as magnesium [7], mannitol [8] and adenosine [9].

NON-CARDIOPLEGIC PROTECTION

Some surgeons prefer fibrillatory arrest to cardioplegic arrest. Most of these operators use mild hypothermia for myocardial protection with venting of the left ventricle, but without cross-clamping the aorta. Atkins has described this method in detail and reports excellent results [10] which are as good as those for procedures performed with cardioplegic arrest. A recent study has shown that intermittent cross-clamp of the aorta with fibrillatory arrest may be superior to antegrade cardioplegia delivery or combined antegrade–retrograde, but this conclusion is controversial [11, 12].

OFF-PUMP CORONARY SURGERY (OPCAB)

In the last few years an old method of revascularization has been revived [13–15]. This procedure is surgical myocardial revascularization without the use of cardio-pulmonary bypass. The procedure is performed on the beating heart, without use of cross-clamps; as a result the ischemic time is eliminated and cardioplegia is no longer necessary. The proponents of this method claim that it is safer and it is especially suitable for high-risk cases. The method is suitable for a selected population with significant limitations of good quality distal vessels, patients without hemodynamic instability and relatively normal size hearts [16, 17]. Some authors recommend the use of perfusion assisted systems [17] for myocardial protection in OPCAB surgery while others recommend the use of assist devices [18] or intra-aortic balloon pump for 'difficult' cases [19, 20].

THE AWESOME STUDY: OUR EXPERIENCE AT THE BOSTON VA MEDICAL CENTER, WEST ROXBURY CAMPUS

The patients enrolled in the AWESOME study were high-risk patients who meet the criteria described in Chapter 16. In an earlier Veterans Administration multiple center study on high-risk non-Q wave myocardial infarction patients [21], the mortality for patients undergoing surgical revascularization was 7.7%. This was a non-risk adjusted mortality. In comparison, the 'crude' and adjusted mortalities were significantly lower for the AWESOME study.

There were a total of 312 patients who underwent CABG surgery in the randomized trial and registry of AWESOME at the West Roxbury campus. There were three surgeons dividing the workload (a, b, c,) with the results shown in Table 34.1.

The conduct of the myocardial preservation was done differently by all three surgeons. Surgeon (a) used crystalloid cardioplegia for all coronary revascularization cases. The patient was not cooled actively, and usually the temperature drifted to 34°C–35°C. Once the cross-clamp was applied, cold crystalloid cardioplegia at 10°C was delivered to the aortic root until arrest was achieved. Ice slush was not used, since reduced temperature is not a good indicator of myocardial protection [22]. In selected cases intramyocardial tissue pH monitoring was

Table 34.1 Breakdown of myocardial preservation performed by three surgeons at the West Roxbury campus

	Randomized	Registry	Cross-over PTCA → CABG	Cross-over Medical → CABG	Total	Death within 30 days
(a)	10	114	16	5	145	3 (2.17%)
(b)	6	111	4	0	121	5 (3.90%)
(c)	2	42	1	3	46	2 (4.30%)

used for myocardial protection [23]. (The temperature measured here is just for pH adjustment.) Once complete arrest was achieved the antegrade cardioplegia was stopped and the heart vented via the aortic root. Then, a venous graft was constructed to the vessel which was most severely diseased (often the right coronary artery; so the graft was constructed to the posterior descending artery). Once the graft was completed, the flow to the graft was measured: any flow over 100 cc/min is acceptable [24], and a small amount of cardioplegia 50–100 cc was delivered directly to the graft to ensure adequate delivery to remote areas. Next, other vein grafts were constructed, and small amounts of cardioplegia were delivered each time until all venous grafts were complete. The left internal mammary artery graft (and/or right internal mammary artery whenever used) was constructed last. A single clamp technique was used on a selective basis for calcified aortic root, short aortic root and reoperations. In the majority of the cases the heart came back to sinus rhythm once the cross-clamp was released and the weaning of cardiopulmonary bypass was performed easily with small amounts of nitroglycerin and renal dose dopamine. The other surgeons (b and c) both used continuous antegrade blood cardioplegia. Surgeon (b) let the patient's temperature drift and vented the aortic root as surgeon (a), and used a terminal 'hot-shot' with blood only.

Surgeon (c) routinely used warm bodies at 37°C and vented the left ventricle via the right superior pulmonary vein.

The conduct of the rest of the surgery, including the routines of the graft construction, was similar for all three surgeons. None of the three surgeons used substrate-enhanced cardioplegia, since our data do not support it [25]. None of the surgeons is routinely using retrograde coronary sinus cardioplegia; instead all preferred cardioplegia applied directly to the grafts as mentioned earlier.

All cardioplegic solutions in our institution are similar except the potassium content:

Solvent	1000 cc 2.5% dextrose 0.45% sodium chloride
Buffer	5 mEq sodium bicarbonate
Additive	100 mg lidocaine
	2 g magnesium
Potassium chloride	90 mEq for blood cardioplegia diluted 1:4
	30 mEq for crystalloid cardioplegia induction
	10 mEq for crystalloid cardioplegia maintenance

CONCLUSIONS

This chapter presents a short summary of several alternative methods of myocardial protection. Alternatives are practiced in our institution. In spite of the differences in myocardial protection the results are quite similar in a relatively high-risk group. The expected mortality at 30 days in this group by the Veterans Administration Cardiac Surgery Consultant Committee criteria was 5.7%, while the observed was only 3.2% with an observed/expected (o/e) ratio of 0.56 which is reassuring. Similar results were obtained in two other studies of high-risk patients. The caseload distribution per surgeon and myocardial protection method were similar to the AWESOME study. The first study, presented at Chest 2000, demonstrated a mortality of 5.2% in a group of 95 patients with a reduced EF of 25% or below, while the expected mortality was 7.2%, leading to an o/e of 0.72 [26]. The second study is to be presented at the 2nd International Congress on Heart Disease [27], and had a mortality rate of 5.4% and 6.1% with expected mortality of 9.29% and 10.1%, resulting in o/e ratios of 0.5 and 0.6 respectively, in two high-risk reoperation CABG groups. These studies are examples of continuously monitoring one's own data in an effort to improve performance. In this manner one can revise procedural conduct so as to obtain the best results possible. Our conclusion is that myocardial protection complements:

- meticulous preoperative work-up of the patient;
- judgment;
- meticulous intraoperative technique; and
- excellent postoperative care.

REFERENCES

1. Melrose DC, Dreyer B, Bentall HH, Baker JBE. Elective cardiac arrest, *Lancet* 1955; **2**:21–22.
2. Buckberg GD, Brazier JR, Nelson RL et al. Studies on hypothermia on regional myocardial flow and metabolism during cardiopulmonary bypass: I. The adequately perfused beating fibrillating and arrested heart, *J Thorac Cardiovasc Surg* 1977; **73**:87.
3. Warner KG, Josa M, Butler MD. Regional changes in myocardial acid production during ischemic arrest: a comparison of sanguinous and asanguinous cardioplegia, *Ann Thorac Surg* 1998; **45**:75–81.
4. Buckberg GB, Beyersdorf F, Allen BS et al. Integrated myocardial management: background and initial application, *J Card Surg* 1995; **10**: 68–89.
5. Buckberg GD. Update on current techniques of myocardial protection, *Ann Thorac Surg* 1995; **60**:805–814.
6. Atanasuleas CL, Remeer DW, Buckberg GD. The role of integrated myocardial management in reoperative coronary surgery, *Sem Thorac Cardiovasc Surg* 2001; **13** (1):33–37.
7. Caputo M, Bryan AJ, Calafiore AM et al. Intermittent antegrade hyperkalemic warm blood cardioplegia supplemented with magnesium prevents myocardial substrate derangement in patients undergoing coronary artery bypass surgery, *Eur Cardiothorac Surg* 1998; **14**: 596–601.
8. Ferreira R, Burgos M, Liesui S et al. Reduction of reperfusion injury with mannitol cardioplegia, *Ann Thorac Surg* 1989; **48**:77–83.
9. Mentzer RM Jr, Birjiniuk V, Khuri S et al. Adenosine myocardial protection. Preliminary results of a phase II clinical trial, *Ann Surg* 1999; **229** (5):643–650.
10. Akins CW. Cardiac arrest by ventricular fibrillation. In: Piper HM, Preuss CJ, eds, *Ischemia-reperfusion in cardiac surgery* (Dordrecht: Kluwer Academic Publishers, 1993) 267–278.
11. Casthly PA, Shah C, Mekhjian H et al. Left ventricular diastolic function after coronary artery bypass grafting. A correlative study with three different myocardial protection techniques, *J Thorac Cardiovasc Surg* 1997; **114**:254–260.
12. Sunderdiek U, Feindt P, Gams E. Aortocoronary bypass grafting: a comparison of HTK cardioplegia vs intermittent aortic cross-clamping, *Eur J Cardiothorac Surg* 2000; **18**:393–399.
13. Murray G, Porcheron R, Hilano J et al. Anastomosis of a systemic artery to the coronary, *Can Med Assoc J* 1954; **71**:594–597.
14. Kolesov V. Mammary artery–coronary artery anastomosis as a method of treating angina pectoris, *J Thorac Cardiovasc Surg* 1967; **54**:535–544.
15. Stamou SC, Corso PJ. Coronary revascularization without cardiopulmonary bypass in high-risk patients: a route to the future, *Ann Thorac Cardiovasc Surg* 2001; **71**:1056–1061.
16. Wait MA. OPCAB Selection bias, *Ann Thorac Surg* 2001; **71**:1731.
17. Puskas JD, Vinten-Johansen J, Muraki S, Gyton R. Myocardial protection for off-pump coronary artery bypass surgery, *Sem Thorac Cardiovasc Surg* 2001; **13** (1):81–88.
18. Myens B, Sergeant P, Nishida T et al. Micropumps to support the heart during CABG, *Eur J Cardiothorac Surg* 2000; **17**:169–174.
19. Carver JM, Murrah PC. Elective intra-aortic balloon counterpulsation for high-risk off-pump coronary artery bypass operations, *Ann Thorac Cardiovasc Surg* 2001; **71**:1220–1223.
20. Kim KB, Lim C, Ahn H et al. Intra-aortic balloon therapy facilitates posterior vessel off-pump coronary artery bypass grafting in high risk patients, *Ann Thorac Surg* 2001; **71**:1964–1968.
21. Boden WE, O'Rourke RA, Crawford MH et al. Outcomes in patients with acute non-Q wave myocardial infarction randomly assigned to an invasive as compared with a conservative management strategy, *N Engl J Med* 1998; **338**: 1785–1792.
22. Dearani JA, Axford TC, Patel MA et al. Routine measurement of myocardial temperature is not reflective of myocardial metabolism during cardiac surgery, *Surgical Forum* 1990; **XLI**:228–230.
23. Tantillo MB, Khuri SF. Myocardial tissue pH in the assessment of the extent of myocardial ischemia and adequacy of myocardial protection. In: Piper HM, Preusse CJ, eds, *Ischemia-*

reperfusion in cardiac surgery (Dordrecht: Kluwer Academic Publishers, 1993) 335–352.

24. Sharma GV, Khuri SF, Folland ED et al. Prognosis of aorta coronary graft patency. A comparison of pre-operative and intra-operative assessment, *J Thorac Cardiovasc Surg* 1983; **85**: 570–576.

25. Wallace AW, Ratcliffe MB, Nose PS et al. Effect of induction and reperfusion with warm substrate enriched cardioplegia on ventricular func-

tion, *Ann Thorac Surg* 2000; **70**:1301–1307.

26. Birjiniuk V, Rocco T, Sharma GVRK et al. Surgical coronary revascularization in patients with low ejection fraction: outcomes in high-risk patients, *Chest* 2000; **188** (suppl 4):S108.

27. Birjiniuk V, Rocco T, Hossein MM et al. Is prophylactic intra-aortic balloon counterpulsation necessary, 2nd International Congress on Heart Disease; Washington, DC, USA July 21–24, 2001.

Section VII: What can be done after the revascularization to discourage recidivism?

35

Cardiac rehabilitation

Shefali Vora and Victor Froelicher

CONTENTS • **Introduction** • **Infarct severity** • **Cardiac rehabilitation** • **Early studies of progressive ambulation post-MI** • **Randomized trials of early ambulation** • **Patients with left ventricular dysfunction** • **Summary: changes due to economic forces** • **Future directions in the United States** • **Summary**

INTRODUCTION

Cardiac rehabilitation was conceived in the 1960s as a treatment for patients who had suffered a myocardial infarction. Before the 1970s, the patient who suffered a myocardial infarction (MI) was almost completely immobilized for six weeks or more and was even washed, shaved and fed in order to keep the work of the heart to a minimum (Table 35.1). It was thought that this approach provided the heart with the opportunity to form a firm scar as if the beating heart could rest. Also, the patient was told not to expect to be able to return to a normal life. These were incorrect beliefs particularly in the situation of an uncomplicated MI. Prolonged immobilization not only did not speed healing but also exposed the patient to the additional risks of venous thrombosis, pulmonary embolism, muscle atrophy, lung infections, and deconditioning. Equally serious was the psychological result of such an approach, often leading to psychological impairment.

Today, the physician's approach to the acute MI has completely changed [1]. A relatively brief period of time being monitored is followed by early mobilization, sitting at the bedside, walking and in the uncomplicated patient,

discharge from the hospital in less than a week. Psychological rehabilitation takes place in the doctor's office along with prescribing exercise and education. Certainly all patients do not need all rehabilitative interventions, but exercise programs, educational sessions, group therapy, and psychological and vocational counseling are available in most communities for those who need them.

Hospital admission for an acute MI is a stressful experience but it must be remembered that hospital discharge can be equally stressful. Discharge into an uncertain future and to home and work where one is considered damaged, can be as damaging to one's self-esteem as the acute event itself. The physician is faced with the difficult task not only of supervising the physical recovery of the patient but of maintaining morale, providing education, helping the family cope and provide support, and facilitating the return to a gratifying lifestyle. Cardiac rehabilitation can be considered the conservation of human life. Its goal is to restore the patient to optimal physiological, psychological, and vocational status.

Atherosclerotic cardiovascular diseases (ASCVD) are also the leading cause of activity limitation and disabled worker benefits in the

Table 35.1 A review of previous textbook recommendations for bed rest in acute myocardial infarction

Author	Publication	Weeks of bed rest
Lewis, T	*Diseases of the Heart* (New York: The Macmillan Company, 1937)	8 weeks bed rest
White, PD	*Heart Disease*, 3rd edn (New York: The Macmillan Company, 1945)	4 weeks bed rest
Wood, P	*Diseases of the Heart and Circulation*, 2nd edn (London: Eyre and Spottiswoode, 1960)	3–6 weeks in bed
Friedberg, CK	*Diseases of the Heart*, 3rd edn (Philadelphia: W B Saunders Company, 1966)	2–3 weeks minimum bed rest
Wood, P	*Diseases of the Heart and Circulation*, 3rd edn (London: Eyre and Spottiswoode, 1968)	2 weeks in bed

US, and the fourth leading cause of days lost from work. In fact, ASCVD alone is responsible for almost one out of five disability allowances paid by the Social Security Administration. However, the total economic impact of the disability related to cardiovascular diseases results from the combination of Social Security benefits, welfare support, disability insurance income, unemployment compensation, loss of taxable revenue, and reduced worker productivity related to these diseases. Therefore, from a purely economic standpoint, it is essential that patients with ASCVD be rehabilitated as quickly and efficiently as possible to enable their return to employment. Just as important, however, is the psychosocial impact of heart disease, which cannot be measured in dollars lost. Clearly, therefore, improved quality of life, including lessened depression and an expedient return to pre-illness social roles in the family and community, should be another important goal in the effective rehabilitation of patients with heart disease.

With the addition of thrombolysis and acute catheter interventions to MI treatment the disability incurred by an MI has been decreased. Approximately 85% of MI patients undergo cardiac catheterization and many receive catheter intervention. Because of the functional benefits observed in cardiac rehabilitation, physicians have extended services to other groups of patients. These patients include those who have undergone interventions (percutaneous transluminal coronary angioplasty [PTCA], coronary artery bypass grafts [CABG], pacemakers, transplantation and valve surgery) as well as those limited by angina or congestive heart failure or whose heart disease is complicated by additional diseases such as diabetes and renal disease. Next, the pathophysiology of MI that relates to rehabilitation will be reviewed.

INFARCT SEVERITY

Myocardial infarctions are divided basically into those that evolve Q waves and result in transmural myocardial cell death and those that do not evolve Q waves and only result in subendocardial cell death [2]. Subendocardial MI cannot be localized while transmural MI can be roughly localized by the Q wave pattern. Attempts have been made to judge MI severity or size electrocardiographically by Q wave and R wave scores and even by utilizing body surface mapping, but these methods only provide

Table 35.2 The presence of any one or more of the following criteria classify a myocardial infarction as complicated

- Prior MI
- Continued cardiac ischemic (pain, late enzyme rise)
- Left ventricular failure (congestive heart failure)
- New murmurs (chest x-ray changes)
- Shock (blood pressure drop, pallor, oliguria)
- Important cardiac dysrhythmias (PVCs greater than 6/min, atrial fibrilation)
- Conduction disturbances (bundle branch block, A-V block, hemiblock)
- Severe pleurisy or pericarditis
- Complicating illnesses
- Marked enzyme rise without a noncardiac explanation
- Age greater than 75
- Stroke or TIAs

rough estimates. In general, the greater the number of areas with Q waves and the greater the R wave loss, the larger the MI. Non-Q wave MIs are usually less likely associated with complications such as congestive heart failure (CHF) or shock, but they can be complicated particularly when a prior MI has taken place. Their prognosis is particularly good if they do not have prior MIs or a decreased ejection fraction. Because more myocardium has survived, patients with non-Q wave MIs are more likely to suffer ischemic events. Anterior Q wave MIs are usually larger than inferior infarcts and are more likely to be associated with congestive heart failure and cardiogenic shock. Anterior infarcts are more likely to cause aneurysms and a greater decrease in ejection fraction. Surprisingly however, in follow-up they have a similar or not much poorer prognosis than Q wave inferior MIs [3]. Fifteen percent of patients with Q wave MI lose their Q waves over the following year but still have the same prognosis as those who do not lose their Q waves.

It is well known that morbidity and mortality in post-infarction patients who have complicated courses are much higher than in those with uncomplicated MIs. Diabetes doubles the mortality with any type of MI. The criteria for a complicated MI are listed in Table 35.2. The progressive ambulation program should be delayed until such individuals reach an uncomplicated status, and even then progressive ambulation should be slower.

There has been some controversy over the relative long-term risk of subendocardial versus transmural myocardial infarction. Some of this difficulty has been due to whether or not prior MIs occurred which raises the risk in both types. Estimation of the severity of an MI requires consideration of clinical findings and test results other than the ECG to judge a patient's risk and infarct size. Clinical findings, hemodynamic monitoring, the level of enzyme elevation, and the presence of congestive heart failure or shock or both should judge the severity of an infarction. The concept that a subendocardial infarction is 'uncompleted' and poses an increased post-discharge risk has not been substantiated; however, they are more likely to be associated with post-infarction angina. A study done at the Mayo clinic demonstrated that in the patient with a first MI, prognosis is much better in follow-up for a non-Q wave MI than for a Q wave MI [4]. The recent VANQWISH trial demonstrated that acute intervention does not improve survival in all non-Q wave MI patients [5].

Certain clinical features during a patient's immediate post-myocardial infarction convalescence identify a higher risk for future cardiac events or death, and mandate coronary angiography for consideration of coronary revascularization (PTCA or CABG). Ross and colleagues developed one of the early schemes for deciding which patients should undergo coronary angiography post-myocardial infarction [6]. If a patient manifests any spontaneous ischemia during hospitalization, they have an increased risk of 18–20% mortality in the first year post-myocardial infarction, and should be referred for diagnostic coronary angiography prior to discharge. If a patient has had a previous myocardial infarction and clinical or radiographic evidence of left ventricular failure, their projected mortality risk is 25% in the first year, and they should undergo coronary angiography as well. In those patients who are unable to exercise, a resting evaluation of ventricular function is recommended. Given that ventricular function is the most powerful predictor of prognosis in patients under the age of 70, patients with left ventricular ejection fractions between 20 and 40% would be classified as high risk (12% first-year mortality) [7].

It is estimated that for every 100 people that suffer an acute myocardial infarction and survive their hospitalization, ten will manifest spontaneous ischemia/angina, 20 will have evidence of diminished ventricular function, and an additional ten patients will have probable ischemia on pre-discharge exercise testing and be identified at higher risk [8]. Klein and colleagues studied 198 patients who survived a myocardial infarction and underwent pre-discharge submaximal exercise testing and followed them for two years [9]. They found that patients who had exercise-induced ST-depression had a risk ratio two times that of patients without ST-depression for suffering reinfarction or death. However, if the pretest electrocardio-

gram did not have diagnostic Q waves, the risk increased to 11 times for an abnormal ST-segment response. This suggests that the pre-discharge exercise test is an even more powerful predictor of risk in the patient who has suffered an acute non-Q wave myocardial infarction. This is in agreement with Krone and co-workers who found that non-Q wave myocardial infarction patients with exercise induced ischemia (angina and/or ST-depression) had a three fold higher incidence of cardiac events in the year following their infarction compared to those with a normal pre-discharge exercise test [10].

The invasive strategy of pre-discharge diagnostic coronary angiography to consider PTCA in patients with clinical evidence of reperfusion by thrombolytic therapy, but no evidence of spontaneous or residual ischemia, has been found to offer no benefit over a conservative strategy [11–13]. In spite of these studies, nearly 85% of patients receive a heart catheterization at the time of their infarction. Benefits from thrombolysis appear to extend for 10 years [14].

CARDIAC REHABILITATION

Animal experiments

Hammerman designed a study to evaluate the effect of early exercise on late scar formation in an MI animal model [15]. After occlusion of the proximal left coronary artery, infarct extent was assessed 24 hours later by ECG criteria. They concluded that short-term swimming during the first week after an MI had effects on scar formation when assessed two weeks later. Two similar studies with rats forced to swim seven days post-MI reported the same results [16, 17].

Bed rest: lack of activity or gravity

There are definite hemodynamic alterations due to deconditioning including a 20 to 25% decrease in maximal oxygen uptake. Other than decreased functional capacity, prolonged bed rest can result in orthostatic hypotension and venous thrombosis through a loss of blood volume, in which plasma loss exceeds red blood cell mass loss. Pulmonary function is decreased, and the patient can be in negative nitrogen and calcium balance.

There are at least four reasons supporting the concept that much of these alterations are due to loss of the upright exposure to gravity: (1) supine exercise does not prevent the deconditioning effects of being in bed; (2) there is both less and a slower decline in maximal oxygen consumption with chair rest than with bed rest; (3) there is a greater decrease in maximal oxygen uptake after a period of bed rest measured during upright exercise versus supine exercise; and, (4) a lower body positive pressure device decreases the deconditioning effect of bed rest [18]. Perhaps intermittent exposure to gravitational stress during the bed rest stage of hospital convalescence from surgery or MI may obviate much of the deterioration in cardiovascular performance that can follow these events.

Post-discahrge activity recommendations have had little basis for their enforcement. Return to work, return to driving, and return to sex have been based on clinical judgements rather than physiological assessments [19]. Because of this, physicians have left much of this up to their patients—allowing them to see how they respond symptom-wise—rather than the older very conservative approach, which can foster invalidism. These decisions should be made considering the consequence of the coronary event and the nature of the activities.

Allen and colleagues researched and summarized 39 trials for 15 different conditions (total patients 5777) were found [20]. In 24 trials investigating bed rest following medical procedure no outcomes improved significantly and eight worsened significantly in some procedures (lumber puncture, spinal anesthesia, radioculography, and cardiac catheterization). In 15 trials investigating bed rest as a primary treatment, no outcomes improved significantly and nine worsened significantly for some conditions (acute lower back pain, labour, proteinuric hypertension during pregnancy, myocardial infarction, and acute infectious hepatitis).

According to this study, patient discomfort with prolonged bed rest following cardiac catheterization was a significant nursing problem [21]. Safely reducing the time required for supine bed rest could improve patient comfort and reduce nursing care needs. A review of the literature was conducted and decision was made to implement two hours of bed rest, a significant decrease from the previous practice of six hours. Vascular complications were closely monitored in the first 50 patients, as a means of implementing the research-based change in practice. No significant vascular complications occurred.

EARLY STUDIES OF PROGRESSIVE AMBULATION POST-MI

In 1961, Cain and colleagues [22] reported one of the first studies of the use of a progressive activity program for acute MI patients. They reported 335 patients with an uncomplicated myocardial infarction who were at least 15 days post-infarction. The electrocardiogram was monitored after the patient performed activities such as climbing stairs and walking up a grade. In 1964, Torkelson [23] reported results in ten patients with an uncomplicated MI. On the sixth week of his in-hospital rehabilitation program, a low-level treadmill test was performed using 1.7 mph at a 10% grade. Sivarajan, Bruce, and colleagues [24] described 12 patients with an acute MI whose symptoms, signs, and hemodynamic and ECG responses during and after three activities were assessed. Activities included sitting upright, walking to the toilet, and walking on a treadmill done at three, six, and ten days after infarction. These observational studies set the stage for the following randomized trials.

RANDOMIZED TRIALS OF EARLY AMBULATION

Hayes and colleagues studied 189 patients with an uncomplicated myocardial infarction selected at random for early or late mobilization and discharge from the hospital [25]. Patients were admitted to the study after 48 hours in a coronary care unit if they were free of pain and showed no evidence of heart failure or significant dysrhythmias. One group of patients was mobilized immediately and discharged home after a total of nine days in the hospital, and the second group was mobilized on the ninth day and discharged on the sixteenth day. At six weeks after admission, no significant differences were observed between the groups in terms of morbidity or mortality.

In a randomized study, Bloch and colleagues studied the effects of early mobilization after uncomplicated MI [26]. One hundred fifty-four patients under 70 years of age who were hospitalized for an acute MI and had no complications on day one or day two were randomly assigned to two treatment groups. In the early mobilization group, patients were treated by a physical therapist with a progressive activity program that began on day two or day three after infarction. In the control group, the patients underwent the traditional hospital regimen of strict bed rest for three or more weeks. The mean duration of hospitalization was 21 days for active patients and 33 days for the control group. There were no significant differences between the two groups and on follow-up there was actually greater disability in the control than in the active group.

Sivarajan and colleagues have reported the effects of early supervised exercises in preventing deconditioning after an acute MI [27]. Eighty-four patients were randomized to a control group, 174 to an exercise group. The exercise program began at an average of 4.5 days after admission. The mean discharge was ten days after admission for both groups. There were no differences between the two groups in the clinical, hemodynamic, or ECG responses to a low-level treadmill test performed on the day before hospital discharge. Nor was there any significant difference between the two groups for the incidence of complications or death. These three randomized studies of patients with uncomplicated infarctions have demonstrated that the risks of early ambulation are minimal and that progressive mobilization during the early stages of an acute MI is recommended.

Exercise testing before hospital discharge

The low-level exercise test early after an acute MI (from three days to three weeks) has been shown to be safe. Today, it is a standard part of the treatment for MI patients in many hospitals. This test has many benefits including clarification of the response to exercise and the work capacity, determination of an exercise prescription, and recognition of the need for medications or surgery. It appears to have a beneficial psychological impact on recovery and is an effective part of rehabilitation.

Exercise prescription

Exercise training can be an important part of cardiac rehabilitation for returning a patient to their formerly active lifestyle, or as functional a lifestyle as possible, after an acute cardiac event. Cardiac rehabilitation is defined by the World Health Organization as 'the sum of activities required to ensure them the best possible physical, mental, and social conditions so that they may, by their own efforts resume as normal a place as possible in the life of the community ... and that ... rehabilitation cannot be regarded as an isolated form of therapy, but must be integrated into the whole treatment of which it constitutes only one facet' [28]. The explicit details of exercise protocols/equipment, absolute and relative contraindications to exercise, warm-up and cool-down periods, guidelines for terminating exercise, are all outlined by the American College of Cardiology and the American Heart Association [29].

In prescribing exercise, two basic physiological principles should be considered. Myocardial oxygen consumption is the amount of oxygen required by the heart to maintain itself and do the work of pumping blood to the other organs. It cannot be measured directly without catheters but can be estimated by the product of systolic blood pressure and heart rate (double product). The higher the double product, the higher the myocardial oxygen consumption and vice-versa. Patients usually have their angina at the same double product, unless affected by other factors such as catecholamine level, left ventricular end-diastolic volume, hemoglobin-oxygen disassociation as affected by acid-base balance, and coronary artery spasm.

The second consideration is ventilatory oxygen consumption (VO_2), which is the amount of oxygen taken in from inspired air by the body to maintain itself and to do the work of muscular activity. Measuring VO_2 requires the collection of expired air, gas analyzers and skilled technical help. However, it can be estimated from knowing the workload of various activities. Since the body's mechanical efficiency is relatively constant, estimates of the oxygen cost of various activities without using gas analysis can be applied between individuals. There are many tables giving the approximate oxygen cost of different activities. Since oxygen consumption is equal to arteriovenous oxygen difference (a-vO_2) times cardiac output, and a-vO_2 difference is roughly a constant at maximal exercise, maximal oxygen consumption can be an approximation of maximal cardiac output. However, patients with diseased hearts will often have a wider a-vO_2 difference, a lower cardiac output, and lower VO_2 than normal subjects performing the same submaximal workload.

Another important physiological concept of exercise is the type of work the body is performing. Dynamic work (bicycling, running, jogging) requires the movement of large muscle masses and requires a high blood flow and increased cardiac output. Since this movement is rhythmic there is little resistance to flow and in fact, there is a 'milking' action that returns blood to the heart. The other type of muscular work is isometric work such as lifting a weight or squeezing a ball. Isometric activities involve a constant muscular contraction that limits blood flow. Instead of a cardiac response to increased cardiac output and blood flow, as during dynamic exercise, blood pressure must be increased in order to force blood into the active, contracting muscles. Pressure work demands much more oxygen by the heart than flow work, and since coronary artery blood flow depends upon cardiac out-put, the myocardial oxygen supply can become inadequate. Also, dynamic exercise is more easily controlled or graded so that myocardial oxygen consumption can be gradually increased whereas isometric exercise can increase myocardial oxygen consumption needs very quickly. In addition, though isometric exercise is good for peripheral muscle tone and function, it does not result in the same beneficial cardiac and hemodynamic effects as dynamic exercise.

Weight training

Kelemen and colleagues [30] performed a prospective, randomized evaluation of the safety and efficacy of 10 weeks of weight training in coronary disease patients, aged 35–70 years. Circuit weight training was safe, and resulted in significant increase in aerobic endurance and musculoskeletal strength compared with traditional exercise used in cardiac rehabilitation programs. In a six-month study of 16 men, there was a 22% gain in strength without an increase in blood pressure or untoward events [31].

Intervention studies (Table 35.3)

Kallio and colleagues were part of a World Health Organization coordinated project to assess the effects of a comprehensive rehabilitation and secondary prevention program on morbidity, mortality, return to work, and various clinical, medical, and psychosocial factors after an MI [32]. The study included 375 consecutive patients under 65 years of age treated for acute MI from two urban areas in Finland between 1973 and 1975. On discharge, the patients were randomly allocated to an intervention or to a control group, both of which were followed for three years. Patients in the control group were followed by their own doctors and were seen by the study team only once a year during the three-year follow-up. The program for the intervention group was started two weeks after hospital discharge. An exercise prescription was determined from a bicycle test, and for most patients the program was supervised. After the three-year follow-up, the cumulative coronary mortality was significantly smaller in the intervention group than in the controls (18.6% versus 29.4%). Of the intervention group and the controls, 18.1% and 11.2% respectively, presented with non-fatal infarctions. Total mortality was 21.8% in the intervention group and 29.9% in the control group. Kentala studied 298 consecutive males less than 65 years of age admitted to the University of Helsinki Hospital in 1969 with a diagnosis of acute MI [33]. There was no difference in morbidity or mortality between the groups.

Palatsi's study was a non-randomized trial of 380 patients less than 65 years old recovering from MI [34]. The first 100 patients were allocated to an exercise program and the second were the controls. Exercise training was begun 10 weeks after the MI and included breathing and relaxation exercises, calisthenics of all muscle groups and walking which progressed to running in places. The authors concluded that home training was not as effective as continual supervised programs, but still accelerated recovery of aerobic capacity. There was no group difference in symptoms, smoking habits, serum cholesterol, or return to work.

Wilhelmsen's study included patients born in 1913 or later and hospitalized for an MI between 1968 and 1970 in Goteborg, Sweden [35]. Patients were randomized to a control group ($n = 157$) or an exercise group ($n = 158$). The exercise group trained three times a week for 30 minutes a session. Calisthenics, cycling and running were performed at 80% of the maximal age predicted heart rate. After one year the exercise group showed increased work capacity, lower blood pressure, but no difference in blood lipids. At one year only 39% continued to come to the hospital to exercise, while 21% trained elsewhere. No significant differences were seen with respect to cause of death, type of death, or place of death.

The National Exercise and Heart Disease Project (NEHPD) included 651 men post-MI enrolled in five centers in the US [36]. It was a randomized three-year clinical trial of the effects of a prescribed supervised exercise program starting two to 36 months after MI (80% were more than eight months post-infarction). In this study, 323 randomly selected patients performed exercise three times a week that was designed to increase their heart rate to 85% of the individual maximal heart rates achieved during treadmill testing, and 328 patients served as controls. The three-year mortality rate was 7.3% (24 deaths) in the control group versus 4.6% (15 deaths) in the exercise group. Neither difference was statistically significant. The need for coronary artery surgery and hospitalization was equal in both groups. This study suggests a beneficial effect of cardiac rehabilitation, but insufficient participants due to financial limitations and drop-outs prevented a definitive conclusion.

The Ontario Study included seven Canadian centers that collaborated in a randomized prospective trial [37]. Seven hundred thirty-three post-MI males underwent random stratified allocation to either a high-intensity group or a low-intensity exercise group. This contin-

Table 35.3 Summary of the major randomized trials of cardiac rehabilitation assessing cardiac events, mortality, or both in patients with coronary disease

Investigator	Total	Cntrl	Ex	Exclusions (> yrs)	% women	Mean no. months entry after MI	Mean age	Years follow-up	Dropouts Cntrl %	Dropouts Ex %	Return to work Cntrl %	Return to work Ex %	RE-MI Cntrl %	RE-MI Ex %	Sudden Cntrl %	Sudden Ex %	Cardiac Cntrl %	Cardiac Ex %	Total Cntrl %	Total Ex %
Kentala 1972	158	81	77	> 65	0	1.75	53	2			5	8	5	8			12	10	14	14
Wilhelmsen 1975	315	157	158	> 57	11	3	51	4		46			21	18			18	16	22	18
Palatsi 1976	380	200	180	> 65	19	2.5	52	2.5		35	33	36	15	12	3	6	14	10	14	10
Kallio 1979	357	187	188	> 65	19	3	55	3					11	18	14	6	29	19	30	22
Mayou 1981	129	42	44	> 60	0	1	51	1.5	25	25	30	57					6	4	7	5
NEHDP 1981	651	328	323		0	14	52	3	31	23			7	5						
Carson 1982	303	152	151	> 70	0	1.5	52	2.1					7	8					14	8
Ontario 1982	761	371	390	> 54	0	6	48	3.3	45	46			10	9			4	4	7	10
Sivarajan 1982	172	84	88	> 70	20	0.13	56	0.50	13	15							2	4		
Bengtsson 1983	171	90	81	> 65	0	1.5	51	1	6		73	75	4	2					7	10
Carson 1983	303	152	151	> 70	0	1.5	55	3.5	4	17	81	7	7						8	14
Roman 1983	193	100	93		10	2	49	9		4			23	17	7	4	17	10	24	14
Vermeulen 1983	98	51	47	> 55	0	1.75	53	5	14	17			18	9			10		10	4
Froelicher 1984	146	74	76	> 65	0	4	55	1	7				1	1			3	0	0	1
Hung 1984	53	23	30	> 70	0	0.75	57	0.5		9			7	9					3	0
Hedback 1985	297	154	143	> 65	15	1.5		1		45	59	66	16	5			8	8	8	9
Marra 1985	167	83	84	> 65		2		4.5					11	6			5	6	6	7
Hamalainen 1989	375	187	188	> 65	20	< 1		10	12	15			19	26	23	13	47	35	52	44
DeBusk 1994	585	292	293	> 70	21	0.10	57	1					7	3			3	4	3	4

Cntrl = controls; Ex = exercised; MI = myocardial infarction.

ued for eight weeks after which they trained four times a week on their own. The low-intensity group trained once a week with relaxation exercises, volleyball, bowling, or swimming for one hour. They attempted to keep their heart rate at less than 50% of maximal oxygen uptake. Both groups were encouraged to stop smoking and control their weight. They found that the high-intensity exercise program had similar results to one designed to produce a minimal training effect and did not reduce the risk of reinfarction.

Bengtsson reported on 171 MI patients under the age of 65 who were randomized to a control and exercise group [38]. The rehabilitation program consisted of an outpatient exam, supervised exercise (large muscle group interval training by use of bicycles, calisthenics and jogging for 30 minutes, two days a week for three months at 90% of the maximal heart) and counseling. There were no reported differences between groups for age, sex, number of infarcts, highest enzyme, heart size, number of days in the hospital, number of admissions, angina, CHF, arrhythmia, or depression or hypochondriasis on the MMPI.

Carson et al performed their 3.5-year study in a population of 1311 male MI patients [39]. The exercise group trained in a gym two times a week for twelve weeks at 85% of the exercise-test determined maximal heart rate or until symptoms of angina, shortness of breath, or a poor systolic blood pressure response. They concluded that the difference in fitness between the exercise and control patients after completion of the study was highly significant. There was no significant decrease in mortality for the exercise group except for those with an inferior wall MI.

Vermeulen described a prospective randomized trial with a five-year follow-up [40]. Approximately one month after MI, patients underwent a symptom-limited exercise test and then entered a six-week rehabilitation program. Mortality and morbidity was 50% lower in the rehabilitation group.

Roman reported on 139 patients including 19 females who entered into their cardiac rehabilitation study [41]. The exercisers trained thirty minutes, three times a week at 70% of maximum heart rate for an average of 42 months. At the nine-year follow-up, the mortality rate was 5.2% for the control group and 2.9% for the rehabilitation group. There was a significant decrease in angina in the exercise group.

Mayou and colleagues studied 129 men, 60 years of age or less, admitted with an MI [42]. They were sequentially allocated to either normal treatment, exercise training, or counseling groups. The control group received standard inpatient care, advice booklets and one to two visits as outpatients. The exercise group received the normal treatment plus eight sessions (two times a week) of circuit training in groups, written reminders and reviews of their results. The 'advice group' received normal treatment plus discussion groups, kept a daily activity diary, had couples therapy and three to four follow-up sessions. The three groups were comparable socially, medically, and psychologically. At 18 months the only significant findings were a better outcome in terms of overall satisfaction, hours of work, and frequency of sexual intercourse for the counseled group. There was no group difference with compliance to advice in smoking, diet or exercise.

Hedback's study in Sweden was retrospective with a control group of 154 patients and an intervention group of 143 patients [43]. Both groups were treated the same during their acute hospitalization. Training began six weeks after MI following a bicycle test. One year following the MI, there was no group difference in mortality, but the exercise group had a significantly lower rate of non-fatal reinfarction, fewer uncontrolled hypertensives and fewer smokers. Goble et al found similar benefits from a low-level program compared to a high level [44].

Meta-analysis of the cardiac rehab studies

Although not every single-center study has

shown definitive differences between participants in exercise programs compared with controls in regard to physiological or psychosocial variables, the overall benefits of cardiac rehabilitation are accepted. Because of the time and expense involved in conducting controlled studies with large numbers of patients, few such trials have been performed. We are left with numerous studies showing significant benefits in exercise capacity, and often psychosocial benefits, but usually only trends toward improved morbidity and mortality. Meta-analysis is a method of combining separate but similar studies. O'Connor and colleagues performed a meta-analysis of 22 randomized trials of cardiac rehabilitation involving 4554 patients [45]. They found a 20% reduction of risk for total mortality, a 22% reduction for cardiovascular mortality, and a 25% reduction in the risk for fatal reinfarction. Oldridge and associates performed a similar meta-analysis with ten randomized trials including 4347 patients and found a similar reduction for all-cause death and cardiovascular death in the patients undergoing cardiac rehabilitation [46].

Complications during exercise training

Haskell surveyed 30 cardiac rehabilitation programs in North America using a questionnaire to assess major cardiovascular complications [47]. This survey included approximately 14,000 patients for 1.6 million exercise-hours. Of 50 cardiopulmonary resuscitations (CPR), eight resulted in death, and of seven MIs, two resulted in death. Exercise programs resulted in four other fatalities occurring after hospitalization. Thus, there was one non-fatal event per 35,000 patient-hours and one fatal event per 160,000 patient-hours. The complication rates were lower in ECG monitored programs. These programs reported a 4% annual mortality rate during exercise, which is a rate not different from that expected for such patients. Other programs have reported rates of cardiopulmonary

resuscitations ranging from one in 6000 to one in 25,000 man-hours of exercise. Such events are difficult to predict, can occur in patients with only single-vessel disease, and can occur at any time after being in a program.

A Seattle cardiac rehabilitation program (CAPRI) reported the highest rate of one CPR in 6000 exercise hours [48]. Of 15 patients requiring defibrillation, the CAPRI group successfully resuscitated all of them. Eleven had angiography, which showed single-vessel disease in four patients and multi-vessel disease in seven. Subsequently, the CAPRI record improved and they have had experience with defibrillating two patients simultaneously; on another occasion, a physician monitoring an exercise class was defibrillated. Of 2464 patients observed during a 13-year period, 25 cardiac arrests occurred during 375,000 hours of supervised exercise, a rate of one arrest per 15,000 hours. The same incidence rate was reported in Toronto and in Atlanta where five arrests occurred in 75,000 hours of exercise, and a similar rate of one arrest per 12,000 hours (total of 36,000 gymnasium hours) was reported in Connecticut. In CAPRI, 12 of the 25 victims had been enrolled for 12 or more months. Fibrillation was recorded in 23 cases and ventricular tachycardia in two. Prompt defibrillation was carried out and all patients survived. Each cardiac arrest was a 'primary' arrhythmic event, and none were associated with acute MI. Eighteen of the 25 patients had ST-segment depression, and five had developed hypotension with prior exercise testing.

Van Camp and Peterson obtained statistics from 167 randomly selected outpatient cardiac rehabilitation programs and found that the incidence rate for cardiac arrest was 8.9 per million patient hours [49]. Of these cardiac arrests, 86% were successfully resuscitated, giving an incidence rate for death of 1.3 per million patient hours. This compares favorably with the estimated fatality rate for unselected joggers at 2.5 per million person-hours of jogging [50]. There also was no significant difference in cardiac event rate between rehabilitation programs with or without electrocardiographic monitoring [51].

The incidence of exertion-related cardiac arrest in cardiac rehabilitation programs is small, and because of the availability of rapid defibrillation, death rarely occurs. Using an annual 10% incidence rate of sudden arrhythmic deaths during any activity (one per 88,000 man-hours), the risk is one-sixth that observed during participation in exercise programs. The majority of sudden deaths are temporally associated with routine activities of daily life and not with exercise. Exertion related cardiac arrest is usually due to ventricular fibrillation or tachycardia and exercise may increase its risk by 100 times [52, 53].

Improved exercise capacity due to cardiac rehabilitation

In a comprehensive review, Greenland and Chu analyzed eight controlled studies of supervised exercise programs and their effect on physical work capacity [54]. In all the studies reviewed, exercise capacity improved after the intervention, whether the patients were in a control or active intervention group. This suggests that either a patient's exercise capacity is artificially limited by the patient himself or by the physician's caring for them, or there is a spontaneous improvement in exercise capacity as time passes from time of infarction. However, the exercise groups always had a greater exercise capacity than the control groups after the interventions 20–25%. Studies that failed to show any benefit may have been limited by inadequacies of the exercise programs and also by compliance with the exercise prescription.

Cardiac changes due to exercise progress in cardiac patients

The NIH funded a study called PERFEXT (PERFusion, PERFormance, EXercise Trial) [55]. Male coronary heart disease patients were recruited for a free exercise program and encouraged to accept randomization by being promised that if randomized to the control group they could join the exercise classes after the one-year study was completed. Disease stability was assured by careful history taking and by not allowing the patient to enter the study until at least four months after a cardiac event, a change in symptoms, or surgery. Of 146 patients randomized, 72 were in the training group and 74 in the control group. The patients randomized to the exercise intervention group began training in a continuous electrocardiographic monitored class. The initial training intensity was progressed throughout the year. Patients randomized to the control group were offered a low-intensity walking program. The distribution of patients is illustrated in Figure 35.1.

The decrease in their resting and submaximal heart rates, as well as the significant increase in the measured and estimated maximal oxygen uptake was evidence of a significant training effect in the intervention group. The control group showed a significant decrease in exercise capacity. The significant increase in estimated (18%) and measured (8.5%) VO$_2$ max is similar to most studies.

Radionuclide ventriculography demonstrated a baseline increase in both end-systolic and end-diastolic volume in response to supine exercise. There were no significant differences at rest, during the three stages of exercise or the percent change from rest to exercise between the control and trained group at one year in ejection fraction, end-diastolic volume, stroke volume, or cardiac output.

The PERFEXT exercise intervention group experienced a significant improvement in the exercise thallium images following the year using the Atwood scoring system [56] as well as using computer techniques [57]. However, comparing thallium scans side-by-side failed to demonstrate improved perfusion. Exercise induced ST-segment changes did not show an improvement nor did they agree with the thallium changes [58].

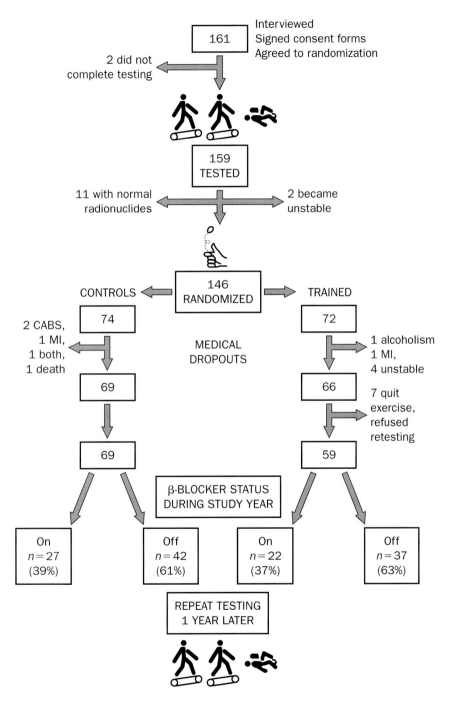

Figure 35.1 Patient distribution and flow in the PERFEXT study.

One criticism might be that our patients did not exercise hard enough and that if they had, more definite improvements might have been possible. However, even if we chose those that trained the most intensely or had the highest exercise class attendance, we did not find greater changes. Surprisingly, there was a poor correlation between the intensity or attendance and change in aerobic capacity or the radionuclide changes; in fact there was a poor correlation between the change in aerobic capacity and changes in the radionuclide tests. A paradox now exists regarding this. While impressive cardiac changes have been reported in highly selected groups of cardiac patients with asymptomatic ST-segment depression exercised at very high levels [59], the question remains whether the usual cardiac patient can be exercised safely at higher levels and if so, whether more definite cardiac changes can be demonstrated.

The effect of beta-blockers on exercise training

There is evidence that a functioning sympathetic nervous system may be necessary to achieve the beneficial hemodynamic alterations of training. In addition, the limitation in cardiac output due to beta-blockade may result in fatigue and reduce the intensity of training or compliance to exercise. Also, if ischemia (the major stimulus for collateral development), is lessened by beta-blockade, this potential benefit of training could also be impeded.

In 1974, Malmborg and colleagues first reported that a training effect could not be obtained in coronary patients with angina on beta-blockers [60] but Obma and colleagues reported a conflicting result was published in 1979 [61]. Pratt and colleagues retrospectively studied 35 patients with coronary heart disease who underwent a three-month walk-jog cycle training program [62]. Vanhees and colleagues compared two groups of post-MI patients without angina pectoris; 15 were receiving beta-blockers and 15 were not receiving them [63].

Both studies showed lower heart rates, systolic blood pressures, and rate pressure products after training, at rest and during submaximal exercise in the patients receiving beta-blockers. Peak measured oxygen uptake increased an average of about 35% in both groups but maximal heart rate and rate pressure product were also higher.

To help resolve these questions, we performed an analysis of patients in PERFEXT who exercised for one year versus controls, in which patients were placed on beta-blockers at the prerogative of their physicians [64]. Our findings and the last two studies above support the beneficial effects of exercise training in coronary patients taking beta-blocker medication.

Compliance

The success and benefits of any exercise training program are obviously directly related to the amount of exercise actually performed by the patient; in other words, their compliance with the exercise prescription. Kentala reported that only 13% of his patients carried out their assigned exercise prescription at least 70% of the time. As time progresses, compliance fell. At three months, compliance was 80%, one year later compliance was only 45–60%, and at four years it was only 30–55% [65]. Several options are available to improve compliance behavior—reduce the waiting time, expert supervision, tailoring of the exercise prescription to avoid physical discomfort and/or frustration, use of variable activities including games, incorporation of social events, recalling absent patients, involving the patient's family or spouse in the program, and involving the patients in monitoring themselves and their progress.

PATIENTS WITH LEFT VENTRICULAR DYSFUNCTION

Not long ago, patients with left ventricular dysfunction were thought to be poor candidates for exercise programs. This was out of concern for safety and the general thinking that they were unable to benefit from training. This has been dispelled, however, by a number of studies performed over the last decade. Squires and colleagues studied 20 post-MI patients with left ventricular ejection fractions less than 25% in a supervised cardiac rehabilitation program. There was substantial improvement in exercise capacity in most patients, and a favorable trend was observed in performing desired activities and returning to work [66]. Conn and associates studied ten patients with a history of prior myocardial infarction and left ventricular ejection fractions of less than 27% [67]. They found that with a cardiac rehabilitation program their exercise capacity increased from a mean of 7.0 METs to 8.5 METs and there was no exercise-related morbidity or mortality.

The controversy was re-ignited in 1988 when Judgutt and co-workers reported 13 patients with anterior Q wave myocardial infarctions using echocardiography before and after supervised low-level exercise training [68]. They found that patients with left ventricular asynergy (akinesis or dykinesis), had more detrimental ventricular shape distortion, with expansion and thinning of their left ventricle after exercise training. Several randomized trials have shown training not only improves exercise capacity, but reverses skeletal muscle metabolic derangement [69], increases maximal cardiac output, and improves measures of quality of life in these patients.

Giannuzzi and colleagues [70] completed a multicenter controlled trial of exercise training in Italy. After six months, patients in both the trained and control groups whose ejection fractions were < 40% demonstrated some degree of additional global and regional dilation. Importantly however, training had no effect on this response, and there was no effect in either group among patients with ejection fractions > 40%. More recently, these investigators completed a larger randomized trial in patients with left ventricular dysfunction after a myocardial infarction [71]. After six months, patients in the control group demonstrated increases in both end-systolic and end-diastolic volumes, and a worsening in both wall motion abnormalities and regional dilatation relative to patients in the exercise group. The latter study was the first to suggest that an exercise program may actually attenuate abnormal remodeling in patients with reduced ventricular function.

The data from Switzerland using magnetic resonance imaging (MRI) confirm that exercise training in patients with reduced left ventricular function following a myocardial infarction is effective in improving exercise capacity [72]. These data support the recent Agency for Health Care Policy and Research recommendations that exercise is a useful adjunct to medical therapy in these patients [73]. Training did not cause further myocardial damage (i.e., wall thinning, infarct expansion, changes in ejection fraction, or increases in ventricular volume), nor were there any long-term changes in these measures assessed using MRI. The application of MRI represents a significant advance in precision over previous studies. Another study to investigate the effect of exercise training on central hemodynamic responses in men with reduced left ventricular function showed substantial increases in VO_2 max by way of an increase in maximal cardiac output with widening of arteriovenous oxygen difference, but no change in contractility [74]. Training did not worsen the hemodynamic status or cause further myocardial damage. Myers et al investigated ventilatory response to exercise in patients with reduced ventricular function [75]. Exercise training resulted in systematic improvement in ventilatory response. Training increased cardiac output, tended to lower Vd/Vt, and markedly improved the efficacy of ventilation.

Exercise training alters sympathovagal control of heart rate variability (HRV) towards parasympathetic dominance in patients with acute myocardial infarction. Dubach's group [76] designed a trial with eight weeks of supervised high intensity exercise training in a regional rehabilitation center. The results of trial showed no change in HRV index. A significant decrease in standard R-R and high-frequency power in the control group suggested an ongoing process of sympatho-vagal imbalance in favor of sympathetic dominance in untrained patients after MI with new-onset left ventricular dysfunction.

Reinhart and colleagues conducted a randomized trial to investigate influence of exercise training on blood viscosity in patients with coronary artery disease and impaired left ventricular function [77]. Twenty-five patients with chronic heart failure (ejection fraction < 40%) after myocardial infarction were randomly assigned to either eight-week intensive exercise program at a residential rehabilitation center or eight weeks of sedentary life at home. There was no change in blood viscosity. Exercise training improves vasodilatory capacity in normal subjects but not in those post-MI.

Peripheral vascular resistance increases after congestive heart failure. Exercise may induce production of endothelial relaxing factors such as nitric oxide (NO). Nitric oxide also inhibits production of endothelin-1 a potent vasoconstrictor (ET-1). Dubach's group in Switzerland designed a study to investigate the influence of intensive physical training on urinary nitrate elimination and plasma endothelin-1 level in patients with acute MI and CHF [78]. After eight weeks the urinary nitrate elimination in the control group decreased while it was unchanged in the exercise group. Plasma endothelin level did not change in both groups. Nitrate elimination mirrors endogenous NO production, and so these results suggest that training may positively influence endothelial vasodilator function.

The Leipzig group conducted a prospective study of the effect of exercise training on endothelial function in patients with coronary artery disease [79]. They randomly assigned 19 patients with coronary endothelial dysfunction, indicated by abnormal acetylcholine-induced vasoconstriction, to an exercise-training group (10 patients) or a control group (nine patients).

To reduce confounding, patients with coronary risk factors that could be influenced by exercise training were excluded. In an initial study and after four weeks, the changes in vascular diameter in response to the intracoronary infusion of increasing doses of acetylcholine were assessed. The mean peak flow velocity was measured by Doppler velocimetry, and the diameter of epicardial coronary vessels was measured by quantitative coronary angiography. After four weeks of exercise training, coronary-artery constriction in response to acetylcholine at a dose of 7.2 micrograms per minute was reduced by 54% (from a mean [±SE] decrease in the luminal diameter of 0.41 ± 0.05 mm in the initial study to a decrease of 0.19 ± 0.07 mm at four weeks; $p < 0.05$ for the comparison with the change in the control group). In the exercise-training group, the increases in mean peak flow velocity in response to 0.072, 0.72, and 7.2 micrograms of acetylcholine per minute were 12 ± 7, 36 ± 11, and 78 ± 16 percent, respectively, in the initial study. After four weeks of exercise, the increases in response to acetylcholine were 27 ± 7, 73 ± 19, and $142 \pm 28\%$ ($p < 0.01$ for the comparison with the control group). Coronary blood-flow reserve (the ratio of the mean peak flow velocity after adenosine infusion to the resting velocity) increased by 29% after four weeks of exercise (from 2.8 ± 0.2 in the initial study to 3.6 ± 0.2 after four weeks; $p < 0.01$ for the comparison with the control group). Exercise training improved endothelium-dependent vasodilatation both in epicardial coronary vessels and in resistance vessels in patients with coronary artery disease.

Another study was conducted by the Leipzig group to determine if regular physical exercise corrects the endothelial dysfunction in patients with chronic heart failure [80]. In this study, 22 patients were prospectively randomized to training or control group. At baseline, and after six months, peak flow velocity was measured in the left femoral artery using a Doppler wire; vessel diameter was determined by angiography. Peripheral blood flow was calculated from average peak velocity (APV) and cross sectional area. After exercise training, nitroglycerin-induced endothelium-independent vasodilatation remained unaltered (271% vs 281%). Peripheral blood flow improved significantly in response to 90 micrograms per minute; acetylcholine by 203% (from 152 ± 79 to 461 ± 104 mL/min, $p < 0.05$ versus control group) and the inhibiting effect of L-NMMA increased by 174% versus control group. The increase in peak oxygen uptake was correlated with the endothelium-dependent change in peripheral blood flow ($r = 0.64$, $p < 0.005$). Regular physical exercise improved basal endothelium-dependent vasodilatation of skeletal muscle vasculature in patients with CHF. The correction of endothelium dysfunction is associated with a significant increase in exercise capacity.

The Leipzig group [81] designed a study to investigate if apoptosis occurs in skeletal muscle myocytes and its relation to exercise intolerance in patients with CHF. Skeletal muscle (m. *vastus lateralis*) biopsies of 34 CHF patients (NYHA II and III) and eight age-matched control subjects were analyzed by terminal deoxyribonucleotidyl transferase-mediated deoxyuridine triphosphate nick end-labeling for the presence of apoptosis, and by immunohistochemistry and videodensitometrical quantification for inducible nitric oxide synthase (iNOS) and Bcl-2 (tumor suppressor gene) expression. VO_2 max was determined by ergospirometry. The results indicated that apoptosis was frequently found in skeletal muscle obtained from CHF patients and was associated with significant impairment of functional capacity (Table 35.6). In skeletal muscles of these patients, iNOS and Bcl-2 were possibly involved in regulation of apoptosis. Apoptosis leads to loss of myocytes and loss of contractile function. Nitric oxide has been reported to function as pro- and anti-apoptotic factor. A condition associated with high levels of NO elaborated by iNOS seems to favor apoptosis. This study demonstrated that apoptosis is present in 50% of skeletal muscle biopsies obtained

from patients with CHF. The increased expression of iNOS and reduced expression of Bcl-2 are possible factors for induction of apoptosis. Occurrence of apoptosis diminishes exercise capacity. A recent study conducted by the same group was designed to analyze the effect of iNOS on mitochondrial creatine kinase (mi-CK) expression and exercise capacity in CHF [82]. This study showed increased expression of iNOS in skeletal muscle of patients with CHF inversely correlated with mi-CK expression and exercise capacity. It also confirmed causal relationship with NO.

Hambrecht and colleagues [83] conducted a study to determine the effect of exercise and oral L-arginine in patients with CHF. Dietary supplementation of L-arginine as well as regular physical exercise improved agonist-mediated, endothelium-dependent vasodilatation to a similar extent. Both interventions together seemed to have additive effects.

Patients with right ventricular dysfunction

Haines and colleagues studied 61 patients after they had suffered an acute inferior or true posterior myocardial infarction [84]. Right ventricular dysfunction was determined to be none, moderate, or severe by blinded, subjective readings of gated equilibrium blood pool images at rest. They found no significant differences in exercise tolerance as assessed by treadmill time or METs, at pre-discharge or three months post-discharge testing, between patients with and without right ventricular dysfunction. There also was no difference in exercise-induced ST-segment depression, chest pain, thallium-201 defects, medically refractory angina, reinfarction rate, or cardiac mortality. No attempt was made to standardize cardiac rehabilitation, other than usual care by the patient's own physicians. Crosby and associates studied five patients who had suffered a hemodynamically significant right ventricular infarction and found an improvement in exercise capacity with cardiac rehabilitation similar to that of

Table 35.4 Effects of cardiac rehabilitation and exercise training on exercise capacity, obesity index and lipids

Value	Very elderly (n = 54)				Younger (n = 229)			
	Before rehabilitation	After rehabilitation	% Change	p value	Before rehabilitation	After rehabilitation	% Change	p value
Exercise capacity (estimated METs)	4.4 ± 1.6	6.2 ± 2.6	39	< 0.0001	7.6 ± 3.1	10.0 ± 3.8	31	< 0.0001
Body mass index (kg/m²)	24.8 ± 3.7	24.7 ± 3.6	0	0.25	28.5 ± 4.6	28.1 ± 4.3	−1.5	< 0.001
Percent body fat	26.0 ± 17.8	24.3 ± 6.5	−7	0.13	24.6 ± 6.3	23.5 ± 6.5	−4	< 0.0001
Total cholesterol (mg/dl)	198 ± 50	189 ± 49	−5	0.01	204 ± 39	201 ± 35	−1.5	0.13
Triglycerides (mg/dl)	140 ± 64	118 ± 51	−16	< 0.001	186 ± 112	163 ± 85	−12	< 0.001
HDL Cholesterol (mg/dl)	43.7 ± 11.5	46.3 ± 16	6	0.05	36.5 ± 99	38.3 ± 10.0	5	< 0.0001
LDL Cholesterol (mg/dl)	126 ± 42	120 ± 39	−6	0.04	131 ± 37	130 ± 30	−1	0.76
LDL/HDL	3.0 ± 1.0	2.7 ± 0.9	−8	0.02	3.78 ± 1.4	3.62 ± 1.2	−4	0.03

Improvement was greater ($p = 0.06$) in the very elderly group than in the younger cohort. HDL = high-density lipoprotein; LDL = low-density lipoprotein.

patients without right ventricular infarction [85].

Elderly patients

Williams and associates studied 361 patients grouped according to age with 76 patients being 65 years of age or older, all of whom had acute myocardial infarction or CABG enrolled in a 12-week exercise program. They found that the improvement in physical capacity by the elderly group was the same as for the younger groups, and that benefits from cardiac rehabilitation were unrelated to age [86].

Wielenga et al [87] designed a prospective trial to evaluate exercise training in elderly patients with chronic heart failure. Patients with CHF (NYHA Class II and III) were randomly assigned to a training group and a control group. Patients in the training group performed additional exercise three times a week, while patients in the control group continued regular treatment. To analyze the influence on age, both groups were subdivided in subjects younger and older than 65. Quality of life aspects were evaluated with the help of Heart Patients Psychological Questionnaire and a single-question Self Awareness of General Well-Being test. Comparison of changes between groups revealed that training increased the exercise capacity and improved quality of life in the trained patients both younger and older than 65 years.

Lavin and Milani investigated effects of cardiac rehabilitation and exercise training programs in patients > 75 years of age [88]. They studied 54 consecutive patients ⩾ 75 years of age (mean 78 ± 3 years; 72% men) and 229 younger patients (< 60 years; mean 51 ± 6 years; 85% men) referred to their program. After their cardiac rehabilitation and exercise training program, the very elderly patients had modest, although statistically significant, improvements in lipids, including reductions in total cholesterol, triglycerides, low density lipoprotein (LDL) cholesterol, LDL/HDL ratio,

and increased in high-density lipoprotein (HDL) cholesterol (6%; $p = 0.05$) (Table 35.5). Body mass index did not change significantly. In addition, the very old patients demonstrated a marked 39% increase in estimated exercise capacity greater than the 31% improvement noted in the younger patients. In subgroup of patients in whom behavioral characteristics and quality of life components were assessed, the very elderly patients demonstrated significant improvements (Table 35.6). Behavioral improvement was associated with significant reduction in scores of depression, anxiety, somatization and hostility. Another trial was conducted to investigate the benefits of cardiac rehabilitation and exercise training in secondary coronary prevention in the elderly. This trial showed significant improvements in exercise capacity, obesity index and lipids. The results were similar in young and old patients. These studies emphasize that elderly patients should not be denied secondary coronary prevention including formal cardiac rehabilitation and supervised exercise training.

Exercise programs for patients post-coronary artery bypass surgery (CABS)

Adams and colleagues were the first to report a study of exercise training for CABS patients [89]. They entered four male CABS patients into a training program with 45 sedentary normal males and 11 post-MI patients. After three months of walking and jogging at least three days a week, 40 minutes a day at a heart rate 75–85% of maximum, the bypass patients had exercise capacities equal to the trained post-infarction patients, and had shown an 11% increase in maximal oxygen uptake.

Oldridge and colleagues conducted a study of the effects of an exercise program of 32 months duration among post-CABS patients [90]. Twenty-one patients with angina were given maximal treadmill tests one week prior to CABS and again 16 weeks after surgery. Six of these patients then entered a program of 45–60

Table 35.5 Effects of cardiac rehabilitation and exercise training on behavioral characteristics and quality of life parameters

Value	Very Elderly (n = 33)				Younger (n = 93)			
	Before rehabilitation	After rehabilitation	% Change	p value	Before rehabilitation	After rehabilitation	% Change	p value
Behavioral characteristics, units*								
Anxiety	3.8 ± 5.5	1.3 ± 2.1	−66	< 0.01	5.8 ± 5.3	3.8 ± 4.4	−34	< 0.001
Depression	2.7 ± 3.7	1.2 ± 2.3	−56	0.04	4.5 ± 5.3	3.3 ± 4.8	−27	0.01
Somatization	7.3 ± 3.9	4.2 ± 3.0	−42	< 0.0001	7.0 ± 4.3	4.2 ± 3.9	−40	< 0.0001
Hostility	2.0 ± 3.7	0.7 ± 1.3	−65	< 0.05	4.5 ± 5.1	3.7 ± 4.8	−18	0.10
Quality-of-life parameters, unit†								
Mental health	23 ± 7	27± +3	17	< 0.01	23 ± 4	24 ± 4	4	< 0.01
Energy	13 ± 4	16 ± 4	23	< 0.0001	14 ± 4	17 ± 4	21	< 0.0001
General health	20 ± 3	33 ± 4	65	< 0.001	21 ± 5	22 ± 5	5	< 0.01
Function	30 ± 9	38 ± 8	27	< 0.0001	35 ± 9	42 ± 7	20	< 0.0001
Well-being	44 ± 1	52 ± 7	18‡	< 0.0001	44 ± 9	50 ± 9	15	< 0.0001
Total quality of life	94 ± 19	113 ± 15	20ξ	< 0.0001	101 ± 19	115 ± 18	14	< 0.0001

* Lower score indicates improvement in behavioral characteristics. † Higher score indicates improvement in quality of life parameters. Improvement appeared greater (‡ $p < 0.05$; ξ $p = 0.09$) in the very elderly cohort than the younger cohort.

Table 35.6 Clinical parameters in apoptosis-positive or negative patients

	CHF patients		
	Apoptosis-positive (n = 16)	Apoptosis-negative (n = 18)	p value
Etiology			
DCM	10	14	
ICM	6	4	
Age (yr)	60.1 ± 7.1	55.9 ± 9.5	0.20
Weight (kg)	76.4 ± 14.1	82.6 ± 12.7	0.21
LVEF (%)	19.6 ± 7.9	19.6 ± 8.1	0.90
VO_2 max (ml/kg/min)	12.0 ± 3.7	18.2 ± 44	0.0005*
Duration (months)	64.3 ± 60.2	25.8 ± 42.7	0.02*
Decompensations (events/patient)	1.1 ± 1.4	0.8 ± 1.0	0.60
Medication			
ACE inhibitors (%)	100	100	
Diuretics (%)	100	83.3	
Digitalis (%)	81.2	72.2	
Amiodraone (%)	6.2	38.8	

* Statistically significant. Data presented are mean value ± SD or percent of patients. DCM = dilated cardiomyopathy; ICM = ischemic cardiomyopathy; VO_2 max = maximal oxygen consumption; LVEF = left ventricular ejection fraction; ACE = angiotensin-converting enzyme.

minutes of exercise, three times a week, at heart rates 65–75% of their post-operative functional capacity. Treadmill tests were performed on the exercise subjects 32 months after training began, and 28–34 months after surgery in the control group. Maximal oxygen uptake increased by 28% in the exercisers, with only a 3% increase observed in the controls. The exercise group had also been tested after four months of exercise, and by that time 90% of the total improvement in functional capacity observed at the end of 32 months had already occurred.

Soloff conducted a non-randomized study of the effect of rehabilitation on mood and physical performance in 27 post-bypass and 18 post-infarction patients [91]. The post-bypass patients significantly improved maximal oxygen uptake and maximum heart rate after an inpatient program of bedside exercise and early ambulation, followed by six weeks of monitored, three times weekly calisthenics and 20 minutes of bicycle ergometry.

In Ireland, Horgan and colleagues exercised 51 patients three times a week, in a program, which began 8–10 weeks after CABS [92]. These patients exercised 16 minutes each session at 85% of their maximal heart rate. After eight weeks of exercise, duration of exercise and maximum workload were increased.

Dornan et al reported 210 men who were referred consecutively to a rehabilitation program following CABS [93]. The program involved submaximal exercise testing at eight weeks with an intervening 12-week exercise program and a repeat exercise test. A retrospective analysis showed 50% of the patients to be on no medication throughout their rehabilitation while the others were on medications likely to affect cardiac performance. Age and the extent of revascularization did not appear to influence exercise tolerance. Following the 12-week exercise program, patients in both groups had improved significantly.

Fletcher retrospectively studied 22 patients who had undergone CABS [94]. Group I (mean age 53 years) was currently enrolled in the rehabilitation program. They concluded that the CABS patients in their program had greater maximal oxygen uptake, smoked less, were less often rehospitalized, and were more often fully employed than those who dropped out.

A study by Nakai and associates showed that physical exercise improved graft patency rate at seven weeks post-CABS (98% patency in exercise group versus 80% patency in control group) documented by coronary angiography [95]. Perk et al demonstrated less medication use and hospitalizations in CABS patients who participated in an exercise program [96].

PERFEXT CABS patients
Analysis of the CABS patients in our randomized exercise trial included 53 CABS patients who were randomized, resulting in 28 in the exercise-intervention group and 25 in the control group [97]. The mean time from surgery until entry into the study was two years. Favorable training effects were observed, however, which were similar to the larger group, but no radionuclide changes were significant. The available studies demonstrate that exercise programs can improve the exercise capacity of patients who have undergone CABS [98, 99].

Rehabilitation after PTCA

Fitzgerald and associates have shown that despite the minimal invasiveness of PTCA and lack of any physical contraindications, some patients have found it difficult to return to work because of low self-confidence [100], and only 81% of PTCA patients actually return to work [101]. It would therefore seem practical to offer cardiac rehabilitation to these patients in order that they too can benefit from the improvement in exercise capacity.

Ben-Ari and co-workers studied the effects of cardiac rehabilitation in patients post-PTCA and compared them to a group of matched patients who received usual care post-PTCA without rehabilitation [102]. They found a higher physical work capacity and ejection fraction in the rehabilitation group compared to controls, and a lower total cholesterol, lower LDL, and higher HDL as well. There was no difference in the rate of restenosis, though, at 5.5 months of follow-up. Further work by this group documented a higher return to work after their program [103].

Return to work

The presumed inability to resume gainful employment can contribute greatly to a patient's loss of self-esteem and perceived economic impotence. A concerted effort by the medical/rehabilitation team must be directed to allay these concerns [104]. A symptom-limited exercise test, if normal, can do much to encourage and re-instill confidence in the patient to resume their job-related activities. On the other hand, an exercise test showing a lower exercise capacity can be used to guide a patient's level of activity at work.

Occupational evaluation and counseling was shown to be of benefit by Dennis and co-workers who decreased the time interval between infarction and return to work by an average of 32% with counseling low risk patients [105]. Cost benefit analysis of these same patients revealed that total medical costs per patient in the six months post-myocardial infarction were lower by $502, and their occupational income was greater in this same time period was $2102 greater [106]. The fact that people are working longer into their later years, and 80% of patients under the age of 65 eventually return to work after their myocardial infarction underscores that the majority of post-myocardial infarction patients can benefit from this type of counseling. A rehabilitation program has also been found to lower rehospitalization costs in 580 patients (58% post-CABS and 42% post-MI) followed over three years [107].

Risk factor modification

Given the recurrence rate of reinfarction and overall cardiovascular mortality in survivors of myocardial infarction, theoretical benefits of risk factor modification, in this selected high-risk population, could be very significant [108]. As part of a WHO study, Kallio and associates performed a multi-factorial intervention combined with cardiac rehabilitation in post-myocardial infarction patients beginning two weeks after their event. They found in the treated group a decrease in blood pressure, lower body weight, and improved serum cholesterol and triglycerides; smoking decreased by 50% in both the treated and control groups. The National Exercise and Heart Disease Project showed a reduction in low density lipoprotein (LDL) fractions [109]. The analysis of 10-year mortality from cardiovascular disease in relation to cholesterol level by Pekkanen et al demonstrated the importance of serum cholesterol in men with pre-existing cardiovascular disease [110]. Hamalainen and colleagues noted a reduction in sudden deaths by almost 50% in patients enrolled in an aggressive, multi-factorial intervention program for 10 years post-myocardial infarction [111]. Their interventions included control of smoking, hypertension, and lipids, and the use of antiar-

rhythmic agents in addition to beta-blockers. The demonstration of regression and retarding progression of coronary artery disease [112, 113], the demonstration of cardiac changes due to diet and exercise [114, 115], and the development of the public health recommendations for physical activity rather than physical fitness all have an important impact on how health professionals counsel risk factor modification [116]. The multitude of studies demonstrating a 30–50% reduction in cardiac events in cardiac patients receiving a statin assures the prominent role of statins in rehabilitation.

Predicting outcome in cardiac rehabilitation patients

If a patient's likelihood of improving their work capacity could be predicted on the basis of initial data, much time and money could be saved. Considering VO_2 max and other indicators of a training effect [117], we asked the following questions: (1) Can clinical features prior to training predict whether or not beneficial changes occur with training? (2) Do initial treadmill and/or radionuclide measurements contribute information to improve this prediction? and (3) Does the intensity of training over the year predict beneficial changes? Our major finding was that a patient's success or failure in improving aerobic capacity following a one-year aerobic exercise program was poorly predicted on the basis of initial clinical, treadmill, or radionuclide data. Correlation between initial parameters and outcome were poor. Training intensity had little to do with outcome. Those with ischemic markers (exercise test induced angina, ST depression, or dropping ejection fraction) did not show a different degree of training effect than patients without ischemia; neither did those with markers of myocardial damage.

There was a trend for those who initially showed evidence of the poorest state of fitness (high resting or submaximal heart rate, low estimated maximal oxygen uptake) or high thallium ischemia scores to have the most improvement in the same respective parameter. However, initial measured maximal oxygen uptake, the best measure of aerobic capacity on entry, showed no relationship to any measure of training effect at the end of the year of training. Older patients showed only slightly less benefit than younger ones. Those with characteristics suggesting larger amounts of scar or ischemia did not have significantly different results from those with less. Multivariate analysis did not greatly improve the ability to predict outcome.

A very detailed initial evaluation did not allow accurate prediction of who would train and who would not. Even those patients whose characteristics suggested they had the most ischemia or scar showed as much improvement from training as patients without such characteristics. Van Dixhoorn added psychosocial variables and was able to better predict 'failure' to improve than success [118]. Other investigators of this issue have observed mixed results [119].

SUMMARY: CHANGES DUE TO ECONOMIC FORCES

There are significant changes coming about in the US regarding exercise testing and cardiac rehabilitation. The current wave of changes also includes care provider assessment by regulatory bodies and reimbursement for cognitive interactions, with a decrease in payment for procedures [120, 121]. Influential in this area is the joint commission on accreditation of health care organizations (JCAHO)—hospital accreditation will depend upon the assessment of physician diagnostic and treatment performance. The JCAHO plans a change of agenda from quality assurance (i.e., quality by inspection) to quality assessment [122]. Markers of performance must be utilized to evaluate quality of care and the implementation of guidelines. In an effort to shape these changes, medical associations (such as the AHA, ACP,

ACC, AACVPR, ACSM) are defining and refining guidelines for treatment and the use of technology and are becoming more involved in the accreditation of practitioners. While not put into practice initially as hoped now they are being used as a means of evaluating health organization and physician performance [123, 124]. They are even replacing 'the standard of practice in the community' in legal matters.

The changes that are coming in regard to exercise testing and cardiac rehabilitation are the following:

- Exercise testing will be performed more by family practitioners and internists than by cardiologists. In an American College of Physicians survey, 50% of internists were performing exercise tests [125]. The test will be used to decide which patients need to be referred to the cardiologist. It will serve as the 'gatekeeper' to more expensive and invasive tests. A key need will be to educate these practitioners to do testing properly.
- Cardiac rehabilitation is being accepted as standard of practice in the US. 'In-hospital' programs must be implemented in order for hospitals to be accredited. Physical and occupational therapists are critical in this process. 'Outpatient' programs are being greatly curtailed by declining reimbursement. No longer can they generate revenue by charging for ECG monitoring of patients who really do not need it. Guidelines have greatly limited the percentage of patients who are to receive the ECG monitored component. Each hospital has had its own outpatient program in order to compete with nearby hospitals but eventually centralized programs responsible for a region will be the best approach. The practitioners are changing as well. It is much more practical and realistic to teach cardiology and exercise physiology to physical medicine rehabilitation physicians and to family practitioners than to expect cardiologists to perform cardiac rehabilitation. In addition, research has demonstrated that exercise

programs can be safely carried out in selected low-risk patients in the home setting [126]. The Multi-Fit program tested in the HMO setting by Debusk and colleagues demonstrates that trained nurses can save health care costs using computer algorithms and telephone surveillance methods.

Some of the problems of modern medicine can be explained by the imposition of technology between practitioners and patients. Cardiac rehabilitation can insure that humanistic concerns reverse these problems. It may well be that the guise of our implementation of these goals is changing and we should become part of 'outcome assessment' plan proposed by JCAHO. The three or four phases of cardiac rehabilitation were largely directed to the exercise goals at different time points of myocardial infarction. With the in-hospital phase shortened to 3–5 days, phase 1 has all but disappeared and now applies only to patients with complications. Interventions including coronary artery bypass surgery (CABG) and percutaneous transluminal coronary angioplasty (PTCA) have also affected the early phases. There are two factors responsible for lessening the need for formal later phases: (1) the public health emphasis on increasing levels of moderate physical activity rather than promoting fitness; and (2) the fact that patients now experience less deconditioning with shorter hospital stays.

FUTURE DIRECTIONS IN THE UNITED STATES

Cardiac rehabilitation professionals must continue to develop innovative means to deliver their services and to document what they are doing by using outcome assessment and cost control. They must gather evidence on consequences of care, not just at completion of formal treatment, but downstream and with assessment tools that are sensitive to life-style factors associated with disease risk and progression, as well as quality of life. Their services must have a focus that is population based with a primary responsibility to manage capitated enrollees. Rather than respond to hospital directors, they must relate to executives responsible for managing primary care. Re-engineering is critical. Cardiac rehabilitation professionals must start asking, 'Do we really need this particular aspect of rehabilitation?,' 'Is there a better and cheaper way to deliver this service?,' and 'Which patients really need and benefit from a particular component?' No longer can each hospital or clinic have a program just to be competitive. One or two centers will be sufficient for each community. The following sections describe suggestions for the survival of cardiac rehabilitation.

Reinventing cardiac rehabilitation: implementing restructuring

As suggested by Ribisl, a new era requires a new model [127]. The old model of a standard, fixed 36-session program in which every patient receives the same intervention, regardless of specific needs or characteristics, is outmoded and a disservice to patients. Part of the reason for adhering to the old model was failure to interact with third-party payers in the design of appropriate programs that met patient needs. The security of a 'safe' and reliable means of obtaining reimbursement was the driving force behind this approach—and programs have been reluctant to make any change because of a fear that revenues would be lost. Some observations/suggestions follow and then recommendations of several models for consideration that are based on impressions of current trends and opportunities that exist today.

Initiate patient contact early

Too many patients are leaving the inpatient setting without any contact with the cardiac rehabilitation specialists. Efforts must be intensified to ensure an early contact at the inpatient setting. The cardiac rehabilitation team must be integrated into the clinical pathway to work with these patients at this ideal time. Waiting until well after discharge has been proven to be ineffective. The current trend is to reduce the length of both the hospital stay and the follow-up period as a method of cost saving. Thus, it becomes even more important that these patients be provided with an opportunity to interact with rehabilitation specialists who can assist them in their recovery. Practitioners must be more active in educating primary care physicians, managed care administrators, and consumers about the value of rehabilitation. Under a capitated system, they must be convinced that low technology alternatives are in place to minimize costs. They also must be able to readily access services so admissions occur at acceptable rates when appropriate cases arise. With cardiac rehabilitation care serving approximately 15–20% of eligible patients today, utilization is low.

Reach a more diverse pool of patients

The treatment plan for patients with cardiovascular disease is really limited to a single diagnosis. It is unusual to find an older patient who is free of other diagnoses of chronic disease. It is likely that many patients with cardiac disease have one or more additional disease such as obesity, diabetes, chronic obstructive pulmonary disease (COPD) [128], arthritis, or other complications that must be taken into account in the intervention plan. Yet few programs market their services to patients with these other diagnoses and thereby lose a key opportunity to serve the widest client base with a common set of interventional strategies applicable to the treatment of multiple diseases. For instance, weight control is an important intervention in the treatment of those chronic diseases that are aggravated by obesity. Dietary modification, including a reduction of fat and cholesterol

intake, and an increase in complex carbohydrates in the form of whole grains, fresh fruits, and vegetables is not only essential in clinical efforts to slow the progress of atherosclerotic lesions, but also helps the diabetic, arthritic, and the obese. The benefits of exercise to each of these chronic disease groups are well documented, as is the use of relaxation and cognitive strategies in behavior change. Cardiac rehabilitation needs to consider a new and broader identity and expand its scope of practice to include all chronic disease—especially as the aged segment of our patient population continues to grow requiring the most costly services available in the health-care system.

Increase physician awareness

There is a clear lack of awareness among those in the medical profession who are responsible for making decisions regarding the treatment options available to their patients in the community. It is a well-recognized fact that physicians infrequently counsel their patients regarding healthful behaviors even though most would agree to the benefits. Whether it is a lack of awareness of the availability of these services or whether it is simply negligence, ignorance, or skepticism—the fact remains that few patients are being referred to rehabilitative programs. The critical step in any effort to change this pattern rests with the primary care physician who now serves as a 'gatekeeper' to these potential services. The primary care physician must become an integral part of the treatment plan for their patients who are most likely to benefit from cardiac rehabilitation. They must become educated about the short and long-term benefits; otherwise, without this collaborative treatment planning and consequent increase in clientele it is unlikely that these programs can survive in the future. Since training in preventive strategies has never been an integral part of medical education, efforts must be made to convince current practitioners and medical students about the benefits to patients.

Expand utilization

Less than 20% of all eligible cardiac patients are referred to cardiac rehabilitation programs; 100% of all eligible patients could benefit from some form of cardiac rehabilitation. One reason for this discrepancy may be a physician belief system that fails to incorporate secondary prevention (i.e., cardiac rehabilitation) into the patient's treatment plan. Physicians should become more familiar with alternatives to their current practice and utilize other health care professionals to efficiently and economically extend their capacity to treat their patients. Ideally specialists who would determine their needs and individualize a program would see every patient at a rehabilitation center. All of the modalities of rehabilitation would be considered (home-based to monitored groups) without outside pressures to enter patients into expensive approaches. In addition, eligibility should be expanded to the elderly and patients with congestive heart failure and post-surgical intervention. In some circumstances, all the rehabilitation needed or available might be counseling by a primary care physician. Patients who are more successful in changing their lifestyle behaviors report that the physician's recommendation had a strong influence on their willingness to change. Physicians who are confident and have good counseling skills are more effective in changing the behavior of their patients. Physicians with good personal health habits and positive health beliefs are also more likely to have a positive influence on their patient's lifestyles. It has been suggested that the traditional physical exam in apparently healthy persons is a waste of physician and patient time—time that could better be spent on counseling regarding better life-style habits.

Highlight potential reduction in mortality

Cardiac rehabilitation is successful, as demonstrated by two independent meta-analyses; these rigorous analyses collectively demonstrated a 25% reduction in CV mortality but no reduction in morbidity. Numerous studies have documented the benefits of lowering serum cholesterol using drugs. Angiographic studies have shown regression or stopping of progression while a follow-up study found a 25% reduction in mortality and a 42% reduction in coronary artery bypass surgery. Since the recent studies of regression of coronary disease and decrease in events with cholesterol lowering using statins underscore the benefits of rehabilitation, the control of lipid abnormalities must be a key part of any rehabilitation program.

Document cost efficacy

Like all clinical interventions today, cardiac programs must demonstrate to hospital administrators that they are cost effective. While such documentation is likely to exist for many if not most programs, few have made the effort to publish such data. There has been a proliferation of research methodologies in recent years that consider alternative ways of conducting economic evaluation of health care [129]. Although this has added some uncertainty of approach, standardization is coming and decision makers are beginning to consider these findings, as they reformulate the scope of their health insurance coverage. Importantly, recent studies clearly demonstrate that cardiac rehabilitation is cost-effective. Oldridge et al performed an economic evaluation of patients one-year after randomization to either an eight-week rehabilitation intervention or usual care and revealed that cardiac rehabilitation is an efficient use of health care resources [130]. Ades et al presented the results of a three-year economic evaluation of patients undergoing 12 weeks of rehabilitation, which revealed that per-capita hospitalization charges for rehab participants were $739 lower than for non-participants [131]. Bondestam et al described the effects of early rehabilitation that relied totally upon the primary health care system on consumption of medical care resources during the first year after acute myocardial infarction in patients 65 years of age or older [132]. Patients from one primary health care district were assigned to a rehabilitation program, while patients from a neighboring district constituted a control group. The rehabilitation measures were initiated very early after the infarction with individual counseling in the home of the patient and later in the local health center, where 21% of the patients also joined a low-intensity exercise group. During the first three months there was a significantly lower incidence of rehospitalization in the intervention group, expressed both in terms of percentage of patients and days of rehospitalization. Visits to the emergency department without rehospitalization were also significantly lower in the intervention group. After 12 months the differences still remained, with the exception of no intergroup difference in follow-up relative to days of rehospitalization. In the matched groups the same result was seen. While re-admissions and emergency department visits generally were well justified in the intervention group, vague symptoms dominated among the controls. Levin et al presented the results of an economic evaluation of patients followed five years after rehabilitation intervention or usual care which demonstrated that mean patient costs were $8800 lower in the rehab group [133].

Implement restructuring

Cardiac rehabilitation needs to be restructured by adding newer cost-effective techniques to survive the current reformation of health care. Traditional rehabilitation will be best delivered at centers in the community rather than the current fragmented approach where each hospital has a competitive program. Newer models involve the use of other medical and paramedical professionals, volunteers and communication with patients via telephone, internet and the postal service. Four specific models with

research documenting their efficacy are presented below.

1. Center-based model
Physician referral could be improved as general practitioners become more responsible for triage and have the option of directing patients to a center with multi-disciplinary specialists available. Health care managers must be convinced that cardiac rehabilitation is effective. The necessary components of this triaging approach include initial assessment by a team of specialists, risk stratification, exercise prescription (often just a walking program, with indirect supervision, when medically appropriate), dietary instruction, lipid abnormality classification and treatment, psychological and vocational counseling, education, and a discharge plan.

The center-based model is the classic model that was the prototype for the majority of the programs in recent history. Its major shortcomings are lack of adequate referral; physician referral could be improved if general practitioners become more responsible for triage and have the option of directing patients to a center with multi-disciplinary specialists available. In addition, health care managers must be convinced that cardiac rehabilitation is as effective yet less expensive than interventional cardiology.

2. Home-based model
This model has been in place for over a decade and numerous studies in the literature have documented its effectiveness. This model has been validated at Stanford in a one-year randomized clinical trial including 160 women and 197 men aged 50–65 years who were sedentary and free of cardiovascular disease [134]. It included physician referral, assessment, prescription, and multiple interventions. There was regular feedback and home visits to prevent relapses. The main outcomes measured were treadmill exercise performance, exercise participation rates, and CVD risk factors. Compared with controls, subjects in all three

exercise training conditions showed significant improvements in VO$_2$ max at both six and 12 months. Lower-intensity training achieved training changes comparable with those of higher-intensity training. Twelve-month exercise adherence rates were better for the two home-based exercise training conditions in comparison to the group-based exercise training condition. This community-based exercise training program improved fitness but not CHD risk factors among sedentary, healthy older adults. Home-based exercise was as effective as group exercise in producing these changes. Lower-intensity exercise training was as effective as higher-intensity exercise training in the home setting.

3. Volunteer community model

The Volunteer community model is a unique approach that was developed by Lorig and colleagues in patients with arthritis [135]. These investigators trained non-medical lay volunteers (who themselves had arthritis) to direct educational programs of self-management in the community to help patients with arthritis deal with their disease outside of a medical setting. Lorig et al have since expanded this model to include four chronic disorders (CHD, COPD, stroke, and arthritis). After physician referral there was assessment, prescription, and multiple intervention as in the center-based model but utilizing an eight-week educational training program off-site. There was regular monitoring of behaviors as well as regular feedback and modification of intervention to prevent relapses. The program was two hours/week for seven weeks and was taught by two lay leaders in small interactive groups. The processes taught included problem solving, cognitive symptom management, design of exercise programs, fatigue and sleep management, anger and depression management, appropriate use of medications, patient/physician communications, proper use of advanced directives, self-efficacy enhancement, skills mastery, modeling, and reinterpretation of symptoms. The patients developed self-confidence, understood symp-tom management, and learned how to solve problems.

4. Health risk appraisal model

A randomized 12-month trial comparing claims data was performed in a large insured population. After assessment with a Health Risk Appraisal (HRA) instrument accomplished via mail, feedback on risk factors and recommendations for change was provided again by mail using an educational packet of self-management materials [136]. This study demonstrated a considerable cost trend reduction from a simple mail-based health promotion program. The insurance company was so pleased with the reduction in claims that the program has been continued.

SUMMARY

Cardiac rehabilitation is going through the same type of dramatic metamorphosis as the entire health care system. However, its principles have become part of good medical practice. The emphasis on the health benefits of physical activity rather than physical fitness and the lessening of iatrogenic deconditioning have decreased the emphasis on exercise prescription and the phased approach. As our society adopt a 'Patient Bill of Rights', cardiac rehabilitation and exercise-induced prevention programs should be considered for inclusion.

REFERENCES

1. Ryan TJ, Anderson JL, Antman EM et al. ACC/AHA guidelines for the management of patients with acute myocardial infarction: executive summary. A report of the American College of Cardiology/American Heart Association Task Force on Practice Guidelines (Committee on Management of Acute Myocardial Infarction), *Circulation* 1996; **94** (9):2341–2350.
2. Maisel AS, Ahnve S, Gilpin E et al. Prognosis after extension of myocardial infarct: the role of

Q wave or non-Q wave infarction, *Circulation* 1985; **71**:211–217.

3. Maisel AS, Gilpin E, Hoit B, LeWinter M, Ahnve S. Survival after hospital discharge in matched populations with inferior or anterior myocardial infarction, *J Am Coll Cardiol* 1985; **6**:731–736.

4. Connolly DC, Elveback LR. Coronary heart disease in residents of Rochester, Minnesota. VI. Hospital and posthospital course of patients with transmural and subendocardial myocardial infarction, *Mayo Clinic Proceedings* 1985; **60**:375–381.

5. Boden WE, O'Rourke RA, Crawford MH et al. Outcomes in patients with acute non-Q wave myocardial infarction randomly assigned to an invasive as compared with a conservative management strategy. Veterans Affairs Non-Q Wave Infarction Strategies in Hospital (VAN-QWISH) trial investigators, *N Engl J Med* 1998; **338** (25):1785–1792.

6. Ross J, Gilpin EA, Madsen EB et al. A decision scheme for coronary angiography after acute myocardial infarction, *Circulation* 1989; **79**:292–303.

7. Ahnve S, Gilpin E, Ditrich H et al. First myocardial infarction: age and ejection fraction identify a low-risk group, *Am Heart J* 1988; **116**:925–932.

8. Guidelines for risk stratification after myocardial infarction. American College of Physicians, *Ann Intern Med* 1997; **126** (7):556–560.

9. Klein J, Froelicher VF, Detrano R, Dubach P, Yen R. Does the rest electrocardiogram after myocardial infarction determine the predictive value of exercise-induced ST depression? A two-year follow-up study in a veteran population, *J Am Coll Cardiol* 1989; **14**:305–311.

10. Krone RJ, Dwyer EM, Greenberg H, Miller JP, Gillespie JA. The Multicenter Post-Infarction Research Group. Risk stratification in patients with first non-Q wave infarction: limited value of the early low level exercise test after uncomplicated infarct, *J Am Cardiol* 1989; **14**:31–37.

11. The TIMI Study Group. Comparison of invasive and conservative strategies after treatment with intravenous tissue plasminogen activator in acute myocardial infarction. Results of the Thrombolysis in Myocardial Infarction (TIMI) Phase II trial, *N Engl J Med* 1989; **320**:618–627.

12. Simoons ML, Arnold AE, Betriu A et al. Thrombolysis with tissue plasminogen activa-tor in acute myocardial infarction: no additional benefit from immediate percutaneous coronary angioplasty, *Lancet* 1988; **1**:197–203.

13. DeBono DP, for the SWIFT Investigators Group. Should we intervene following thrombolysis? The SWIFT study of intervention versus conservative management after anistreplase thrombolysis, *Eur Heart J* 1989; **10** (suppl):253.

14. Franzosi MG, Santoro E, De Vita C et al. Ten-year follow-up of the first mega-trial testing thrombolytic therapy in patients with acute myocardial infarction: results of the gruppo italiano per lo studio della sopravvivenza nell'Infarto-1 study, *Circulation* 1998; **98** (24):2659–2665.

15. Hammerman H, Schoen FJ, Kloner RA. Short-term exercise has a prolonged effect on scar formation after experimental acute myocardial infarction, *J Am Coll Cardiol* 1983; **2**:979–982.

16. Kloner RA, Kloner JA. The effect of early exercise on myocardial infarct scar formation, *Am Heart J* 1983; **106**:1009–1014.

17. Hochman JS, Healy B. Effect of exercise on acute myocardial infarction in rats, *J Am Coll Cardiol* 1986; **7**:126–132.

18. Convertino VA. Effect of orthostatic stress on exercise performance after bed rest: relation to in-hospital rehabilitation, *J Cardiac Rehab* 1983; **3**:660–663.

19. DeBusk RF. Sexual activity triggering myocardial infarction. One less thing to worry about, *JAMA* 1996; **275** (18):1447–1448.

20. Chris A, Paul G, Chris D. Bed rest: a potentially harmful treatment needing more careful evaluation, *Lancet* 1999; **354** (9186):1229–1233.

21. Vlasic W, Almond D. Research-based practice: reducing bedrest following cardiac catheterization, *Can J Cardiovasc Nurs* 1999; **10** (1–2):19–22.

22. Cain HD, Frasher WG, Stivelman R. Graded activity program for safe return to self-care after myocardial infarction, *J Am Med Assoc* 1961; **177**:111–120.

23. Torkelson LO. Rehabilitation of the patient with acute myocardial infarction, *J Chronic Disability* 1964; **17**:685–704.

24. Sivarajan ES, Snydsman A, Smith B et al. Low-level treadmill testing of 41 patients with acute myocardial infarction prior to discharge from the hospital, *Heart & Lung* 1977; **6**:975–980.

25. Hayes MJ, Morris GK, Hampton JR. Comparison of mobilization after two and nine

days in uncomplicated myocardial infarction, *BMJ* 1974; **3**:10–13.

26. Bloch A, Maeder J, Haissly J, Felix J, Blackburn H. Early mobilization after myocardial infarction. A controlled study, *Am J Cardiol* 1974; **34**:152–157.

27. Sivarajan E, Bruce RA, Almes MJ et al. *New Eng J Med* 1981, **305**:357–362.

28. World Health Organization (WHO), Report of Expert Committee. Rehabilitation of patients with cardiovascular diseases. Technical report no. 270. Geneva: WHO, 1964.

29. Fletcher GF, Balady G, Blair SN et al. Statement on exercise: benefits and recommendations for physical activity programs for all Americans. A statement for health professionals by the Committee on Exercise and Cardiac Rehabilitation of the Council on Clinical Cardiology, American Heart Association, Dallas, TX 75231-4596, USA, *Circulation* 1996; **94** (4):857–862.

30. Kelemen MH, Stewart KJ, Gillilan RE et al. Circuit weight training in cardiac patients, *J Am Coll Cardiol* 1986; **7**:38–42.

31. Sparling PB, Cantwell JD, Dolan CM, Niederman RK. Strength training in a cardiac rehabilitation program: a six-month follow-up, *Arch Phys Med Rehabil* 1990; **71**:148.

32. Kallio V, Hamalainen H, Hakkila J, Luurila OJ. Reduction in sudden deaths by a multifactorial intervention programme after acute myocardial infarction, *Lancet* 1979; **2**:1091–1094.

33. Kentala E. Physical fitness and feasibility of physical rehabilitation after myocardial infarction in men of working age, *Ann Clin Res* 1972; **4**:1–25.

34. Palatsi I. Feasibility of physical training after myocardial infarction and its effect on return to work, morbidity, and mortality, *Acta Med Scand* 1976; **599**:1–100.

35. Wilhelmsen L, Sanne H, Elmfeldt D et al. A controlled trial of physical training after myocardial infarction, *Preventive Med* 1975; **4**:491–508.

36. Shaw LW. Effects of a prescribed supervised exercise program on mortality and cardiovascular mortality in patients after a myocardial infarction, *Am J Cardiol* 1981; **48**:39–46.

37. Shepard, RJ. Exercise regimens after myocardial infarction: rationale and results, *Cardiovasc Clinics* 1985; **14**:145–157.

38. Bengtsson K. Rehabilitation after myocardial infarction, *Scand J Rehab Med* 1983; **15**:1–9.

39. Carson P, Phillips R, Lloyd M et al. Exercise after myocardial infarction: a controlled trial, *J Royal Col Phys London* 1982; **16**:147–151.

40. Vermeulen A, Liew KI, Durrer D. Effects of cardiac rehabilitation after myocardial infarction: changes in coronary risk factors and long-term prognosis, *Am Heart J* 1983; **105**:798–801.

41. Roman O. Do randomized trials support the use of cardiac rehabilitation? *J Cardiac Rehab* 1985; **5**:93–96.

42. Mayou RA. A controlled trial of early rehabilitation after myocardial infarction. *J Cardiac Rehab* 1983; **3**:397–402.

43. Hedback B, Perk J, Perski A. Effect of a post-myocardial infarction rehabilitation program on mortality, morbidity, and risk factors, *J Cardiopulmonary Rehabil* 1985; **5**:576–583.

44. Goble AJ, Hare DL, Macdonald PS et al. Effect of early programmes of high and low intensity exercise on physical performance after transmural acute myocardial infarction, *Br Heart J* 1991; **65**: 126–131.

45. O'Connor GT, Buring JE, Yusuf S et al. An overview of randomized trials of rehabilitation with exercise after myocardial infarction, *Circulation* 1989; **80**:234–244.

46. Oldridge NB, Guyatt GH, Fischer ME, Rimm AA. Cardiac rehabilitation after myocardial infarction. Combined experience of randomized clinical trials, *J Am Med Assoc* 1988; **260**:945–950.

47. Haskell WL. Cardiovascular complications during exercise training of cardiac patients. *Circulation* 1978; **57** (5):920–924.

48. Hossack KF, Hartwig R. Cardiac arrest associated with supervised cardiac rehabilitation. *J Cardiac Rehab* 1982; **2**:402–408.

49. Van Camp SP, Peterson RA. Cardiovascular complications of outpatient cardiac rehabilitation programs. *J Am Med Assoc* 1986; **256**: 1160–1163.

50. Thompson PD, Funk EJ, Carleton RA, Sturner WQ. Incidence of death during jogging in Rhode Island from 1975 through 1980, *J Am Med Assoc* 1982; **247**:2535–2538.

51. Thompson PD. The benefits and risks of exercise training in patients with chronic coronary artery disease, *J Am Med Assoc* 1988; **259**: 1537–1540.

52. Cobb LA, Weaver DW. Exercise: a risk for sudden death in patients with coronary heart disease, *JACC* 1986; **7**:215.

53. Cantwell J. Exercise and the heart: current management of severe exercise-related cardiac events. *Chest* 1988; **93** (6):1264–1269.

54. Greenland P, Chu JS. Efficacy of cardiac rehabilitation services. With emphasis on patients after myocardial infarction, *Ann Intern Med* 1988; **109**:650–666.

55. Froelicher VF, Jensen D, Genter F et al. A randomized trial of exercise training in patients with coronary heart disease, *J Am Med Assoc* 1984; **252**:1291–1297.

56. Atwood JE, Jensen D, Froelicher VF et al. Agreement in human interpretation of analog thallium myocardial perfusion images, *Circulation* 1981; **64**:601–609.

57. Sebrechts CP, Klein JL, Ahnve S, Froelicher VF, Ashburn WL. Myocardial perfusion changes following one year of exercise training assessed by thallium-201 circumferential count profiles, *Am Heart J* 1986; **112**:1217–1226.

58. Myers J, Ahnve S, Froelicher V et al. A randomized trial of the effects of one year of exercise training on computer-measured ST-segment displacement in patients with coronary artery disease, *J Am Coll Cardiol* 1984; **4**:1094–1102.

59. Ehsani AA, Martin WH, Heath GW, Coyle EF. Cardiac effects of prolonged and intense exercise training in patients with coronary artery disease, *Am J Cardiol* 1982; **50**:246–254.

60. Malmborg R, Isaccson S, Kallivroussis G. The effect of beta-blockade and/or physical training in patients with angina pectoris, *Curr Ther Res* 1974; **16**:171.

61. Obma RT, Wilson PK, Goebel ME, Campbell DE. Effect of a conditioning program in patients taking propranolol for angina pectoris, *Cardiology* 1979; **64**:365–371.

62. Pratt CM, Welton DE, Squired WG et al. Demonstration of training effect during chronic beta-adrenergic blockade in patients with coronary artery disease, *Circulation* 1981; **64**:1125–1129.

63. Vanhees L, Fagard R, Amery A. Influence of beta-adrenergic blockade on the hemodynamic effects of physical training in patients with ischemic heart disease, *Am Heart J* 1984; **108**:270–275.

64. Froelicher VF, Sullivan M, Myers J, Jensen D. Can patients with coronary artery disease receiving beta-blockers obtain a training effect? *Am J Cardiol* 1985; **55**:155D–161D.

65. Rechnitzer PA, Cunningham DA, Andrew CM et al. Relation of exercise to recurrence rate of myocardial infarction in men. Ontario Exercise-Heart Collaborative Study, *Am J Cardiol* 1983; **51**:65–69.

66. Squires RW, Lavie CJ, Brandt TR, Gau GT, Bailey KR. Cardiac rehabilitation in patients with severe ischemic left ventricular dysfunction, *Mayo Clin Proc* 1987; **62**:997–1002.

67. Conn EH, Williams RS, Wallace RG. Exercise responses before and after physical conditioning in patients with severely depressed left ventricular function, *Am J Cardiol* 1982; **49**:296–300.

68. Judgutt BI, Michorowski BL, Kappagoda CT. Exercise training after interior Q wave myocardial infarction: importance of regional left ventricular function and topography, *J Am Coll Cardiol* 1988; **12**:363–372.

69. Adampouls S, Coats AJS, Brunotte F et al. Physical training improves skeletal muscle metabolism in patients with chronic heart failure, *J Am Coll Cardiol* 1993; **21**:1101–1106.

70. Giannuzzi P, Tavazzi L, Temporelli PL et al. Long-term physical training and left ventricular remodeling relative to infarct size, *Circulation* 1995; **92**:S2041.

71. Giannuzzi P, Corra U, Gattone M, Giordano A, Tavazzi L. Attenuation of unfavorable remodeling by exercise training in postinfarction patients with left ventricular dysfunction: results of the Exercise in Left Ventricular Dysfunction (ELVD) trial, *Circulation* 1997; **96** (6):1790–1797.

72. Dubach P, Myers J, Dziekan G et al. Effect of exercise training on myocardial remodeling in patients with reduced left ventricular function after myocardial infarction, *Circulation* 1997; **95**:2060–2067.

73. Agency for Health Care Policy and Research Clinical Practice Guidelines. Cardiac rehabilitation. Washington, DC: US Department of Health and Human Services, 1995.

74. Dubach P, Myers J, Dziekan G et al. Effect of high intensity exercise training on central hemodynamic responses to exercise in men with reduced left ventricular function, *J Am Coll Cardiol* 1997; **29**:1591–1598.

75. Myers J, Dziekan G, Goebbels U, Dubacj P. Influence of high-intensity exercise training on the ventilatory responses to exercise in patients with reduced ventricular function, *Med Sci Sports Exerc* 1999; **31** (7):929–937.

76. Duru F, Candinas R, Dziekan G et al. Effect of exercise training on heart rate variability in patients with new-onset left ventricular dysfunction after myocardial infarction, *Am Heart J* 2000; **140**:157–161.

77. Reinhart W, Dziekan G, Goebbels U, Myers J, Dubach P. Influence of exercise training on blood viscosity in patients with coronary artery disease and impaired left ventricular function. *Am Heart J* 1998; **135**:379–382.

78. Callaerts-Vegh Z, Wenk M, Goebbels U et al. Influence of intensive physical training on urinary nitrate elimination and plasma endothelin-1 levels in patients with congestive heart failure, *J Cardiopulmonary Rehabil* 1998; **18**: 450–457.

79. Hambrecht R, Wolf A, Gielen S et al. Effect of exercise on coronary endothelial function in patients with coronary artery disease, *N Engl J Med* 2000; **342** (7): 454–460.

80. Hambrecht R, Fiehn E, Weigl C et al. Regular physical exercise corrects endothelial dysfunction and improves exercise capacity in patients with chronic heart failure, *Circulation* 1998; **98**: 2709–2715.

81. Volker A, Jiang H, Yu J et al. Apoptosis in skeletal myocytes of patients with chronic heart failure is associated with exercise intolerance, *J Am Coll Cardiol* 1999; **33**:959–965.

82. Hambrecht R, Adams V, Gielen S et al. Exercise intolerance in patients with chronic heart failure and increased expression of inducible nitric oxide synthase in the skeletal muscle, *J Am Coll Cardiol* 1999; **33**:174–179.

83. Hambrecht R, Hilbrich L, Erbs S et al. Correction of endothelial dysfunction in chronic heart failure: additional effects of exercise training and oral L-arginine supplementation, *J Am Coll Cardiol* 2000; **35**:706–713.

84. Haines DE, Beller GA, Watson DD et al. A prospective clinical, scintigraphic, angiographic, and functional evaluation of patients after inferior myocardial infarction with and without right ventricular dysfunction, *J Am Coll Cardiol* 1985; **6**:995–1003.

85. Crosby L, Paternostro-Bayles M, Cottington E, Pifalo WB. Outpatient rehabilitation after right ventricular infarction, *J Cardiopulmonary Rehabil* 1989; **7**:286–291.

86. Williams MA, Maresh CM, Esterbrooks DJ, Harkbrecht JT, Sketch MH. Early exercise training in patients older than age 65 years compared with that in younger patients after acute myocardial infarction or coronary artery bypass grafting, *Am J Cardiol* 1985; **55**:263–266.

87. Wielenga R, Huisveld IA, Bol E et al. Exercise training in elderly patients with chronic heart failure, *Coronary Artery Dis* 1992; **9**:765–770.

88. Lavine C, Milani R. Effect of cardiac rehabilitation and exercise training programs in patients > 75 years of age, *Am J Cardiol* 1996; **78**:675–677.

89. Adams WC, McHenry MM, Bernauer EM. Long-term physiologic adaptations to exercise with special reference to performance and cardiorespiratory function in health and disease, *Am J Cardiol* 1974; **33**:765–775.

90. Oldridge NB, Nagle FJ, Balke B, Corliss RJ, Kahn DR. Aortocoronary bypass surgery: effects of surgery and 32 months of physical conditioning on treadmill performance, *Arch Phys Med Rehabil* 1978; **59** (6):268–275.

91. Soloff PH. Medically and surgically treated coronary patients in cardiovascular rehabilitation: a comparative study, *Int J Psychiat Med* 1980; **9**:93–106.

92. Horgan JH, Teo KK, Murren KM, O'Riordan J, Gallagher T. The response to exercise training and vocational counselling in post-myocardial infarction and coronary artery bypass surgery patients, *Irish Med J* 1980; **74**:463–469.

93. Dornan J, Rolko AF, Greenfield C. Factors affecting rehabilitation following aortocoronary bypass procedures, *Can J Surg* 1982; **25**:677–680.

94. Fletcher BJ, Lloyd A, Fletcher GF. Outpatient rehabilitative training in patients with cardiovascular disease: emphasis on training method, *Heart Lung* 1988; **17**:199–205.

95. Nakai Y, Kataoka Y, Bando M et al. Effects of physical exercise training on cardiac function and graft patency after coronary artery bypass grafting, *J Thorac Cardiovasc Surg* 1987; **93**: 65–72.

96. Perk B, Hedback E, Engvall G. Effects of cardiac rehabilitation after CABS on re-admissions, return to work, and physical fitness, *Scand J Soc Med* 1990; **18**:45–53.

97. Froelicher VF, Jensen D, Sullivan M. A randomized trial of the effects of exercise training after coronary artery bypass surgery, *Archives of Internal Medicine* 1985; **145**:689–692.

98. Robinson G, Froelicher VF, Utley JR. Rehabilitation of the coronary artery bypass graft surgery patient, *J Cardiac Rehabil* 1984; **4**: 74–86.

99. Foster C. Exercise training following cardiovascular surgery, *Exerc Sport Sci Rev* 1986; **14**: 303–323.

100. Fitzgerald ST, Becker DM, Celentano DP, Swank R, Brinker J. Return to work after percutaneous transluminal coronary angioplasty, *Am J Cardiol* 1989; **64**:1108–1112.

101. Meier B, Gruentzig AR. Return to work after coronary artery bypass surgery in comparison to coronary angioplasty. In: Walter PJ, ed, *Return to work after coronary bypass surgery: psychosocial and economic aspects*, (New York: Springer-Verlag NY Inc, 1985) 171–176.

102. Ben-Ari E, Rothbaum DA, Linnemeir TJ et al. Benefits of a monitored rehabilitation program versus physician care after percutaneous transluminal coronary angioplasty: follow-up of risk factors and rate of restenosis, *J Cardiopulmonary Rehab* 1989; **7**:281–285.

103. Ben-Ari E, Rothbaum DA, Linnemeir TA et al. Return to work after successful coronary angioplasty: comparison between a comprehensive rehabilitation program and patients receiving usual care, *J Cardio Rehab* 1992; **12**:20–24.

104. Haskel WL. Restoration and maintenance of physical and psychosocial function in patients with ischemic heart disease, *J Am Coll Cardiol* 1988; **12**:1090–1121.

105. Dennis C, Houston-Miller N, Schwartz RG et al. Early return to work after uncomplicated myocardial infarction: results of a randomized trial, *J Am Med Assoc* 1988; **260**:214–220.

106. Picard MH, Dennis C, Schwartz RG et al. Cost-benefit analysis of early return to work after uncomplicated acute myocardial infarction, *Am J Cardiol* 1989; **63**:1308–1014.

107. Ades P, Huang D, Weaver SO. Cardiac rehabilitation participation predicts lower rehospitalization costs, *Am Heart J* 1992; **123** (4):916–920.

108. Siegel D, Grady P, Browner WS, Hulley SB. Risk factor modification after myocardial infarction, *Ann Intern Med* 1988; **109**:213–218.

109. LaRosa JC, Clearly P, Muesing RA et al. Effect of long-term moderate physical exercise on plasma lipoproteins. The National Exercise and Heart Disease Project, *Arch Int Med* 1982; **142**:2269–2274.

110. Pekkanen J, Linn S, Heiss G et al. Ten year mortality from cardiovascular disease in relation to cholesterol level among men with and without pre-existing cardiovascular disease, *N Engl J Med* 1990; **322**:1700–1707.

111. Hamalainen H, Luurila OJ, Kallio V et al. Long-term reduction in sudden deaths after a multifactorial intervention programme in patients with myocardial infarction: 10-year results of a controlled investigation, *Eur Heart J* 1989; **10**:55–62.

112. Brown G, Albers JJ, Fisher LD et al. Regression of coronary artery disease as a result of intensive lipid-lowering therapy in men with high levels of apolipoprotein B, *New Engl J Med* 1990; **323**:1289–1298.

113. Schuler G, Hambrecht R, Schlierf G, Hoberg E, Grunze M. Progression of coronary stenoses in patients on intensive physical exercise and low-fat diet, *Circulation* 1990; **82**:III–238.

114. Ornish D, Brown SE, Scherwitz LW et al. Can lifestyle changes reverse coronary heart disease? *Lancet* 1990; **336**:129–133.

115. Schuler G, Shlierf G, Wirth A et al. Low-fat diet and regular, supervised physical exercise in patients with symptomatic coronary artery disease: reduction of stress-induced myocardial ischemia, *Circulation* 1988; **77**:172.

116. McHenry PL, Ellestad MH, Fletcher GF et al. A position statement for health professionals by the committee on exercise and cardiac rehabilitation of the Council on Clinical Cardiology, American Heart Association, *Circulation* 1990; **81**:396–398.

117. Hammond KH, Kelly TL, Froelicher VF, Pewen W. Use of clinical data in predicting improvement in exercise capacity after cardiac rehabilitation, *J Am Coll Cardiol* 1985; **6**:19–26.

118. Van Dixhoorn E, Duivenvoorden H, Pool G. Success and failure of exercise training after myocardial infarction: Is the outcome predictable? *J Am Coll Cardiol* 1990; **15**:974–980.

119. Myers J, Froelicher VF. Predicting outcome in cardiac rehabilitation, *J Am Coll Cardiol* 1990; **15**:983–985.

120. Detsky AS, Naglie IG. A clinician's guide to cost-effectiveness analysis, *Ann Int Med* 1990; **113**:147–154.

121. Hadorn DC. The future of the American health care system, *New Engl J Med* 1990; **10**:752.

122. Clinical Outcomes, *Managing Patients and the Total Cost of Care* 1990; **1**:1–8.

123. McGuire LB. A long run for a short jump: understanding clinical guidelines, *Ann Int Med* 1990; **113**:705–708.

124. Audet AM, Greenfield S, Field M. Medical practice guidelines: current activities and future directions. *Ann Int Med* 1990; **113**:709–714.

125. Wigton RS, Nicolas JA, Blank LL. Procedural skills of the general internist: a survey of 2500 physicians, *Ann Intern Med* 1990; **111**:1023–1034.

126. DeBusk FR, Haskell WL, Miller NH et al. Medically directed at-home rehabilitation soon after clinically uncomplicated acute myocardial infarction: a new model for patient care, *Am J Cardiol* 1985; **55**:251.

127. Froelicher VF, Herbert W, Myers J, Ribisl P. How cardiac rehabilitation is being influenced by changes in health-care delivery, *J Cardiopulmonary Rehabil* 1996; **16** (3):151–159.

128. Ries AL, Kaplan RM, Limberg TM, Prewitt LM. Effects of pulmonary rehabilitation on physiologic and psychosocial outcomes in patients with chronic obstructive pulmonary disease, *Ann Intern Med* 1995; **122**:823–832.

129. Drummond M, Brandt A, Luce B, Rovira J. Standardizing methodologies for economic evaluation in health care. Practice, problems and potential, *Int J Tech Assess Health Care* 1993; **9** (1):26–36.

130. Oldridge N, Furlong W, Feeny D et al. Economic evaluation of cardiac rehabilitation soon after acute myocardial infarction, *Am J Cardiol* 1993; **72**:154–161.

131. Ades PA, Huang D, Weaver SO. Cardiac rehabilitation participation predicts lower rehospitalization costs, *Am Heart J* 1992; **123**:916–921.

132. Bondestam E, Breikss A, Hartford M. Effects of early rehabilitation on consumption of medical care during the first year after acute myocardial infarction in patients 65 years of age or older, *Am J Cardiol* 1995; **75**:767–771.

133. Levin LA, Perk J, Hedback B. Cardiac rehabilitation: a cost analysis, *J Intern Med* 1991; **230**:427–434.

134. King AC, Haskell WL, Taylor CB, Kraemer HC, DeBusk RF. Group versus home-based exercise training in healthy older men and women: a community-based clinical trial, *JAMA* 1991; **266**:1535–1542.

135. Lorig K, Holman H, Sobel D et al. *Living a healthy life with chronic conditions: self-management of heart disease, arthritis, stroke, diabetes, asthma, bronchitis and emphysema* (Palo Alto, CA: Bull Publishing, 1994).

136. Fries R, Long M, Forsythe D. Randomized controlled trial of cost reductions from a health education program, *Am J Health Promotion* 1994; **8**:216.

Section VIII: Medicine vs PCI vs CABG in 2001 for high-risk unstable angina

36

Cost comparisons of PTCA vs CABG

Kevin T Stroupe

CONTENTS • **Introduction** • **Cost analyses** • **Discussion**

INTRODUCTION

Coronary revascularization is an expensive technique and among the most frequently performed in the US, with about 428,000 percutaneous transluminal coronary angioplasty (PTCA) procedures and 501,000 coronary artery bypass grafts (CABG) performed per year. Estimated health care costs associated with revascularizations range from $12–$20 billion each year [1]. A patient receiving a single PTCA procedure is expected to require fewer resources and to cost less than a patient revascularized by CABG. However, to compare total resource utilization and cost of PTCA and CABG, the costs of follow-up care must also be included to determine whether PTCA follow-up costs offset the lower initial PTCA costs.

There is growing attention in the medical literature to the costs and cost-effectiveness of health care provision. Definitions of cost analyses conflict, and methods for conducting studies and reporting results are discrepant. A Panel on Cost-Effectiveness in Health and Medicine, convened by the US Public Health Service, has published guidelines for the conduct and presentation of such studies [2–5]. To consider costs for all relevant stakeholders, the Panel on Cost-Effectiveness has recommended that costs

be calculated from the societal perspective. To compare the complete ramifications of choosing one treatment or another, it is recommended that all health care costs be considered and not just the costs of the particular intervention being examined. In addition, because the choice of treatments may impact health care utilization into the future, the Panel on Cost-Effectiveness recommends examining long-term costs over multiple years following the intervention. When examining costs and health outcomes over multiple years, costs and outcomes should be discounted to take into account society's preference for events in the present over events in the future. To maintain equivalent treatment of the measures of costs and effectiveness over time, costs and outcomes should be discounted at the same rate, which the Panel on Cost-Effectiveness recommends at 3%.

There have been six randomized control trials since the late 1980s comparing PTCA and CABG that have reported cost results: EAST [6, 7], RITA [8, 9], ERACI I [10], BARI [11], ERACI II [12], and ARTS [13]. Although these cost analyses vary considerably in the extent to which they conform to the recommendations of the Panel on Cost-Effectiveness, they paint a consistent picture that costs are substantially less initially for patients receiving PTCA. However, due to the greater need for revascularization among the patients randomized to PTCA, the cost differences narrow or are eliminated after three to eight years.

Table 36.1 presents the characteristics of these trials, and the following section describes the economic results of these trials in more detail.

Table 36.1 Characteristics of RCTs reporting costs analyses

Trial	Recruitment period	Sample size	Sites	Follow-up period	Exclusion criteria
EAST	1987 to 1990	CABG = 189 PTCA = 197	1 site in US	8 years	1) Prior PTCA or CABG; 2) left main CAD; 3) multiple chronic total occlusions; 4) old chronic occlusions (> 8 weeks duration) of bypassable arteries serving viable myocardium and an ejection fraction ≤ 25%; 5) Insignificant myocardium at risk to warrant CABG; 6) MI within 5 days; 7) another illness threatening survival.
RITA	March 1988 to November 1991	CABG = 501 PTCA = 510	17 sites in UK	5 years	1) More than 3 vessels requiring treatment; 2) previous MI; 3) left main-stem disease; 4) hemodynamically significant valve disease; 5) or non-cardiac disease likely to limit long-term prognosis.
ERACI I	June 1988 to December 1990	CABG = 64 PTCA = 63	1 site in Argentina	3 years	1) Severe main left trunk stenosis; 2) left ventricular ejection fraction ≤ 35%; 3) associated severe valvular or hypertrophic heart disease, or both; 4) evolving acute MI; 5) and limited life expectancy.
BARI*	August 1988 to August 1991	CABG = 469 PTCA = 465	7 sites in US	5 years	1) No angina or objective evidence of myocardial ischemia severe enough to warrant coronary revascularization; 2) stenosis < 50%; 3) not technical suitable for both angioplasty and bypass surgery; 4) prior coronary revascularization procedure.
ERACI II	October 1996 to September 1988	CABG = 225 PTCA = 225	7 sites in Argentina	Mean of 18.5 months	1) Single-vessel disease; 2) previous CABG; 3) previous PCA in the past year; 4) previous stenting; 5) acute MI during the last 24 hours,; 6) left ejection fraction ≤ 35%; 7) more than 2 chronic total occlusions; 8) concomitant severe valvular heart disease; 9) or limited life expectancy because of older age or concomitant illness.
ARTS	April 1997 to June 1998	CABG = 605 PTCA = 600	Sites in 19 countries internationally	1 year	1) Left ventricular ejection fraction of ≤ 30%; 2) overt CHF; 3) a history of cerebrovascular accident; 4) a transmural MI in the previous week; 5) severe hepatic or renal disease; 6) diseased saphenous veins neutropenia or thromboctopenia, or an intolerance or contraindication to acetylsalicylic acid or ticlopidine; 7) or a need for concomitant surgery.

* Seven out of 18 sites and 934 out of 1829 patients participated in the economic substudy.

COST ANALYSES

There are two methods for estimating health care costs. One is to determine the units of health care utilization and then apply a cost per unit. Another method is to adjust the amount that health care facilities charge the patient (or the patient's designated third-party payer) using cost-to-charge ratios, which facilities in the US are required to report annually to the Centers for Medicare and Medicaid Services (formerly the Health Care Financing Administration (HCFA)) [14]. Both costing methods have been used by the RCTs comparing PTCA and CABG. All costs described below are reported per patient on an intent-to-treat basis.

EAST: Emory Angioplasty versus Surgery Trial

As shown in Table 36.1, EAST was the first of these RCTs to begin recruiting patients. EAST was a single-center RCT to evaluate PTCA and CABG for patients with multi-vessel disease. Patients were randomized in EAST from 1987 through 1990 within strata of disease severity [6]. The primary end-point was a composite of death, Q wave myocardial infarction, and a large reversible thallium defect [6]. Outcomes were reported at three and eight years of follow-up. At three years, there was no significant difference in mortality or the composite end-point. Mortality was 7.1% among patients randomized to PTCA and 6.2% among the CABG group, and the occurrence of the composite primary outcome was 28.8% among the PTCA group and 27.3% among the CABG group [6]. At eight years, mortality was 17.3% for the CABG group and 20.7% for the PTCA group ($p = 0.4$) [7].

The cost analyses from the EAST study included the costs of the initial revascularization procedure and the costs of follow-up revascularization procedures. Hospital charges for revascularizations at Emory hospital were obtained from the UB92 (UB82 before 1993) forms, which are the uniform billing forms used by third-party insurance carriers, and costs were estimated using department-specific cost-to-charge ratios [6, 7]. Physician's fees were obtained from Emory administrative records, and costs for follow-up revascularizations at non-Emory hospitals were imputed based on Emory's costs [6, 7]. Costs were inflated to 1997 dollars using the medical care component of the Consumer Price Index and discounted at 3% [7]. It was reported that the initial costs of a revascularization (hospital costs plus physician's fees) were $27,793 ($\pm$ $21,236 SD) for patients randomized to PTCA and $41,972 ($\pm$ $11,276 SD) for patients randomized to CABG ($p < 0.0001$). At three years, costs were $39,706 ($\pm$ $25,764 SD) for PTCA patients and $43,584 ($\pm$ $12,814 SD) for CABG patients ($p = 0.051$), and at eight years the costs were $43,758 ($\pm$ $26,950 SD) for PTCA patients and $46,225 ($\pm$ $14,526 SD) for the CABG patients ($p = 0.29$) [7].

Thus, initially the cost of revascularization for PTCA patients was only 66% of the cost for CABG patients. However, by three years the total costs of revascularization for patients randomized to PTCA was 91% of the cost for patients randomized to CABG, and by eight years, revascularization costs for the PCTA group was 94.7% of the costs for the CABG group. The narrowing cost difference was due to the greater need for revascularizations among the PTCA group over the follow-up period. The PTCA group also had more hospitalizations for angina and used more anti-anginal medications during follow-up. Had these costs been included, the cost difference between patients randomized to PTCA and CABG would have been reduced even further [6].

RITA: Randomized Intervention Treatment of Angina

The RITA trial took place at 17 sites in Britain and was the only trial described here that included patients with single-vessel (45%) or multi-vessel disease (55%) [9]. Patients were recruited from March 1988 to November 1991, and the primary end-point was a composite of death or non-fatal myocardial infarction [8, 9]. At five years of follow-up, mortality was 7.6% among patients randomized to PTCA and 9.0% among patients randomized to CABG ($p = 0.51$), and death or non-fatal myocardial infarction occurred in 17.1% of the PTCA group and 16% of the CABG group [9].

The reported cost analysis included the costs of the initial revascularization, the cost of subsequent revascularizations, the cost of other inpatient admissions, and the costs of anti-anginal drugs. Costs were estimated by multiplying the number of units of health care utilized by a per unit cost obtained from a London and non-London site [8, 9]. Costs were inflated to 1997 prices using the British Health Service Cost Index, and costs were discounted at 6% [9]. The initial costs of revascularization (in British pounds) were £3592 (± £1962 SD) for the PTCA group and £6912 (± £2971 SD) for the CABG group [9]. After five years of follow-up, the costs of subsequent revascularizations were £2656 (± £4520 SD) for the PTCA group and £435 (± £1655 SD) for the CABG group. Other hospitalizations were £2338 (± £3754 SD) for the PCTA group and £1750 (± £3797 SD) for the CABG group, and anti-anginal medications were £332 (± £274 SD) for the PCTA group and £155 (± £211 SD) for the CABG group ($p < 0.05$ for all preceding cost comparisons). At five years, the total costs were £8842 (± £7516 SD) for the PCTA group and £9268 (± £5384 SD) for the CABG group ($p = 0.30$) [9].

Thus, initially the cost of revascularization for PTCA patients was only 52% of the cost for CABG patients. However, by five years the cost for patients randomized to PTCA was 95.4% of the cost for patients randomized to CABG.

ERACI I: Argentine Randomized Trial of Percutaneous Transluminal Coronary Angioplasty versus Coronary Artery Bypass Surgery in Multi-vessel Disease

ERACI I was a single-center RCT in Argentina that recruited patients from June 1988 to December 1990 [10]. The primary end-point was event-free survival (survival with freedom from myocardial infarction, angina, and repeat revascularization). At three years of follow-up, there were no differences in mortality (4.7% versus 9.5%; $p = 0.5$) or in the frequency of myocardial infarction (7.8% versus 7.8%; $p = 0.8$) for the CABG versus the PTCA group [10]. However, CABG patients were more frequently free of angina (79% vs 57%; $p < 0.001$) and needed fewer repeat revascularizations (6.3% vs 37%; $p < 0.001$). Thus, event-free survival occurred in 77% of CABG patients compared with 47% of PTCA patients ($p < 0.0005$) [10].

The reported costs included only the costs of the revascularization procedures and were estimated using the number of revascularizations and the unit cost per revascularization. The unit costs per revascularization were the patients from the medical system of Argentina ($4000 and $5000 for a non-complex and complex PTCA and $12,000 and $15,000 for a non-complex and complex CABG in US dollars). The year in which these prices apply was not reported. On average, the initial cost for patients randomized to PTCA was $4286 and the cost for patients randomized to CABG was $12,813 ($p = 0.01$). However, the cost for subsequent revascularizations was on average $3238 for the PTCA group and $188 for the CABG group [10]. Over the three year follow-up period the total costs of revascularization were $7524 for PTCA patients and $13,000 for the CABG group ($p = 0.02$) [10].

Thus, the initial cost for the PCTA group was only 33% of the costs for the CABG group, but by three years of follow-up the total cost of the revascularizations for the PTCA group were 57% of the costs for the CABG group. However, as with the EAST study, the follow-up costs only included the costs of the revascularization procedures. Since the PTCA group had significantly more angina the costs of hospitalizations for angina and anti-anginal medications would likely narrow the cost difference during the follow-up period by even more.

BARI: Bypass Angioplasty Revascularization Investigation

BARI was a multicenter RCT at 18 sites in the US [11]. From August 1988 through August 1991, 1829 qualifying patients with multi-vessel disease suitable for either procedure were randomized to PTCA or CABG [15]. At seven of the 18 sites, an economic substudy was conducted involving 934 patients. At five years of follow-up there was no significant difference in death or a composite of death and Q wave myocardial infarction. It was found that mortality among the PTCA patients was 14% compared with 11% for the CABG patients, and the portion of death or Q wave myocardial infarction was 21% for PTCA patients compared with 22% for CABG patients [11].

The BARI study conducted the most comprehensive economic analysis of the trials discussed. The costs estimated were the costs of the initial procedure (including hospital costs and physician's fees), all subsequent hospitalizations (regardless of length or diagnosis), visits to physicians and other health care providers, and outpatient cardiac tests and procedures, nursing home stays, and anti-anginal medications. Charges were obtained from hospital bills and were adjusted to costs using department specific cost-to-charge ratios in the hospital's Medicare cost reports, which are sent annually to the Centers for Medicare and Medicaid Services (formerly HCFA). When hospital bills were not available, the Medicare reimbursement for the diagnostic related group was used. Physician's inpatient charges were obtained from hospitals, and physician's charges for office visits were based on Medicare

reimbursement rates. Costs for cardiac medications were based on 1995 Red Book prices. All costs were converted to 1995 dollars using the Consumer Price Index, and costs were discounted at 3% annually [11].

The initial procedure costs were $21,113 for the PTCA group and $32,347 for the CABG group ($p < 0.001$). During five years of follow-up, subsequent hospital costs (including physicians' fees) were $27,439 for the PTCA group and $29,529 for the CABG group, and anti-anginal medications cost $4948 for the PTCA group and $3670 for the PTCA group [11]. The total health care cost at five years of follow-up was $56,225 for the PTCA group and $58,889 for the CABG group ($p = 0.047$). With a higher cost for the CABG group and with a slightly higher survival (0.1 life-year added with CABG), the cost-effectiveness ratio is $26,117 per year of life added [11]. However, the cost-effectiveness ratio should be interpreted with caution. The estimate is fairly imprecise due to considerable variation in long-term costs and relatively small differences in mortality, and cost-effectiveness ratios > $100,000 per life year added could not be excluded ($p = 0.13$). Moreover, the cost-effectiveness of CABG versus PTCA varied considerably from $478,609 per life year added after the first year to $26,117 after five years [11].

The cost difference was related to patients' severity of illness. Costs for patients with two-vessel disease were significantly different ($52,930 for the PTCA versus $58,498 for the CABG group; $p < 0.05$) but not for patients with three-vessel disease ($60,918 for the PTCA versus $59,430 for the CABG group) [11].

Thus, the initial cost among the PTCA group was 65% of the cost of the CABG group. However, by five years of follow-up the total health care costs for the PTCA group were 95% of the costs of the CABG, owing largely to the greater need for revascularization among PTCA patients.

ERACI II: Argentine Randomized Study of Coronary Angioplasty with Stenting versus Coronary Bypass Surgery in Patients with Multiple-Vessel Disease

ERACI II was a multicenter trial at seven sites in Argentina that recruited patients from October 1996 to September 1998. ERACI II differed from ERACI I and other previous RCTs in that the angioplasty included stents. The composite primary end-point was occurrence of a major adverse cardiac event: death, Q wave myocardial infarction, or stroke within 30 days or need for repeat revascularization within 30 days [12]. At 30 days, mortality was 0.9% in the PTCA group and 5.7% in the CABG group ($p = 0.012$), and the composite end-point occurred in 3.6% of the PTCA group and 12.3% of the CABG group ($p = 0.002$). At follow-up (mean 18.5 months), survival was 96.9% in the PTCA group versus 92.5% in the CABG group ($p < 0.017$), freedom from Q wave myocardial infarction was in 97.7% in the PTCA group versus 93.4% in the CABG group. However, repeat revascularizations were higher in the PTCA group 16.8% versus 4.8%. Event-free survival (death, myocardial infarction, and repeat revascularization) were similar in both groups. There was more frequent angina in the PTCA group (92% versus 84.5%) [12].

The reported costs included only the costs of revascularizations and were estimated from hospital charges, procedural resources (stents, abxicimab, etc.) and physician's fee [12]. Costs were estimated by multiplying the units of utilization by a per unit cost in US dollars. The year for which the per unit prices were obtained was not reported. The 30-day costs for the revascularization procedures were $11,327 for the PTCA group and $10,736 for the CABG group ($p = 0.9$) [12]. The average follow-up (mean 18 months) costs for revascularization procedures were $993 for the PTCA group and $424 for the CABG group ($p = 0.04$). The overall costs for revascularizations at follow-up were $12,320 for the PTCA and $11,160 for the CABG group ($p > 0.05$) [12].

Thus, ERACI II actually reports the costs among the PTCA group to be higher than for the CABG group. However, there are issues to consider when interpreting these results. Unlike the other RCTs, the initial procedure costs were not reported. Rather, results for a 30-day period are reported. In addition, it was found that the PTCA group had more frequent angina. Consequently, there are likely to be differences in the hospitalizations for angina and use of anti-anginal medications that would further impact cost differences between the two groups.

ARTS: Arterial Revascularization Therapies Study

ARTS was an international study that recruited patients in 19 countries from April 1997 to June 1998. As with the ERACI II trial, ARTS also used stents in the angioplasty procedure. The primary end-point was freedom at one year after randomization from death; stroke, transient ischemic attacks, and reversible ischemic neurologic deficits; documented non-fatal myocardial infarction; and repeat revascularization by PTCA or CABG [13]. The percent of patients who died (2.5% for the PTCA versus 2.8% for the CABG group), had a cerebrovascular accident (1.7% for the PTCA versus 2.1% for the CABG group), and myocardial infarction (6.2% for the PTCA versus 4.8% for the CABG group) were similar. However, the need for repeat revascularizations was greater in the PTCA group (21% versus 3.8%, $p < 0.05$). So, for the composite end-point, 26.2% of the PTCA versus 12.2% for the CABG group ($p < 0.05$) had an event [13].

Costs per patient were estimated from the hospital's perspective. Costs were calculated as the number of resources used multiplied by the cost per unit, which were estimated from costs in a Dutch hospital. The year from which the unit prices came were not reported. The resources included: the initial revascularization procedure, outpatient visits, hospital days,

Table 36.2 Cost comparisons between RCTs

Trial	Utilization and costs included in follow-up	Base year of costs	Discount rate	Initial costs of revascularization	Ratio of PTCA to CABG	Total follow-up costs (Follow up period)	Ratio of PTCA to CABG
EAST	1) Revascularization procedures	1997	3%	PTCA = $27,793 CABG = $41,972	0.66	PTCA = $43,758 CABG = $46,225 (8 years)	0.95
RITA	1) Revascularization procedures 2) Other hospital admissions 3) Antianginal medications	1997	6%	PTCA = £3592 CABG = £6912	0.52	PTCA = £8842 CABG = £9268 (5 years)	0.95
ERACI I	1) Revascularization procedures	Not reported	0%	PTCA = $4286 CABG = $12,813	0.33	PTCA = $7524 CABG = $13,000 (3 years)	0.58
BARI	1) Revascularization procedures 2) Other hospital admissions 3) Outpatient visits 4) Outpatient testing 5) Cardiac medications 6) Nursing home admissions	1995	3%	PTCA = $21,113 CABG = $32,347	0.65	PTCA = $56,225 CABG = $58,889 (5 years)	0.95
ERACI II	1) Revascularization procedures	Not reported	0%	PTCA = $11,327 CABG = $10,736	1.06*	PTCA = $12,320 CABG = $11,160 (Mean 18.6 months)	1.10
ARTS	1) Revascularization procedures 2) Other hospital admissions 3) Transfusions 4) Vascular surgery 5) Thrombolysis 6) Angiography 7) Computed tomographic scanning 8) Other procedure-related resources 9) Outpatient visits 10) Rehabilitation services 11) Medications	Not reported	0%	PTCA = EUR 6441 CABG = EUR 10,653	0.60	PTCA = EUR 10,665 CABG = EUR 13,638 (1 year)	0.78

* Costs are reported for a 30-day period rather than strictly the initial revascularization procedure.

postoperative intensive care, coronary care, non-intensive and non-coronary care, diagnostic tests, therapeutic procedures measured in terms of their duration (e.g., PTCA and surgery), materials consumed (e.g., supplies used in revascularization), drugs, and rehabilitation services. The same data were also obtained for patient's health care at facilities not in the study [13].

The cost (in EUROs) of the initial revascularization was EUR 6441 for the PTCA group and EUR 10,653 for the CABG group ($p < 0.001$). At one year of follow-up, the cost of subsequent revascularization was EUR 1020 for the PTCA group and EUR 151 for the CABG group ($p < 0.001$), and the cost of medications was EUR 925 for the PTCA group and EUR 642 for the CABG group [13]. Total health care costs at one year of follow-up were EUR 10,665 for the PTCA group and EUR 13,638 for the CABG group ($p < 0.001$) [13].

Thus, the initial costs for the PTCA group with stenting were 60% of the cost of the CABG group. By one year the costs of the PTCA group were 78% of the CABG group.

DISCUSSION

A comparison of the costs for these trials is presented in Table 36.2. These studies found that for patients randomized to PTCA the cost of an initial revascularization procedure was typically 33% to 65% of the cost for patients randomized to CABG (ERACI II examines costs over a 30-day period rather than strictly costs of the initial procedure). The larger initial cost for CABG reflects the greater length of time needed to perform the procedure and the longer time patients spend in the hospital. For example, in the ARTS trial it was found that an average of 2.56 minutes in the catheterization laboratory and 234.41 minutes in the operating room were required for patients randomized to CABG compared with 97.79 minutes in the catheterization laboratory and 1.94 minutes in the operating room for patients randomized to

PTCA [13]. In addition, it was found in the ARTS trial that patients in the CABG group spent an average of 8.45 days in the hospital compared with 2.93 days for the PTCA group [13]. Moreover, it was reported from the BARI trial that CABG patients spent an average of 13.25 days in the hospital for the initial procedure compared with 9.03 days for PTCA patients [11].

However, these studies have consistently found that at three to eight years of follow-up the cost differences narrow or disappear. For example, the EAST, RITA, and BARI trials all report that at five to eight years of follow-up the health care costs of patients randomized to PTCA are 95% of the costs of patients randomized CABG due largely to the greater need to revascularizations among the PTCA group [7, 9, 11]. The BARI trial, which performed the most comprehensive economic analysis, also reported that costs at five years were significantly lower in the PTCA group for patients with two-vessel disease, but costs were not significantly different for patients with three-vessel disease [11]. Thus, the implications of severity of illness on the costs of treatment with PTCA versus CABG remain an area for further examination.

REFERENCES

1. Faxon DB. Myocardial revascularization in 1997: angioplasty versus bypass surgery. *Am Fam Phys* 1997; **56** (5):1409–1420.
2. Gold MR, Siegel JE, Russell LB, Weinstein MC, eds, *Cost-effectiveness in health and medicine* (New York (NY): Oxford University Press, 1996).
3. Russell LB, Gold MR, Siegel JE, Daniels N, Weinstein MC. The role of cost effectiveness analysis in health and medicine, *JAMA* 1996; **276**: 1172–1177.
4. Weinstein MC, Segel JE, Gold MR, Kamlet MS, Russell LB. Recommendations on cost effectiveness in health and medicine, *JAMA* 1996; **276**:1253–1258.
5. Siegel JE, Weinstein MC, Russell LB, Gold MR. Recommendations for reporting cost effec-

tiveness analyses, *JAMA* 1996; **276**:1339–1341.

6. Weintraub WS, Mauldin PD, Becker E, Kosinski AS, King SB. A comparison of the costs and quality of life after coronary angioplasty or coronary surgery for multivessel coronary artery disease: results from the Emory Angioplasty Versus Surgery Trial (EAST), *Circulation* 1995; **92** (10): 2831–2840.

7. Weintraub WS, Becker E, Mauldin PD et al. Costs of revascularization over eight years in the randomized and eligible patients in the Emory Angioplast Versus Surgery Trials (EAST), *Am J Cardiol* 2000; **86**:747–752.

8. Sculpher MJ, Seed P, Henderson RA et al. Health service costs of coronary angioplasty and coronary artery bypass surgery: the Randomized Intervention Treatment of Angina (RITA) trial, *Lancet* 1994; **344**:927–930.

9. Henderson RA, Pocock SJ, Sharp SJ et al. Long-term results of RITA-1 trial: clinical and cost comparisons of coronary angioplasty and coronary-artery bypass grafting, *Lancet* 1998; **352**: 1419–1425.

10. Rodriguez A, Mele E, Peyregne E et al. Three-year follow-up of the Argentine Randomized Trial of Percutaneous Transluminal Coronary Angioplasty Versus Coronary Artery Bypass Surgery in Multivessel Disease (ERACI), *J Am Coll Cardiol* 1996; **27** (5):1178–1184.

11. Hlatky MA, Rogers WJ, Johnstone I et al. Medical care costs and quality of life after randomization to coronary angioplasty or coronary bypass surgery, *N Engl J Med* 1997; **336** (2):92–99.

12. Rodriguez A, Bernardi V, Navia J et al. Argentine randomized study: coronary angioplasty with stenting versus coronary bypass surgery in patients with multiple-vessel disease (ERACI II): 30-day and one-year follow-up results, *J Am Coll Cardiol* 2001; **37** (1):51–58.

13. Serruys PW, Unger F, Sousa JE et al. Comparison of coronary-artery bypass surgery and stenting for the treatment of multi-vessel disease, *N Engl J Med* 2001; **344** (15):1117–1124.

14. Hlatky MA. Analysis of costs associated with CABG and PTCA, *Ann Thorac Surg* 1996; **61**: S30–S32.

15. Rogers WJ, Alderman EL, Chaitman BR et al. Bypass Angioplasty Revascularization Investigation (BARI): baseline clinical and angiographic data, *Am J Cardiol* 1995; **75** (9):9C–17C.

37

High-risk myocardial ischemia in 2002: medicine, PCI and CABG

Douglass A Morrison and Jerome Sacks

This text has attempted to review the evidence-based approaches available for the treatment of patients with high-risk myocardial ischemia, as of 2002. The text is subdivided into sections based upon 7 themes:

- Theme 1: Treat myocardial ischemia with the medical therapy supported by randomized clinical trials (RCTs).
- Theme 2: Either established form of revascularization (coronary artery bypass graft surgery or CABG; percutaneous coronary intervention or PCI) is at its 'best' when it is applied to patients receiving RCT-based medical therapy.
- Theme 3: For patients whose symptoms of myocardial ischemia are not controlled with medical therapy, there are two *different* methods of revascularization: CABG and PCI. Because the advantages, disadvantages, and applicabilities are different, these methods are *complementary*, not primarily competitive.
- Theme 4: There are subsets of patients, for which caregivers and patients will not permit random allocation in a revascularization RCT. Accordingly, the decisions regarding revascularization for these patients must be an individual judgement, made without the benefit of RCT data.

- Theme 5: In the era of chronic diseases, most patients have more than one clinical problem and often, more than one organ system at risk. Disease of other organ systems complicates the weighing of risks versus benefits for nearly every diagnostic and therapeutic option.
- Theme 6: Anything we do to increase the likelihood of success in one area may come at increased hazard in another.
- Theme 7: Neither CABG nor PCI, in their current state, represent a fundamental interruption of the biologic process of atherosclerosis. An attempt to interrupt the atherosclerotic process, primarily by risk-factor modification, is necessary to avoid repetitive revascularization.

Theme 1. Treat myocardial ischemia with the medical therapy supported by randomized clinical trials (RCTs).

1. Medically refractory now must include *both forestalling adverse clinical events*, such as cardiac death and/or myocardial infarction (MI), *and relieving symptoms*, such as angina or its equivalents. Optimal management of coronary artery disease (CAD) includes: blood pressure control, lipid-lowering to guidelines, smoking cessation, treatment of

post-MI patients with beta-blockers to RCT doses, treatment of patients with reduced left ventricular ejection fraction (LVEF) with RCT doses of angiotensin-converting enzyme (ACE) inhibition, and antiplatelet treatment with aspirin and/or clopidogrel. Medically refractory includes both the components of optimal CAD treatment and anti-anginal drugs to either symptom relief and/or vital sign tolerance.

2. In the absence of objective contraindications, post-myocardial infarct patients should receive both acute and chronic (at least one year) beta-blocker therapy. Beta-blockade titration is also indicated for treatment of patients with left ventricular systolic dysfunction, who are receiving RCT doses of angiotensin-converting enzyme inhibition. Beta-blockers are a preferred antihypertensive category for patients with angina, prior MI, or LV dysfunction.

3. Lipid lowering to target (LDL < 100 for patients with prior MI and/or revascularization; LDL < 130 for subjects with multiple risk factors, but no prior cardiac event) is now part of optimal medical therapy and 'medically refractory'. Patients undergoing either a PCI or CABG should have a fasting lipid panel and the initiation of lipid lowering if they are not at target.

4. Patients with left ventricular ejection fraction (LVEF) < 0.40 should receive titrated doses of angiotensin-converting enzyme inhibition toward RCT doses, unless contraindicated. ACE-I are a preferred category of antihypertensive agent for subjects with LV systolic dysfunction defined as LVEF < 0.40.

5. Aspirin, and/or clopidogrel is part of optimal treatment for nearly all categories of patients with CAD. Aspirin and/or clopidogrel is/are mandatory for all patients before elective PCI and after stent implantation. Aspirin and/or clopidogrel are of benefit, long-term after CABG. Antiplatelet therapy is part of 'medically refractory'.

6. Some form of heparinoid anticoagulation is mandatory for all acute coronary syndromes. The relative advantages/disadvantages of low molecular weight heparin, and direct thrombin inhibitors relative to unfractionated heparin are under intense current scrutiny.

Theme 2. Either established form of revascularization (coronary artery bypass graft surgery or CABG; percutaneous coronary intervention or PCI) is at its 'best' when it is applied to patients receiving RCT-based medical therapy.

7. RCTs from the 1970s support the revascularization paradox, namely that it is patients at the highest risk of events who appear to have the most to gain from revascularization. Specifically, if risk is expressed in terms of moderately impaired LV systolic dysfunction (0.35 < LVEF < 0.55) and/or severity of extent of CAD (left main > 50% and/or three vessels with > 70%), patients at-risk appeared to have a survival benefit of CABG as compared with medical therapy in that era. Components of risk which were not evaluated in the 1970s RCTs include: recent or on-going infarction, severely reduced LVEF, prior CABG, extreme old age, hemodynamic instability, prior CABG, or comorbidity.

8. Both CABG and PCI relieve myocardial ischemia and in so doing, relieve angina or angina-equivalent. A consequence of relief of limiting symptoms is extension of exercise tolerance.

9. Primarily as a result of extending exercise capacity, patients are able to live more fully, specifically to work and to love.

10. Patients with prior myocardial infarction (MI) are among the highest risk groups for further cardiac events. As discussed at length in Section 1, a number of medical therapies have been shown to reduce cardiac events among post-MI patients *regardless of whether they have symptoms or not.* Alternatively, most of the available data

suggest that *revascularization is likely to reduce events only among those post-MI patients who have reversible ischemia and perhaps primarily among post-MI patients who have medically refractory symptoms.* Medically refractory symptoms are an objective reason to consider a revascularization effort, *without having to invoke reduction of events.*

Theme 3. For patients whose symptoms of myocardial ischemia are not controlled with medical therapy, there are two different methods of revascularization: CABG and PCI. Because the advantages, disadvantages, and applicabilities are different, these methods are largely complementary, not primarily competitive.

11. To date, at least nine 'pre-stent' and five 'stent-era' trials have randomly allocated CAD patients between CABG and PCI. The 'pre-stent' trials include BARI, CABRI, RITA I, EAST, ERACI I, GABI, MASS I, Lausanne and Toulouse. The 'stent-era' trials include ARTS, SOS, ERACI II, MASS II, and AWESOME.

12. With the exception of diabetic patients with multi-vessel disease, revascularized without benefit of either stents or glycoprotein IIb/IIIa receptor blocking agents, in the PCI arms, there has been no consistent demonstration of a survival benefit of one revascularization option relative to the other.

13. There has been no consistent demonstration of prevention of MI or other non-fatal cardiac events by either CABG or PCI, relative to the other.

14. Symptom relief has been somewhat more favorable with CABG but only recently have attempts been made to 'standardize' medical therapy, particularly based upon RCT data.

15. Repeat revascularization has always favored CABG in trials of PCI versus CABG, but the gap is closing with the use of both stents and glycoprotein IIb/IIIa receptor blockers.

16. There are clearly groups, which are at higher risk or have greater potential gain with one of the two revascularization options. *Most of these groups have been carefully excluded from most previous RCTs.*

17. AWESOME specifically attempted to include several groups that are likely 'differential' between risks/benefits of CABG versus PCI Specifically, patients with on-going MI and/or hemodynamic instability are likely much higher risk for CABG than PCI. Patients who have had prior CABG, patent conduits and discrete lesions in native vessels are likely much more favorable for PCI. Conversely, patients with only total occlusions, or unprotected left main and favorable runoff, are likely much more favorable for CABG. As discussed in Section 5, co-morbidity is a whole new collection of 'wild-cards'.

Theme 4. There are subsets of patients, for which caregivers and patients will not permit random allocation in a revascularization RCT. Accordingly, the decisions regarding revascularization for these patients must be an individual judgement, made without the benefit of RCT data.

18. Numerous large databases have provided the data from which it has been possible to identify clinical and angiographic risk factors for short and long-term mortality and/or various morbidities with CABG. Surgical registries include the Veterans Affairs Continuous Improvement in Cardiac Surgery, state of New York, Society of Thoracic Surgeons, Duke database, and the Northern New England registry. In every iteration of every large database, the following have emerged and reemerged as predictors of CABG-associated mortality: prior CABG, hemodynamic instability, including shock, on-going infarction. Prior CABG is not a high-risk factor for PCI, if the 'ischemia-causing lesion' is a relatively 'favorable' lesion in a native vessel (and pump function is normal). Conversely, a

prior-CABG patient whose 'ischemia-producing lesion' is limited to old, degenerated vein grafts, is high-risk for either PCI or CABG. In both cases, new strategies are needed.

19. Since the first VA medical therapy versus CABG trial, unprotected left main has been considered 'surgical territory'. Is this changing with stents and glycoprotein IIb/IIIa receptor blockers? Investigators from Korea, Argentina and France seem to think so.

20. A specific subset of medical therapy versus PCI RCTs has been the thrombolytic versus primary PCI literature. Where logistically feasible, PCI appears to accord a survival advantage for acute MI patients, relative to fibrinolytic therapy.

21. Shock is the most extreme intersection of the sets of acutely infarcting and hemodynamically unstable patients.

22. Despite the difficulties implicit in conducting an RCT, it appears that PCI affords a survival advantage.

23. Clearly, there are patients who are too far along (sustained metabolic acidosis) and too elderly, for revascularization to have much hope of reversing the underlying problem.

24. Chronic total occlusions have been nearly 'impenetrable' for the PCI operator.

Theme 5. In the era of chronic diseases, most patients have more than one clinical problem and often, more than one organ system at risk. Disease of other organ systems complicate the weighing of risks versus benefits for nearly every diagnostic and therapeutic option.

25. Chronic pulmonary disease, especially when it entails, chronic hypoxemia (such as in the case of patients needing chronic home oxygen), chronic hypercarbia, and/or chronic steroid medication use, increase the risk of perioperative mortality. Also increased are the risks for mediastinitis and/or prolonged mechanical ventilation.

PCI may offer considerable help for patients whose coronary anatomy is only mildly unfavorable but whose pulmonary co-morbidity places them at high risk.

26. Cerebral adverse outcomes (stroke or neuropsychologic impairment) are among the most feared complications of any procedure. Risk factors for adverse cerebral outcomes with CABG include, ascending aortic disease, carotid disease, elderly, atrial fibrillation and left atrial or ventricular thrombi. As with MI, patients with prior cerebrovascular events are at greatly increased risk of subsequent events. All of these factors may make PCI, off-pump, or even hybrid procedures attractive alternatives to conventional CABG. Peripheral vascular disease is also a risk factor for CABG-associated adverse outcomes in its own right. PVD also limits the options for support devices and access.

27. The liver is intimately involved in metabolism of sedatives and other medications, as well as wound healing, hemostasis and a host of other reparative processes relative to the recovery from either revascularization. Cirrhosis, and hepatitis especially complicated by encephalopathy, ascites, and/or synthetic functional impairment may all constitute contraindications to CABG, and reasons to consider PCI.

28. Renal impairment is a risk factor for adverse outcome with either CABG or PCI. Dialysis and/or transplant may be part of the revascularization risk/benefit equation.

29. Diabetes mellitus is associated with advanced coronary and peripheral vascular disease and is a risk factor for adverse outcome with both CABG and PCI. As of this point, the BARI survival advantage for CABG does not appear to be maintained in the 'stent-era'.

Theme 6. Anything we do to increase the likelihood of success in one area may come at increased hazard in another.

30. The MIDCAB allows for CABG without the necessity of aortic cross-clamp, thereby potentially reducing the cerebral morbidity. Other modifications may obviate the need for heart-lung bypass. Will the patency of MIDCAB grafts equal conventional CABG? Is complete revascularization possible?

31. Do IABP, femoral-femoral bypass, left-ventricular assist devices extend the scope of PCI to include high-risk subsets who might otherwise be excluded?

32. Stents have changed everything!

33. Glycoprotein IIb/IIIas reduce adverse outcomes. How does one cost-effectively use stents and all of the pharmacologic options?

34. Myocardial protection is one of the CABG breakthroughs but everyone seems to have their own recipe. What is known and what is constant?

Theme 7. Neither CABG nor PCI, in their current state, represent a fundamental interruption of the biologic process of atherosclerosis. An attempt to interrupt the atherosclerotic process, primarily by risk-factor modification, is necessary to avoid repetitive revascularization.

35. Like an MI, a revascularization can be an opportunity to begin to change one's life for the better. Cardiac rehabilitation is a process, and an MI or a revascularization can help the cardiac patient begin to fundamentally change his/her life. Precisely what has made it so hard to study cardiac rehabilitation with RCTs, namely that breaking down into component parts is so impractical, is one of its greatest clinical strengths. *It is hard to systematically increase your physical activity without improving your diet and your attitude and cutting down on your smoking and becoming a little more compliant with your medical regimen.* That is the idea!

36. With so many options, balancing cost/benefit can be as tricky as trying to balance risk/benefit.

Index

abciximab (Reopro) 87–89, 491, 496–497
  in acute coronary syndromes 88–89, 90
  bleeding complications 496
  in failed thrombolysis 294–295
  as PCI adjunct 88–89, 90, 192, 491, 492–494
    in acute MI 16, 296, 299–300, 495
    costs 198
    in diabetes 435, 438
  vs tirofiban 89, 494
acebutolol 28, 29
ACE inhibitors *see* angiotensin-converting enzyme (ACE)
    inhibitors
acetaminophen 390
acetylcholine-induced vasoconstriction 526, 527
acetylcysteine 416
acetylsalicylic acid (ASA) *see* aspirin
ACIP (Asymptomatic Cardiac Ischemia Pilot) study 33,
    104–105
ACME study 122–123, 211
  exercise tolerance benefits 114, 116
  exercise tolerance and degree of stenosis 107–108
  symptom relief 109–112
activated clotting time (ACT) 80
  for PCI in acute MI 300, 303
activity
  after CABG vs PTCA 167
  lack of 514–515
  limitation 155, 511–512
  post-MI increase 515
  see also exercise
ACULYSIS system 298
ACUTE II study 80–81
acute coronary syndromes (ACS) 73–74, 85
  anticoagulants 75–77, 80–81
  antiplatelet agents 74, 86, 88–89, 90
  glycoprotein IIb/IIIa receptor blockers 88–89, 90,
    494–495, 497
  pathophysiology 489–491
  risk factors 89
  terminology 78, 90
  see also acute myocardial infarction; non-Q wave acute
    myocardial infarction; non-ST-segment elevation
    acute coronary syndromes; unstable angina
acute myocardial infarction (AMI)
  ACE inhibitors 61–63
  anticoagulants 73, 77–81
  aspirin therapy 86, 298, 299, 303
  bed rest 80, 511, 512
  beta-blockers 26–28, 35

cardiogenic shock *see* cardiogenic shock
  in diabetes 301, 427–428, 432
  early CABG 188–189, 190–191
  glycoprotein IIb/IIIa receptor blockers 494–495
  left main coronary artery stenting 279
  mechanical complications 338
  medical therapy 16
  off-pump CABG 461
  primary PCI 283–304
    additional benefits 300–301
    adjunctive pharmacotherapy 80–81, 298–300,
      494–495
    atherectomy 296–297
    in congestive heart failure 293–294
    device therapy 295–298
    economics 301
    in elderly patients 291–292
    emergent transfer for 302
    future insights 303–304
    IABP support 472–473
    laser angioplasty 298
    limitations 301–302
    patient selection 302–303
    periprocedural care 302–303
    prior CABG and 294
    rheolytic thrombectomy 297–298
    stenting 295–296, 303
    therapeutic ultrasound 298
    vs thrombolytic therapy 283–291, 562
  recurrent 287, 290
  'rescue' PCI 291, 294–295
  risk stratification 300–301
  stenting 295–296, 297, 303, 481
  terminology 78
  thrombolysis *see* thrombolysis
adhesion molecules, endothelial 431
ADMIRAL trial 300
advanced glycation end products (AGEs) 432
age
  perioperative stroke and 456, 457
  see also elderly
Aggrastat *see* tirofiban
AIRE (Acute Infarction Ramipril Efficacy) trial 64, 65
Air Force/Texas Coronary Artery Prevention Study
    (AFCAPS/TexCAPS) 46, 47, 52, 53
Air-PAMI trial 302
alcohol abuse, screening 390
alcohol-related liver disease 388, 393
Allen's test 260

alteplase 79
American College of Cardiology/American Heart
    Association (ACC/AHA) guidelines 11
  acute MI management 79, 302, 332
  CABG surgery 363
amlodipine 33
analgesics, in liver disease 403–404
anaphylactoid reactions 301
anesthesia
  hemodynamic effects 402–403
  -related pulmonary complications 367–368
angina 73, 107
  chronic stable
    benefits of revascularization 107–118
    beta-blockers 31–32
    CABG 97–105
    CABG vs PCI vs medical therapy 204–212
    medical therapy 16–17
    PCI vs medical therapy 121–133
  in chronic total occlusions 348
  placebo effect 108
  relief 108–114, 560
    CABG vs medical therapy 108–109
    CABG vs PTCA 113–114, 154–155, 158, 165–166, 168, 181
    CABG vs stenting 241, 244
    PCI vs medical therapy 109–112, 172
    stenting in left main disease 274–275
  unstable *see* unstable angina
Angina With Extremely Serious Operative Mortality
    Evaluation trial *see* AWESOME trial
angioplasty *see* percutaneous transluminal coronary
    angioplasty
Angioplasty Compared to Medicine study *see* ACME study
angiotensin II (AII) 61, 490
angiotensin-converting enzyme (ACE) inhibitors 61–69
  in acute MI 61–63
  after revascularization 69
  cardiovascular protection 67–68
  in diabetes 427
  in heart failure 61, 66–67
  in hypertension 67–68
  long-term post-MI 63–66
  mechanism of action 62
  recommended use 15, 16, 17, 560
  target doses 14, 15
angiotensin receptor blockers 17, 69
angiotensin system 61
anti-angina medication *see* anti-ischemic medication
anti-arrhythmic agents, ACE inhibitors as 64
anticoagulants 73–81
  in acute MI 16, 73, 77–81
    morbidity/mortality prevention 78–79
    for PCI 80–81
    systemic embolization prevention 79–80
    venous thrombosis prevention 80
  recommendations 15, 16, 560
  in unstable angina 74–77, 78
  see also heparin
anti-ischemic medication
  CABG vs PTCA studies 155, 166–167
  CABG vs stenting 241, 244
  in COURAGE trial 128, 129
  in RITA-2 study 170, 172
antiplatelet agents 85–90
  in acute coronary syndromes 74, 86, 88–89, 90
  for PCI 87, 88, 90

  in acute MI 298, 299, 303
  recommended use 15, 16
  target doses 14
  see also aspirin; clopidogrel; glycoprotein IIb/IIIa receptor
    blockers; ticlopidine
Antiplatelet Trialists Collaboration 86, 204
antithrombin agents
  in acute MI 79
  in PCI for acute MI 299
  in unstable angina 74, 81, 90
anti-Xa levels 80
aorta
  atherosclerosis
    CABG re-operations 260, 261
    embolization 375, 456
    prevention of embolization 457–458
  calcification (porcelain) 373, 375, 457
  cross-clamping 373–374, 376
  mobile atheroma 457, 458
  no-touch technique 457–458, 459
APACHE (Acute Physiology, Age and Chronic Health
    Evaluation) III score 395
apolipoproteins 43
apoptosis, skeletal muscle myocytes 527, 531
APPLE trial 50, 51
APRES study 69
APSIS (Angina Prognosis Study in Stockholm) 31, 32
APSI study 28, 29
argatroban, in unstable angina 74, 77
Argentine randomized studies 187–200
  see also ERACI I; ERACI II
L-arginine 527
arterial cannulation sites
  alternative 457
  complications 474, 475, 476
arterial conduits
  AWESOME trial 220
  CABG re-operations 260, 262–263
  EAST study 184
  see also internal mammary artery (IMA) grafts
Arterial Revascularization Therapy Study *see* ARTS
arterial thromboembolism
  pathophysiology 489–491, 496
  prevention 77–78
ARTS (Arterial Revascularization Therapy Study) 4, 235–250
  12-month outcome 241, 242, 243, 244
  diabetes subgroup 168, 245, 248
  economic analysis 241–242, 550, 554–556
  methods 236–238
  quality of life 241, 244
  results 238–242
  vs AWESOME 229, 231
  vs ERACI II 191, 192
Asan medical center, stenting in left main stenosis 268–270
ascites
  intraoperative care 401
  postoperative management 400
aspiration (of gastric contents) 368
aspirin 86, 204
  in acute MI 86, 298, 299, 303
  COURAGE trial 128, 131
  in non-ST segment elevation acute coronary syndromes
    141
  recommended use 15, 16, 560
  target dose 14
  in unstable angina 74, 86, 90

ASSENT PLUS trial 79
Asymptomatic Cardiac Ischemia Pilot (ACIP) study 33, 104–105
ATACS trial 75, 77
atelectasis, postoperative 363, 366, 367, 368
atenolol 25–26
  in angina 32
  post MI 26, 27
  in silent ischemia 32–33
  target dose 14
Atenolol Silent Ischemia Study (ASIST) 32–33
atherectomy
  directional
    in acute MI 297
    in left main stenosis 269, 270, 272, 273–274
  extraction, in acute MI 297
  rotational
    in acute MI 296
    IABP support 472
    in left main stenosis 273, 277
  transluminal extraction (TEC) 297
atherosclerosis
  aortic *see* aorta, atherosclerosis
  arterial thrombosis pathophysiology 489–491
  coronary 73
    see also coronary artery disease
  pathophysiology in diabetes 429–432
  vein graft 258–259
atorvastatin 53, 123–124
  secondary prevention 47, 49, 50
  target dose 14
Atorvastatin Versus Revascularization Treatment (AVERT) trial 123–124
atrial fibrillation 373, 375
AUDIT (Alcohol Use Disorders Identification Test) 390
AWESOME trial 4, 12, 217–232, 561
  cardiogenic shock 339, 340, 342
  diabetes subgroup 438–439, 440
  lessons learnt 231–232
  methods 218–220
    outcome variables 220
    patient screening and accrual 218–219
    statistical methods 220
  myocardial protection 504–505
  results 220–224
    baseline characteristics 220, 221–223
    CABG and PCI methods 220–223
    long-term outcomes 224, 225
    short-term outcomes 223–224
  stenting in high-risk cohorts 482–483
  vs BARI 225–228, 229
  vs other trials 229, 230–231

balloon angioplasty *see* percutaneous transluminal coronary angioplasty
BARI 3, 6–7, 145–159, 550
  diabetes subgroup 145, 156–159
    MI events and cardiac mortality 153, 157–158
    current relevance 159, 437–438
    repeat revascularization 154, 158
    survival rates 151–152, 156–158, 197, 425–426
    vs other trials 195–196, 435
  economic substudy 155–156, 157, 158, 553, 555, 556
  limitations 159
  major findings 156–158
  methods 145–147

    data collection 147
    definitions 147
    inclusion and exclusion criteria 146–147
    study design 145–146
  results 148–156
    5- and 7-year outcomes 141, 150–153, 156–158, 168
    baseline characteristics 148–149
    clinical and functional outcomes 113–114, 154–156, 168–169
    patient population 148
    procedural and hospital outcome 149–150
    reintervention 153–154
  second trial in diabetics (BARI 2D) 105, 159
  strengths 158–159
  vs ARTS 243
  vs AWESOME 225–228, 229
Bcl-2 527
BECAIT study 49, 50
bed rest
  in acute MI 80, 511, 512
  adverse effects 514–515
behavior
  exercise training effects 529, 530
  promoting change 537
BENESTENT trial 481
beta-adrenergic system 25–26
Beta-Blocker Heart Attack Trial (BHAT) 28, 29
beta-blockers 25–36
  in acute MI 26–28, 35
  cardiac rehabilitation and 524
  contraindications 26
  heart failure 33–35
  hypertension 36
  long-term post MI 28–29, 35
  mechanism of action 25–26
  recommended use 15, 16, 17, 560
  selectivity 25
  side effects 26
  silent ischemia 32–33
  stable angina 31–32
  target doses 14
  underutilization 35–36
  unstable angina 29–31
bezafibrate 54
  secondary prevention 47, 48, 49, 50
bile acid binding resins 53–54
BIOMACS trial 79
BIP study 47, 48
bisoprolol 33
bivalirudin (hirulog)
  in acute MI 79, 81
  in unstable angina 74, 76, 77
bleeding complications
  glycoprotein IIb/IIIa receptor blockers 496
  PCI vs thrombolysis 287
blood pressure, target 15, 16, 17, 128
blood transfusion
  PCI vs thrombolysis 287
  prior history 390
  supported PCI 474, 476
blood viscosity, exercise training and 526
body mass index, exercise training and 528, 529
bradykinin system 61
breathlessness, after CABG vs PTCA 167
Bypass Angioplasty Revascularization Investigation *see* BARI

bypass conduits
    for CABG re-operations 260, 262, 263
    see also arterial conduits; vein grafts

c7e3 Fab monoclonal antibody *see* abciximab
CABG *see* coronary artery bypass graft (CABG) surgery
CABG Patch Trial database 436
CABRI
    vs ARTS 243, 247
    vs AWESOME 229, 230–231
CAD *see* coronary artery disease
CADILLAC trial 296, 300, 428, 495
CAGE questionnaire 390
calcification
    aorta (porcelain) 373, 375, 457
    coronary artery, in chronic renal failure 418
calcium blockers
    COURAGE trial 131
    recommended use 15, 17
Canadian Amlodipine/Atenolol in Silent Ischemia Study
    (CASIS) 33
Canadian Cooperative Study 86
CAPRIE trial 87
CAPRI trial 521
captopril
    anti-ischemic activity 67
    post MI 63, 64, 65–66
    target dose 14
CAPTURE study 88, 491, 492, 493
cardiac arrest, exertion-related 521–522
cardiac catheterization
    in acute MI 300
    in cardiogenic shock 314, 315, 342
    stroke complicating 376, 377
    see also coronary angiography
cardiac free-wall rupture, post MI 332, 338
cardiac index, in cirrhosis 401
cardiac rehabilitation 511–539, 563
    animal experiments 514
    center-based model 538
    compliance 524
    definition 516
    early ambulation studies 515
    economic forces 534–535
    in elderly 528, 529, 530
    exercise prescription 516–517
    future directions in USA 535–539
    health risk appraisal model 539
    home-based model 538–539
    indications 512
    intervention studies 518–520
    meta-analysis of trials 520–521
    in LV dysfunction 524–527
    outcome prediction 533–534
    post CABG 529–532
    post PTCA 532
    randomized trials 516–524
    restructuring 535, 538–539
    return to work and 532–533
    in right ventricular dysfunction 527–529
    volunteer community model 539
    see also exercise, training
cardiac tamponade
    complicating PCI 352
    post MI 332
cardiogenic shock 311–321, 337–343, 562

in diabetes 330, 331, 428
diagnosis 315, 328, 337–338
early recognition and prevention 321
etiologies and mechanisms 337–338
late 320–321
lessons learnt 340–343
mechanical support devices 320
    see also intra-aortic balloon pump
PCI 292–293, 311–321, 327–332
    complete vs target vessel revascularization 318
    and glycoprotein IIb/IIIa receptor blockers 319–320
    IABP support 472–473
    in left main stenosis 320
    non-randomized studies 311–315
    observational studies 312–313
    randomized controlled trials 293, 315–318
    registry data 313–315
    stenting 319, 481
    VA perspective 338–343
    see also SHOCK trial; SMASH trial
thrombolysis 292–293
cardioplegia 503
    CABG re-operations 259, 261
    methods, AWESOME trial 504–505
    postoperative hypoventilation and 367
cardiopulmonary assist devices 320
cardiopulmonary bypass (CPB)
    CABG re-operations 261
    CABG without *see* off-pump coronary artery bypass
        surgery
    hepatic complications 405
    -induced coagulopathy 396
    in liver disease 396, 397, 402
    pathophysiologic effects 454
    percutaneously inserted *see* percutaneously inserted
        cardiopulmonary bypass
    pulmonary complications 368, 369
    renal dysfunction after 415–416, 459–460
CARE trial 47, 48–49, 52, 53
carotid stenosis
    CABG re-operations and 260
    post-CABG neurological impairment and 373, 376
CARP (Coronary Artery Revascularization in Peripheral
    disease) study 378
carvedilol
    in acute MI 27
    in heart failure 34–35
    target dose 14
CASS (Coronary Artery Surgery Study) 100–101, 108, 114,
    115, 203–204
CATS (captopril and thrombolysis study) 65–66
CCAIT study 49–50
CCS-1 study 61–62, 63
center-based model, cardiac rehabilitation 538–539
cerebral edema, post-CABG 456
cerebral emboli, during cardiopulmonary bypass 456
cerebrovascular accident (CVA) *see* stroke
cerebrovascular disease
    CABG risk 376
    see also carotid stenosis
cerebrovascular morbidity/mortality 562
    with CABG 373–376, 436, 454–459
    with PCI 376, 377
    see also neurologic impairment
cerivastatin 53
chest wall compliance, decreased 367–368

Child–Pugh classification 394–395, 397
cholestasis, benign postoperative 405
cholesterol 43, 44
   'hypothesis' 45
   reverse transport 45
   serum 45, 210
      cardiac rehabilitation and 533, 537
      in diabetes 429
cholesterol ester transfer protein, in diabetes 429
cholestyramine 53–54
   primary prevention 46
   secondary prevention 49, 50
chronic obstructive pulmonary disease (COPD)
   CABG risk 363–365
   PCI as alternative to CABG 369
chronic total occlusions (CTO) 347–356, 562
   benefits of recanalization 348
   contraindications for PCI 348–349
   future directions 355
   indications for PCI 347–348
   influence of stenting 353–355
   management of recurrence 353
   patient subsets 355–356
   results of recanalization 351–353, 354
   stenting 347–348, 353–355, 481
   techniques and predictors of PCI success 349–351
chylomicrons 43–44, 45
CIBIS trial 33
CIBIS II trial 33
cilazapril 69
circulatory support devices 320, 469–476
circumflex coronary artery branches, off-pump grafting 461
cirrhosis 388–389, 562
   intraoperative care/cautions 401–402
   postoperative management 399–400
   revascularization options 395–396, 397
   surgical risk 394–395
'classic diet-heart' hypothesis 45
CLASSICS study 299
CLAS trials 49, 50–51
Clinical Outcomes Utilizing Revascularization and
      Aggressive druG Evaluation trial *see* COURAGE
      trial
clofibrate 54
   primary prevention 46, 54
   secondary prevention 47–48
   target dose 14
clopidogrel 87, 90
   COURAGE trial 128, 131
   for PCI in acute MI 298, 299
   recommended use 15, 16, 560
   target dose 14
coagulation
   alterations in diabetes 430
   defects (coagulopathy)
      cardiopulmonary bypass-induced 396
      in liver disease 396, 398, 399
   postoperative assessment 391–392
cognitive dysfunction, post-CABG 455–456
colestipol 53–54
   primary prevention 46
   secondary prevention 49, 50–51
co-morbid disease 562
   cardiac rehabilitation and 536
   stenting 483
   see also specific diseases

compliance, cardiac rehabilitation 524
CONSENSUS 66, 67
CONSENSUS-II 61–62, 63
contrast agents
   adverse effects 301
   injections, in chronic total occlusion 349, 350
contrast-induced nephropathy 301, 398–399, 416
Cooperative CABG Database 377–378
CORAMI (Cohort of Rescue Angioplasty in Myocardial
      Infarction) study 294
coronary angiography
   in acute MI 300, 303
   in acute coronary syndromes 135–136
   CABG re-operations 260
   'index segments' 180
   post-MI 514
   stroke complicating 376, 377
   see also cardiac catheterization
coronary angioplasty *see* percutaneous transluminal
      coronary angioplasty
coronary artery bypass graft (CABG) surgery 5–7, 122
   ACE inhibitors after 69
   in acute MI 188–189, 190–191
   acute renal failure complicating 415–417
   in cardiogenic shock 314–315, 320, 342
      see also SHOCK trial; SMASH trial
   cerebrovascular morbidity/mortality 373–376, 436,
      454–459
   in chronic renal failure 418–419
   in chronic total occlusion (CTO) 347, 348
   in COPD 363–365
   in diabetes *see under* diabetes mellitus
   emergency/urgent
      recanalization of chronic total occlusions 352–353
      re-operations 262
      stenting to prevent 479–480
   exercise programs after 529–532
   high surgical risk 218
   in left main coronary artery disease 275–277, 278
   lipid-lowering therapy after 50–51
   in liver disease 395–399
   in medically refractory high-risk unstable angina
      217–218, 224–225
   medical therapy after 17
   minimally invasive 141, 376, 399
   minimally invasive direct (MIDCAB) 262, 454, 462, 563
   myocardial protection *see* myocardial protection
   in non-ST segment elevation acute coronary syndromes
      136–137, 141, 188–189
   off-pump *see* off-pump coronary artery bypass surgery
   patient selection 561–562
   in peripheral vascular disease 190–191, 193, 377–378
   preoperative evaluation 366, 389–392
   prior, thrombolysis vs PCI in acute MI 294
   pulmonary complications 363–369
   recent advances 104, 248
   recommendations 560–561
   re-operations 257–264
      evolution 259–260
      indications 258
      late outcomes 263
      multiple 263
      off-pump 261–262, 461–462
      pre-operative evaluation 260
      risk 262–263
      technical aspects 260–261

coronary artery bypass graft *continued*
    urgent/emergent/salvage 262
      vs PCI 258–259
  selection of patients for 181, 184
  surgical mortality 188–189, 192–193
  time on waiting list 245–248
  vs medical therapy 5, 6–7, 203–204
    quality of life benefits 108–109, 114, 115
    survival benefits 97–105
    in unstable angina 103–104, 136–137
  vs PCI (including stenting) *see* percutaneous coronary
    intervention (PCI), vs CABG
  vs PTCA *see* percutaneous transluminal coronary
    angioplasty (PTCA), vs CABG
  vs PTCA or medical therapy 104, 123, 203–214
Coronary Artery Bypass Graft Surgery Trialists
    Collaboration 101–102
coronary artery disease (CAD) 73
  in chronic renal failure 417–418
  diffuse ('bad vessels'), CABG re-operations 262
  index 6
  liver disease with 387–389
  pathophysiology in diabetes 429–432
  peripheral vascular disease co-morbidity 376–377
  progression
    ACE inhibitors and 67–68
    in diabetes 434
    EAST study 181–183, 184
    MASS-1 study 210, 211–212
  severity 6
    CABG vs medical therapy and 98
    costs of PTCA vs CABG and 553, 556
    exercise tolerance and 107–108
    see also high-risk patients; low-risk patients; moderate-
      risk patients
  stenosis measurement 108
  see also occlusion, coronary artery
Coronary Artery Surgery Study *see* CASS
Coronary Drug Project 47
coronary sinus retroperfusion 471
corticosteroid therapy, chronic 364
cost benefit analysis, cardiac rehabilitation 532–533
cost-effectiveness
  analysis guidelines 549
  CABG vs PTCA 553
  CABG vs stenting 237–238, 245, 246, 247, 248
  cardiac rehabilitation 537–538
costs
  analysis guidelines 549
  CABG vs PTCA 155–156, 157, 158, 167, 181, 549–556
  CABG vs stenting 196–198, 235, 237–238, 245, 246,
    554–556
  primary PCI in acute MI 301
  PTCA vs medical therapy 173
coumarin derivatives *see* oral anticoagulants
COURAGE trial 121–133, 232
  design overview 124
  eligibility criteria 124, 126, 127
  end-points 125
  hypothesis 124
  intensive medical therapy 127–129
  objectives 124
  PCI 129–132
  post-randomization management 132
  pre-randomization testing 124–125
  review of previous trials 122–124
  risk factor intervention 125, 128, 129, 130

CPB *see* cardiopulmonary bypass
C-reactive protein 85
creatine kinase (CK)
  MB iso-enzyme 240, 241, 245, 248
  mitochondrial (mi-CK) 527
creatinine, elevated serum 418, 460
CRUISE study 272
cryoprecipitate 399
CURE trial 87, 90

dalteparin
  in acute MI 79, 80, 81
  in unstable angina 75
databases 4, 5–7, 561–562
debulking procedures
  in acute MI 296–298
  in chronic total occlusions 351
  in left main stenosis 199–200, 270, 272, 273–274
  see also atherectomy
deconditioning, bed rest-induced 514–515
defibrillation, in exercise-induced cardiac arrest 521
defibrillator, implantable cardiac 436
desmopressin (DDAVP) 399
device therapy
  in acute MI 295–298
  see also atherectomy; stenting, coronary
diabetes mellitus 6–7, 425–439, 562
  BARI 2D trial 105, 159
  CABG risk 435–437
  CABG vs PTCA trials 437–438
    BARI *see* BARI, diabetes subgroup
    EAST 181, 182, 184
    RITA-1 165, 168
  cardiogenic shock 330, 331, 428
  chronic renal failure 417, 418, 420
  COURAGE trial 129
  epidemiology 426
  glycoprotein IIb/IIIa receptor blockers 428, 437–438, 492,
    493
  left main disease 277
  myocardial infarction 301, 426, 427–428, 437
  pathophysiology of coronary artery disease 429–432
  PCI 432–435
    in acute MI 301, 427–428, 432
    AWESOME trial 438–439, 440
    future directions 435
    mortality 435
    vs CABG 194–196, 245, 248
  type II 426
  unstable angina 428, 436, 439
Diabetes Mellitus Insulin Glucose Infusion in Acute
    Myocardial Infarction (DIGAMI) study 427
dialysis
  in acute renal failure 417, 460
  revascularization in patients on 417–420
diaphragmatic paralysis, postoperative 366–367
diet
  Mediterranean 51–52
  as risk factor 45
dietary intervention studies 51–52, 55
dietary modification 536
digoxin 17
dilated cardiomyopathy 33–34
dipyridamole 86
disability 511–512
dissection, coronary artery
  left main 278, 351

recanalized chronic total occlusions 349, 351, 353
   stenting 480–481
dopamine 415–416
drugs
   hepatotoxic 390
   nephrotoxic 415
   see also medical therapy; specific drugs and classes of drugs
Duke Databank for Cardiovascular Diseases 6
duteplase 284
dyslipidemia, in diabetes 429–430

EAST (Emory Angioplasty versus Surgery Trial) 3, 177–185
   8-year follow-up 168, 181, 182–183
   cost analyses 181, 550, 551, 555, 556
   methods 177–178
   progression of disease 181–183
   quality of life 181
   results 178–183
   screening procedures 178
   vs AWESOME 229, 230
echocardiography, after exercise training 525
economics
   CABG vs PTCA 181, 549–556
   cardiac rehabilitation 534–535, 537–538
   cardiovascular disability 512
   COURAGE trial 132, 133
   primary PCI in acute MI 301
   see also cost-effectiveness; costs
ejection fraction see left ventricular ejection fraction
elderly
   CABG re-operations 263
   cardiac rehabilitation 528, 529, 530
   cardiogenic shock 329, 330
   off-pump CABG 462–463
   perioperative stroke 456, 457
   post-CABG neurologic impairment 373
   primary PCI for acute MI 291–292
   stenting 481
electrolyte abnormalities, postoperative 399–400
embolization, systemic
   during CABG 373–374, 375, 376, 456
   during PCI 376, 377
   prevention 79–80, 492
   see also stroke
Emory Angioplasty versus Surgery Trial see EAST
emotional costs, emergency revascularization 342–343
employment status
   CABG vs PCI vs medical therapy 210
   CABG vs PTCA 155, 167
   cardiac rehabilitation and 532–533
   PTCA vs medical therapy 172–173
enalapril
   anti-ischemic activity 67–68
   in heart failure 66
   post MI 63, 64
   target dose 14
encephalopathy
   hepatic 400
   postoperative 373, 374, 455
endothelial dysfunction 68, 489–490
   in diabetes 430–431
   exercise training effects 526–527
endothelin(-1) 437, 490, 526
enflurane 402, 403
enoxaparin
   in acute MI 79
   in acute coronary syndromes 76, 80–81

enteral nutrition 401
EPIC study 300, 491, 492, 495
   bleeding complications 496
   data pooled with EPISTENT/EPILOG 88, 435, 493
EPILOG study 491, 492, 496
   data pooled with EPIC/EPISTENT 88, 435, 493
EPISTENT study 491, 492–493
   data pooled with EPIC/EPOLOG 88, 435, 493
   diabetic patients 184, 299, 438
eptifibatide 88, 90, 491, 497
   as PCI adjunct 493
   in unstable angina 88, 320, 494
ERACI I 189–190, 198
   cost analysis 550, 552–553, 555
   vs AWESOME 229, 230–231
ERACI II 4, 190–198, 200
   30-day and long-term outcome 192
   economic analysis 196–198, 550, 554, 555
   eligibility criteria 190
   late clinical follow-up 193–194
   patient characteristics 190–191
   revascularization techniques 191–192
   subset results 194–196
   surgical mortality 192–193
   vs AWESOME 229, 231
esmolol 30
esophageal varices 400
ESSENCE study 76
European Coronary Surgery Study 99–100, 108
European Esmolol Study Group Trial 30
EuroQol 238
evidence, hierarchy of 11
exercise
   capacity, training effects 522, 525, 528, 529
   -induced ischemia 514
   physiological aspects 517
   testing
      economic forces 535–536
      pre-discharge 514, 516
      see also stress testing
   tolerance 107
      benefits of revascularization 114, 115–118, 560
      CABG vs PTCA studies 114, 118, 155, 167
      PTCA vs medical therapy 114, 117, 172
      severity of disease and 107–108
   training
      beta-blockers and 524
      cardiac effects 522–524
      complications 521–522
      elderly 529
      outcome prediction 533–534
      randomized trials 516–524
      see also cardiac rehabilitation
   see also activity

FAMIS trial 65
FANTASTIC study 299
fat, saturated 51
FATS trial 49
felodipine, in angina 32
FEMINA trial 31, 32
femoral access site complications 474, 476
femoral-femoral bypass see percutaneously inserted
      cardiopulmonary bypass
fenofibrate 54
fentanyl 367–368, 404
fibrates 54, 55

fibrin 490
fibrinolysis, in diabetes 430
FLARE trial 50, 51
fluvastatin 49, 51, 53
foam cells 429, 431, 490
forced expiratory volume in 1 second (FEV1) 363, 364
fosinopril 65
Fragmin and Fast Revascularization during Instability in
    Coronary Artery Disease *see* FRISC
FRAXIS trial 75
free radicals 431, 490
FRESCO trial 295
fresh frozen plasma 399
FRIC trial 75–76
FRISC study 75
FRISC-II study 81, 139, 140–141, 189
fulminant hepatic failure 393, 397

GABI trial 229, 230–231
gastroepiploic artery, CABG re-operations 260, 263
'gatekeeper' concept 535, 536
gemfibrozil 54, 55
    primary prevention 46, 47
    secondary prevention 48
    target dose 14
gender, glycoprotein IIb/IIIa receptor blockers and 493
GISSI-1 trial 292, 293–294
GISSI-2 trial 79
GISSI-3 trial 61–63, 427
Global Use of Strategies to Open Occluded Coronary
    Arteries *see* GUSTO
glucose, blood
    elevated *see* hyperglycemia
    tight control 436–437
glucose–insulin–potassium infusions 332
glycoprotein Ia/Ib receptors, platelet 490
glycoprotein IIb/IIIa receptor blockers 87–89, 489–497, 563
    in acute MI 494–495
    in acute coronary syndromes (ACS) 88–89, 90, 494–495, 497
    in AWESOME trial 220, 228
    bleeding complications 496
    in cardiogenic shock 319–320
    overall picture 491
    as PCI adjunct 88, 89, 174, 484, 491–494
        in acute MI 299–300, 303, 494–495
        in CABG vs PCI studies 192, 229
        in diabetes 428, 437–438, 492, 493
    plus heparin 74–75
    recommended use 15, 16
    see also abciximab; eptifibatide; tirofiban
glycoprotein IIb/IIIa receptors, platelet 87, 489, 490, 496
Goteberg Metoprolol Trial 27
GRAMI trial 295
gravity, effects of 514–515
Gruppo Italiano per Studio della Streptochinasi nell'Infarto
    Miocardio *see* GISSI
guide wires, in chronic total occlusion 349–350, 351
GUSTO-I trial 79, 293–294
    cardiogenic shock 313–315, 320, 332
    diabetic subgroup 427
    elderly patients 291
GUSTO-IIA trial 79
GUSTO-IIB trial
    diabetic subgroup 427–428, 432
    hirudin vs heparin 76, 77, 79
    PTCA vs thrombolysis 287, 292, 301, 302
GUSTO-III trial 315, 495

GUSTO-IV trial 88–89

halothane 402, 403
HARP study 49, 50
health risk appraisal model, cardiac rehabilitation 539
heart failure
    ACE inhibitors 61, 66–67
    beta-blockers 33–35
    in diabetes 427
    exercise training 526–527, 529, 531
    IABP-supported PCI 473
    stenting 481
    thrombolysis vs primary PCI 293–294
    see also left ventricular dysfunction
heart rate
    after cardiac rehabilitation 522
    variability (HRV) 525–526
heart transplant, lipid-lowering therapy after 50–51
Helsinki Heart Study 46, 54
hemodynamics
    in cirrhosis 401–402
    inhaled anesthetics and 402–403
    mechanical support devices 469–476
Hemopump 320, 471
heparin
    low molecular weight (LMWH)
        in acute MI 79, 80–81
        in unstable angina 74, 75–76, 90
        in non-ST segment elevation acute coronary syndromes
            141
    for PCI in acute MI 300, 303
    recommended use 16, 78, 560
    unfractionated (UFH)
        in acute MI 78–79, 80
        in PCI for acute MI 299
        in unstable angina 74, 75, 90
    vs glycoprotein IIb/IIIa receptor blockers 492, 494
Heparin Aspirin Reperfusion Trial (HART-2) 79
heparin-induced thrombocytopenia (HIT) 75, 78
hepatic artery 389
hepatic encephalopathy 400
hepatic failure, fulminant 393, 397
hepatitis 562
    acute 393
    alcoholic 393
    chronic 393–394
    viral 387–388, 390, 393
hepatitis A 387
hepatitis B 387
hepatitis C 387–388, 390
hepatocytes 389
hepatopulmonary syndrome 404
hepatotoxic medications 390
herbal medications 390
HERO-2 trial 79
HEROICS study 320
hibernating myocardium 355–356
high-density lipoprotein (HDL) 44, 45
    cholesterol, serum 45
    in diabetes 429–430
high-risk patients 559–563
    CABG re-operations 259–260
    CABG vs medical therapy 98–99, 100, 102, 103–104
    CABG vs PCI 187–200, 217–232
    CABG vs PCI vs medical therapy 212–214
    CABG vs PTCA 145–159
    cardiogenic shock 321

invasive vs conservative therapy 137–138, 140, 142
off-pump CABG 453–464
primary PCI in acute MI 301, 303
stenting 479–485
supported PCI 471–476
hirudin 78
in acute MI 79
in unstable angina 74, 76–77
hirulog *see* bivalirudin
HIT-3 study 79
HIT-4 study 79
Holland Interuniversity Nifedipine/metoprolol Trial (HINT) 30
home-based model, cardiac rehabilitation 538–539
homocysteine 183
HOPE study 67, 68
hydrophilic wires, in chronic total occlusion 349, 350, 351, 352
3-hydroxy-3-methylglutaryl CoA (HMG-CoA) reductase 43, 53
inhibitors *see* statins
hypercarbia, in liver disease 404–405
hypercoagulable state, in diabetes 430
hyperglycemia
in atherosclerosis pathogenesis 429, 431
myocardial infarction and 427
hyperinsulinemia 430, 432
hypertension 533
ACE inhibitors 67–68
beta-blockers 36
hypokalemia 400
hyponatremia 399–400
hypoperfusion
clinical signs 331, 337–338
neurologic impairment risk 375–376
hypotension
in cardiogenic shock 337–338
percutaneously inserted cardiopulmonary bypass 470–471
hypothermia (cooling) 471, 503
phrenic nerve injury 366–367
hypoventilation
chronic 364
perioperative 363, 366–368
hypoxemia/hypoxia
in liver disease 404
perioperative 368–369

IABP *see* intra-aortic balloon pump
ileal bypass 49, 50
immobilization *see* bed rest
IMPACT II study 491, 493
implantable cardiac defibrillator 436
inagotran, in unstable angina 77
inhaled anesthetics, hemodynamic effects 402–403
insulating pad, phrenic nerve protection 366–367
insulin
intensive therapy 427
precursors 430
Integrilin *see* eptifibatide
intellectual impairment
post-CABG 373, 374, 375
risk factors 375
interleukin-8 437
intermediate-density lipoprotein (IDL) 44, 45
intermediate-risk patients *see* moderate-risk patients
intermittent positive pressure ventilation 368
internal mammary artery (IMA, internal thoracic artery,

ITA) grafts 104
CABG re-operations 260, 261, 262
CABG vs medical therapy 98, 99, 100, 101
CABG vs PCI trials 191–192, 236
CABG vs PTCA 149, 152, 153
in diabetes 437
intraoperative phrenic nerve injury 367
MIDCAB 462
myocardial protection and 505
internal mammary ligation procedure 108
internal thoracic artery *see* internal mammary artery
International Study Group (ISG) trials 292–294
intimal hyperplasia (fibroplasia) 258, 434, 484
intra-aortic balloon pump (IABP) 341, 469, 563
in AWESOME trial 220–223, 339, 340
complications 472
contraindications 472
indications 470, 471
role 320
in SHOCK trial 316, 327, 328
supporting PCI 471–473
vs percutaneously inserted CPB 475–476
intracranial bleeding 287
intravenous drug users 390
intrinsic sympathomimetic activity (ISA) 25
ISAR (Intracoronary Stenting Antithrombotic Regimen) study 299
ISAR-II study 495
ISIS-1 trial 26, 27
ISIS-2 trial 86
ISIS-3 trial 79
ISIS-4 trial 61–62, 63, 64
isoflurane 402, 403
isometric exercise 517
IVUS *see* ultrasound, intravascular

jaundice, postoperative 405, 406
Joint commission on accreditation of health care organizations (JCAHO) 534, 535

labetolol 25
lactulose 400
laser
angioplasty, in acute MI 298
wire recanalization, chronic total occlusion 350–351
LCAS trial 49
LDL *see* low-density lipoprotein
left anterior descending (LAD) coronary artery
proximal stenosis 203
CABG vs medical therapy 99, 100, 101
CABG vs stenting 194–196
off-pump CABG 453
PCI vs CABG vs medical therapy 123, 204–212
repeat grafting 262, 462
stenting 484
vein graft stenosis 258
left atrial thrombus 373, 375
left main coronary artery (LMCA)
acute occlusion, primary stenting 279
anatomy 265–266
dissection 278, 351
left main coronary artery (LMCA) stenosis 265–279
bifurcation area 270, 271–272
CABG vs medical therapy 98, 100, 101
cardiogenic shock, CABG or PCI 320
classification 266
etiology 266

left main coronary artery *continued*
  protected 266, 277–279
    emergency interventions 278–279
    stenting 277, 278
  supported PCI 473
  unprotected 266–277, 562
    PTCA 266
    stenting 198–200, 265, 266–277
left ventricular aneurysm 80
left ventricular assist devices 320, 563
left ventricular dysfunction
  ACE inhibitors 61, 66–67
  CABG vs medical therapy 97–98, 100–102, 103–104
  in cardiogenic shock 331, 332, 338
  medical therapy 17
  off-pump CABG 461
  stenting 482
  supported PCI 473, 475–476
  see also heart failure
left ventricular ejection fraction (LVEF)
  CABG vs PCI vs medical therapy 210
  exercise training and 525
  low
    ACE inhibitors 63–64, 67–68, 560
    CABG benefits 5, 100–101, 103
    stenting 481
    supported PCI 474, 475–476
  stenting in left main stenosis and 267, 268, 269, 270
left ventricular function, supported PCI and 474–475
left ventricular thrombus 373, 375
Leiden Intervention Trial 51
lifestyle behaviors, changing 537
lipid-lowering therapy 43–55
  in cardiac rehabilitation 533, 537
  COURAGE trial 129, 131
  in diabetes post-CABG 437
  for primary and secondary prevention 45–54
  recommendations 16, 560
  target doses 14, 15
Lipid Research Clinics Coronary Primary Prevention Trial
  46, 54
lipids 43–45
  cardiac rehabilitation and 528, 529
LIPID study 47, 49, 52, 53
lipoprotein(a) 44
lipoprotein lipase (LPL) 44, 45
  in diabetes 428
lipoproteins 43–45
lisinopril
  in diabetes 427
  post MI 63
  target dose 14
liver
  architecture 389
  function 389
liver chemistries
  asymptomatic patients with abnormal 392–393, 396
  postoperative changes 405
  postoperative 392
liver disease 387–406, 562
  acute 388
    surgical approach 397
    surgical risk 393
  chronic 388
    surgical approach 397–398
    surgical risk 393–395
  epidemiology 387–389

  estimating surgical risk 392–395
  etiology 388
  intraoperative care/cautions 401–405
  postoperative care/complications 405, 406
  postoperative evaluation 389–392
  postoperative management 399–401
  revascularization options 395–399
liver transplantation 388–389, 393, 396, 401
Lopressor Intervention Trial (LIT) 28, 29
lovastatin 53
  primary prevention 46, 47
  secondary prevention 49–50, 51
  target dose 14
low-density lipoprotein (LDL) 44
  cholesterol 44, 52, 53
    in arterial thrombosis 490
    in diabetes 429
  in diabetes 429–430
  oxidation 429–430
  phenotypes 183
  receptor 44
  small dense 429–430
low-risk patients
  CABG vs medical therapy 98, 99, 102, 103
  invasive vs conservative therapy 138, 140, 142
  primary PCI in acute MI 300–301, 303
  PTCA vs medical therapy 169–173
Lyon Diet Heart Study 51–52

MAAS trial 49
macrophages 490
magnetic resonance imaging (MRI), after exercise training
  525
Magnum wire 349, 351
malnutrition, in liver disease 400–401
MARCATOR study 69
MARS trial 49, 50
MASS (Medicine, Angioplasty or Surgery Study)
  203–214
  first (MASS-1) 104, 123, 204–212
    anginal symptom relief 209
    atherosclerosis progression 210, 211–212
    employment status 210
    event-free survival 206–209
    statistical analysis 206
    ventricular function 210
  second (MASS-2) 212–214
MATTIS study 299
Mayo Clinic study of PTCA vs thrombolysis (Gibbons et al)
  284, 292, 301
mechanical ventilation, postoperative 363, 369
median sternotomy, repeat 261
mediastinal infection, postoperative 365, 366
medically refractory 11–17, 559–560
  after revascularization 17
  definition 218–219, 231–232
  importance of concept 11–12
  prior to revascularization 12–17
medical therapy
  in CABG vs PCI studies 229
  in chronic renal failure 418
  in COURAGE trial 127–129, 232
  in non-ST segment elevation acute coronary syndromes
    136–137
  for PCI support *see* percutaneous coronary intervention
    (PCI), pharmacological support
  recent advances 104, 122, 174

recommendations 15, 16–17, 559–561
vs CABG *see* coronary artery bypass graft (CABG)
  surgery, vs medical therapy
vs CABG or PTCA 104, 123, 203–214
vs PCI 121–133
vs PTCA 109–112, 114, 116, 117, 169–173
vs revascularization in cardiogenic shock 315–318,
  327–332
see also specific drugs and drug classes
Medicine, Angioplasty or Surgery Study *see* MASS
Mediterranean diet 51–52
MELD (Model for End-Stage Liver Disease) 395
meperidine 404
MERCATOR study 69
MERIT-HF trial 34
metformin 301
metoprolol 25
  in MI 26–27, 28, 29
  in angina 30–31, 32
  in heart failure 33–34
  recommended use 16
  target doses 14
Metoprolol in Dilated Cardiomyopathy (MDC) trial
  33–34
MI *see* myocardial infarction
MIAMI trial 26–27
Mid American Heart Institute (Kansas City) study 284
minimally invasive coronary artery bypass graft (CABG)
  surgery 141, 376, 399
minimally invasive direct coronary artery bypass grafting
  (MIDCAB) 262, 454, 462, 563
MIRACL study 47, 49
mitral regurgitation, in cardiogenic shock 331
MOCHA trial 35
moderate-risk patients
  CABG vs medical therapy 98, 99, 102, 103
  CABG vs PTCA 163–169, 177–185
  invasive vs conservative therapy 138, 140
  primary PCI in acute MI 303
monocytes 431, 490
morphine 404
mortality rate 4
Multicenter Investigation of Limitation of Infarct Size
  (MILIS) study 292
multi-vessel disease
  CABG re-operations 461–462
  CABG vs PCI/stenting 187–200, 235–250
  CABG vs PTCA 3, 145–159, 163–169, 177–185, 225–228
  and chronic total occlusion 348
  in diabetes 425, 435, 437–438
  stenting 3–4, 484
  supported PCI 475
  see also three-vessel disease; two-vessel disease
Munich Mild Heart Failure (MHFT) trial 66
myocardial infarction (MI)
  acute *see* acute myocardial infarction
  complicated 513
  in diabetes mellitus 301, 426, 427–428, 437
  long-term medical therapy after
    ACE inhibitors 63–66
    anticoagulants 78
    beta-blockers 28–29, 35
  non-Q-wave *see* non-Q wave acute myocardial infarction
  non-ST segment *see* non-ST segment elevation myocardial
    infarction
  prior 560–561
  PTCA procedure-related 171, 173

Q wave 73, 512–513
  rehabilitation after *see* cardiac rehabilitation
  risk prediction after 137–138, 514
  severity 512–514
myocardial ischemia
  definition 218
  exercise-induced 514
  medical therapy 16–17
  recurrent, thrombolysis vs PCI 287, 290
  silent
    beta-blockers 32–33
    in diabetes 427
  symptoms *see* symptoms, myocardial ischemia
  see also angina
myocardial perfusion imaging, in acute coronary
  syndromes 136
myocardial protection 503–506, 563
  AWESOME study 504–505
  CABG re-operations 259
  non-cardioplegic 503–504
  off-pump CABG 504
  see also cardioplegia
myocardium
  hibernating 355–356
  oxygen consumption 517
  viability studies, CABG re-operations 260

Na⁺–H⁺ exchanger inhibition 332
nadolol 25
nadroparin, in acute coronary syndromes 75, 76
naloxone 368
narcotics, in liver disease 404
National Cooperative Study 136–137
National Exercise and Heart Disease Project (NEHPD)
  518
National Health and Nutrition Examination Survey
  (NHANES I) 426
National Heart, Lung and Blood Institute (NHLBI)
  CABG study (1972–1976) 103
  Dynamic Wave Registry 480, 482
  Registry of angioplasty 177, 181, 184, 433, 480
National Registry of Myocardial Infarction (NRMI 2) 35
neomycin 400
nephrotoxic drugs 415
neurocognitive dysfunction, post-CABG 455–456
neurohumoral system dysregulation, in cirrhosis 401–402
neurologic impairment 562
  post-CABG 368, 373–376
    approaches to prevention 376
    in diabetes 436
    off-pump surgery 454–459
    pathophysiologic mechanisms 375–376
    problems in identifying 374–375
    risk factors 373, 375
    in specific patient groups 374
  post-PCI 376, 377
  see also stroke
neuromuscular blocking agents, in liver disease 404
neuropsychologic complications 373
New York State Database 6–7
NHLBI *see* National Heart, Lung and Blood Institute
niacin 54, 55
  COURAGE trial 129
  secondary prevention 47, 49, 50, 51
  target dose 14
nicotinic acid 54
nifedipine, in angina 30–31, 32

nitrates
target doses 14, 15
urinary elimination 526
nitric oxide (NO) 431, 490
exercise training and 526, 527
nitric oxide synthase, inducible (iNOS) 527
nitroglycerin 14, 368–369
nitroprusside 368–369
nitrous oxide 402, 403
non-Q wave acute myocardial infarction (AMI) 73–74,
513–514
early intervention vs conservative therapy 137–140,
188–189
glycoprotein IIb/IIIa receptor blockers 494
risk prediction 137–138, 514
non-ST segment elevation acute coronary syndromes 85,
135–142
cardiogenic shock 320
early intervention vs conservative therapy 137–140,
188–189
differences between trials 140–141
tailoring to risk profile 141–142
medical therapy 16
antiplatelet agents 87, 88, 90
vs CABG 136–137
non-invasive and invasive testing 135–136
see also non-Q wave acute myocardial infarction; non-ST-
segment elevation myocardial infarction; unstable
angina
non-ST-segment elevation myocardial infarction (NSTEMI)
85
acute management 342
cardiogenic shock 331, 338
medical therapy 16, 87, 88, 90
Norwegian Timolol Trial 28, 29
nutritional status, in liver disease 400–401
nutritional support, postoperative 401

OASIS-1 pilot study 76–77
OASIS-2 study 77
OASIS-4 trial 87
OASIS registry 428
obesity
cardiac rehabilitation 528
postoperative hypoventilation 363
occlusion, coronary artery
acute thrombotic 73, 74
glycoprotein IIb/IIIa receptor blockers and 491–492
stents to prevent/treat 480–482
chronic total (CTO) see chronic total occlusions
in diabetes 434
see also re-occlusion
off-pump coronary artery bypass surgery (OP-CAB)
453–464
acute MI/LV dysfunction 461
completeness of revascularization 461, 463–464
in elderly 462–463
limitations 463–464
myocardial protection 504
neurological injury and 376, 454–459
origins 453–454
renal impairment and 416, 459–460
for re-operations 261–262, 461–462
OPUS/TIMI 16 study 89
oral anticoagulants (coumarin derivatives), in unstable
angina 74, 75, 77
Organization to Assess Strategies for Ischemic Syndromes

see OASIS
osteal lesions, stenting 481
over-the-wire systems, in chronic total occlusion 349, 351
oxidant stress, in diabetes 431
oxygen consumption
myocardial 517
ventilatory (VO$_2$) 517
oxygen therapy, home 364, 369
oxygen uptake, maximal (VO$_{2max}$) 517, 522, 525, 534

PAMI 1 trial 283–284, 287, 291–292, 301
PAMI 2 trial 287, 292, 294, 301, 302
PAMI No Surgery on Site (No SOS) trial 292, 294, 302
PAMI Stent Pilot trial 295
Panel on Cost-Effectiveness in Health and Medicine 549
papillary muscle rupture 338
PARAGON B study 89
PASTA trial 295
PCI see percutaneous coronary intervention
percutaneous coronary intervention (PCI) 3–4
in acute MI see under acute myocardial infarction
in cardiogenic shock see cardiogenic shock, PCI
cerebrovascular morbidity/mortality 376, 377
in chronic renal failure 419–420
in chronic total occlusions 347–356
COURAGE trial 129–132
in diabetes see under diabetes mellitus
in left main stenosis 265–279
in liver disease 395–399
in medically refractory high-risk unstable angina
217–218, 224–225
new developments 248
in non-ST segment elevation acute coronary syndromes
136, 141
patient selection 561–562
pharmacological support 17, 489–497
ACE inhibitors 69
in acute MI 80–81, 298–300
antiplatelet therapy 87, 88, 90
glycoprotein IIb/IIIa receptor blockers 88, 489–497
lipid-lowering therapy 50–51
in pulmonary disease 369
recommendations 560–561
risk determinants 469–470
supported 471–476
comparison trials 475–476
with IABP 471–473
with percutaneously inserted CPB (PCPS) 473–475
in vein graft stenosis 258–259
vs CABG 4, 5–7, 187–200, 235–250
see also ARTS; AWESOME trial
vs medical therapy 121–133
see also atherectomy; percutaneous transluminal coronary
angioplasty; stenting, coronary
percutaneously inserted cardiopulmonary bypass (PCPS)
469, 470–471, 563
complications 474
contraindications 474
indications 471, 473
PCI support 473–475
vs IABP 475–476
percutaneous transluminal coronary angioplasty (PTCA) 3
in acute MI 80, 81, 283–295
prevention of cardiogenic shock 311
see also acute myocardial infarction (AMI), primary PCI
cardiac rehabilitation after 532–533
in cardiogenic shock see cardiogenic shock, PCI

in chronic renal failure 419–420
in diabetes *see under* diabetes mellitus
in left main disease 266, 277
plus stenting *see* percutaneous coronary intervention
procedure-related MI 171, 173
recent advances 184, 210–211
risk determinants 469–470
'salvage' 218
supported *see* percutaneous coronary intervention (PCI),
    supported
vein graft stenoses 258
vs CABG 3, 104–105, 113–114, 163–169
    cost comparisons *see* costs, CABG vs PTCA
    see also BARI; EAST
vs CABG or medical therapy 104, 123, 203–214
vs medical therapy 109–112, 114, 116, 117, 169–173
PERFEXT study 522–524, 532
perforation, coronary artery
atherectomy-associated 270
in chronic total occlusion 349, 351, 352
peripheral vascular disease (PVD) 376–378, 562
    CABG re-operations and 260
    CABG risk 190–191, 193, 377–378
peritoneal dialysis 417
peritonitis, spontaneous bacterial 400
phrenic nerve injury 363, 366–367
physical activity *see* activity
physicians
awareness of cardiac rehabilitation 536, 538
changing patients' behavior 537
placebo effect 108
PLAC study 49, 50
plaque, atherosclerotic 73, 74, 490
rupture/erosion 481, 489, 490–491
plasma, fresh frozen 399
plasmapheresis, exchange 399
plasminogen activator inhibitor type 1 (PAI-1), in diabetes
    430
platelets
activation 490, 496
aggregation 87, 489, 490, 496
altered function in diabetes 430
glycoprotein Ia/Ib receptors 490
glycoprotein IIb/IIIa receptors 87, 489, 490
in thrombosis pathogenesis 489–490, 496
transfusions 399
pleural effusion 368
pneumonia, nosocomial 365, 366
portal vein 389
POSCH study 49, 50
positron emission tomography 260
Possis AngioJet device 297–298
postoperative care, in liver disease 405
postoperative complications
acute renal failure 415–417
in diabetes 436
in liver disease 405, 406
pulmonary *see* pulmonary complications, postoperative
pravastatin 53
primary prevention 46–47
secondary prevention 47, 48–49, 50, 51
target dose 14
PRECISE trial 34–35
PREDICT study 50, 51
postoperative evaluation
in liver disease 389–392
in pulmonary disease 366

Primary Angioplasty in Myocardial Infarction *see* PAMI
primary care physicians 536
primary prevention, lipid-lowering agents 45–54
PRISM-PLUS study 88, 89, 428, 494
PRISM study 88, 494
probucol 51
proinsulin 430
propranolol 25
in MI 27, 28, 29
in angina 30
target dose 14
prostacyclin (PGI$_2$) 431
proteins
dietary restriction 400, 401
glycation 431
proteinuria 435
prothrombin time, postoperative correction 399
prothrombotic state, in diabetes 429, 430
psychological rehabilitation 511
psychosocial impact 512
PTCA *see* percutaneous transluminal coronary angioplasty
pulmonary complications, postoperative 363–369
mechanisms 363, 366–368
pneumonia or mediastinal infection 365, 366
postoperative evaluation 366
strategies to decrease 369
pulmonary congestion, in cardiogenic shock 331
pulmonary disease, chronic 363–369, 562
CABG risk 363–365
PCI as alternative to CABG 369
pulmonary edema, perioperative 368
pulmonary embolism 80, 368, 369
pulmonary function
in liver disease 404–405
postoperative testing 366
pulmonary hypertension 369
PURSUIT study 88, 320, 494

quality of life (QOL)
benefits of revascularization 107–118
CABG vs PTCA 155–156, 158, 167, 181
CABG vs stenting 241, 244
cardiac rehabilitation benefits 529, 530
COURAGE trial 133
PTCA vs medical therapy 172
quinapril(at) 67, 68

radial artery, CABG re-operations 260, 263
radiation therapy
in left main disease 275
recanalized chronic total occlusion 355
radiocontrast agents *see* contrast agents
ramipril
after PCI or CABG 69
HOPE study 67, 68
post MI 64, 65
target dose 14
randomized clinical trials (RCT) 11
Randomized IABP Study Group 472
Randomized Interventional Treatment of Angina *see* RITA
RAPPORT study 300, 491, 493, 495
reactive oxygen species (ROS) 431
REGRESS trials 49, 50
rehabilitation *see* cardiac rehabilitation
renal disease, end-stage (ESRD) 417–420
renal failure 562
acute (ARF) 415–417, 460

renal failure *continued*
  chronic (CRF) 415, 417–420, 460
  contrast-induced 301, 398–399, 416
renal function 415–420
  after cardiopulmonary bypass 415–416, 459–460
  liver disease and 399–400
renal replacement therapy
  in acute renal failure 417
  see also dialysis
renal transplant recipients 419
re-occlusion
  recanalized chronic total occlusions 353, 354, 355
  thrombolysis vs primary PCI 291
  see also restenosis
Reopro *see* abciximab
repeat revascularization 561
  CABG vs PTCA 3, 153–154, 158, 180, 181, 183, 189–190
  CABG vs stenting 193–194, 241
  chronic total occlusion 353
  in diabetes 433
  stenting in left main disease 275
  see also coronary artery bypass graft (CABG) surgery, re-
    operations
RESCUE trial 294
restenosis 3–4, 204
  ACE inhibitors and 69
  in diabetes 433–434
  EAST study 182–183
  left main coronary artery stents 270, 272, 274, 275, 276
  lipid-lowering therapy and 50, 51
  recanalized chronic total occlusions 353, 354, 355
  stenting and 484
  vein graft 259
  see also re-occlusion
RESTORE study 491, 493
reteplase 79
revascularization
  ACE inhibitors after 69
  in cardiogenic shock 311–321, 327–332
  in chronic renal failure 417–420
  completeness, in off-pump CABG 461, 463–464
  cost comparisons 549–556
  emotional costs 342–343
  lipid-lowering therapy after 50–51
  in liver disease 395–399
  in medically refractory high-risk unstable angina
    217–218, 224–225
  in non-ST segment elevation acute coronary syndromes
    137–141
  quality of life effects 107–118
  recommendations 560–561
  repeat *see* repeat revascularization
  selection of procedure 561–562
  symptom relief 108–114
  see also coronary artery bypass graft (CABG) surgery;
    percutaneous coronary intervention; percutaneous
    transluminal coronary angioplasty; stenting, coronary
right ventricular dysfunction
  CABG risk 369
  cardiac rehabilitation 527–529
RISC study 75, 86
risk factors 105
  goals, COURAGE trial 128
  modification 533, 563
risk scores
  CABG vs medical therapy and 98–99, 102
  see also TIMI risk score

RITA 163–176
  first study (RITA-1) 163–169
    cost analysis 167, 550, 551–552, 555, 556
    exercise tolerance 114, 118, 155, 167
    protocol 163–164
    results 164–167
  second study (RITA-2) 123, 163, 169–173
    angina relief 111–112, 172
    exercise tolerance 114, 117, 172
    protocol 169–170
    results 170–173
  vs AWESOME 229, 230–231

S-100 neuropeptide 456
saphenous vein grafts (SVGs) 104
  CABG re-operations 260, 263
  CABG vs medical therapy 97–98, 99, 100, 101
  CABG vs PCI trials 152, 153, 236
  stenting 481
  thrombotic occlusion 294
  see also vein grafts
SAVE (Survival and Ventricular Enlargement) trial 63–64,
    65, 66, 67
Scandinavian Simvastatin Survival Study (4S) 47, 48, 52, 53,
    204
SCAT study 49, 50
secondary prevention 533, 563
  lipid-lowering therapy 45–54
  see also cardiac rehabilitation
sedatives, in liver disease 403–404
self-esteem, loss of 532
SEQOL *see* Study of Economics and Quality of Life
SHOCK registry 327
  lessons learnt 331–332
  results 331
SHOCK trial 327–332, 337, 338
  design 315, 327–328
  interventions 315, 316, 329
  lessons learnt 331–332
  results 293, 317, 328–331
    diabetic subgroup 330, 331, 428
    subgroup analyses 329–330
    success of angioplasty 330–331
  vs SMASH 314, 315–318
simvastatin 53
  COURAGE trial 129
  secondary prevention 47, 48, 49, 50, 67–68
  target dose 14
Simvastatin/Enalapril Coronary Atherosclerosis Trial
    (SCAT) 67–68
single-vessel disease
  CABG re-operation 262, 461, 462
  PTCA 3, 110–111
  PTCA vs CABG 163–169, 211, 229
SMASH trial 315–318, 337, 338
  baseline characteristics 314
  design 315
  inclusion and exclusion criteria 314
  interventions 315, 316
  results 318
  vs SHOCK 314, 315–318
SMILE (Survival of Myocardial Infarction Long-term
    Evaluation) study 61–62, 63, 64
smoking cessation 15, 51, 533
Society for Cardiac Angiography Intracoronary
    Streptokinase Registry 292
Society for Thoracic Surgery (STS) cardiac surgery

database 4, 377
COPD definition 364
postoperative renal impairment 416, 460
reoperative CABG 262, 461
SOLVD (Survival of Left Ventricular Dysfunction) studies
66, 67
d-sotalol 28, 29
STARS trial 49, 50
statins 15, 43–55, 537
mechanism of action 43, 53
primary and secondary prevention 45–54
target doses 14
stenting, coronary 3–4, 479–485, 563
in acute MI 295–296, 297, 303, 481
in acute occlusions 480–482
adjunctive therapy 484, 492–493
ACE inhibitors 69
antiplatelet agents 87, 89
Argentine (ERACI) studies 189–200
ARTS study 168, 235–250
AWESOME trial 217–232, 482–483
in CABG vs PCI studies 229
in cardiogenic shock 319, 481
in chronic renal failure 419, 420
in chronic total occlusions 347–348, 353–355, 481
in co-morbid conditions 483
in coronary dissection 480–481
costs analyses 554–556
current role 184, 210–211, 479–480
in diabetes 433–434, 435, 437–438
in acute MI 427–428
ARTS study 245, 248
ERACI II 196
in high-risk clinical settings 480
in LV dysfunction 482
in non-ST segment elevation acute coronary syndromes
140–141
practical aspects 483–484
in protected left main stenosis 277–279
in emergency situations 278–279
outcomes 277, 278
radiation therapy after 355
restenosis 484
RITA-1 study 165
in unprotected left main stenosis 198–200, 265, 266–277
angiographic restenosis after 274
Asan medical center experience 268–270
current recommendation 277
debulking before 273–274
device selection and techniques 270–272
IVUS guidance 272, 273
long-term outcomes 274–275
ULTIMA experience 198, 266–267
vs CABG 275–277
vein graft stenoses 258–259
Stent PAMI trial 292, 294, 295–296
stents, coronary 174
drug eluting 355
left main disease 270–272
selection 483
stent thrombosis 248, 319
in diabetes 432–433
in left main stenosis 270
prevention 492, 495
sternotomy, repeat median 261
STICH (Surgical Treatment for IsChemic Heart Failure)
Trial 7

Stockholm Ischaemic Heart Disease Study 47–48
streptokinase 79, 284–287
stress testing
after cardiac rehabilitation 522
for CABG re-operations 260
in vein graft stenosis 258
see also exercise, testing
STRESS trial 433, 481
stroke (cerebrovascular accident, CVA)
complicating CABG 373, 455, 456–459
alternative surgical techniques 457–458
identification problems 375
incidence 374, 456
off-pump surgery and 458–459
re-operations 260
risk factors 375, 456–457
complicating PCI 376, 377
hemorrhagic 287, 288
post-MI
prevention 79–80
thrombolysis vs PCI 287, 288
risk in diabetes 436
ST-segment elevation myocardial infarction 6–7, 85
acute management 342
cardiogenic shock 338
medical therapy 16, 79
PCI with abciximab 493
Study of Economics and Quality of Life (SEQOL) 146,
155–156, 157, 158
sudden cardiac death 64, 85, 522
sulfinpyrazone 86
Swiss Multicenter Angioplasty for SHock trial *see* SMASH
trial
SWORD study 28, 29
symptoms, myocardial ischemia 107
benefits of revascularization 108–114, 116–117, 561
placebo effect 108
see also angina

TACTICS TIMI-18 study 89, 140, 320
TAMI (Thrombolysis and Angioplasty in Myocardial
Infarction) trial 427
TARGET study 89, 90, 493–494
tattoos 390
TECBEST study 297
tenecteplase 79
thienpyridine therapy 87
see also clopidogrel; ticlopidine
three-vessel disease
CABG vs medical therapy 98, 99, 100, 101, 103–104
CABG vs PCI vs medical therapy 212–214
CABG vs PTCA or PCI 194–196, 197, 229
PTCA vs medical therapy 111–112
thrombectomy, rheolytic 297–298
thrombin 430, 490
thrombin inhibitors, direct
for PCI in acute MI 299
in unstable angina 76–77
thrombocytopenia, heparin-induced (HIT) 75, 78
thrombolysis 283
anticoagulation and 79
in diabetes 427
enhanced (with IABP) 320
failed, 'rescue' PCI 291, 294–295
prevention of cardiogenic shock 311
in SHOCK trial 327
vs primary PCI 283–291, 562

Thrombolysis in Myocardial Infarction *see* TIMI
thrombosis
  pathophysiology 489–491, 496
  stent *see* stent thrombosis
  tendency, in diabetes 429, 430
thrombotic thrombocytopenic purpura (TTP) 299
thrombus
  aspiration, in acute MI 297–298
  formation 73, 74, 489
    inhibition of further 77, 79–80, 489, 491
  intracardiac, embolization 375
  lysis, in acute MI 298
  occlusive, stenting 481
TIBET (Total Ischemic Burden European Trial) 31, 32
ticlopidine 87, 299
TIMI-IIB study 27–28, 140
TIMI-IIIB trial 137–138, 140–141
TIMI 4 study 294
TIMI-9A study 79
TIMI-9B trial 79
TIMI 18 study 89, 140, 320
TIMI risk score 89, 140
timolol, in MI 27, 28, 29
tirofiban (Aggrastat) 88, 90, 491, 497
  in acute coronary syndromes 88, 89, 140, 494
  in diabetes 428
  as PCI adjunct 88, 493
  vs abciximab 89, 494
tissue factor 490
tissue plasminogen activator (tPA) 79, 284, 287
TOPIT study 297
TOTAL trial 350–351
TRACE trial 64, 65
trandolapril
  post MI 64, 65
  target dose 14
TREND (Trial on Reversing Endothelial Dysfunction) study
    68
triglycerides 43–44
  in diabetes 429, 437
troponin 85, 89, 139
two-vessel disease
  CABG vs medical therapy 98, 99
  CABG vs PTCA or PCI 229
  PTCA vs medical therapy 111–112

ULTIMA registry 198, 266–267, 279
ultrasound
  intravascular (IVUS)
    in diabetes 431–432
    stenting in left main disease 272, 273
  therapeutic, in acute MI 298
United States Renal Data System database 418, 419–420
unstable angina (UA) 73, 85, 90
  anticoagulants 74–77, 78
  antiplatelet agents 74, 86, 88
  appropriate revascularization options 217–218,
    224–225
  aspirin 74, 86
  beta-blockers 29–31
  CABG vs medical therapy 103–104, 136–137
  CABG vs PCI 189–198, 200
  COURAGE trial 128, 130
  in diabetes 428, 436, 439

early intervention vs conservative therapy 137–140,
    188–189
  glycoprotein IIb/IIIa receptor blockers 494, 497
  medical therapy 16
  non-invasive and invasive testing 135–136
  see also non-ST-segment elevation myocardial infarction

VA-HIT study 47, 48, 53, 54
ValPREST study 69
valsartan 69
VANQWISH trial 105, 138–139, 514
  vs other trials 140–141, 188–189
vascular remodeling, in diabetes 431–432
vasodilation, in diabetes 431
Vein Graft AngioJet Study, second (VeGAS 2) 297–298
vein grafts
  atherosclerosis 258–259
  CABG re-operations 262–263
  myocardial protection and 505
  stenosis 257–258
    early 258
    late 257–258
    PCI 258–259
  see also saphenous vein grafts
venous thromboembolism 515
  prevention 78, 80
ventilation/perfusion mismatching 368
ventilatory oxygen consumption (VO$_2$) 517
ventricular septal rupture, post MI 331–332
very low-density lipoproteins (VLDL) 43–44, 45
  in diabetes 429
Veterans Administration Angioplasty Compared to
    Medicine Study *see* ACME study
Veterans Administration CABG study 364
Veterans Administration Cooperative Study
  CABG in stable angina 97–99, 102–103, 108, 109, 114
  unstable angina 86, 103, 136–137
Veterans Affairs High-density lipoprotein Intervention
    Trial *see* VA-HIT study
Veterans Affairs hospitals, cardiogenic shock cases 338–339
Veterans Affairs Non-Q Wave Infarction Strategies in
    Hospital *see* VANQWISH trial
VHeFT (Vasodilator Heart Failure Trial) II 64, 66, 67
vitamin K 399
volunteer community model, cardiac rehabilitation 539
Von Willebrand factor 490
warfarin
  post-MI 78
  in unstable angina 75, 77
weight control 536
weight training 517
West of Scotland Primary Prevention Study (WOSCOPS)
    46–47, 52, 53
work
  return to 532–533
  see also employment status
World Health Organization (WHO) trial 45–46, 54
WOSCOPS 46–47, 52, 53

zofenopril
  post MI 63, 65
  target dose 14
ZWOLLE trial 284–287, 291–292, 301